ROUTLEDGE INTERNATIONAL HANDBOOK OF CRITICAL ISSUES IN HEALTH AND ILLNESS

The *Routledge International Handbook of Critical Issues in Health and Illness* is a multidisciplinary reference book that brings together cutting-edge health and illness topics from around the globe. It offers a range of theoretical and critical perspectives to provide contemporary insights into complex health issues that can offer ways to address inequitable patterns of illness and ill health.

This collection, written by an international pool of expert academics from a range of disciplinary backgrounds, is unique in providing theoretical and critical analyses on key health topics, considering power and broader social structures that influence health and illness outcomes. The chapters are organised into three parts. The first covers medical contexts; here, chapters provide commentary and critical analysis of the history of medicine, medicalisation, pharmaceuticalisation, services and care, medical technology, diagnosis, screening, personalised medicine, and complementary and alternative medicine. The second part covers life contexts; chapters include a range of life contexts that have implications for health, including gender, sexuality, reproduction, disability, ethnicity, indigeneity, inequality, ageing, and dying. The third part covers shifting contextual domains; chapters consider contemporary areas of life that are rapidly changing, including bioethics, digital health, migration, medical travel, geography and "place", commercialisation, globalisation, and climate change.

The *Routledge International Handbook of Critical Issues in Health and Illness* is a key contemporary reference text for scholars, students, researchers, and professionals across disciplines, including sociology, psychology, anthropology, geography, medicine, public health, and health science.

Kerry Chamberlain is Emeritus Professor of Social and Health Psychology at Massey University and Senior Research Fellow at Te Herenga Waka, Victoria University of Wellington, New Zealand. He is editor-in-chief of the journal *Methods in Psychology* and co-editor (with Antonia Lyons) of the book series *Critical Approaches to Health*.

Antonia Lyons is Professor of Health Psychology and Head of School of the School of Health, Te Herenga Waka, Victoria University of Wellington, New Zealand. She is co-editor for *Qualitative Research in Psychology*, Associate Editor for *Psychology and Health*, and co-editor (with Kerry Chamberlain) of the book series *Critical Approaches to Health*.

ROUTLEDGE INTERNATIONAL HANDBOOK OF CRITICAL ISSUES IN HEALTH AND ILLNESS

Edited by Kerry Chamberlain and Antonia Lyons

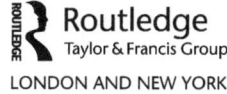

Routledge
Taylor & Francis Group

LONDON AND NEW YORK

First published 2022
by Routledge
2 Park Square, Milton Park, Abingdon, Oxon OX14 4RN

and by Routledge
605 Third Avenue, New York, NY 10158

Routledge is an imprint of the Taylor & Francis Group, an informa business

British Library Cataloguing-in-Publication Data
A catalogue record for this book is available from the British Library

Library of Congress Cataloging-in-Publication Data
Names: Chamberlain, Kerry, editor. | Lyons, Antonia C., editor.
Title: Routledge international handbook of critical issues in health and illness/[edited by] Kerry Chamberlain, Antonia Lyons.
Other titles: International handbook of critical issues in health and illness
Description: Milton Park, Abingdon, Oxon; New York, NY: Routledge, 2021. | Includes bibliographical references and index.
Identifiers: LCCN 2021001933 (print) | LCCN 2021001934 (ebook) | ISBN 9781032027951 (hardback) | ISBN 9781003185215 (ebook)
Subjects: LCSH: Medicine–Research–Social aspects. | World health. | Health services accessibility. | Social medicine. | Health and race.
Classification: LCC R853.S64 R68 2021 (print) | LCC R853.S64 (ebook) | DDC 362.1–dc23
LC record available at https://lccn.loc.gov/2021001933
LC ebook record available at https://lccn.loc.gov/2021001934

ISBN: 978-1-032-02795-1 (hbk)
ISBN: 978-1-032-03982-4 (pbk)
ISBN: 978-1-003-18521-5 (ebk)

Typeset in Bembo
by Deanta Global Publishing Services, Chennai, India

CONTENTS

EDITORS

Kerry Chamberlain is Emeritus Professor of Social and Health Psychology at Massey University, Auckland, New Zealand, and an Adjunct Professor and Senior Research Fellow in the School of Social and Cultural Studies at Te Herenga Waka Victoria University of Wellington, New Zealand. He is a critical social scientist who has published widely on health issues and qualitative research and methodologies. His research has focused on critical approaches to health and illness, with a particular interest in disadvantage, medications, everyday life, media, materiality, food, and innovative qualitative research methodology. He is co-editor (with Antonia Lyons) of the book series *Critical Approaches to Health* (Routledge), editor-in-chief of *Methods in Psychology*, and serves on the editorial boards of several health journals.

Antonia Lyons is Professor of Health Psychology and Head of School in the School of Health at Te Herenga Waka Victoria University of Wellington, New Zealand. Her research has focused on the social and embodied contexts of behaviours related to health and wellbeing, particularly alcohol consumption, youth drinking cultures, and social media marketing. Her latest research project uses the concept of "limbic capitalism" to explore mobile social media and the marketing of unhealthy products. Antonia is currently co-editor for *Qualitative Research in Psychology,* associate editor for *Psychology and Health,* and is also co-editor (with Kerry Chamberlain) of the book series *Critical Approaches to Health* (Routledge). She co-edited (with Tim McCreanor, Ian Goodwin, and Helen Moewaka Barnes) the book *Youth Drinking Cultures in a Digital World* (Routledge, 2017).

CONTRIBUTORS

Peter J. Adams is Professor at the School of Population Health and an Associate Director of the Centre for Addiction Research, both at the University of Auckland, New Zealand. He was trained initially as a clinical psychologist and has practised in hospital, community, and private practice settings for over 13 years. He has published seven sole-authored books: *How to Talk about Spiritual Encounters* (Palgrave Macmillan, 2020) *Reflecting on the Inevitable: Mortality at the Crossroads of Psychology, Philosophy and Health* (Oxford University Press, 2020), *Navigating Everyday Life: Exploring the Tension Between Finitude and Transcendence* (Lexington Books, 2018), *Moral Jeopardy: Risks of Accepting Money from the Tobacco, Alcohol and Gambling Industries* (Cambridge University Press, 2016), *Masculine Empire: How Men Use Violence to Keep Women in Line* (Dunmore, 2012), *Fragmented Intimacy: Addiction in a Social World* (Springer, 2008), and *Gambling, Freedom and Democracy* (Routledge, 2007). His research interests include social theory, family impacts of addictions, industry conflicts of interest, and public health approaches to gambling.

Gavin J. Andrews is Professor in the Department of Health, Aging and Society at McMaster University, in Canada, and an Associate Member of the School of Geography and Earth Sciences at the same institution. He is a health geographer with wide-ranging empirical interests, including ageing, holistic medicine, phobias, healthcare work, fitness cultures, health histories, and arts. Much of his work is theoretical, considering the progress and future of health geography. In recent years he has become interested in the potential of posthumanist and non-represen-tational theories for conveying the vitality, immediacy, and practice of health and wellbeing. His recent books – most with collaborators – include *Non-Representational Theory and Health* (Routledge, 2018), *Geographical Gerontology* (Routledge, 2018), *Routledge Handbook of Health Geography* (Routledge, 2018), *Health Geographies: A Critical Introduction* (Blackwell, 2018), and *An Introduction to Mental Health and Illness* (Oxford, 2020).

Natalie Armstrong is Professor of Healthcare Improvement Research in the Social Science Applied to Healthcare Improvement Research (SAPPHIRE) Group, Department of Health Sciences, University of Leicester, UK. A medical sociologist by background and specialising in qualitative research, her work uses social science theory and methods to tackle problems in the delivery of high-quality healthcare. Natalie's work covers a number of healthcare topics, although she has a longstanding special interest in women's and children's health and in pre-ventative healthcare, particularly population-based screening. Her work has included two edited collections of special issues for the journal *Sociology of Health & Illness*: one in 2012 on "The Sociology of Medical Screening" (with Helen Eborall) and another in 2020 on "Understanding and Managing Uncertainty on Healthcare" (with Nicola Mackintosh).

Erica Borgstrom is Lecturer in Medical Anthropology and End-of-Life Care at the Open University in the UK, where she leads Open Thanatology and teaches across health and social care. She is co-editor of the journal *Mortality* promoting the interdisciplinary study of death and dying. She sits on the council for the Association for the Study of Death and Society (ASDS) and is a fellow of the Royal Anthropological Institute. She has co-edited *Researching Death, Dying and Bereavement* (2017) with Julie Ellis and Kate Woodthorpe. Her research uses anthropological skills to disrupt the normative concepts in end-of-life care by foregrounding people's everyday experiences and the structural and discursive elements that shape how care is provided. For example, as a co-investigator, she has been involved in the Forms of Care project, examining the concept of "non-interventions" through an ethnographic study of palliative and end-of-life care (UKRI-ESRC ES/P002781/1).

Hannah Bradby is Professor in the Sociology Department at Uppsala University, Sweden. Hannah has a longstanding interest in disrupting professionally centred understandings of health and illness through sociological and anthropological enquiry. Her research focusses on the implications of ethnicity, religion, and culture when contextualised in global migration regimes, for health and healthcare, and is published in leading sociological and public health journals. Her latest co-authored book is entitled *Exploring Welfare Bricolage in Europe's Superdiverse Neighbourhoods* (Routledge, 2021). She blogs at "Cost of Living" and is the chief editor of *Frontiers in Sociology*. She leads the Welfare Research Group at the Sociology Department of Uppsala University, where she has been Professor since 2013.

Toba Bryant is Associate Professor in the Faculty of Health Sciences at Ontario Tech University in Oshawa, Canada. She is the author of *Health Policy in Canada* and has published numerous book chapters and articles on policy change, housing, employment, health within a population health perspective, and community quality of life. She is editor of *Critical Studies*, a peer-reviewed journal located at the Faculty of Health Sciences, Ontario Tech University. She is co-author with Dennis Raphael of *The Politics of Health in the Canadian Welfare State* and co-editor of *Staying Alive: Critical Perspectives on Health, Illness, and Health Care*.

Heide Castañeda is Professor of Anthropology at the University of South Florida in the USA. Her research areas include political and legal anthropology, law and society, medical anthropology, borders, migration, migrant health, citizenship, and policing, focusing on the US/Mexico border, United States, Mexico, Germany, and Morocco. She is the author of *Borders of Belonging: Struggle and Solidarity in Mixed-Status Immigrant Families* (Stanford University Press, 2019) and co-editor of *Unequal Coverage: The Experience of Health Care Reform in the United States* (NYU Press, 2018). Her latest book is *Migrant Health: Cross-Disciplinary and Critical Perspectives* (Routledge, 2021). Dr Castañeda has also published dozens of research articles on migration and healthcare access for immigrant populations. Her work has been funded by the National Science Foundation, National Institutes of Health, the Fulbright Programme, the German Academic Exchange Service (DAAD), and the Wenner-Gren Foundation for Anthropological Research.

Catharine Coleborne is Professor of History and Head of the School of Humanities and Social Science/Dean of Arts at the University of Newcastle, Australia. Her research into the histories of medicine and mental health, the regulation of human mobility, and colonial societies and cultures is internationally recognised. Her books include *"Madness" in the family: Insanity and*

Institutions in the Australasian Colonial World 1860s–1914 (Palgrave Macmillan, 2010) and *Insanity, Identity and Empire: Colonial Institutional Confinement in Australia and New Zealand, 1870–1910* (Manchester University Press, 2015). Her most recent book is *Why Talk about Madness? Bringing History into the Conversation* (Palgrave Pivot, 2020) and with Elizabeth Roberts-Pedersen she is writing *Making Mental Health: A Global History*, for the Routledge Series *Critical Approaches to Health*. Catharine is the President of the Australia and New Zealand Society for the History of Medicine (2020–2021).

Angus Dawson is Professor of Bioethics and Director of Sydney Health Ethics at the University of Sydney, Australia. His main research interests are in public health ethics, research ethics, and the methodology of bioethics. His work is increasingly focused on working with organisations to embed ethics into policy and everyday practice. He is working currently on a series of papers about "socially-embedded" concepts that he believes would be useful to extend discussions in bioethics, including sustainability, solidarity, community, and trust. He is the joint editor-in-Chief of the journal *Public Health Ethics* and was one of the editors of the casebook *Global Perspectives on Public Health Ethics*, which has been downloaded in full or in part over 738,000 times. You can download it for free here: www.springer.com/gp/book/9783319238463.

Sarah de Leeuw was awarded a Canada Research Chair (Humanities and Health Inequities) in 2018 and was appointed in 2017 to the Royal Society of Canada's College of Emerging Scholars, Artists, and Scientists. Sarah de Leeuw is a poet, essayist, activist, and scholar working in the Northern Medical Programme with the University of Northern British Columbia, a distributed programme with the University of British Columbia's Faculty of Medicine. Her research focuses on anticolonial feminist and arts-based methodologies to address health inequities, especially in northern, rural, and remote geographies. Author or co-editor of eleven books, her creative writing was shortlisted in 2017 for a Governor General's Literary Award in non-fiction. She holds a Western Magazine Gold Award (2013) for top-ranked feature essay writing and a Dorthey Livesay Award (2013) for the best book of poetry in British Columbia. Her health-focused academic social science and humanities research appears in over 135 journals, textbooks, and encyclopaedias.

Kevin Dew is Professor of Sociology at Victoria University of Wellington, New Zealand. He is a founding member of the Applied Research on Communication in Health (ARCH) group. Current research activities include studies of cancer survivorship, complementary and alternative medicine, and cancer care decision-making in relation to health inequities. His books include *The Cult and Science of Public Health: A Sociological Investigation, Social, Political and Cultural Dimension of Health* (with Anne Scott and Allison Kirkman), *Sociology of Health in New Zealand* (with Allison Kirkman), *Public Health, Personal Health and Pills: Drug Entanglements and Pharmaceuticalised Governance*, and the forthcoming *Complementary and Alternative Medicine: Containing and Expanding Therapeutic Possibilities*. He has authored or co-authored over 100 articles and book chapters, is an Advisory Board member on a number of journals including *Sociology of Health and Illness* and the *Journal of Sociology* and is associate editor for the Australasia/Asia region for *Critical Public Health*.

May Farrales is a Filipinx interdisciplinary scholar whose research centres on the embodied and lived experiences of people of colour in settler-colonial urban geographies. She is Assistant Professor in Urban Social Change in Geography, cross-appointed with the Department of Gender, Sexuality and Women's Studies at Simon Fraser University, Canada, located on the unceded territories of the Squamish (Sḵwx̱wú7mesh Úxwumixw), Tsleil-Waututh (səlilw̓ətaʔɬ),

Kwikwetlem (kwikwəƛ̓ əm), and Musqueam (xwməθkwəy̓ əm) Nations. Before joining SFU, she completed a postdoctoral fellowship as a Michael Smith Foundation for Health Research Trainee at the University of Northern British Columbia. She holds a PhD (2017) in Geography from the University of British Columbia.

Jonathan Gabe is Emeritus Professor of Sociology in the School of Law and Social Sciences, Royal Holloway, University of London, UK. He has research interests in pharmaceuticals, healthcare organisation, and chronic illness, and has published widely in these areas. His most recent publications are *Health and Illness in the Neoliberal Era in Europe* (Emerald, 2020; co-edited with Mario Cardano and Angela Genova) and *Key Concepts in Medical Sociology* (Sage, 3rd edition, 2021; co-edited with Lee Monaghan). He has been a co-editor of the international journal *Sociology of Health and Illness* twice, and is a former President of the International Sociological Association Research Committee 15, Sociology of Health, and the European Sociological Association Research Network 16, Sociology of Health & Illness. He is a Fellow of the UK Academy of Social Sciences.

Dan Goodley is Professor of Disability Studies and Education at the University of Sheffield in the UK and co-director of iHuman (the Research Institute for the Study of the Human).

Margo Greenwood, Academic Leader of the National Collaborating Centre for Indigenous Health, is an Indigenous scholar of Cree ancestry with years of experience focused on the health and wellbeing of Indigenous children, families and communities. She is also Vice-President of Indigenous Health for the Northern Health Authority in British Columbia and Professor in both the First Nations Studies and Education programmes at the University of Northern British Columbia, Canada. While her academic work crosses disciplines and sectors, she is particularly recognised for her work in early childhood care and education of Indigenous children and for public health. Margo has undertaken work with UNICEF, the United Nations, the Canadian Council on Social Determinants of Health, Public Health Network of Canada, and the Canadian Institute of Health Research, specifically, the Institute of Population and Public Health.

Johanna Hanefeld is the Director of the Centre for International Protection Department at the Robert Koch Institute, the national public health institute for Germany. She has been leading the department's response to COVID-19, amongst other health topics. She is Associate Professor in Health Policy and Systems Research at the London School of Hygiene and Tropical Medicine and the academic lead of their Berlin office. Her academic work is situated within the field of health policy and systems and focuses on the political economy of global health. A policy analyst by training, she has a diverse background, and has a decade long history working on health inequities and the social determinants, including for WHO, Amnesty International, amongst others. She has written about globalisation and health, including editing the book *Globalization and Health* (2015).

Flis Henwood is Professor of Social Informatics in the School of Applied Social Science and the Centre for Digital Media Cultures at the University of Brighton in the UK. She is a social scientist whose research combines medical sociology and science and technology studies (STS) to explore the socio-technical contours of digital health. She has published widely on the relationship between information, digital technologies and care, most recently co-editing *Digital Health: Sociological Perspectives* (Wiley Blackwell, 2019; with Benjamin Marent). She is joint Chief Editor of the Wiley journal *Sociology of Health and Illness*.

Stuart Hogarth trained in the history of medicine, but his research now focuses on the political economy of biomedical innovation in the 21st century. His primary interest is the diagnostics sector, with a particular focus on regulatory governance, intellectual property rights, and the impact of genomic science. His work uses an international comparative methodology to explore the continued salience of national institutions (regulatory regimes, healthcare systems, research networks, and commercial infrastructure) in a bioeconomy which is increasingly characterised by global governance structures, international scientific collaborations and transnational flows of capital and scientific labour.

Annemarie Jutel is Professor of Health at Te Herenga Waka/Victoria University of Wellington in New Zealand. After a first career in nursing, and a long engagement in elite sport, she became a critical diagnosis scholar, which means she studies clinical diagnosis from cultural, social and creative perspectives. Her book, *Putting a Name to It: Diagnosis in Contemporary Society* (JHUP) was the first to provide an in-depth look at the sociology of diagnosis. In recent years, she has been interested in the interface between medicine and the arts, and organised *Mataora: Encounters between Medicine and the Arts*, and has written *Diagnosis: Truths and Tales* (UTP), an exploration of the narrative portrayal of the diagnostic moment

Dharmi Kapadia is Lecturer at the Department of Sociology, University of Manchester, UK, and a member of the ESRC Centre on Dynamics of Ethnicity (CoDE). With expertise in social statistical methods, her main areas of research are ethnic inequalities in health and access to health services. She has also conducted research on ethnic inequalities in the labour market, and on the relationships between poverty, ethnicity and social networks. She has published in journals including the *British Medical Journal* and *Ethnicity and Health*.

Robin A. Kearns is Professor of Geography in the School of Environment at the University of Auckland, New Zealand. His doctoral study took him to Canada supported by a Commonwealth Scholarship where he examined the inner-city experience of impoverished psychiatric patients. In the three decades since, he has maintained an interest in the links between health and place and is an editor of the journal of the same name. Papers on the nature of place in medical/health geography in *The Professional Geographer* (1993) and *Progress in Human Geography* (2002; with Graham Moon) are among the most cited in the scholarly field. Robin has collaborated with a wide range of geographers and other social scientists with funding from agencies such as the Health Research Council of NZ and the NZ National Science Challenges. He is a qualitative methodologist with a particular interest in experiential and observational approaches. His current research centres on islands, ageing, and home environments. His most recent book is the co-edited *Blue Space, Health and Wellbeing: Hydrophilia Unbounded* (Routledge, 2019).

Susan Kelly is Emeritus Professor at the University of Exeter, UK, where she has a longstanding involvement with Egenis, the Centre for the Study of the Life Sciences. Throughout her scholarly career, Susan Kelly has been passionately interested in how new technologies are received by patients and physicians alike, with an interest in how they affected work practices as well as everyday actions. Her best-known works are "Choosing Not to Choose", about prenatal technologies, published in the *Sociology of Health and Illness*, and "the Maternal Foetal interface and Gestational Chimerism: The Emerging Importance of Chimeric Bodies", published in *Science as Culture*.

Rebecca Lawthom is Professor of Community Psychology at the University of Sheffield, UK, where she is Head of the School of Education.

Supuni Liyanagunawardena is a PhD candidate at the School of Social and Cultural Studies, Victoria University of Wellington, New Zealand, and Lecturer at the Faculty of Medical Sciences, University of Sri Jayewardenepura, Sri Lanka. Her doctoral thesis explores everyday therapeutic practices in a Sri Lankan community from a praxeological lens. Supuni's research interests include therapeutic diversity, healthcare interactions in the Global South, and postcolonial/decolonial theories.

Sara MacBride-Stewart is Reader in Health Medicine and Society, School of Social Sciences, Cardiff University, UK. Her research in environmental sociology addresses social inequalities (gender, geospatial) and problems for health and wellbeing that emerge from changes to the natural landscape (biodiversity loss, socio-cultural change), and the social affects (affordances) of protected nature. She has projects on Kauri dieback, placed-based citizen science for water SDGs, post-coloniality, and nature. Her approach conceptualises and co-constructs social solutions that address problems between the natural and social world (citizen social science). She has published on recreational and wellbeing uses of the natural environment, access to nature-based and outdoor recreation, and global sustainable development, in international journals (*Health*; *GeoForum*; *Journal of Transport and Health, Gender Work and Organization*).

Kathryn MacKay is Lecturer at Sydney Health Ethics, at the University of Sydney, Australia. Kate completed her Master's degree in Philosophy with a specialisation in Bioethics at McGill University, Canada, in 2009, and then worked in health promotion for 5 years. In 2014, Kate began doctoral studies at the University of Birmingham, UK, funded by a Wellcome Trust Fellowship, and was awarded her PhD in 2017. Kate's research focusses on issues of human flourishing at the intersection of feminist theory, ethics, and political philosophy. She is particularly interested in questions related to power, health and wellbeing, identity and group relations, and personal and group agency. She is currently working on the nature of compassion and its possibilities for public health ethics and practice, and is Chief Investigator of an ARC Discovery Grant (2020) exploring theories of autonomy in the context of expanding genetic and assisted reproductive technologies.

Benjamin Marent is Assistant Professor of Digital Technologies at Work in the University of Sussex Business School in the UK. With a background in sociology and science and technology studies he explores the co-evolution of digital technologies and health practices. By facilitating co-design spaces with diverse stakeholders, his research aims to stretch the imagination of practitioners, policymakers, and scholars to contribute towards value-centric innovation in healthcare delivery. His publications have highlighted the complexities of citizen participation and the ambivalence of digital health. Recently, he served as co-editor (with Flis Henwood) for the special issue Digital Health: Sociological Perspectives in *Sociology of Health & Illness*, 2019: 41(s1).

Paul Martin is Professor of the Sociology of Science and Technology at the Department of Sociological Studies, University of Sheffield, UK. He is co-director of iHuman, the Institute for the Study of the Human, which seeks to develop innovative multidisciplinary research on what it means to be human in the 21st Century. He has a first training in molecular biology and works at the interface of STS and medical sociology. Recent research interests include the clinical and commercial development of genome editing, the role of science in (social) policy, and the governance of biomedical technologies. In 2020 he was awarded a major 5-year Wellcome Trust Investigator Award to study the contemporary development of very high-priced orphan drugs and their impact on the pharmaceutical industry and access to medicines.

Fiona A. Miller is Professor of Health Policy; she holds the Chair in Health Management Strategies and is the Founding Director of the Centre for Sustainable Health Systems in the Institute of Health Policy, Management and Evaluation in the Dalla Lana School of Public Health at the University of Toronto, Canada. Fiona's research programme is concerned with health technology and innovation policy and how health systems support population health and health equity. She is particularly interested in the regulatory institutions that condition the adoption of technologies within collectively financed health systems, such as health sector procurement and health technology assessment, viewing these as instruments of demand-driven innovation.

Lisa Jean Moore is Medical Sociologist and SUNY Distinguished Professor of Sociology and Gender Studies in the School of Natural and Social Sciences at Purchase College, State University of New York, USA. Her books include an urban ethnography of NYC beekeeping called *Buzz: Urban Beekeeping and the Power of the Bee* (NYUP; co-authored with Mary Kosut). *Catch and Release: The Enduring, yet Vulnerable, Horseshoe Crab* (NYUP) investigates the interspecies relationships between humans and *Limulus polyphemus* (Atlantic Horseshoe Crabs). Her most recent book project *The Transgenic Animal: Spider Goats, Synthetic Biology, and Imminent Obsolescence* explores the invention of goats modified with spider DNA to lactate spider silk protein.

Tracy Morison is Senior Lecturer in Health Psychology in the School of Psychology at Massey University, Aotearoa, New Zealand. She is an associate editor for *Feminism & Psychology* and an Honorary Research Associate of the Critical Studies in Sexualities and Reproduction programme at Rhodes University (South Africa), where she obtained her PhD. Her postdoctoral work was conducted at the Human Sciences Research Council in South Africa, where she subsequently worked as Senior Researcher before returning to the academy. Dr Morison's research is located at the intersection of health psychology, critical psychology, and feminism. Her work is driven by a social justice orientation and seeks to explore how the socio-political context shapes and constrains sexual and reproductive decision-making, relations, and practices. A key focus in her work is on gender, sexualities, and their interrelationship with other social locations. She draws on feminist and other critical theories and in-depth qualitative methodologies to illuminate the multiple, complex processes in which sexualities and reproduction are embedded.

Michael Morrison is Senior Researcher in Sociology with the Centre for Health, Law and Emerging Technologies (HeLEX) and Associate Fellow at the Institute for Science, Innovation and Society at the University of Oxford, UK. His work deals with the dynamics of innovation in biomedical technologies, where he has worked on a range of topics, including human enhancement, biobanking, and regenerative medicine. Michael's most recent work investigates how potential clinical applications of new technologies are shaped by scientific, regulatory, economic, and cultural factors through three interrelated case studies of induced pluripotent stem cells, genome editing, and 3D printing of living biological material. Michael obtained his MA and PhD from the Institute for Science and Society, University of Nottingham, and has worked in the Science and Technology Studies Unit (SATSU) at the University of York and the ESRC Centre for Genomics in Society (Egenis) at the University of Exeter before moving to Oxford in 2012.

Alex Müller is Adjunct Associate Professor at the Gender Health and Justice Research Unit at the University of Cape Town, South Africa, and currently a Humboldt Fellow at the Department of Medical Ethics and History of Medicine at the University of Göttingen, Germany. Together with community organisations and activists, she researches the health and wellbeing of queer people in Southern and East Africa, and informs health policy, strategic litigation, and health professions education. With the Qintu Collab, she has published the graphic anthology *Meanwhile ... Graphic Short Stories about Everyday Queer Life in Southern and Eastern Africa.*

Rebecca E. Olson is Reader in Sociology at the University of Queensland, Australia, Program Director of the Bachelor of Social Science, and Co-Director of SocioHealthLab, an interdisciplinary research collective that pursues social transformation in health and healthcare through applied socio-cultural research. Her research intersects the sociologies of health and emotion. As a leading innovative qualitative researcher, funded by competitive grants (e.g. NHMRC, Arthritis Australia, Cancer Australia), Olson employs video-based, participatory, reflexive, post-qualitative, and post-paradigmatic approaches to inform translational inquiry. Her recent books include *Towards a Sociology of Cancer Caregiving: Time to Feel* (Ashgate, 2015) and *Emotions in Late Modernity* (Routledge, 2019; co-edited with Patulny, Bellocchi, Khorana, McKenzie, and Peterie).

Dennis Raphael is Professor at the School of Health Policy and Management at York University in Toronto, Canada. He is editor of *Social Determinants of Health: Canadian Perspectives, Tackling Health Inequalities: Lessons from International Experiences,* and *Immigration, Public Policy, and Health: Newcomer Experiences in Developed Nations,* and author of *Poverty in Canada: Implications for Health and Quality of Life* and *About Canada: Health and Illness.* He is co-author with Toba Bryant of *The Politics of Health in the Canadian Welfare State,* and co-editor of *Staying Alive: Critical Perspectives on Health, Illness, and Health Care.*

Katherine Runswick-Cole is Professor of Education and Director of Research in the School of Education at the University of Sheffield, UK.

Christine Stephens is Professor of Social Science Research in the School of Psychology at Massey University, New Zealand, where she co-leads the cross-disciplinary Health and Ageing Research Team. The focus of the team's activity is a longitudinal study of health in ageing (health, work, and retirement study) which has conducted bi-annual surveys of a population sample of older people for 14 years. The research also includes qualitative studies on topics such as informal caregiving, palliative care, the experience of cancer, and housing needs. Christine's research is located at the intersection of health psychology and gerontology. She has authored or co-authored over 175 peer-reviewed papers in these areas. She is the author of *Health Promotion: A Psychosocial Approach* (Open University Press, 2008) and her latest book, co-authored with Mary Breheny, is *Healthy Ageing: A Capability Approach to Inclusive Policy and Practice* (Routledge, 2018).

Angelina Taylor is Research Associate in the Department for Infectious Disease Epidemiology at the Robert Koch Institute, the national public health institute in Germany. She is currently coordinating the WHO AMR Surveillance and Quality Assessment Collaborating Centres Network to support the global improvement of surveillance of antimicrobial resistance. She is also working on anti-discrimination and public health, as well as on COVID-19. Angelina's career has focused on health policy, strategy and public health practice. She has previously worked in public health in local government, the Health Foundation, the Royal College of Surgeons of England, and the National Health Service (NHS) in the UK. She has an MSc in Public Health from the London School of Hygiene and Tropical Medicine.

Jonathan N. Torres is from Brooklyn, New York, USA. They are pursuing a Master's Degree in International Affairs and Global Justice at the City University of New York, Brooklyn College. Their undergraduate thesis focused on the health and lived experiences of queer persons of colour. Current interests include LGBTQ+ research, policy, and media.

Felicity Thomas is Senior Research Fellow at the University of Exeter, UK, and Director of the WHO Collaborating Centre for Culture and Health. Much of her work seeks to understand how health "conditions" become pathologised and medicalised, and to explore how this interrelates with, and can reinforce, poverty, and inequality. Felicity leads a programme of research examining how lived experiences of health inequalities can inform more effective clinical practice and applied health and social policy.

Cecilia Vindrola-Padros is a medical anthropologist interested in applied health research and the development of rapid approaches to research. She works across five interdisciplinary teams, applying anthropological theories and methods to study and improve healthcare delivery in the UK and abroad. She has written extensively on the use of rapid qualitative research and currently co-directs the Rapid Research Evaluation and Appraisal Lab (RREAL) with Dr Ginger Johnson. Cecilia works as a Senior Research Fellow in the Department of Targeted Intervention, University College London, UK, and as a Social Scientist at the NIAA Health Services Research Centre, Royal College of Anaesthetists.

ACKNOWLEDGEMENTS

We would like to give particular thanks to all of the 41 authors who contributed chapters to this handbook. Finding experts with critical perspectives on research who were willing to write chapters on the wide range of topics we wanted to cover in the handbook proved daunting at times but, in the end, we obtained a great cohort of authors who provided outstanding contributions. We also thank them for their patience as they waited, sometimes for long periods, for us to complete our editorial reviews of chapters, suggest revisions, and press deadlines for their completion. It was a pleasure to work with so many accomplished researchers and writers – their abilities made our work, and the work of our reviewers, so much easier. Many of the revisions suggested for initial chapter drafts were quite minor due to the excellent quality of the initial submissions.

We would also like to sincerely thank all of those authors listed below for agreeing to serve on the Advisory Board for the handbook. Their input has been invaluable throughout the development of this handbook. They have offered advice on potential authors for chapters, provided in-depth reviews of chapter drafts, and contributed their expertise to improve the overall quality of this handbook.

We would also like to thank everyone at Routledge who has been involved with this handbook. The idea for a critical handbook on health issues was first proposed by Russell George, who also initiated the Routledge book series *Critical Approaches to Health*, which we edit. Russell argued the need for such a handbook, growing out of the work on the series. Like all academics, we were very busy, and procrastinated about developing the handbook for some time. By the time we agreed to proceed, and to draft a proposal for the handbook, the Routledge editorial role had passed to Lucy Kennedy, who assisted greatly in getting the handbook underway. Soon after the project started, her Editorial Assistant, Charlotte Mapp, came on the scene, and carried the bulk of the work, meeting our enquiries, tolerating our changes in deadline, and providing very helpful advice. When Charlotte moved on to take up other opportunities, Lucy returned to carry the final work through into production, and we again benefitted from her considerable knowledge and support. We are grateful to them all, for their guidance, assistance, and good cheer along the way; without them standing behind us, this handbook would most likely never have appeared.

We would also like to thank the School and Faculty of Health at Te Herenga Waka, Victoria University of Wellington, where Antonia has been based over most of the course of this project, and the School of Psychology at Massey University, where Kerry was working until his recent retirement, and where his connection continues as Emeritus Professor. We have had the benefit of being surrounded by outstanding scholars, colleagues and friends in both institutions, and we would like to acknowledge their advice, support, and friendship throughout our handbook journey.

Finally, sincere thanks to Vivienne and Ian, for their continued support of all that we do.

Kerry Chamberlain & Antonia Lyons

December 2020

Handbook Advisory Board Members

Peter Adams
Hannah Bradby
Heidi Castañeda
Cathy Coleborne
Angus Dawson
Sarah de Leeuw
Kevin Dew
Jonathan Gabe
Flis Henwood
Annemarie Jutel
Robin Kearns
Supuni Liyanagunarwardena
Kathryn MacKay
Fiona Miller
Lisa Jean Moore
Alex Müller
Christine Stephens
Felicity Thomas
Cecilia Vindrola-Padros

1

CRITICAL PERSPECTIVES ON HEALTH AND ILLNESS

Antonia Lyons and Kerry Chamberlain

Introduction

Health and illness are significant concerns around the world, and garner enormous amounts of research attention, funding, and scholarship across many disciplines and fields. Most health and illness topics and issues have strong contemporary relevance internationally. The *Routledge International Handbook of Critical Issues in Health and Illness* aims to provide a current, multidisciplinary, international reference handbook that covers an important, and comprehensive, range of topics and issues that are central to health and illness. Research and analysis on these topics cut across many disciplines (sociology, psychology, anthropology, geography, medicine, public health, nursing, health science, sport and exercise, etc.), and consequently our plan for this handbook was for content to be multidisciplinary and inclusive, and comprehensive to a wide audience of readers from different disciplinary backgrounds.

There are many excellent handbooks that are concerned with health (e.g. *Handbook of Global Urban Health*, edited by Vojnovic et al., 2019; *Routledge Handbook of Health Geography*, edited by Andrews, Pearce, & Crooks, 2018; *The Oxford Handbook of Global Health Politics*, edited by McInnes, Lee, & Youde, 2020; *The Oxford Handbook of Stigma, Discrimination, and Health*, edited by Major, Dovidio, & Link, 2018), and some that take explicitly critical perspectives (e.g. *Health Inequalities: Critical Perspectives*, edited by Bambra, Smith, & Hill, 2016; *Staying Alive: Critical Perspectives on Health, Illness, and Health care*, edited by Raphael, Rioux, & Bryant, 2019; *Routledge International Handbook of Critical Mental Health*, edited by Cohen, 2017). However, currently none are designed to address key contemporary health and illness topics using critical perspectives across disciplines and fields ranging from medicine to globalisation and climate change.

As co-editors of the Routledge series *Critical Approaches to Health*, we have had the pleasure of working with a range of authors, from different backgrounds and disciplines, who have written books for this series. Over the past eight years we have identified many potentially relevant topics, and possible authors, who could contribute excellent books for this series, leading us to realise that what was missing for researchers and students was a comprehensive overview of critical approaches to specific health and illness topics from a range of different disciplinary perspectives. This was the impetus for the current handbook; we saw the potential for it to make a distinctive contribution to the field. This is a large remit that traverses many fields and is integrated by a particular approach to scholarship, namely theorising and conceptualising critical perspectives on particular health and illness topics. The work presented in specific chapters often sits within its own disciplinary boundaries yet has high relevance to scholars working on these health issues across many different disciplines.

What do we mean by taking critical perspectives on health and illness topics? As we have outlined elsewhere (Chamberlain & Lyons, 2020, p. 431), critical perspectives mean "explicitly considering the nature of knowledge generation, the paradigms in which it was generated, and the consequences of this in terms of what knowledge is produced, with whom, and who benefits from this knowledge". Critical perspectives seek to locate an "object" or topic of investigation, such as health, within its historical, social, and cultural contexts and, in particular, to understand how social and material conditions shape, influence, or constrain the object or topic under consideration. They involve reflexive considerations of how cultural understandings, social structures, and social and material practices operate to determine, shape, and limit the object of study, with an ambition to change practices in ways that can remove or limit disparities and benefit the disadvantaged. In the case of health, this necessarily involves a critical examination of the roles of the different actors and systems involved in health and healthcare – ill people, patients, carers, health professionals, hospitals, clinics, treatments, commercial companies, and so on – to understand and reflexively interpret their influences on health – their interests and involvements, and their power. Critical perspectives usually orient to issues of power, and its distribution and exercise, in the widest sense, including political and economic power, social and cultural power, access to power, and resistance. This can extend to exploring who benefits from the research and practice in the field. In the broadest sense, critical perspectives challenge and unsettle taken-for-granted views on health and illness, or views that might be considered "common-sense" (Cohen, 2017). Often, critical perspectives broaden our view of issues through providing analyses from multiple, diverse, and intersectional standpoints, including gender, ethnicity, sexuality, or marginalised positions. Such analyses can identify ideologies, and the way systems work, how meanings are produced, and how resistance or change may come about. There are, of course, different kinds of critical perspectives and debates about what should be emphasised and even how critical scholarship should be conducted. In this handbook our overarching objective is to render critical perspectives on contemporary health and illness topics more visible and accessible.

Many critical perspectives on health and illness align with the United Nations' (UN) 17 Sustainable Development Goals (SDGs). These were adopted by the member states of the UN in 2016 to address global challenges, including to end poverty, protect the planet, and ensure well-being for all around the world. The SDG agenda has set specific global targets to be achieved by 2030. Goal 3, to "ensure healthy lives and promote well-being for all at all ages", is clearly relevant for scholars who are working on critical issues in health, although other goals include a range of determinants of health. In fact, all of the 17 SDGs[1] can be viewed as highly relevant to – and indeed are critical issues involved in – health, illness and well-being. Addressing social and global issues such as poverty, hunger, climate change, sustainability, gender equality, education, reduced inequalities, and clean water and sanitation will, without doubt, lead to better health outcomes. The SDGs are integrated and indivisible, with targets across social, environmental, and economic spheres (Nunes, Lee, & O'Riordan, 2016).

Health is influenced by all of the SDGs, but it is worth noting that health and illness reciprocally influence the goals as well. These links between health and broader social, economic, political, and cultural factors operate across levels (individual, societal, global) and lie at the heart of health inequities within and between countries (Lin, Kickbusch, & Baer, 2017). The Director-General of the World Health Organization, Dr Tedros Adhanom Ghebreyesus, has previously noted that the importance of a global commitment to sustainable development enshrined in the

SDGs "offers a unique opportunity to address the social, economic and political determinants of health and improve the health and well-being of people everywhere" (Government of South Australia & WHO, 2017). Integration across the SDGs is important, as is the consideration that health and well-being are both preconditions and outcomes of sustainable development (Nune et al., 2016). The World Health Organisation (n.d.) continues to highlight the importance of the social determinants of health for influencing health and illness outcomes, noting that these are

> the conditions in which people are born, grow, work, live, and age, and the wider set of forces and systems shaping the conditions of daily life. These forces and systems include economic policies and systems, development agendas, social norms, social policies and political systems.

About the handbook

The handbook is not focused on specific diseases or illnesses but is organised into three parts to capture the different contexts in which health and illness play out, namely medical contexts, life contexts, and other contemporary contextual domains that are rapidly changing (we have labelled these "shifting contextual domains"). Each of the 26 chapters provides a stand-alone contribution that can be utilised as a separate reading, but each has similar structures and aims. Chapter authors provide an overview of the topic, introduce and discuss the main arguments on the topic, including coverage of the relevant theory and research on the topic, take critical and multidisciplinary perspectives, and conclude by proposing some implications for the topic – for research and for practice where relevant – drawn from the arguments and discussion within the chapter.

Authors come from a range of countries, including the UK, USA, Canada, Sweden, Germany, South Africa, Australia, and New Zealand. This does produce a focus on Western research and scholarship, although the chapters bring diverse critical perspectives to bear on their specific topics. Also, we have made an effort to be inclusive of diverse views across the globe where this has relevance. Authors also come from a wide range of disciplines and backgrounds, including sociology, public health, history, geography, health policy, anthropology, science and technology studies, and psychology. The emphasis on cross-disciplinary and multidisciplinary approaches provides the handbook with a broad, diverse range of epistemic and theoretical frames, adding depth to the ways in which the complexity of health and illness issues can be understood, including how these vary across different life and geographical contexts, and from different worldviews. There are thematic, conceptual, and theoretical links between many of the chapters, within and across the three parts of the handbook. We have organised the handbook in a way that will make it a useful and easily accessible resource for a range of readers, including students, academics, researchers, health professionals, policymakers, and non-governmental organisations.

Part I: Medical contexts

In Part I, each chapter focuses on a key issue relating to medicine, moving from broader and more general issues to more focused ones. These chapters together provide critical considerations of the authority of medicine in society, the operation of power dynamics within institutions, disciplines, clinical practice, and the over-riding commercial imperatives that underlie much of the medical realm.

This section begins (Chapter 2) with an historical discussion, by Catharine Coleborne, of the development of medicine in terms of its social and cultural histories and the significant

ways in which medicine has changed. This is followed by several chapters which discuss changing aspects of medicine. The first of these examines medicalisation (Chapter 3), where Felicity
Thomas examines the diverse ways in which medicalisation is conceived and experienced, and
how it creates controversial and competing agendas. Then Jonathan Gabe and Paul Martin
discuss pharmaceuticalisation (Chapter 4) as a complex socio-technical process, involving the
global pharmaceutical industry alongside networks of related institutions, organisations, actors,
and artefacts, that functions to translate human conditions and capabilities into opportunities
for pharmaceutical intervention. Next, Stuart Hogarth and Fiona Miller (Chapter 5) examine
the role of health technology in modern medicine, and particularly changes and innovation
around medical devices and how they are adopted. Chapter 6 explores health services and care,
where Rebecca Olson highlights how political, economic, gendered, raced, and affective forces
interconnect and underpin the organisation of formal health services and informal family care.
Annemarie Jutel (Chapter 7) considers diagnosis as a social action that is shaped by historical,
political, and other social processes that exist outside of the body.

Population-based screening for identifying health and disease is discussed by Natalie
Armstrong in Chapter 8, including an overview of the discussions and debates in this field
about potentials for harms and benefits. The rapidly growing field of personalised medicine
is outlined in Chapter 9, and implications of the changing technologies, datasets, and associated promises for individual identities, behaviours and social cohesion are critically explored by
Michael Morrison and Susan Kelly. The final chapter in this section, by Kevin Dew and Supuni
Liyanagunarwardena (Chapter 10), considers complementary and alternative medicine, including trends in its uptake and use, how it is positioned in different medical landscapes, and how it
relates to biomedicine.

Part II: Life contexts

Part II focuses on a range of important life contexts where issues of health and illness appear
sharply, and where contexts impact the type of health experienced and the access to treatment
and care for illness. Each of these contexts has significance for health and illness in different ways,
providing a space for critical engagement with the relevant issues arising. These chapters all take
a critical approach to exploring this diversity of situating contexts – age, gender, sexual orientation, reproductive rights, ethnicity, indigeneity, (dis)ability, social setting – and how they work
to locate people in context, affecting how they live, how they experience health and illness, and
how they die. The chapters discuss how these particular life contexts affect health outcomes
and access to healthcare, located within a critical examination of the dynamics of inequality,
disadvantage, oppression, discrimination, and social justice, which form common threads across
chapters. The chapters also discuss how these key issues function to shape and constrain the
development of relevant policy and appropriate interventions, with many chapters offering suggestions for improvements in these areas.

In the opening chapter of Part II (Chapter 11), Dennis Raphael and Toba Bryant consider
the unfair and unjust differences in health outcomes across the world that have their sources
in peoples' living and working conditions. They argue that these social determinants of health
and their distribution are determined by government public policy decisions and shaped by
dominant ideological frameworks, and that identifying health inequalities and responding to
them should be a moral imperative. Then Lisa Jean Moore and Jonathan Torres consider how
gender is a primary social determinant of health status and outcomes (Chapter 12), and critically
discuss how health inequities exist between genders, race, class, and location. They promote a
contemporary perspective on gender and health research that draws from the interdisciplinary

contributions of queer theory and transgender studies. This is followed by a consideration of sexual orientation and gender identity (Chapter 13), by Alex Müller, who discusses how these terms are pathologised and limit access to healthcare for sexual and gender minorities, and how global legal frameworks governing sexual orientation and gender identity affect the health of sexual and gender minorities. Tracy Morison utilises the radical cross-disciplinary feminist framework of Reproductive Justice (Chapter 14) to illuminate the nuanced, multi-dimensional power dynamics that are embedded within reproductive health issues and identifies areas for further research in this field.

Next, Dharmi Kapadia and Hannah Bradby consider ethnic inequities in healthcare across the lifecourse (Chapter 15) and argue that the key reasons for these inequalities are racism and socioeconomic inequalities. They suggest how researchers can theorise ethnicity responsibly in their research without compounding racialisation and essentialisation and ensure that their research leads to progressive policy and practice. Sarah de Leeuw, Margot Greenwood, and May Farrales (Chapter 16) use anticolonial frameworks to critically examine how Indigenous peoples' health and illness have been framed and produced, and suggest ways to reconsider understandings about Indigenous peoples' health. They offer concrete ways to transform the languages, methods, methodologies, and pedagogies pertaining to Indigenous health and illness. Dan Goodley, Rebecca Lawthom, and Katherine Runswick-Cole (Chapter 17) explore the relationship between disability, technology, and health, arguing that considerations of the place of people with disabilities in advanced capitalist societies must attend to the systemic discrimination they experience. They then discuss some contemporary technologies that can enable the lives of people with disabilities. Then Christine Stephens (Chapter 18) considers the homogenising effects of treating "older age" as a category, and the damaging effects of ageism in healthcare, health promotion, and health-related public policy. She highlights the diversity of older people's social and environmental circumstances and emphasises that theoretical and policy frameworks need to focus on health in terms of people's capability to function in ways that they value. In the final chapter in this part, Erica Borgstrom (Chapter 19) utilises the concept of "good death" to critically examine end-of-life care, assisting both life-extension and dying, and changing mortality trends, to illustrate the diversity of death and dying in different contexts, arguing that the social context of death is neither as universal nor as equalising as is often presumed.

Part III: Shifting contextual domains

In Part III, we take a much broader focus on health matters, to examine some of the important, evolving social, environmental, and global contexts where health and illness are heavily implicated in various ways. The topics of these chapters – ethics, digital technology, migration, travel and tourism, place, climate change, globalisation, and commercialisation – may initially be viewed as sitting outside the specific domain of health, but as each chapter demonstrates, these are large, important, overarching concerns for health and healthcare. The application of critical perspectives to these major concerns brings issues of power, identity, disadvantage, and inequality explicitly into view. The chapters all take a broad global or ecological perspective on health, and consequently illustrate, in different ways, how people are highly interconnected, and how health and healthcare can be reconfigured by these global processes.

This part opens with a chapter on bio-ethics (Chapter 20). Here, Kathryn MacKay and Angus Dawson provide a critical review of this field, and discuss a range of innovative approaches, including feminist, public health, and global ethics drawing from African ethics and First Nations ethics. These are all focused around notions of community and connection, and provide a broader set of ethical issues for scholars to consider, which relate to health systems, public health, and global health, as well as urgent environmental matters. In the following chapter (Chapter 21), Benjamin Marent and Flis Henwood provide an overview and critique of the role of digital technologies in health, and discuss how these (re)configure healthcare, in terms of knowledge about health and illness, relationships between patients and healthcare professionals, and new forms of control that shift between technologies and people in practices of care. Next, Heide Castañeda delivers a critical account of migrant health (Chapter 22), showing how this is affected by exclusionary policies, discrimination and racism, employment in marginal and dangerous jobs, the high cost of healthcare, inadequate housing, and poor access to transportation and other resources. She argues that addressing migrant health requires an understanding of structural factors underlying displacement and recognition of processes of institutional, economic, and political marginalisation, which shape understandings of migrants as deserving or undeserving. This is followed by a consideration of medical travel – journeys undertaken to obtain medical treatment, therapies or medication in a different locality – by Cecilia Vindrola-Padros (Chapter 23). This chapter unpacks relations of power, the consequences of global and local health structures, and the (re)production of inequalities in access to care. Continuing with the concept of location, the following chapter by Robin Kearns and Gavin Andrews (Chapter 24) critically reviews the concept of place in health research. Drawing on examples that range from clinic waiting rooms to health-promoting postage stamps, they argue that the "where-ness" of place is important, but also that connections to identity and felt place-in-the-world are indelibly etched into the experience of health and illness.

The final three chapters in the handbook take up more complex and large-scale issues, commercialisation, climate change, and globalisation, as they relate to health. In Chapter 25, Peter Adams provides an overview of how commercial organisations have negatively influenced health promotion agendas through different chains of influence, illustrated by case studies of commercialisation processes involving smoking, alcohol consumption, gambling, food consumption, and the marketing of pharmaceutical and gun products. The chapter concludes with strategies for weakening industry influence on health-related matters. In Chapter 26, Sara MacBride-Stewart discusses how health is affected by climate change, and how climate change is shaping critical understandings of health. She argues for an ecosystem approach to health, discussing eco-health, one health, and planetary health as different critical lenses that raise complex questions about the nature of health, and provide opportunities to consider how the health of individuals and groups is interconnected to the health of an ecosystem. Chapter 27, by Angelina Taylor and Johanna Hanefeld, takes up the issue of globalisation, arguing that as the world becomes more interconnected and interdependent, globalisation is increasingly relevant to all aspects of health. They document how the global interconnection between transnational corporations, the movements of people, goods and diseases, and the interconnection of people around the world are important for health, producing the need for increased global coordination, health policies, and governance.

Concluding comments

This handbook focuses on many major contemporary health and illness issues that require not just attention but critical examination. As Cohen has previously argued (2017), there is an urgency for critical thinking in the academy. While he has applied this view specifically to mental health and illness (see the *Routledge International Handbook of Critical Mental Health*, 2017), we agree with his contention that the neoliberal university system often functions to discourage and displace critical and theoretical work for an emphasis on work that can be straightforwardly applied to specific situations and contexts (Cohen, 2017). But critical, conceptual, and deeply theoretical scholarship does lead to socially useful research that has tangible and important benefits. Furthermore, critical perspectives are needed now more than ever as we face unprecedented challenges to health and well-being around the globe, including climate change, social injustice, and global pandemics, including (as we write this) COVID-19. These all invoke practices that reinforce the individualising nature of neoliberalism, reinforce capitalism and the conglomeration of power and wealth in the hands of fewer people and companies, and create and sustain systems that perpetuate health inequalities, difficulties and challenges.

We trust that this handbook will provide a stimulating and vibrant collection of chapters, with its range of different positions on key issues in health and well-being in the 21st century, and its engagement with a broad set of theoretical perspectives to address oftentimes complex – or overlooked – aspects of the realities of the worlds in which people live.

Note

1 The specific goals include: Sustainable Cities and Communities; Poverty; Hunger; Health and Wellbeing; Quality Education; Gender Equality; Clean Water and Sanitation; Affordable and Clean Energy; Decent Work and Economic Growth; Industry, Innovation and Infrastructure; Reduced Inequalities; Responsible Consumption and Production; Climate Action; Life below Water; Life on Land; Peace, Justice and Strong Institutions; and Partnerships.

References

Andrews, G., Pearce, J., & Crooks, V. (Eds.). (2018). *Routledge handbook of health geography*. London: Routledge.

Bambra, C., Smith, K. E., & Hill, S. E. (Eds.). (2016). *Health inequalities: Critical perspectives*. Oxford: Oxford University Press.

Chamberlain, K., & Lyons, A. (2020). Critical and qualitative approaches to behavior change. In M. S. Hagger, L. Cameron, K. Hamilton, N. Hankonen, & T. Lintunen (Eds.), *The handbook of behavior change* (pp. 430–442). Cambridge: Cambridge University Press.

Cohen, B. M. (Ed.). (2017). *Routledge international handbook of critical mental health*. London: Routledge.

Government of South Australia & World Health Organization. (2017). *Progressing the sustainable development goals through health in all policies: Case studies from around the world*. Adelaide: Government of South Australia.

Lin, V., Kickbusch, I., & Baer, B. (2017). Introduction. In Government of South Australia & World Health Organization (Ed.), *Progressing the sustainable development goals through health in all policies: Case studies from around the world*. Adelaide: Government of South Australia.

Major, B., Dovidio, J., & Link, B. (Eds.). (2018). *The Oxford handbook of stigma, discrimination, and health*. Oxford: Oxford University Press.

McInnes, C., Lee, K., & Youde, J. (Eds.). (2020). *The Oxford handbook of global health politics*. Oxford: Oxford University Press.

Nunes, A. R., Lee, K., & O'Riordan, T. (2016). The importance of an integrating framework for achieving the sustainable development goals: The example of health and well-being. *BMJ Global Health*, 1(3), 1:e000068.

Raphael, D., Rioux, M. H., & Bryant, T. (Eds.). (2019). *Staying alive: Critical perspectives on health, illness, and health care* (3rd ed.). Toronto: Canadian Scholars.

Vojnovic, I., Pearson, A. L., Asiki, G., DeVerteuil, G., & Allen, A. (Eds.). (2019). *Handbook of global urban health*. London: Routledge.

World Health Organisation. (n.d.). *Social determinants of health*. Retrieved from https://www.who.int/health-topics/social-determinants-of-health#tab=tab_1

PART I

Medical contexts

2

THE SOCIAL AND CULTURAL HISTORIES OF MEDICINE

Catharine Coleborne

The most rapid changes in medical science took place in the 20th century when vast improvements in human health were witnessed across the world's populations. This idea of the 20th century as an era of fast-paced change affecting more people is the premise of the fascinating documentary series *People's Century*, a co-production between the British Broadcasting Corporation (BBC) and Boston's Public Broadcasting Service (PBS), which uses thousands of hours of oral interviews and video footage. The episode "Living Longer, 1954" examines the theme of health and medicine from the 1950s.[1] It features interviews with people who experienced hospitalisation and contemporary management of lung function in cases of polio, such as the iron lung, and it explores the radical advances in human health made as a result of penicillin used during World War Two and manufactured for the widespread treatment of tuberculosis in the 1950s as part of a combined therapy. The episode shows that a combination of public health measures put in place across different nations – including vaccination campaigns in India to eradicate polio from 1978 – resulted in a new world order of health across successive decades. Not only that, but with medical knowledge, the common imagery of disease as linked to dirt, poverty, and deprivation was beginning to be replaced by a better understanding of disease transmission and control.

This story of health and medicine is one of progress and improvement. Yet such a teleological account of medical advances can easily be critiqued. In 2020, the global pandemic known as COVID-19 has once again challenged societies, communities and governments to respond to the "threat" of disease, and not for the first time. The global influenza pandemic of 1918–1919 is now held up as an example of public health in action: how did the flu spread, and what practices contained it? What lessons from that terrible experience might translate into our present? This and other experiences of illness shows that historical interpretations of health and medicine continue to provide us with a deep sense of public community awareness.

This chapter sets out a social and cultural history of medicine to lay the groundwork for the current volume, which by nature has a broad audience and reach. It positions major ideas in the social and cultural histories of health and medicine for readers of subsequent chapters. The field of medical history is now so immense (see Porter, 1999; Huisman & Warner, 2004; and Jackson, 2011) that any attempt to provide a pithy account of it will necessarily disappoint (Waddington, 2011, p. 339). Therefore, this chapter focuses on themes pertinent to the volume as a whole and asserts the relevance of medical history to a critical reading of health and illness in the present.

It touches on global problems in health history, as well as describing some specific changes in methodologies and theories of health and illness used by historians interested in health and medicine.

Relevant themes in the field include national and local policy shifts; the politics of medicine inside welfare states; health and human rights; and finally, the changing imagination of the body in sickness and health. The way that 21st-century sensibilities now shape our understandings of the body also influences how historians think, write, and practice their research around questions of immunity, medical technology, the role of the carer, and future societies and medical interventions. Inherently interdisciplinary, the social history of medicine reaches across into histories of the environment, and the emergent field of global and planetary health. It is at the forefront of complex interpretations of the body, dialogue between actors in a health relationship, cultural specificity in understandings of disease and treatment, as well as consumer and activist groups and health economies.

By the late 20th century, the social history of medicine had assumed the mantle of a highly regarded and successful field of historical research and educational studies at large. Supported by research funding from the Wellcome Trust in the United Kingdom, and by institutional and philanthropic funds in the United States and Europe, the social history of medicine has provided generations of scholars with the impetus to link historical thinking with current problems of policy, public interest or debate, and with local and regional heritage and healthcare projects. These factors make the social history of medicine an important source of relevance for the humanities in an increasingly technological world, and allow historians to find commonality and purpose, as well as collaborative potential, with medical science researchers and practitioners. Scholars of the medical humanities argue that the arts, humanities and social sciences are "best viewed not as in service or in opposition to the clinical and life sciences, but as productively entangled with a biomedical culture" (Viney, Callard, & Woods, 2015, p. 2). The formulation of the medical humanities should therefore be understood as one intellectual context for the wider relevance of the medical history approach.

Importantly, this chapter shows that the historiographical field of the social history of medicine has been challenged by waves of changing analytical models from the middle of the 20th century, making historians attune to questions of social class, gender, ethnicity, sexuality and difference, as well as power, institutions, authority, professionalisation, and the attendant themes of specialisation and practice. Ultimately, the critical historian of health and medicine faces the deeper problems of subjectivity and objectification. How did "we" become the subjects of medicine? What is the effect of medical language – diagnoses, aetiologies, framings – on people?

Polio – a disease with successive outbreaks over the course of the 20th century – was seen as a disease of the poor. Visual representations of lurking and stalking polio, broadcast as public health messages from the early part of the 20th century, were frightening and created panic during epidemics, such as the 1916 outbreak of polio in the north-eastern United States (Rogers, 1992, p. 29). The stigma attached to a disease could, time and time again, limit the shaping of effective social responses to it, from polio outbreaks across the 20th century to the impact of HIV/AIDs in the 1980s. Charles Rosenberg's important argument about the "framing" of disease as set out in Rosenberg and Golden's edited collection underpins the ideas provided in this chapter's account of the history of medicine (Rosenberg & Golden, 1992). Read in the light of the rise of biomedical discourses, which had become entrenched from the early 20th century (Warner, 2013, p. 323), this body of work is all the more remarkable: it asked that we scrutinise all medical knowledge very carefully, evaluating language and context. We need to continue to open up medical power and authority for historical scrutiny. Here, I suggest that the history of medicine is a multiplicity of histories of health and healing, boundaries, relationships, and understandings.

Being prepared to interrogate medical histories in these ways can help the historian establish different understandings of clinical knowledge and practice for our present.

The chapter starts with a reflection on world history and disease.[2] It then moves on to describe the way medical education, another impetus for the work of the medical historian, frames some of the debates about the relevance of the field. Social medicine becomes the focus of a brief historiography of the social history of medicine before the chapter examines methodologies and approaches in the field, including those that reshaped the scholarship from the 1980s. Vital areas of inquiry, such as health encounters and medical authority, space and geographies, and the patient's voice, all sprang from new theoretical strands in the wider discipline of historical studies. Finally, the chapter foreshadows future histories of health and medicine, and shows how far the field has moved: from the "disease and society" model to global histories of health and biomedicine, including the profound question of ecological change and human survival.

World history and disease

The relationship between world history and disease provides a useful starting point to examine health and illness over time. The exploration and conquest of new lands by Europeans inevitably led to the spread of diseases fatal to Indigenous populations everywhere. Combined with disruption to traditional food sources, environments, and outright violence, disease spread by contact with the carriers of new pathogens played a significant role in the depopulation of peoples in North America, Australia, and the Pacific islands (see Crosby, 1992). The 1789 outbreak of smallpox in Port Jackson, New South Wales, was described by British marine officer, Watkin Tench (Tench, 1789), who called it "an extraordinary calamity", and documented the pain and suffering of the people he called "Indians", their "bodies … in all the coves and inlets of the harbour":

> Pustules, similar to those occasioned by the smallpox, were thickly spread on the bodies; but how a disease to which our former observations had led us to suppose them strangers could at once have introduced itself, and have spread so widely, seemed inexplicable.
>
> *(Tench, 1789)*

In the middle of the 20th century, historians became interested in a post-war narrative of humanity. They contested the model of "Western civilisation" and began to think about the way the world's economic, trade, and political networks were also opportunities to think about cultural exchanges between peoples. Disease, too, was an outcome of human contact and mobility. William McNeill's epidemiological history *Plagues and Peoples* (1976) was the culmination of his thinking about world history modes, and it became an exemplar of thinking about infectious disease as an actor in historical change over the long period between 1300 and 1700 – a time of enormous global expansion through both exploration and trade, as well as conquest, the migration of peoples, and of germs. Medicine was inextricably linked with imperialism (MacLeod & Lewis, 1988).

Global histories produced in the 21st century now include the uneven histories of health, the role of technologies of medicine, and the question of bioethics. Later in this chapter I briefly examine the emergent field of planetary health as an extension of global histories of health, medicine, and disease, but also as a newer form of historical thinking that combines scientific, medical, and environmental knowledge with the work of physician-historians.

Medical education

Medical education was multiple and dispersed before the modern era. The world of healers in premodern times was characterised by different types of practitioners, known for their specific contributions to surgery, the diagnosis of illnesses using various methods, and the treatment of common illnesses with potions, drugs, and remedies. Popular healers were part of a medical marketplace plying their trades, and until at least the 18th-century healers peddled good and bad practices and competed for recognition. As historian Roy Porter noted of the century or so to 1800:

> Thousands of people made a living, or topped up their incomes, from medicine at this time. Grocers and pedlars sold drugs. Blacksmiths and farriers drew teeth and set bones. Itinerants toured the country, selling bottles of brightly coloured "wonder cures". Some were probably simply rogues. Other travelling doctors possessed genuine skills is treating eye, teeth or ear complaints.
>
> *(Porter, 1992, p. 94)*

Porter went on to suggest that many more people looked after neighbours, "well-versed" in herbal medicine; there was also an important role for parish communities.[3]

Between 1550 and 1640, over 700 unlicensed medical practitioners had some contact with the London College of Physicians (Pelling, 1995, p. 254–255). Formal university training for male physicians was based on an apprenticeship model with family connections; before the 15th century, students were clerics and were trained in the arts before they studied medical knowledge. By the 19th century, centres of medical education were located in Scotland, England, the Netherlands, Germany, as well as attracting medical migrants from the colonies, ensuring the flow of medical knowledge between the imperial centre and colonial sites. Western medicine was, then, formed in a Judeo-Christian context and carried with it the assumptions about knowledge created in this tradition.

Medical education itself has a long history and occupies its own place in the wider history of medicine (Nutton & Porter, 1995, p. 2). Distinct bodies of knowledge relate to the fields of anatomy and surgery (Waddington, 2011, pp. 117, 123) and the increasing significance of the medical laboratory (Waddington, 2011, p. 199), which pushed the boundaries of hospital training and added new impetus for scientific experimentation inside institutional spaces, as Foucault also wrote (Foucault, 1963,). Historians writing in the latter part of the 20th century focused on the politics of medical training and education, including equitable access to medical education; issues of humanising medical students' understandings of the practice of medicine, including medical ethics; and the impact of social constructionist approaches to historical thinking (Huisman & Warner, 2004; Jordanova, 1995; Waddington, 2011, p. 11).

Canadian historian Jacalyn Duffin crafted accessible, practical narratives for medical education (see Duffin, 1999), which rest on the premise that knowing history helps medical students to question positivist knowledge in their scientific training (Duffin, 1999, p. 7). Yet the "struggle" to retain historical perspectives in the medical curriculum has frustrated medical historians (Jones, Greene, Duffin, & Warner, 2015, p. 623) with frequent conversations among historians about positive models and well-argued justifications for the inclusion of humanities knowledge (Jones et al., 2015, p. 638–639). Special issues and conference panels on this topic show this problem has persisted. For example, in 1999, *Radical History Review* included an array of articles focused on the role of teaching medical students about racism. By 2011, this topic was still worthy of two panels at the Utrecht meeting for the European Association for the Histories of

Health and Medicine (EAHHM), with papers describing challenges in European, British, and US medical curricula. Historians reported the use of case studies, such as the Tuskegee syphilis experiment with African-American peoples (Washington, 2006), to underscore medical human ethics as well as the problem of racism in medicine.

Communicating scientific knowledge to public audiences runs parallel to medical education. Medical museums, which once played a role in medical education, can also be reinterpreted. Their static presentation of medical and anatomical objects in glass bottles and cases has given way to a more dynamic and accessible representation of health and bodies, such as displays in exhibitions that combine visual and material objects with touch screens, and contemporary theories of disease and bodily functions. Such displays blur the lines between expert and lay understandings of health science; for instance, The Health Museum, Houston, Texas or the Wellcome Science Gallery with its focus on medicine.[4] These are both examples of highly current entry points for museum visitors to a world of biomedical expertise, raising the stakes for the museum experience.

The role of the physician in the conceptualisation of medical history is critical to understanding its reach. The historical training of medical students in universities was one powerful impetus for the development of the scholarship in the histories of medicine. Physicians have held special roles in the cultural imagination, and their positions of authority in Western societies have allowed doctors to cultivate and wield political, social, and economic influence. It follows, then, that understanding how doctors have advocated for specific causes should be seen as an important aspect of their histories. Health policy and the role of the state has remained a powerful theme for early 21st-century scholarship. Paul Weindling's exhortation to medical historians to perform an ethical, "scientific", and public role in debates over clinical medicine, access to patient records, evidence-based treatments, and standards of care reminds us of the necessity to lay bare the past failures of medicine, the egregious mistakes and abuses of health systems, not least the darker impact of medicine during the Holocaust (see Weindling, 2014, 2015).

Social medicine

In the post-war era, doctors were part of a new generation of professional practice, a generation that thought deeply about the role of medicine in society. The "physician-historians" who sparked an "important new current" in medical history in the 1930s and 1940s, the field of social medicine, were at the forefront of arguing for the relevance of social understandings of health and medicine (Warner, 2013, p. 326). This was, as John Harley Warner writes, a "sociologically-inflected historical focus" on the many problems and issues swirling around medicine, especially where it intersected with inequalities (Warner, 2013, p. 326). Historical work published in the 1950s and 1960s was the outcome of an intellectual tradition in thinking about medicine and humanity, tackling themes such as diseases and occupations, and the economic context for illness (Warner, 2013, p. 326). By this time, in both North America and Britain, "historically minded medical educators ... promoted the view that physicians must assume leadership in the struggle for the improvement of social conditions" (Dolan, 2010, p. 396).

The significant social changes following World War Two, including a new era for university education, meant that different generations of students entered colleges and institutions, propelled by widening participation in post-secondary learning, including in medicine and allied health, but also in humanities. By the 1970s and 1980s, social historians started to revise earlier traditions of historical research and writing, opening the door to "history from below" as well as the influences of other disciplines, although the history of medicine is a field that has always been intrinsically interdisciplinary in its nature and scope, if not its methodologies. The social history of medicine was arguably transformed by more critical approaches to questions of gender, power, ethnicity, and "race", prompting historians to scour the archive for different sources and records related to health and illness. Now it picked up on the concerns of earlier proponents of social medicine, and reinvigorated questions about the potential for the medicine to be "humanised", a quest which took on new urgency as a more radical critique of the medical establishment was underway (Warner, 2013, p. 326).

Medicalisation and health encounters

In the 20th century, the widespread "medicalisation" of everyday life, which had happened over the course of the 19th century, became the target of fresh analysis. The definition of medicalisation provided by Ann Goldberg in her work about the pathologisation of the Jewish people is especially useful: it was the "process by which medicine and medical thinking increased its prestige" and social problems, as well as populations, came to be viewed as "medical problems" (Goldberg, 1996, p. 265). Medicalisation is a particularly useful concept to unpack in terms of the histories of people and groups. The "othering" of different peoples – that is, different to the Anglo-European norm – tended to work along racial and ethnic lines as well as across the class divide. If whole populations could be pathologised or treated as "sick" or "diseased", it was obvious that medicine itself was a language inflected by specific judgements and lacked objectivity.

Sometimes this had the result of identifying health improvements, but ones tinged by paternalistic health policy. In New Zealand, Māori people were identified as a specific health population from the 1940s following decades of neglect, and new investigations into outbreaks of infectious disease among Māori in remote communities were undertaken. By the 1950s and 1960s, when Māori rural–urban migration was noticeable, along with the large number of Pacific migrants in the city of Auckland, changing perceptions of health and housing combined to force greater awareness of health disparities between Māori, Pasifika and European populations (Coleborne, 2009, p. 507).

Social movements of the 1960s and 1970s influenced the way academic fields were reshaped. The Boston Women's Health Book Collective interventions into women's health challenged some precepts of medical treatment, including the idea that women's bodies were not their own. The publication of *Our Bodies, Ourselves* followed an initial pamphlet publication in 1970. The book has been reprinted continuously, showing the powerful reach of feminist activism for women's health. Similar activism took hold in other places (see Coleborne, 2009, p. 508). The women's movement outside the academy spawned a new generation of women's histories, including the scholarship of women and medicine. Gender difference, conceptualised as a set of norms relating to biological sex difference, became a major analytical tool in the hands of historians interested in the language of medicine and its rendering of biological difference, which impacted the health experiences of women and men (Jordanova, 1989).

Medical power had always been challenged by women: from the early modern contestation over childbirth and the roles of midwives, to the control over women's bodies in the matters of contraception or abortion in the 20th century. What was increasingly clear was the way many health populations had been made subject to medical power over time. The new "sexual politics" of illness highlighted by researchers and activists in the 1970s pointed to the historically contingent experiences of women, such as middle-class women who occupied a "sick role" in the 19th century (Ehrenreich & English, 1973, p. 22). Debates about the role of the midwife were central to the gendering of the history of medicine. Midwives were replaced by male practitioners during the 18th and 19th century, with the surrounding context of medical professionalisation, a recasting of the knowledge about women's bodies, and the introduction of new technologies of childbirth by male obstetricians – the forceps and stirrups – which forced women out of the birthing chamber over time, especially for middle-class and upper-class women (Marland, 2011, pp. 492–493).

The story of the world's peoples – their power, protest, and political advocacy – shaped much new historical writing. By the late 1990s, the subfield of colonial medicine was a fast-growing and exciting addition to the array of new, critical interventions in the social history of medicine. The question "what is colonial about colonial medicine?" (Marks, 1997) hit on the emerging work of a bright generation of scholars tackling imperial medicine and colonial worlds who were seeking out the colonial archive and interrogating medicine as a tool of empire. These histories of colonial encounters were not just "from below", they also symbolised a radical politics of health and empire that promised to de-centre Western historiographies, especially if authored by Indigenous writers. Writing about the Hawaiian peoples' resistance to colonisers, Haunani-Kay Trask pointed to the social determinants of Hawaiian health (Trask, 1993, p. 49). Postcolonial histories of medicine, as imagined by this generation of thinkers, would encourage a return to the earlier framing of health and disease in different spaces and geographical locations (Anderson, 2004, p. 285).

Health encounters over time also point to ideas about cross-cultural understandings of health shaped by power relations. This new slant on critical histories of power, including the power of the medical experts, also highlighted the complexity of the medical encounter. Where did medical authority lie? What knowledge constituted medicine and medical expertise? The dialogue between the sick, their healers, and families and communities, is one of the most important aspects of the social and cultural history of medicine. Diagnoses could be contested, and so too could the language used to frame illness and experience.

Several original works of history captured the imagination of scholars in the 1980s and 1990s. Michael MacDonald's *Mystical Bedlam* (1983) examined the life and work of early modern physician Richard Napier (1559–1634) through extant casebooks.[5] These records show that Napier was consulted thousands of times by people from all walks of life seeking solutions to a range of ailments, including melancholia, making these an early record of treatments for "madness", rich with ideas about mental health filtered by the ideas of the period. This study allowed modern historians to glimpse a pre-asylum world of anxiety, stress, trauma, and distress, as well as mere frustration, as experienced by ordinary people. As MacDonald writes:

> The frustrations that troubled Napier's humble clients reflect the expectations of ordinary men and women, but they naturally tell us more about the vexations endured by wives and daughters than about the difficulties of husbands and sons. … Love and marriage, death and money are their principal themes.
>
> *(MacDonald, 1983, pp. 74–75)*

Similarly, Barbara Duden's *The Woman Beneath the Skin* (1998) gave readers access to the casebooks of an 18th-century German male midwife Johann Storch, and his many consultations as he supported women through their "complaints". Storch also wrote his autobiography and, like Napier, was a prolific healer. These two accounts of the worlds of health and medicine are revealing: Napier's world of mental distress was much like ours, but his insights into healing were filtered by an early modern understanding of astrological medicine and a religious world view. Duden's work, on the other hand, suggests that Storch's accounts tell us that women in the 18th century understood their bodies in an entirely different way to women of a later historical period; the body itself was the construct of time, place and culture.

Anthropological insights provided additional rich dimensions to the historical research, which was interrogating medical culture and practices of medicine. Emily Martin's work on immunology is a good example of medical anthropology that uses historical thinking. Martin's work looks at the way popular conceptions of health and immunity in American culture changed as scientific concepts of the immune system transformed representations of, for instance, the human body's capacity to heal itself or to fend off disease (Martin, 1994). Based on ethnographic research, Martin set out to show that historical specificity could challenge people's thinking about the body and immunity, as evidenced by the HIV/AIDs crisis from the early 1980s. The power of medical imagery to explain a body at "war" with itself was a high point from the 1970s in the United States with the "war on cancer" pronouncements by the Republican President Richard Nixon, and the funding poured into the National Institutes for Health that signalled this military-like campaign to end certain pathogenic cancers, among other illnesses.

Susan Sontag's late 1970s conceptualisation of "illness as metaphor", which she expanded to include AIDS as a metaphor in 1989, explained how cancer and AIDS were understood through metaphorical images and symbols that linked to social ideas about sufferers (Sontag, 1978). These strands of writing have been important to some medical historical writing and research, especially in cultural histories of illness interested in language, narratives of health and sufferers, and in the significance of cultures of health and medicine in different places.

As well as offering care and spaces for recuperation, institutions developed as intricate systems of power and control of the sick, and in some cases isolation, separation, and segregation. The central figure of Thomas Mann's novel *The Magic Mountain*, Hans Castorp, becomes a witness to the tuberculosis sanatorium when he visits his ill cousin in a sanatorium in Davos, Switzerland. What he encounters there is a strange and rarefied world of the institution which asks its members to submit to its regimes and practices, and to its hierarchies. The institutions of health and medicine have taken different forms over time. Rosenberg called this development the "care of strangers", writing about the growth of America's hospitals from their early years as charitable institutions to their roles as teaching institutions and clinical environments (Rosenberg, 1995).

Hospitals for the insane were a largely 19th-century solution to mental breakdowns in communities. By looking at the growth of the asylum system in an Anglo-American context, historian Nancy Tomes was able to point to the shared history of a transition from household care in the early 18th century to a medicalisation or at least "hospitalisation" of insanity over time (Tomes, 1988, p. 6). The "painful domestic problem" of madness, writes Tomes, "offered an institutional alternative" for families dealing with chronic mental illness in an era before more widespread solutions existed (Tomes, 1988, p. 19). Interestingly, the experiences of extra-institutional care, including family care, boarding-out, and community care has been the focus of a late 20th-century historical exploration of alternatives to the large institutions in societies around the world, in part driven by a post-institutional landscape in the present (Coleborne, 2020). Yet institutions − small, large, rural, metropolitan − dominated the landscape of mental healthcare for over a century, also generating vast histories of institutional worlds, populations, and patient or inmate narratives, replete with clinical knowledge and sources of information about experiences of mental illness.

The patient's voice

The patient's voice has been all but obscured in many medical histories. However, histories of psychiatry somewhat paradoxically tend to record the stories of those institutionalised (McCarthy, Coleborne, O'Connor & Knewstubb, 2017). Confined in public mental hospitals, places that were often hidden from view, men and women who suffered mental breakdowns could languish far from friends and families. In hospitals for the insane in most countries, inmates were provided with moral therapies – religious worship, gardening, household work, and other forms of labour – and they also wrote letters. Writing from Toronto Hospital for the Insane sometime in the 1910s, patient Henrietta alternated between reflections on art, and descriptions of her loneliness and memories of violence and abuse (Reaume, 2010, p. 127). Sadly, institutions could both protect inmates from familial violence at home, but also perpetuate painful and abusive relationships common to large institutional environments.

In the 1980s public health systems in the Western world were under scrutiny. How did they stand up inside models of economic rationalisation as conservative governments in many countries challenged older concepts of the welfare state? Responses were mixed, but all involved the highly politically engaged concept of the "patient as consumer". Forcing health consumers to take responsibility for their own health put the spotlight on health behaviours, with individualism one outcome of the shift in thinking about the role of the state in healthcare. By the late 1990s, this was referred to as a "new political economy of health" (D. Porter, 1999).

The wider context was an opportunity for historians interested in public health systems and health institutions, but other historians also focused on the role of the patient. The significance of Roy Porter's work on the patient's voice (Porter, 1985) has endured though critiques of his stance, and his evidentiary base for understanding the world of the patient has been useful (see Bacopoulos-Viau & Fauvel, 2016). This strand of scholarship has in practice spawned a rich inquiry into the many partners to medical and health dialogue, as noted earlier: the emphasis has shifted to looking at communities of care, practice, and treatment, including the roles of families and others in institutional care (see, for example, Mooney & Reinharz, 2009).

The future of the history of health and medicine

What, then, is the future for the history of health and medicine? In the late 1990s, what we knew about the state of the world's health, as well as our own personal experiences of illness and medical treatment, was vastly different from the knowledge and experiences of previous generations. The hopeful narrative of medicine and its potential to cure the diseases of earlier periods of history, including polio, smallpox, and tuberculosis, was threatened by new viruses like HIV/AIDS. Public health systems groaned under the weight of state spending, under-funded institutions and programmes, and global inequalities showed the limitations of a mid-20th-century hopefulness about health and human rights. In the present, anxiety about the future of global mobility in the post-COVID era has created new conversations about health and human behaviours. Roy Porter predicted some of this in his book of 1997 when he reflected that "new" diseases "are not unlucky accidents, but part of the political and economic system that the West pursues" (Porter, 1999, pp. 710–711).

As this chapter has detailed, the social history of medicine is no longer a history of heroic medicine, scientific progress, doctors, or even of disease. It is now an array of perceptions of institutions, people who are experiencing illness, the roles of carers, diagnostic labels and contested treatments, the politics of health, state policy, and interventions into inequalities in the provision of healthcare. Within this busy frame, several futures for the field have emerged as more significant than others.

First, a critical history of biomedicine and its failures – as well as the successes of medical scientific breakthroughs – has become a project for most historians of health and medicine in the first decades of the 21st century. Where research into immunology, stem cell therapies, pharmacological experimentation and advances, and reproductive technologies melds with social change and debates about the future of humanity, historians are needed to provide a measured assessment of the realities of the potential biomedical transformation of human life and ageing or the defeat of diseases. Being broadly attendant to the return of "old diseases" through war, conflict, poverty, and other factors is a reminder of the fragility of medical progress; in the same vein, politically-charged campaigns such as anti-vaccination movements threaten to confront populations with outbreaks of diseases once assumed to be "cured", including measles and polio. Outbreaks of influenza are monitored globally, and vaccines are always in development. But all of this is contingent on social cohesion, good public health, and practical considerations in the prevention of pandemics.

Second, health activism, broadly defined, allows topics and narratives about medicine and the role of the physician-advocate to again come to the fore as we look, for instance, at the late 20th-century episode of HIV/AIDS, or at mental health. Critical disability studies inform this work and places the consumer of health services, including those with lived experiences of illness, at the centre of the narrative. The disability rights movement has a long history, which dates back to the 19th century. For example, deaf and blind people campaigned for access to employment, also challenging ideas about public perceptions of disability and citizenship (Patterson, 2018, pp. 440–441). Returning to the example of polio, it was polio sufferers in the United States from the 1930s who recognised the value of the organised "crusade" for rights, a model taken up by successive generations of Americans with physical disabilities (Patterson, 2018, p. 441).

Planetary health (Dunk, Jones, Capon, & Anderson, 2019) emerges as a third frontier in medical histories. This area takes us back to the potency of the role of the physician-historian. James Dunk and colleagues suggest that the "ailing planet" – evidenced by recent crises in climate change, bushfires in Australia, and political protest around the world – is now the sick patient requiring intervention from doctors and public health experts (Dunk et al., 2019, p. 778). The weight of evidence now of environmental degradation dates at least from the 1960s and has reached a fever pitch. The implications for human health given the seriousness of climate change and its impact on weather, food supplies, air quality, and respiratory disease, as well as everyday health for people living in precarious settings threatened by rising sea levels, are now at a critical stage. Where the social histories of health and medicine and studies of global planetary health collide with a common purpose is promising a new form of contemporary and historical thinking.

Climate change is now one of a growing list of contextual threats to our resilience and mental health, especially for young people who face an uncertain future. Global mental health provides a final strand of the history of health and medicine which continues to situate cultures, peoples and places in relation to the state and its policies and practices (Coleborne & Roberts-Pedersen, forthcoming). As the following chapters in this volume show, the critical appraisal of health, illness, models of treatment and care, belief systems, and the politics of medicine continues to be central to understanding humanity and our place in the world.

Acknowledgements

My teaching of the social and cultural histories of medicine in New Zealand for around 15 years from 2000 allowed me to explore a narrative of the field with students who conducted their own research projects situated in New Zealand histories of health. I was fortunate to learn from their work, including masters and doctoral student research projects during this period. Thanks to Dr Jan McLeod at the University of Newcastle, Australia, for her excellent bibliographical research assistance with this chapter.

Notes

1 See *People's Century*, Episode 19: "Living Longer, 1954", https://www.bbc.co.uk/programmes/b0 0742qp, URL accessed 24 May 2020.
2 Although this chapter takes a global perspective, it focuses on the period from the early modern era to the 21st century and omits any discussion of the ancient or pre-modern world. For this reason, the chapter should be read and understood alongside other texts which take a longer view.
3 This work of neighbours and communities was also common in colonial worlds; see Coleborne and Godtschalk (2013).
4 See https://www.thehealthmuseum.org/, URL accessed 24 May 2020; and https://www.sciencem useum.org.uk/see-and-do/medicine-wellcome-galleries, URL accessed 24 May 2020.
5 Richard Napier's casebooks, along with those of a contemporary, Simon Foreman, have been digitised, and are available to researchers https://casebooks.wordpress.com/about/

References

Anderson, W. (2004). Postcolonial histories of medicine. In F. Huisman and J. H. Warner (Eds.), *Locating medical history* (pp. 285–306). Baltimore: Johns Hopkins University Press.

Bacopoulos-Viau, A., & Fauvel, A. (2016). The patient's turn Roy Porter and psychiatry's tales, thirty years on. *Medical History, 60*(1), 1–18.

Coleborne, C. (2009). Health and illness, 1840s–1990s. In G. Byrnes (Ed.), *The new Oxford history of New Zealand*. Melbourne: Oxford University Press.

Coleborne, C., & Godtschalk, O. (2013). Colonial families and cultures of health: Glimpses of illness and domestic medicine in private records in New Zealand and Australia, 1850–1910. *Journal of Family History, 38*(4), 403–221.

Coleborne, C. (2020). *Why talk about madness? Bringing history into the conversation*. Cham, Switzerland: Springer Nature.

Coleborne, C., & Roberts-Pedersen, E. (forthcoming). *Making mental health: A global history*. London: Routledge.

Crosby, A. W. (1992). Hawaiian depopulation as a model for the Amerindian experience. In T. Ranger & P. Slack (Eds.), *Epidemics and ideas: Essays on the historical perception of pestilence* (pp. 175–201). Cambridge: Cambridge University Press.

Dolan, B. (2010). History, medical humanities and medical education. *Social History of Medicine, 23*(2), 393–405.

Duden, B. (1998). *The woman beneath the skin: A doctor's patients in eighteenth-century Germany*. Cambridge, MA: Harvard University Press.

Duffin, J. (1999). *History of medicine: A scandalously short introduction*. Toronto: University of Toronto Press.

Dunk, J. H., Jones, D. S., Capon, A., & Anderson, W. H. (2019). Human health or an ailing planet – Historical perspectives on our future. *New England Journal of Medicine, 381*(8), 778–782.

Ehrenreich, B., & English, D. (1973). *Complaints and disorders: The sexual politics of sickness*. New York: Feminist Press.

Foucault, M. (1963). *The birth of the clinic: An archaeology of medical perception* (A. M. Sheridan Smith, Trans.). New York: Vintage Books.

Goldberg, J. (1996). The limits of medicalization: Jewish lunatics and nineteenth-century Germany. *History of Psychiatry, vii*, 265–285.

Huisman, F., & Warner, J. H. (Eds.). (2004). *Locating medical history: The stories and their meanings*. Baltimore: Johns Hopkins University Press.

Jackson, M. (Ed.). (2011). *The Oxford handbook of the history of medicine*. Oxford: Oxford University Press.

Jones, D. S., Greene, J. A., Duffin, J., & Warner, J. H. (2015). Making the case for history in medical education. *Journal of the History of Medicine and Allied Sciences, 70*(4), 623–652.

Jordanova, L. (1989). *Sexual visions images of gender and science in medicine between the eighteenth and twentieth centuries*. New York: Harvester Wheatsheaf.

Jordanova, L. (1995). The social construction of medical knowledge. *Social History of Medicine, 8*(3), 361–381.

Marks, S. (1997). What is colonial about colonial medicine? And what has happened to imperialism and health? *Social History of Medicine, 10*(2), 205–219.

Marland, H. (2011). Women, health and medicine. In M. Jackson (Ed.), *The Oxford handbook of the history of medicine* (pp. 484–502). Oxford: Oxford University Press.

Martin, E. (1994). *Flexible bodies: Tracking immunity in American culture from the days of polio to the age of AIDS.* Boston: Beacon Press.

MacDonald, M. (1983). *Mystical Bedlam: Madness, anxiety, and healing in seventeenth-century England.* Cambridge: Cambridge University Press.

MacLeod, R., & Lewis, M. (Eds.). (1988). *Disease, medicine and empire. Perspectives on western medicine and the experience of European expansion.* London: Routledge.

McCarthy, A., Coleborne, C., O'Connor, M., & Knewstubb, E. (2017). Lives in the asylum record, 1864 to 1910: Utilising large data collection for histories of psychiatry and mental health in the British World. *Medical History, 61*(3), 358–379.

McNeill, W. H. (1976). *Plagues and peoples.* New York: Anchor Books.

Mooney, G., & Reinarz, J. (Eds.). (2009). *Permeable walls: Historical perspectives on hospital and asylum visiting.* Amsterdam and New York: Rodopi.

Nutton, V., & Porter, R. (Eds.). (1995). *The history of medical education in Britain.* Amsterdam: Rodopi.

Patterson, L. (2018). The disability rights movement in the United States. In M. Remibis, C. Kudlick, & K. E. Nielsen (Eds.), *The Oxford handbook of disability studies* (pp. 439–457). New York: Oxford University Press.

Pelling, M. (1995). Knowledge common and acquired: The education of unlicensed medical practitioners in early modern London. In V. Nutton & R. Porter (Eds.), *The history of medical education in Britain* (pp. 250–279). Amsterdam: Rodopi.

Porter, D. (1999). *Health, civilization, and the state: A history of public health from ancient to modern times.* London: Routledge.

Porter, R. (1985). The patient's view: Doing medical history from below. *Theory & Society, 14*(2), 175–198.

Porter, R. (1992). The patient in England, c.1660–c.1800. In W. Wear (Ed.), *Medicine in society: Historical essays* (pp. 91–118). Cambridge: Cambridge University Press.

Porter, R. (1999). *The greatest benefit to mankind: A medical history from antiquity to the present.* London: Fontana/Harper Collins.

Reaume, G. (2010). *Remembrance of patients past: Patient life at the Toronto hospital for the insane, 1870–1940.* Toronto: University of Toronto Press.

Rogers, N. (1992). *Dirt and disease: Polio before FDR.* New Brunswick: Rutgers University Press.

Rosenberg, C. (1995). *The care of strangers: The rise of America's hospital system.* Baltimore: Johns Hopkins University Press.

Rosenberg, C. E., & Golden, J. (Eds.). (1992). *Framing disease: Studies in cultural history.* New Brunswick: Rutgers University Press.

Sontag, S. (1978). *Illness as metaphor.* New York: Farrar, Straus & Giroux.

Tench, W. (1789). *A narrative of the expedition to Botany Bay and A complete account of the settlement at Port Jackson.* London: Debrett; T. & J. Swords.

Tomes, N. (1988). The Anglo-American asylum in historical perspective. In C. Smith & J. A. Giggs (Eds.), *Location and stigma: Contemporary perspectives on mental health and mental health care.* Boston: Unwin Hyman.

Trask, H.-K. (1993). *From a native daughter: Colonialism and sovereignty in Hawai'i.* Honolulu: University of Hawai'i Press.

Viney, W., Callard, F., & Woods, A. (2015) Critical medical humanities: Embracing entanglement, taking risks. *Medical Humanities, 41*(1), 2–7.

Waddington, K. (2011). *An introduction to the history of medicine: Europe since 1500.* Basingstoke: Palgrave.

Washington, H. (2006). *Medical apartheid: The dark history of medical experimentation on black Americans from colonial times to the present.* New York: Doubleday.

Warner, J. H. (2013). The humanizing power of medical history: responses to biomedicine in the 20th century United States. *Procedia: Social and Behavioral Sciences, 77,* 322–329.

Weindling, P. (2014, 10–12 July). Opening address, Society for the Social History of Medicine Conference: Disease, Health and the State. Oxford Brookes University and the University of Oxford.

Weindling, P. (2015). *Victims and survivors of Nazi human experiments: Science and suffering in the Holocaust.* London: Bloomsbury.

3

MEDICALISATION

Felicity Thomas

Introduction

Medicalisation is the process by which a growing array of conditions and experiences of human life become defined, understood, and managed through medical and medically-related expertise. As Conrad (2015, p. vii) has stated, research on medicalisation "does not adjudicate whether or not an entity is 'really' a medical problem, but rather how it became to be depicted (and accepted) as a medical problem and with what consequences". The term medicalisation first appeared in the sociology literature with a focus on "deviance as illness" (Pitts, 1968). However, it soon expanded to encompass other human conditions, and over time the increasingly multidisciplinary study of medicalisation has been infused with a wide range of concerns around issues relating to power, domination, freedom, and aspiration.

A range of empirical studies have demonstrated that medicalisation has been driven not only by the work of medical professionals, but also increasingly through pharmaceutical companies and via the efforts of patients or citizens seeking to legitimise their situation, or to acquire treatment to help alleviate their distress. In reviewing the current state of the field, this chapter focuses on core debates surrounding medicalisation, and explores the characteristics, origins and consequences of the phenomenon. Focus is placed on two well-documented areas of medicalisation, namely mental health and gender and health. The final section of this chapter examines the ways that medicalisation can shape, and be shaped by, dominant power structures and inequalities.

The origins of medicalisation

The process of medicalisation dates back to 17th-century Western modernisation, the growing application of positivistic scientific knowledge, and the rising authority of health professionals (Bell & Figert, 2012). The term "medicalisation" itself has its roots in mid- to late 20th-century scholarship in the social sciences and humanities, and originated within a broader socio-political context characterised by the increasing dominance of professionalised biomedicine (Correia, 2017). Here, the expansion of medical authority into the domains of everyday existence was widely linked by social scientists and philosophers such as Foucault (1963), Szasz (1970), and Illich (1975) as a mechanism of social regulation and control. Medical sociologist Irving Zola's

(1972) classic paper "Medicine as an institution of social control" was particularly influential, arguing that as a "new repository of truth", medicine was beginning to replace the more conventional institutions of religion and law as "the place where absolute and often final judgements are made by supposedly morally neutral and objective experts" (1972, p. 187). Defining medicalisation as the process of "making medicine and the labels 'healthy' and 'ill' relevant to an ever-increasing part of human existence" (p. 487), Zola hinted at the social construction of illness, whilst the use of the suffix "-isation" also indicated medicalisation to be a process, or series of changes in itself, much in the same way as with terms such as urbanisation or globalisation.

Peter Conrad, whose writings date back to the 1970s, has also been a leading proponent of the concept and consequences of medicalisation, and like others at that time also wrote specifically about the medicalisation of deviance. His work on the introduction of hyperactive syndrome or "hyperkinesis" (now known as attention deficit hyperactivity disorder, ADHD), for example, examined the medicalisation of what had previously been widely viewed as disruptive behaviour amongst children.

Processes of medicalisation are seen as constitutive of wide-ranging changes within contemporary society, including globalisation, the emergence of new forms of political and economic power, and the reshaping of social, cultural, and moral practices. Linked with these changes, the past three decades have seen a shift in the drivers of medicalisation, from a core focus on the medical profession, social movements, and interest groups, to a focus on biotechnology, and the role of consumers and managed care (Conrad, 2007). Whilst physicians remain as key gatekeepers for many drugs, the pharmaceutical industry has become an increasingly major player in driving medicalisation. Changes in drug and advertising regulations and the role of the internet mean that aggressive marketing and advertising can now be targeted at the public, reaching directly into everyday domestic spaces and with emphasis placed on medicines as consumer goods (Fox & Ward, 2008; Dew et al., 2014).

Much attention has also been placed on the "over-medicalisation" of society, very often focusing on the potential for harm that this may induce (Kaczmarek, 2019). In an attempt to reduce what it saw as "unnecessary" care, for example, The Academy of Medical Royal Colleges in the UK recently identified a range of tests and treatments that should no longer be pursued by doctors, including giving antibiotics for flu and X-rays for back pain. This, they felt, would help bring an end to a "culture of over-medicalisation", in which doctors felt pressured to prescribe treatment even when they knew that it was unlikely to work (Campbell, 2015).

Whilst medical sociologists have been concerned with understanding the process of medicalisation, and the emergence of medical categories and diagnoses, a range of other disciplines, such as anthropology, geography, history, and bioethics, have also made important contributions to the field. Considerable attention has been paid within medical anthropology, for example, to understanding lived experience, focusing on individual, household and community experiences of medication use, meaning making around bodily norms, health conditions and the relevance and implications of various treatments and responses (Conrad & Bergey, 2015). Similarly, scholars in human geography have highlighted the ways that medicalisation plays out across space and context (Dyck, 1995; Brown & Bell, 2007). Both disciplines have also played an important role in providing insight into the concept and manifestation of medicalisation in non-Western settings.

Features of medicalisation

Medicalisation takes place globally and often involves a range of common factors and experiences. However, it is also influenced by local socio-cultural context, meaning that there is no one way, or set of ways, in which it manifests and plays out (Scamell et al., 2017). Indeed, how a problem or condition is defined, and by who, is often key in determining what is done – or what people perceive "should" be done about it. There are also varying "degrees" of medicalisation, with some problems being almost entirely medicalised, such as schizophrenia, some being only partly medicalised, like gaming addiction, and others, such as obesity, being seen as influenced by a range of socio-cultural, economic, behavioural, and biophysical factors, and therefore falling somewhere in between these extremes.

It is important to recognise that categories of medicalisation are dynamic rather than static, and that they very often reflect broader socio-cultural, political, and economic circumstances and agendas. Conrad's (2007) work on ADHD, for example, has shown how what for many years was seen as a disorder of children, has evolved into a disorder affecting people across the lifespan. At the same time, and as part of a broader trend of increased use in performance-enhancing drugs for sport and mental functioning (see Sauter & Gerlinger, 2014), research has shown how "smart drugs" used for ADHD in the US have also long been used as an academic performance-enhancing drug amongst college and university students (Marsh, 2017). A recent study undertaken across Europe found that whilst the majority of university students surveyed believed it was the social norm to use drugs like Ritalin to enhance academic performance, very few had actually used stimulants themselves. Such findings not only point to the pressures students face to succeed in their studies, but, argue the authors, may also lead to an increase in the use of such drugs as they, and academic success, are considered the norm (Helmer et al., 2016).

Whilst some medical categories have evolved, others, such as hysteria, a common diagnosis in the late 19th century, have now almost disappeared. Medicalisation is therefore bidirectional, with some issues or conditions becoming medicalised whilst others are, albeit less commonly, demedicalised. Most scholars define demedicalisation simply as the obverse of medicalisation when a problem is no longer defined in medical terms and medical personnel are no longer deemed appropriate or necessary. Research on medicalisation far outweighs that on demedicalisation or on the limits and resistance to medicalisation, and it is fair to say that there have been many more instances of medicalisation than demedicalisation in the past few decades.

There are only a few well-documented examples of complete demedicalisation. The most well-recognised case being that of homosexuality, which was officially demedicalised and removed from the Diagnostic and Statistical Manual of Mental Disorders (DSM) following a vote by the American Psychiatric Association in 1974. Cases of *re*classification also exist; a recent example being transgenderism, which in 2019 was reclassified in the WHO's International Classification of Diseases as "gender incongruence" under "conditions related to sexual health", and removed from its original and more controversial categorisation as a mental disorder.

In the past four decades, many thousands of academic papers and articles in the popular media have been written on medicalisation, and the term itself has become frequently used within common parlance. At times, the term "medicalisation" is used in a deprecatory manner, with an assumption that medicalisation is in itself, a "bad" or negative entity. Much of this work has drawn on notions of "disease mongering", whereby organisations and institutions, such as the pharmaceutical and wellness industries who have profit to make, actively promote the existence of diseases, afflictions, or conditions that then require the purchase and consumption of particular treatments (Moynihan et al., 2002). A recent legal case in Oklahoma in which Johnson and Johnson were found to have run a "false and dangerous" sales campaign that caused opioid addiction and death can be seen as a case in point (McGreal, 2019). The integrity of pharmaceutical regulatory bodies has also been called into question (Williams et al., 2011) and the "science" underpinning the development of new medicines been accused of being biased in a way that exaggerates the benefits of treatments (Goldacre, 2013).

However, most academic proponents of the term recognise that medicalisation is neither good nor bad. Indeed, the many examples of beneficial medicalisation clearly undermine any arguments that are wholly against it. The medicalisation of pregnancy and childbirth, for example, has involved shifts towards clinical monitoring and intervention that have helped greatly reduce maternal and infant mortality, albeit alongside arguments that point quite clearly to the more contentious implications of extreme medicalisation, such as options for sex selection, and the very high rates of caesarian sections in countries such as India (see Ghosh, 2010) and Brazil (see Barros et al., 1991). In a similar manner, many sufferers of chronic fatigue syndrome (CFS/ME) have welcomed increased medicalisation of the condition, particularly in the US, where an increase in the availability of biomedical treatments is reported to have alleviated symptoms, and importantly provided legitimacy to what has been a much-maligned and controversial issue (see, for example, Fitzpatrick, 2002). Whilst it can be countered that these are not examples of "good" medicalisation, but examples of overcoming past mistakes and aligning practice with improved scientific or medical knowledge, such examples do also underline the problems inherent in assumptions that see medicalisation as inherently negative.

The medicalisation of mental health

The medicalisation of mental health is an area that has received particularly high levels of attention from across a diverse array of academic disciplines. A significant early influence on thinking around the pathologisation and medicalisation of mental distress can be found in Szasz's (1960) classic critique of psychiatry and his conceptualisation of mental illness as "problems in living". More recently, focus has been centred on the power and influence of diagnostic manuals, most notably the Diagnostic and Statistical Manual (DSM) and the International Classification of Diseases (ICD), with DSM-III, the "bible of psychiatry" launched in 1980, attaining particular repute for setting in place crucial distinctions between what should be defined as "normal" and what should not (Frances, 2013).

Whilst these manuals do not explicitly advocate a "biomedically diseased brain" concept, much discourse within psychiatric literature (though note exceptions such as Moncrieff et al., 2013) has fuelled the idea of an underlying pathology at the neuronal level, in turn undermining previously influential understandings of the human mind drawn from fiction, scientific investigation and philosophical and religious writings, and reshaping understandings of how the mind works (Whitaker, 2015).

Others have analysed how psychiatry has transformed behaviours and emotions previously considered normal into mental "disorder", in what Conrad (2007) has referred to as the "pathologisation of everything". Within this analysis, authors such as Conrad (2007, on ADHD), Frances (2013, on PTSD) and Moncrieff (2014, on bipolar disorder) have demonstrated how behaviours once considered as part of normal social variation have become diagnosable as a mental disorder. Further work has explored how boundaries of mental disorder have been officially reconfigured, so that, for example, emotions such as sadness have become recast as clinical depression (Horwitz & Wakefield, 2007); and how terms with distinct meanings in psychiatry, for example, "anxiety" and "depression", have now become part of people's everyday vocabularies to explain behaviours, reactions, and emotions that might once have been considered unremarkable (Brinkmann, 2014).

The lowering of thresholds for some diagnostic categorisations, in particular, the removal of the bereavement exclusion clause from the criteria for major depressive disorder within DSM-5, have been a further cause for concern, leading Dowrick and Frances (2013, p. 3) to lambast the recasting of grief as a mental disorder as a "medical intrusion into private emotions". This, it is suggested, may "cultivate vulnerability" through encouraging people to feel depressed by experiences that were once regarded as routine (Furedi, 2004), and in turn, replace deeply embedded cultural rituals and emotive norms with a dubious and potentially stigmatising medical response. Others have argued that, over time, disorders that first became medicalised in the United States have been "exported" to other parts of the globe (Watters, 2010). There is growing recognition of the ways that common mental health conditions such as depression and anxiety, for example, have become commonplace across much of Asia and Africa, with people increasingly turning to antidepressants rather than continuing with embedded traditions that perceive suffering and sadness as a part of spiritual growth and resilience (Gopalkrishnan 2018).

Bringing an increasing array of "conditions" and behaviours into the purview of psychiatry has invariably resulted in the massive increase in prescribing of antidepressant medications witnessed globally in recent years (OECD, 2015), accompanied by a parallel upturn, particularly in the Global North, towards the use of psychological "talking therapies". These trends towards what many see as the medicalisation of emotional norms has, perhaps not surprisingly, led to a wide and growing range of literature debating the advantages and disadvantages of this form of medicalisation.

Gender and medicalisation

A considerable body of research has examined the gendered implications of medicalisation, although very often with a focus on Western settings. Much feminist writing has lamented the medicalisation of women's bodies, from childbirth (Henley-Einon, 2003; Clesse et al., 2018), to menstruation (Mamo & Fosket, 2009), and menopause (McCrea, 1983), as well as highlighting the pressures placed upon women to undergo surgical procedures to enhance their bodies according to changing societal norms and expectations (see, for example, Veale et al., 2014 on labiaplasty, and Gillespie, 1997 on diverse forms of cosmetic surgery).

Much literature in this field has critiqued the power of the biomedical profession, seeing medicine as a patriarchal institution that exploits women's bodies through various technological interventions. Polzer and Knabe's (2012) analysis of media and public information around HPV vaccination for girls in Canada, for example, describes how the emergence of sexual relationships is constructed as a time fraught with risks to future health that must be managed through biotechnological intervention in the form of vaccination. This, they argue, positions the emergence of female sexuality as the basis of risk and pathologisation that needs management and control. Cacchioni's (2015) work similarly explores how the expectations of normative heterosexuality influence the medicalisation of female sexuality, with the author testifying twice at the US Federal Drug Administration against an ineffective sexual desire drug with several harmful side-effects.

Other researchers (e.g. Reismann, 1983; Bell, 1987; Gunson, 2010) have challenged the idea that medicalisation is an entirely top-down process, and refute implications that posit women as passive recipients of medicalisation by a primarily male medical profession, arguing instead that the process is much more nuanced. Drawing on women's accounts of the use of extended oral contraception for menstrual suppression, for example, Gunson's (2010) work explores how medicalisation occurs within a particular social and cultural moment, and is a dynamic process where dominant social relations can be both reproduced and challenged. Such work points to a broader recognition that a blanket condemnation of medicalisation fails to acknowledge how it can be enabling, through the ways in which people use medical technologies to gain control over their lives, as well as in enabling them to achieve forms of advancement or independence.

Recent feminist and gender scholarship has also started to reimagine what medicalisation is, how it affects men and women, and, drawing on developments in sexuality studies, examines how gendered medicalisation is more complicated and diverse than dichotomous views allow (Clarke et al., 2003; Narrain & Chandran, 2016; Johnson, 2019). Work has shown, for example, how the medicalisation of trans identities has been overly reliant on binary divisions between male and female, placing an onus on trans people to prove themselves "trans enough" to the gatekeepers who oversee trans-specific healthcare, whilst delegitimising trans identities and experiences that do not conform to medical diagnostic criteria (Pearce, 2015).

Contexualising medicalisation

Since its initial conception, the concept of medicalisation has frequently been used to articulate a normative position of defence or criticism of medical power in relation to lay users, other health professionals, and regulators. Considerable attention has been placed on the power relations inherent within biomedicine, with literature focusing on the dominance of biomedicine with its scientifically construed and legitimated evidence over alternative health systems that may in many cases, provide effective and more culturally sensitive options for local populations (World Health Organization, 2017).

Other research has focused on the power structures *within* biomedicine, and the implications of this and associated cultures of working practice in which medicalisation is shaped. Research has shown, for example, that hospital cultures can valorise autonomous decision-making and independent work, and accentuate social hierarchies between junior doctors and senior consultants. A study by Ledingham et al., 2019) on the cultural contexts of antibiotic resistance, for example, reported that this power discrepancy can lead to junior doctors overprescribing broad-spectrum antibiotics rather than consulting with their seniors on what to prescribe, or whether to prescribe at all. Social hierarchies have also been found to contribute to the existence of local "bubbles" of culture, where junior doctors adopt the prescribing practice and preferences of their seniors as a form of social etiquette and fraternal obligation, again, potentially medicalising conditions that may be better treated or attended to in other ways (Broom et al., 2014, 2015; Charani et al., 2013).

Research has also highlighted how existing power structures and inequalities influence people's experiences of medicalisation. A growing body of research, for example, highlights how marginalised populations can struggle to access biomedical options, or may face limitations in the types of options available to them. Joynt et al. (2013), for example, found that patients presenting to emergency departments from lower socioeconomic status (SES) regions of the US were less likely to receive opioids for equivalent levels of pain than those from more affluent areas. Black and Hispanic patients were also less likely to receive opioids for equivalent levels of pain than white patients, regardless of SES. Conversely, a recent study by Public Health England (2019) found high levels of long-term opioid painkillers being used in areas of high deprivation, despite known addiction issues meaning that guidelines did not support their use in this. Furthermore, research suggests that not only do prescribing rates differ, but that the *types* of medications and treatments prescribed for particular conditions vary across socioeconomic status. In their study in Ireland, for example, Zaharan et al. (2014) found that newer, more costly diabetes treatments were being prescribed to patients from higher socioeconomic groups despite all patients receiving free prescriptions.

Debates elsewhere, however, show that whilst lower socioeconomic status may correlate with reduced access to biomedicine, this is not always the case. Studies on ADHD, for example, have drawn links between socioeconomic disadvantage and the likelihood of ADHD diagnosis and treatment (Russell et al., 2014). Prescribing of ADHD drugs has risen markedly in recent years; in the UK, for example, prescriptions rose from 700,000 in 2007 to 1.6 million in 2017 (Reed, 2018). Such figures have fed into the widespread debate over the impact of stereotyping and "labelling" on the likelihood of children (usually boys) being diagnosed with ADHD. Much research in this area has raised concerns over the ways that certain "disruptive" behaviours or actions by children and young people are increasingly being judged as evidence of mental disorders, and used to justify an official diagnosis and drug treatment with stimulants, antipsychotics, and antidepressants (Conrad, 2006; Whitely, 2014). Furthermore, evidence suggests that the risk of such psychopathologisation is greatest for particular ethnic groups, and that children living in poorer households are four times more likely than other groups to be diagnosed with ADHD (Allan & Harwood, 2014). Concerns over the ways in which ADHD diagnosis and treatment are being globalised have also been raised (Lusardi, 2019).

Studies linking medicalisation and mental health have also highlighted health inequalities, emphasising how the medicalisation of poverty-related distress can individualise blame and responsibility whilst masking the broader root causes of deprivation and social injustice that are known to sustain poverty and underpin the erosion of wellbeing (Friedli, 2013; Thomas et al., 2018; see also Chapter 18, this volume). Recent studies have also drawn links between punitive processes of welfare reform and the need for people living in hardship to medicalise the socially and structurally induced distresses of poverty in order to legitimate their welfare claims (Hansen et al., 2014 in the US, Thomas et al., 2020 in the UK). Literature has also shown how health professionals may prescribe antidepressants as an "act of compassion" for poverty-related distress when they feel they have little else to offer their patients, and when they feel that patients from particular backgrounds will not be able to invest sufficient time, energy, and commitment to non-medical alternatives such as talking therapy (Thomas et al., 2019, 2020).

Disparities have also been reported on the medicalisation of infertility, where work has focused on its treatment as a pathological, rather than a natural or social condition. Bell's (2010) work in the US, for example, found that the huge increase in infertility treatments in recent decades was disproportionately benefiting those from higher-income backgrounds, despite the higher prevalence of infertility amongst lower-income groups. Whilst this was in part an outcome of high treatment costs, she provides compelling evidence to show how the process of medicalisation naturalises dominant representations regarding what and who constitutes a "good mother", and how this in turn serves as a gatekeeper to treatment access.

Scholarship on the power dynamics of medicalisation remains crucial in understanding who is affected by the process and in what ways. However, as has been forcefully argued (see, for example, Busfield, 2017), a sole focus on medical dominance risks overlooking the agency of the populace, as well as more general shifts in thinking in which patients are cast as experts in their own health and wellbeing. Recent research has therefore helped refocus analysis to consider the active participation of individual patients and consumers (Figert, 2010), exploring, for example, the role and activism of patients and pressure groups as they seek to challenge medicalisation (e.g. anti-psychiatry groups), or alternatively to directly encourage forms of medicalisation. In their study of non-legal cannabis use in Norway, for example, Pederson and Sandberg (2013) examine how people using the drug for conditions such as multiple sclerosis and rheumatism, as well as for improved quality of life, deploy strategies to gain medical acceptance of its use. Other work has shown how the continuing growth in biomedical enhancements through cosmetic surgery in countries where the largest number of procedures are carried out, are a product of consumer-driven demand, albeit in response to expectations and value agendas set by the fashion and wellness industries (Edmonds, 2007; Davies & Han, 2011; Dworkin & Wachs, 2009).

The future of medicalisation

Attempts to adapt the concept of medicalisation to the complexity of contemporary societies has resulted in growing attention to what Williams et al. (2017) call "co-evolving processes", which call into question the continued relevance of the concept. Clarke et al. (2003), for example, argue that the concept of biomedicalisation better reflects what they see as increasingly complex and technoscientific shifts in modern society. Others have focused on the convergences and distinctions between medicalisation and pharmaceuticalisation, arguing that the latter concept provides more specific insight into the growing use of pharmaceuticals and the power of the pharmaceutical industry to effect and shape-changing attitudes, behaviours, and expectations (Abraham, 2010), and that it can be more usefully used to examine shifts between different types of treatment (Williams et al., 2017; see also Chapter 4, this volume).

Despite these debates, there is wide recognition of the ongoing value of the concept of medicalisation, with a vast number of researchers across the humanities, social sciences, and medical sector still using the term and undertaking research in the field. Given the continuing expansion of medicine alongside advances in technology and ever-changing notions of what it means to live and be healthy and well, it seems likely that medicalisation will remain a relevant concept which continues to shape everyday understandings of human behaviour, experiences and challenges.

Conclusion

This chapter has examined the origins and characteristics of medicalisation, as well as the core debates that it has engendered in recent decades. Drawing on examples focusing on mental health and gender and health, the chapter has shown the diverse ways in which medicalisation is conceived, experienced, and used to bolster an array of often controversial and sometimes competing agendas. Attention has also been given to highlighting the ways in which medicalisation can shape, and be shaped by, dominant power structures and inequalities and the implications of this for healthcare and treatment accessibility, associated cultures of working practice, and societal norms, values and expectations. This chapter also reiterates the ongoing value of the concept of medicalisation in light of medical and technological expansion, and evolving notions of health and wellbeing.

References

Allan, J., & Harwood, V. (2014). *Psychopathology at school: Theorizing mental disorders in education*. Routledge, London.

Abraham, J. (2010). Pharmaceuticalization of society in context: theoretical, empirical and health dimensions. *Sociology, 44*(4), 603–622.

Barros, F. C., Victora, C. E., Vaughan, J. P., & Huttly, S. R. A. (1991). Epidemic of caesarean sections in Brazil. *The Lancet, 338*(8760), 167–169.

Bell, A. V. (2010). Beyond (financial) accessibility: Inequalities within the medicalisation of infertility. *Sociology of Health and Illness, 32*(4), 631–646.

Bell, S. E. (1987). Changing ideas: The medicalisation of menopause. *Social Science and Medicine, 24*(6), 535–542.

Bell, S. E., & Figert, A. E. (2012). Gender and the medicalisation of healthcare. In E. Kuhlmann & E. Annandale (Eds.), *The Palgrave handbook of gender and healthcare* (pp. 127–142). Palgrave Macmillan, London.

Brinkmann, S. (2014). Languages of suffering. *Theory and Psychology, 24*(5), 630–648.

Broom, A., Broom, J., & Kirby, E. (2014). Cultures of resistance? A Bourdieusian analysis of doctors' antibiotic prescribing. *Social Science and Medicine, 110*(Supplement C), 81–88.

Broom, A., Broom, J., Kirby, E., & Scambler, G. (2015). The path of least resistance? Jurisdictions, responsibility and professional asymmetries in pharmacists' accounts of antibiotic decisions in hospitals. *Social Science and Medicine, 146*, 95–103.

Brown, T., & Bell, M. (2007). Off the couch and on the move: Global public health and the medicalization of nature. *Social Science and Medicine, 64*(6), 1343–1354.

Busfield, J. (2017). The concept of medicalisation reassessed. *Sociology of Health and Illness, 39*(5), 759–774.

Cacchioni, T. (2015). *Big pharma, women, and the labour of love.* University of Toronto Press, Toronto.

Campbell, D. (2015). Doctors to withhold treatments in campaign against "too much medicine". *The Guardian*, 12 May 2015.

Charani, E., Castro-Sanchez, E., Sevdalis, N., Kyratsis, Y., Drumright, L., Shah, N., et al. (2013). Understanding the determinants of antimicrobial prescribing within hospitals: The role of "prescribing etiquette". *Clinical Infectious Diseases, 57*(2), 188–196.

Clarke, A., Mamo, E. L., Fishman, J. R., Shim, J. K., & Fosket, J. R. (2003). Biomedicalization: Technoscientific transformations of health, illness, and US biomedicine. *American Sociological Review, 68*, 161–194.

Clesse, C., Lighezzolo-Alnot, J., de Lavergne, S., Hamlin, S., & Scheffler, M. (2018). The evolution of birth medicalisation: A systematic review. *Midwifery, 66*, 161–167.

Conrad, P. (2006). *Identifying hyperactive children: The medicalization of deviant behavior.* Ashgate Publishing, Aldershot.

Conrad, P. (2007). *The medicalization of society: On the transformation of human conditions into treatable disorders.* Johns Hopkins University Press, Baltimore.

Conrad, P., & Bergey, M. (2015). Medicalization: Sociological and anthropological perspectives. *International Encyclopedia of the Social and Behavioral Sciences, 15*, 105–109.

Conrad, P. (2015). Foreword. In Bell, S., & Figert, A. E. (Eds.), *Reimagining (bio)medicalization, pharmaceuticals and genetics: Old critiques and new engagements.* Routledge, London.

Correia, T. (2017). Revisiting medicalisation: A critique of the assumptions of what counts as medical knowledge. *Frontiers in Sociology*, 19 September 2017.

Davies, G., & Han, G. S. (2011). Korean cosmetic surgery and digital publicity: Beauty by Korean design. *Media International Australia, 141*(1), 146–156.

Dew, K., Norris, P., Gabe, J., Chamberlain, K., & Hodgetts, D. (2014). Moral discourses and pharmaceuticalised governance in households. *Social Science and Medicine, 131*, 272–279.

Dowrick, C., & Frances, A. (2013). Medicalising unhappiness: New classification of depression risks more patients being put on drug treatment from which they will not benefit. *British Medical Journal, 347*: f7140.

Dworkin, S. L., & Wachs. F. L. (2009). *Body panic: Gender, health and the selling of fitness.* New York University Press, London.

Dyck, I. (1995). Hidden geographies; the changing lifeworlds of women with multiple sclerosis. *Social Science and Medicine, 40*(3), 307–320.

Edmonds, A. (2007). "The poor have the right to be beautiful": Cosmetic surgery in neoliberal Brazil. *Journal of the Royal Anthropological Institute, 13*(2), 363–381.

Figert, A. E. (2010). The consumer turn in medicalisation: Future directions with historical foundations. In Pescosolido, B., Martin, J., McLeod, J., & Rogers, A (Eds.), *The handbook of the sociology of health, illness and healing: Blueprint for the 21st century*, Springer, New York.

Fitzpatrick, M. (2002). The making of a new disease. *The Guardian*, 7 Feb. 2002, accessed online at https://www.theguardian.com/education/2002/feb/07/medicalscience.healthandwellbeing.

Friedli, L. (2013). "What we've tried, hasn't worked": The politics of assets based public health. *Critical Public Health, 23*(2), 131–145.

Foucault, M. (1963). *The birth of the clinic*, Tavistock, London.

Fox, N. J., & Ward, K. J. (2008). Pharma in the bedroom… and the kitchen…. The pharmaceuticalisation of daily life. *Sociology of Health and Illness, 30*, 856–868.

Frances, A. (2013). *Saving normal*, HarperCollins, New York.

Furedi, F. (2004). *Therapy culture: Cultivating vulnerability in an uncertain age.* Routledge, London.

Hansen, H., Bourgois, P., & Drucker, E. (2014). Pathologizing poverty: New forms of diagnosis, disability, and structural stigma under welfare reform. *Social Science and Medicine, 103*, 76–83.

Ghosh, S. (2010). *Increasing trend in caesarean section delivery in India: Role of medicalisation of maternal health*, Working Paper 236, Institute for Social and Economic Change, Bangalore.

Gillespie, R. (1997). Women, the body and brand extension in medicine: Cosmetic surgery and the paradox of choice. *Women's Health, 24*(4), 69–85.

Goldacre, B. (2013). *Bad pharma: How medicine is broken, and how we can fix it.* Fourth Estate, London.

Gopalkrishnan, N. (2018). Cultural diversity and mental health: Considerations for policy and practice. *Frontiers in Public Health*, 6, 179, doi: 10.3389/fpubh.2018.00179

Gunson, J. S. (2010). "More natural but less normal": Reconsidering medicalisation and agency through women's accounts of menstrual suppression. *Social Science and Medicine*, 71(7), 1324–1331.

Helmer, S. M., Pischke, C. R., Van Hal, G., Vriesacker, B., Dempsey. R. C., Akvardar, Y., et al. (2016). *Drug and Alcohol Dependence, 168*(1), 128–134.

Henley-Einion, A. (2003). The medicalisation of childbirth. In Squire, C. (Ed.), *The social context of birth*, Radcliffe Medical Press Ltd, Abingdon.

Horwitz, A. V., & Wakefield, J. C. (2007). *The loss of sadness: How psychiatry transformed normal sorrow into depressive disorder*, Oxford University Press, New York.

Illich, I. (1975). *Medical nemesis*, Marion Boyars, London.

Johnson, A. H. (2019). Rejecting, reframing, and reintroducing: Trans people's strategic engagement with the medicalisation of gender dysphoria. *Sociology of Health and Illness*, 41(3), 517–532.

Joynt, M., Train, M. K., Robbins, B. W., Halternam, J. S., Caiola, E., & Fortuna, R. J. (2013). The impact of neighbourhood socioeconomic status and race on the prescribing of opioids in emergency departments throughout the United States. *Journal of General Internal Medicine*, 28(12), 1604–1610.

Kaczmarek, E. (2019). How to distinguish medicalisation from over-medicalisation. *Medicine, Health Care and Philosophy*, 22, 119–128.

Ledingham, K., Hinchlife, S., Jackson, M., Thomas, F., & Tomson, G. (2019). Antibiotic resistance: Using a cultural contexts of health approach to address a global health challenge, WHO, Copenhagen, accessed online at http://www.euro.who.int/en/data-and-evidence/cultural-contexts-of-health-and-well-bei ng/publications/antibiotic-resistance-using-a-cultural-contexts-of-health-approach-to-address-a-glob al-health-challenge-2019

Lusardi, R. (2019). Current trends in medicalization: Universalising ADHD diagnosis and treatments. *Sociology Compass*, 13(6), e12697.

Mamo, L., & Fosket, J. R. (2009). Scripting the body: Pharmaceuticals and the (re)making of menstruation. *Signs, 34*(3), 926–949.

Marsh, S. (2017). Universities must do more to tackle use of smart drugs say experts. *The Guardian*, 10 May 2017.

McCrea, F. (1983). The politics of menopause: The "discovery" of a deficiency disease. *Social Problems, 31*(1), 111–123.

McGreal, C. (2019). Johnson and Johnson to pay $572m for fueling Oklahoma opioid crisis, judge rules. *The Guardian*, 26 August 2019, accessed online (10 September 2019) at https://www.theguardian.c om/us-news/2019/aug/26/johnson-and-johnson-opioid-crisis-ruling-responsibility-oklahoma-latest.

Moncrieff, J., Cohen, D., & Porter, S. (2013). The psychoactive effects of psychiatric medication: The elephant in the room. *Journal of Psychoactive Drugs, 45*(5), 409–415.

Moncrieff, J. (2014). The medicalization of "ups and downs": The marketing of the new bipolar disorder. *Transcultural Psychiatry, 51*(4), 581–598.

Moynihan, R., Heath, C. G. P., & Henry, D. (2002). Selling sickness: The pharmaceutical industry and disease mongering: Commentary. *BMJ, 324*(7342), 886–891.

Narrain, A., & Chandran, V. (2016). *Nothing to fix: Medicalisation of sexual orientation and gender identity*, SAGE, New Delhi.

OECD. (2015). *Health at a glance 2015: OECD indicators*, OECD Publishing, Paris.

Pearce, R. (2015). *Understanding trans health: Discourse, power and possibility*, Policy Press, Bristol.

Pedersen, W., & Sandberg, S. (2013). The medicalisation of revolt: A sociological analysis of medical cannabis users. *Sociology of Health and Illness, 35*(1), 17–32.

Pitts, J. (1968). Social control: The concept. In Sills, D. L. (Ed.), *International encyclopedia of the social sciences*, MacMillan, New York.

Polzer, J. C., & Knabe, S. (2012). From desire to disease: Human Papillomavirus (HPV) and the medicalization of nascent female sexuality. *Journal of Sex Research, 49*(4), 344–352.

Reed, J. (2018). "Not just for naughty boys": The rise in adult ADHD pills. *BBC News*, accessed online at https://www.bbc.co.uk/news/health-44004922

Reissman, C. K. (1983). Women and medicalization: A new perspective, *Social Policy, 14*(1), 3–18.

Russell, G., Ford, T., Rosenberg, R., & Kelly, S. (2014). The association of attention deficit hyperactivity disorder with socioeconomic disadvantage: Alternative explanations and evidence. *Journal of Child Psychology, 55*(5), 436–445.

Saunter, A., & Gerlinger, K. (2014). *The pharmacologically improved human*, TAB, Berlin.

Scamell, M., Altaweli, R., & McCourt, C. (2017). Sarah's birth: How the medicalisation of childbirth may be shaped in different settings: Vignette from a study of routine intervention in Jeddah, Saudi Arabia. *Women and Birth, 30*, e39–45.

Szasz, M. D. (1960). The myth of mental illness. *American Psychologist, 15*, 113–118.

Thomas, F., Hansford, L., Ford, J., Wyatt, K., McCabe, R., & Byng, R. (2018). Moral narratives and mental health: Rethinking understandings of distress and healthcare support in contexts of austerity and welfare reform. *Palgrave Communications, 4*(1), 1– 8.

Thomas, F., Thomas, F., Hansford, L., Ford, J., Wyatt, K., McCabe, R., & Byng, R. (2019). How accessible and acceptable are current GP referral mechanisms for IAPT for low-income patients? Lay and primary care perspectives. *Journal of Mental Health*, 1–6. doi: 10.1080/09638237.2019.1677876.

Thomas, F., Wyatt, K., & Hansford, L. (2020). The violence of narrative: Embodying responsibility for poverty-related distress. *Sociology of Health and Illness*. doi: 10.1111/1467-9566.13084.

Veale, D., Eshkevari, E., Ellison, N., Costa, A., & Robinson, D. (2014). Psychological characteristics and motivation of women seeking labiaplasty. *Psychological Medicine, 44*(3), 555–566.

Watters, E. (2010). *Crazy like us: The globalization of the American psyche*, Free Press, New York.

Whitaker, R. (2015). *Anatomy of an epidemic: Magic bullets, psychiatric drugs, and the astonishing rise of mental illness in America*, Broadway Books, New York.

World Health Organization. (2017). *Culture matters: Using a cultural contexts of health approach to enhance policy-making*, WHO, Copenhagen.

Whitely, M. (2014). ADHD: How a lie "medicated" often enough became the truth. In Speed, E., Moncrieff, J., & Rapley, M. (Eds.), *De-medicalising misery II: Society, politics and the mental health industry* (pp. 136–153), Palgrave Macmillan, Basingstoke, Ch 9.

Williams, S. J., Martin, P., & Gabe, J. (2011). The pharmaceuticalisation of society? A framework for analysis. *Sociology of Health and Illness, 33*(5), 710–725.

Williams, S. J., Coveney, C., & Gabe, J. (2017). The concept of medicalisation reassessed: A response to Joan Busfield. *Sociology of Health and Illness, 39*(5), 775–780.

Zaharan, N. L., & Bennett, D. W. K. (2014). Prescribing of antidiabetic therapies in Ireland: 10 year trends 2003–2012. *Irish Journal of Medical Science, 183*(2), 311–318.

Zola, I. K. (1972). Medicine as an institution of social control. *Sociological Review, 20*, 487–504.

4

PHARMACEUTICALISATION

Origins, drivers, and new directions[1]

Jonathan Gabe and Paul Martin

There has been a huge growth in pharmaceuticals since the 1980s, giving the companies that make these medicines ever greater importance, economically, politically, and socially. In the face of this development some sociologists suggested we need a new concept – pharmaceuticalisation – to capture these companies' growing power and their ability to bypass the traditional dominance of the medical profession. This chapter begins with a discussion of how the concept of pharmaceuticalisation developed out of dissatisfaction with medicalisation, which had previously been employed to understand the role of pharmaceuticals, and then outlines the key dimensions of pharmaceuticalisation. It then charts the debate, and the subsequent critiques, extensions, and elaborations of the concept.

From medicalisation to pharmaceuticalisation

Medicalisation is a key concept in medical sociology with a history stretching back to the late 1960s. It has been embraced by Marxists and feminists, social constructionists and Foucauldians, and has even found its way into professional and popular culture (see also, Chapter 2, this volume). In the early 2000s, a number of sociologists associated with the concept suggested it needed modification to take account of the increasingly important role of the pharmaceutical industry. Thus Adele Clark and colleagues (2003) proposed that "biomedicalization" might be a more appropriate term because it better captures the transformation of biomedicine since the mid-1980s and the central role of technoscience, including the role of multinational corporations like drug companies. Peter Conrad (2007) responded in turn by arguing that biomedicalisation is too broad a concept and that medicalisation can take account of the role of "Big Pharma" if we see the latter as a driver of the process. In effect, what Conrad was acknowledging was that doctors are no longer the only drivers of medicalisation and that other drivers need to be acknowledged. For him, these included biotechnology companies, and in particular drug companies, alongside consumers, and in the case of the United States (US), also managed care.

For our purposes, the important point to note is that both these researchers agreed that pharmaceutical companies are increasingly powerful players in health and healthcare and that this needs to be acknowledged conceptually. Others, like John Abraham (2007) and Nick Fox and Katie Ward (2009), subsequently took the argument about Big Pharma even further and suggested that a new concept was needed to recognise its growing role, namely pharmaceuticalisation. However, neither of them endeavoured, until later (e.g. Abraham, 2010), to delineate its sociological credentials, compared to medicalisation.

Next, Williams et al. (2011a) sought to identify such credentials. According to these authors pharmaceuticalisation refers to a complex, dynamic, socio-technical process that involves the discovery, development, commercialisation, use, and governance of pharmaceutical products centred on chemically-based technologies. As such, it can be defined as "the translation or transformation of human conditions, capabilities, and capacities into opportunities for pharmaceutical intervention" (Williams et al., 2011a, p. 711). One benefit of such a broad definition is that it encompasses the non-medical use of pharmaceuticals for lifestyle enhancement amongst "healthy" people. Thus, it covers the purchase of such substances over the internet without any direct involvement by a medical practitioner, thereby illustrating that one can have pharmaceuticalisation without medicalisation.

Williams and colleagues also proposed that pharmaceuticalisation is part of a "pharmaceutical regime" made up of the following: "networks of institutions, organisations, actors and artefacts, as well as the cognitive structures associated with the creation, production and use of new therapeutics" (Williams et al., 2011a, p. 711). Such a regime has been developing since the introduction of pharmaceutical products in the 19th century, involving a chemistry-based technology embodied in the pill.

Williams et al. (2011a) suggested that the term should be seen as value-neutral and descriptive, involving both gains and losses, just as Conrad and Schneider (1980a) had argued for medicalisation. Whether the process is occurring is seen as an empirical question that must be established on a case-by-case basis. This allows for the process to be ongoing and as yet partial and incomplete. Like medicalisation, as discussed by Conrad and Schneider (1980b), pharmaceuticalisation can be viewed as occurring on different levels (with drug testing and regulation seen as occurring at a macro level, and the way in which people understand the meaning of drugs conceived as a micro-level phenomenon). As with medicalisation (Conrad, 1992; Halfmann, 2012), there is also the prospect of it being bi-directional (with de-pharmaceuticalisation occurring as well as pharmaceuticalisation) and for some people to be resistant to the process while others may encourage it, by, for example, campaigning for increased access to particular medicines like Herceptin (in the UK, Abraham, 2009a; in New Zealand, Gabe et al., 2012). In sum, pharmaceuticalisation and medicalisation have a lot in common. Both have been viewed as value-neutral terms, both involve a matter of degree, both involve different levels and both can be bi-directional. However, they still need to be distinguished because, as noted above, one can have pharmaceuticalisation without medicalisation, and one can also have cases where drugs are increasingly used to treat an established medical condition without the transformation of a non-medical problem into a medical one. So, for example, obesity might be increasingly treated with weight loss drugs, having previously been treated by diet control or surgery. Thus one can have pharmaceuticalisation without the *expansion* of medicalisation.

Having defined and delineated pharmaceuticalisation and considered its dynamics, we now turn to the six dimensions that Williams et al. (2011a) suggested underpin the process, namely: selling sickness; changing forms of governance; mediation by the mass media; the role of patients and consumer groups; the use of drugs for non-medical purposes; and how expectations about pharmaceutical futures shape the present. These are considered in turn.

"Selling sickness" – redefining health problems as having a pharmaceutical solution

The first way in which "selling sickness" is demonstrated is through the growth of markets for medicines internationally, especially in the United States and Europe. The pharmaceutical industry is one of the most profitable in the world, enjoying profits of around 25% during most of the 1990s and with worldwide spending on medicines forecast to reach $1.3 trillion by 2018, an increase of 30% over 2013 (Salter & Salter, 2018). Sales in middle-income countries such as Brazil, China, and India have been increasing at a faster rate than in the West, but from a lower base (Busfield, 2010), with pharmaceutical market growth predicted of 8–11% up to 2018 (IMS Institute of Healthcare Informatics, 2014). Overall, the global drugs bill has increased 30 times between 1972 and 2005, although growth has been uneven. The West is currently the dominant consumer as a result of its more affluent, ageing population, which is suffering from chronic health problems in need of medication. This suggests that what we are currently witnessing is the westernisation of the pharmaceutical industry rather than its globalisation (Busfield, 2003).

The second means of selling sickness is through the marketing of disorders. Ray Moynihan (2002; Moynihan & Henry, 2006) has been a particular critic in this regard, claiming that drug companies are involved in "disease mongering", by which he means "widening the boundaries of treatable illness in order to expand the market for products" (Moynihan, 2002, p. 886). He argues that pharmaceutical companies "are actively involved in sponsoring the definition of diseases and promoting them to both prescribers and consumers", a process in which the social construction of illness is replaced by "the corporate construction of disease" (Moynihan, 2002, p. 886). This is said to involve turning ordinary ailments into medical problems; seeing mild symptoms as serious; treating personal problems as medical; seeing risks as disease; and using prevalence estimates to maximise potential markets (Moynihan, 2002).

These arguments are undoubtedly important and valuable. However, "disease mongering" is clearly a value-laden term, in contrast to pharmaceuticalisation, which is value-neutral and has positive and negative faces or sides. Which "face" is dominant is an empirical question to be explored on a case-by-case basis.

A third way of selling sickness is through direct-to-consumer advertising. To date this is limited to the US and New Zealand, although there have been a number of attempts to change the rules in the European Union (EU) to enable drug companies to provide more "information" to patients about prescription-only medicines (Geyer, 2011). In the EU, only information approved by a regulatory body, such as the Medicines and Health Care Products Regulatory Agency (MHRA) in the UK, can be made available to patients and only via certain channels, like drug company websites. The dissemination of information by television, radio, or in magazines is not permitted as it is in the US and New Zealand. In both countries, advertising of prescription-only products on television is commonplace and facilitates a direct relationship between a pharmaceutical company and consumer. It encourages consumers to see drugs like any other product available in the marketplace and arguably increases the demand for such drugs. Critics like Angell (2005) have suggested that this is "marketing masquerading as education".

Changing forms of governance

The second dimension of pharmaceuticalisation can be found in the changing relationship between regulatory agencies and pharmaceutical companies. This involves three components: reforms that reduce the regulatory hurdle or increase the dependence of regulators on the industry; policies that increase the role of regulators in promoting drug innovations; and the globalisation of established modes of governance based on the interests of pharmaceutical companies from the developed world. These will be discussed in turn.

Important work by Abraham and colleagues (e.g. Abraham, 1995, 2009a, 2009b, 2010; Abraham & Davis, 2005; Davis & Abraham, 2013) has focused on the regulation of medicines through detailed empirical work. Case studies of anti-inflammatories, antidepressants, diabetes drugs, and sleeping pills amongst others have provided evidence of corporate bias and privileged access by pharmaceutical companies to regulatory bodies such as the Food and Drug Administration in the US and the MHRA in the UK. Others like Daemmrich (2004) have reported how regulators have been responsive to patient demands for accelerated approval of new drugs, for example, Herceptin for breast cancer and anti-retrovirals for HIV/AIDS. This raises the question about whether such accelerated approval is in the best interest of public health more widely as the risks involved in taking these "accelerated" drugs may subsequently be found to outweigh the benefits.

Since the 1990s, the relationship between Big Pharma and the regulators has been getting closer. The industry now has to pay the costs of funding the activities of most regulators, in line with neoliberalism which requires regulatory bodies to pay their way by charging for their services. In return, there has been a significant reduction in review times for new drugs, down by half in the US and Europe since 1993 (Abraham, 2009b). At the same time, new measures have been put in place, such as fast-tracking the approval of drugs for "life-threatening" conditions, with companies being required to provide less data than usual to demonstrate efficacy and safety. As a result, regulators are increasingly vulnerable to pressures of the market, with agencies competing with each other to get the "business" of pharmaceutical companies who are seen as "customers" (Abraham, 2009b).

The second change in governance has involved developing policies that increase the role of regulators in promoting drug innovations. In recent years, bodies such as the FDA and European Medicines Evaluation Agency (EMEA) have streamlined the approval process so that new drugs can be brought to market more quickly. In doing so, these regulators are no longer just the guardians of public health; they are the promoters of innovation. This change has to be understood in the context of a productivity crisis in large pharmaceutical companies (Hopkins et al., 2007), with most innovation coming from small biotechnology companies rather than large multinationals.

The third change involves the globalisation of established modes of governance based on the interests of drug companies from the developed world. This has involved attempts to harmonise regulatory guidelines for drug development and approval between Europe, the US, and Japan, aimed at promoting the Western regulatory model worldwide. Such harmonisation has been driven by a desire to open up new markets for Western drug companies, for example, in India. In addition, this change has been influenced by the attractiveness of outsourcing drug development to developing countries, where the costs of clinical trials are cheaper. However, minimum standards of clinical care and safety still need to be met if data collected in these trials are to be acceptable to Western regulators. Harmonisation of established modes of governance is also being driven by the globalisation of manufacturing, with Western drug companies manufacturing gaining access to markets in developing and middle-income countries, such as India and Brazil (Sariola et al., 2015).

The role of mass media in (re)framing health problems as having a pharmaceutical solution

The mass media are also clearly involved in the process of pharmaceuticalisation, although as a conveyor or amplifier rather than as a creator or catalyst. The clearest example of this process can be seen in direct-to-consumer advertising, where the media in effect have become marketing tools in the service of pharmaceutical companies (Angell, 2005). Techniques used include using the voice of experts and patients, celebrity endorsement, making drugs person-like by giving drugs personalities, and offering symptom-based self-testing. Such self-testing provides diagnostic validity to the condition and offers a pharmaceutical solution. It may come with the proviso – "ask your doctor if drug X is right for you" – but it also creates the impression that this is a condition that could happen to anyone (Conrad, 2007, p. 18).

At the same time we need to recognise that the mass media are not puppets of the pharmaceutical companies. Media coverage can be contradictory or condemnatory, oscillating between extremes, proclaiming the benefits or demonising medicine users (Seale, 2002) and criticising drug companies. Coverage of new drugs is largely uncritical or even celebratory, but if unwanted side effects appear negative or critical portrayals follow. This can be illustrated by the media coverage of benzodiazepine tranquillisers over time. Early coverage by *Time* magazine in 1960 described Librium, the first of the benzodiazepine family, as a "new drug heralding a new era" and claimed that it came close to "producing pure relief from strain without drowsiness or dulling of mental processes" (Time, 1960). By 1980, newspaper coverage was about "the dangers of tranquillity" and "Valium junkies", drawing on an addiction discourse (Gabe & Bury, 1996). On this evidence it seems rare for the media to present a "balanced" portrayal of the risks and benefits of medicines, no doubt a result, in part, of the need to come up with a new angle or a newsworthy story. What is clear though is that the media may both promote and challenge pharmaceutical products and interests.

So far the focus has been on traditional media like newspapers, television, and magazines, but we also need to consider new media in the form of the internet. The worldwide web is particularly important because it provides the opportunity for people to buy pharmaceuticals online, thus bypassing the doctor–patient relationship. According to Fox and Ward (2009), the pharmaceuticalisation of daily life involves two broad processes. The first is the domestication of drug consumption, as computer-mediated access usually occurs at home and drugs are consumed there. They draw particular attention to drugs purchased for the bedroom, such as Viagra for sexual potency, and drugs purchased for the kitchen, such as Xenical for weight loss. The second broad process concerns drugs being presented as magic bullets for a variety of day-to-day life problems. However, the role of new media is far from straightforward, as the internet provides both new channels for pharmaceuticalisation and new spaces and fora for challenging prevailing understandings about medicines. The latter is illustrated by pro-anorexia websites where pro-ana groups appropriate weight-loss drugs to support an anorectic state, thereby subverting the manufacturers' intention (Fox et al., 2005).

The role of patients and consumer groups

Much has been written in recent years about the increasingly active, if not critical, role that patients and consumers play in their own healthcare. This is particularly true of studies of medicines use, which have portrayed users as knowledgeable, reflexive actors. These users have been found to assess the risks and benefits of the drugs they are offered (e.g. Gabe & Lipshitz-Phillips, 1984; Williams & Calnan, 1996) and to make informed choices about which ones to consume (Stevenson et al., 2002, 2009). And these developments have been re-enforced by current health policy in many developed countries in which patients are constructed as experts, especially if chronically ill, and seen as in partnership with healthcare professionals (Taylor & Bury, 2007). These developments have also been re-enforced by broader trends towards a knowledge-based society in which health information and products are readily accessible on-line (Nettleton et al., 2005).

These developments offer contrasting possibilities. On the one hand the rise of the articulate, information-rich consumer suggests the potential for various challenges or forms of resistance to pharmaceuticalisation. On the other hand, these developments may fuel further pharmaceuticalisation through patient-driven demand for medicines, with or without direct-to-consumer advertising. At the same time, it seems that professional expertise is still valued when it comes to people making decisions about medicines. Patients continue to ask pharmaceutical experts for advice, including about medicines bought over the counter in a pharmacy (Stevenson et al., 2009).

Patients may also have a collective voice as well as being individual consumers. They may be members of self-help groups or patient advocacy organisations or health social movements. Furthermore, some of these groups may receive financial support from pharmaceutical companies to press for early access to an as yet unlicensed drug, while others may demand that pharmaceutical companies remove what they feel are unsafe drugs from the market (Gabe et al., 2012).

Overall, the apparent power of consumer activism may depend on whether they are challenging or supporting the interests of drug companies (Abraham, 2009a). Patient groups have been more successful when they have sought access to a new drug with industry support than when they have battled against drug companies around drug injury to patients (Abraham, 2009a). Some have talked about pro-drug industry groups as having been captured by the industry, although this is the subject of ongoing debate (Abraham, 2009a; Jones, 2009). What is clear, however, is that whilst the patient and consumer challenges are possible, the power and influence of the pharmaceutical industry is extensive and should not be underestimated.

The shift from treatment to enhancement: the use of drugs for non-medical purposes

The desire to improve or enhance ourselves in one way or another is as old as human history. What has changed is the means of doing so. Enhancement itself is, however, a contested term as it is frequently used to indicate going beyond treatment or health to become better than well. Peter Conrad (2007) usefully refers to three main types of biomedical enhancement: normalisation, where biomedical enhancements are used to bring the body into line with what doctors and patients feel is normal or socially expected; repair, in which biomedical interventions are used to restore or rejuvenate the body to its previous condition; and augmentation, to improve or boost performance, giving someone a competitive advantage, as in the case of taking steroids in sport.

Context is important, so the notion of enhancement relates to why or how an intervention is used more than the type of intervention per se. Moreover, enhancement needs to be understood in the context of contemporary culture, which values "bigger, faster and more" and where competitive difference among those who are otherwise similar offers personal advantage and social rewards for those who have "an edge" (Conrad, 2007, p. 89).

Of course not all forms of enhancement are for non-medical purposes. The medical profession may use cosmetic surgery or prescribed medicines such as human growth hormone for medical reasons. Pharmaceuticalisation may nonetheless occur in the absence of any medical involvement, for example, when healthy people use drugs for non-medical reasons to enhance their performance. One example which illustrates this point well is the use of cognitive enhancement drugs to improve alertness, cognition, and memory. In academic and media discourse, drugs like modafinil (for narcolepsy) and Ritalin (for attention deficit hyperactivity disorder), are said to be being used off-label for non-medical purposes to improve performance amongst the healthy (Coveney et al., 2019a). University students in particular have been found to be using these drugs to boost their performance (Vrecko, 2015). Given the lack of knowledge about the medical and social risks of using these drugs for non-medical reasons we need to be cautious when evaluating their use. It is clear that any attempt by drug companies to reconstruct the use of these drugs for enhancement represents another case of creating new drug markets involving a direct relationship with consumers outside the control of the medical profession. The prospect of cognitive enhancement thus demonstrates both the potential of consumerism to drive the process of pharmaceuticalisation and how pharmaceuticalisation may take us beyond medicalisation.

Pharmaceutical futures in the making

Recent work in science and technology studies on expectations has drawn attention to the key role of the future in shaping the present. In particular, this work highlights the dynamic role that expectations play in attracting support and investors and building communities of hope and promise for those who have life-threatening conditions (Brown, 2003). It also highlights how such expectations differ between different stakeholders, such as scientists, the drug industry, consumers and patients, and how the futures envisaged are contested and fought over (Hedgecoe & Martin, 2003).

Take, for example, the field of pharmacogenetics – the use of genetic knowledge to predict drug reactions. This field has generated much speculation about the dawn of a new era of personalised medicine, where tailor-made treatments are geared to an individual's genetic profile (see also Chapter 9, this volume). This in turn holds out the promise of more effective drugs and drugs which have far fewer adverse reactions than is the case currently, with one-size-fits-all drug treatments.

Such pharmaceutical innovation also forms the basis for much policy planning (Department of Health, 2003). As a result, alternative futures are overlooked and the search for new medicines is seen as the best way to improve human health. At the same time, despite much talk of a pharmacogenetic revolution, evidence suggests that progress has been slow, and there is currently little evidence of the widespread benefits envisaged by these expectations (Shendure et al., 2019). Added to this there is evidence of a major productivity crisis in the industry. Despite the increase in potential drug targets resulting from genomics, major investment in research and development since the 1970s and the neoliberal acceleration in regulatory approval times noted earlier, pharmaceutical innovation has remained static or has declined since the 1990s, in terms of new clinical entities or new patented drugs launched (Hopkins et al., 2007; Law, 2006).

This is not to say that biotechnology will not deliver in the future. However, rather than producing revolutionary change, what seems to be occurring is incremental technological diffusion (Nightingale & Martin, 2004). Viewed in this light, one might well ask why the belief in the biotechnology revolution remains so influential? The answer is, in part at least, the power of expectations. Claims about the biotechnology revolution act as "rhetorical devices to generate the necessary political, social and financial capital to allow the perceived promise to emerge" (Hopkins et al., 2007, p. 21). In sum, expectations of the future play a key performative role in shaping the present.

In conclusion, as we have discussed, Williams et al. (2011a) argued that pharmaceuticalisation is a dynamic and complex process involving the development of a pharmaceutical regime. This regime is made up of distinct socioeconomic activities and covers a range of actors from clinicians and patients to regulators and pharmaceutical companies. The extent to which such activities can be seen to involve pharmaceuticalisation is context-specific and depends on the interplay between specific actors in any one case. Taken together they reflect a process that is distinct from medicalisation in important respects.

New directions in pharmaceuticalisation

In the period since the publication of Williams et al.'s (2011a) paper, there has been extension, elaboration and critique of the concept of pharmaceuticalisation. The most significant responses can be broken down under a number of headings:

First, several authors have sought to *extend the concept* both theoretically and empirically. For example, Sariola et al. (2015) used the idea of Big-pharmaceuticalisation to capture important changes in the politics and economics of the Indian industry, brought about by the implementation of the World Trade Organisation's Trade-Related Intellectual Property Rights agreement (TRIPS) and the changing international division of pharmaceutical labour. In particular, the increasing outsourcing of clinical trials and research and development, and the growth of contract research organisations (CROs) in India has extended the power and influence of "Big Pharma" companies. This new concentration of capital has given large Western corporations increased market share and greater influence over regulation and governance, often at the expense of smaller domestic firms. This helps to locate pharmaceuticalisation as a driver of globalisation. Cloatre and Pickersgill (2014) also look at the role of international law in the constitution of intellectual property regimes and the dynamics of pharmaceuticalisation in developing countries by exploring how legal measures shape the identities, circulation and use of drugs by states and citizens. For example, the enforcement of certain intellectual property regimes in African countries cements the power of Western pharmaceutical companies and the definition of some health problems as having a medical rather than a public health solution.

In a similar vein, the pharmaceuticalisation of healthcare systems has been identified by Chabrolab et al. (2017) in exploring access to drugs for hepatitis C in Africa and Europe. By comparing the rationing of drugs in Cameroon with the relative abundance of the same drugs in France they highlight the role of pharmaceuticalisation – manifest as the growing use of drugs in healthcare systems – in the social and political construction of scarcity. Here the concept is used in a non-Western setting as a lens to investigate austerity.

The increasing importance of drugs in the pharmaceuticalisation of public health is highlighted by Thomann (2018) in a study of the scale-up of prophylactic treatment and prevention of HIV/ AIDS using pre-exposure prophylaxis (PrEP) based on anti-retroviral medications. Here a public health problem, the control of infection, is reframed as one of the responsible use of pharmaceuticals. Adopting a similar focus on public health and sexuality, Mamo and Epstein (2014) compare the development and use of vaccines to prevent the spread of the hepatitis B virus and the human papillomavirus, both of which can be sexually transmitted. They place these new vaccines within the trajectory of pharmaceuticalisation. The application of these new technologies redefines the nature of health problems, from public to private, and fundamentally shifts the moral discourses that surround them.

Another significant change linked to the concept of pharmaceuticalisation is the increasing diversification of large transnational tobacco companies into pharmaceutical-like nicotine replacement and maintenance products (Hendlin et al., 2017). Here, tobacco firms start to resemble drug companies but without the testing and oversight required of traditional pharmaceutical products.

In addition to extending the conceptual reach of pharmaceuticalisation into public health and international development, pharmaceuticalisation has also provided a lens to understand changing healthcare practices in different national contexts. For example, Towghi (2014) examined the off-label use of the drug misoprostol in managing home births in a resource poor country (Pakistan). Here drugs are used experimentally as a substitute for adequate health services in an attempt to reduce the risk of haemorrhage. Pharmaceuticalisation is also linked to the reshaping of "traditional" forms of medical practice. For example, Gaudillière (2014) explores how Ayurvedic medicine is becoming increasingly industrialised, resulting in the creation of new pharmacy-like professional groups who work alongside Ayurvedic doctors to manage the material (rather than the clinical) dimensions of polyherbal preparations. This conception of pharmaceuticalisation stresses its institutional dimensions, such as the creation of new professions, rather than just reinforcing the cognitive commitment to biomedicine.

The concept of pharmaceuticalisation has also been extended to non-healthcare settings. Nation-states have increased involvement in the development of "medical counter-measures" against bioterrorism and pandemics as part of national security measures (Elbe et al., 2015). Here, new policies, including changes in liability and governance, have been adopted to incentivise the creation and stockpiling of novel antivirals, next-generation vaccines and antibiotics. These processes have accelerated, intensified, and opened up new trajectories of pharmaceuticalisation.

Second, a body of scholarship has sought to increase the empirical detail and specificity of the concept in several domains. In the clinic, Pollock and Jones (2015) examined the therapeutic landscape for coronary artery disease (CAD) in the US and the shifting balance between "lifestyle" interventions, drugs and surgery. They utilised the pharmaceuticalisation concept in considering CAD in the context of major racial disparities, illustrating the pervasiveness and persuasiveness of drug therapy in an increasingly consumer-driven medical system, as well as the limits of its appeal and reach. Davis (2015) also highlights this trend when focusing on the increasingly aggressive pharmacological treatment of patients with advanced, incurable cancer in several countries. Whilst some of this can be justified as addressing unmet needs, a significant part of this expansion represents an inappropriate use of drugs driven by a range of upstream factors, including industry. The value of pharmaceuticalisation is tested empirically and shown to have explanatory value in both studies.

An important dimension of pharmaceuticalisation is the increased international harmonisation of governance and regulation. This enables the expansion of drug markets throughout the developing world and the Global South. For example, the global reach of pharmaceuticalisation is provided by an examination of ethical review of clinical research across South Asia (Simpson et al., 2015). They illustrate the tensions surrounding the work of ethical review committees and the powerful pull towards harmonisation and alignment with international standards that enable the consolidation and extension of the global pharmaceutical industry and its products.

Pharmaceuticalisation involves enhancement and the non-medical expansion of the use of drugs. Some conditions which have not historically been within the purview of medicine have increasingly become defined as having a pharmaceutical solution. For example, the increasing use of drugs such as human growth hormone (hGH) in the treatment of short stature (Morrison, 2015) provides a valuable case study of this. An historical comparison of the development of hGH in the US and UK shows how the dynamics of pharmaceuticalisation vary between countries with some applications of hGH in treating short stature became acceptable and stabilised as legitimate "therapies" whilst others remain contested as "enhancements".

Similarly, Brown et al. (2015) elaborate the salience of expectations in further entrenching pharmaceuticalisation by looking at the construction of hope and trust around trials for novel therapies for patients suffering from advanced-stage cancer. In doing so, they illuminate the depth and texture of pharmaceuticalisation at the micro-level and highlight how such discourses make disengagement from trials problematic.

However, there have also been critiques of the use and value of pharmaceuticalisation. One is to do with how expansive the definition of pharmaceuticalisation should be. Abraham (2011) has argued that Williams et al.'s (2011a) definition is too expansive as it could include taking heroin or cocaine or overdosing to commit suicide. The latter have defended their position and suggested that the definition needs to be expansive in order to include the use of medicines outside of medical authority. However, they argued that the illicit use of heroin or cocaine is excluded because these drugs are not produced by pharmaceutical companies. Another concern relates to the amount of emphasis given to de-pharmaceuticalisation. Abraham (2011) has suggested that Williams et al. (2011b) have underplayed the possibility of de-pharmaceuticalisation. The latter (2011b) have responded by suggesting that pharmaceuticalisation has so far outstripped de-pharmaceuticalisation and that there are few if any areas of life which, once pharmaceuticalised, have subsequently become fully de-pharmaceuticalised. Their underplaying of de-pharmaceuticalisation was therefore intentional. A further argument revolves around whether pharmaceuticalisation is better understood as a postmodern or modern development. For Bell and Figert (2012a, 2012b), medicalisation, the forerunner to pharmaceuticalisation, is grounded in the modern world, which focuses on progress, mass production, and consumption, whereas pharmaceuticalisation is best understood in terms of postmodern characteristics such as contingency, fragmentation, and volatility. Others have questioned the assumption that only a postmodern standpoint can take account of contingency and complexity (Williams et al., 2012). Finally some (e.g. Busfield, 2017) have suggested that pharmaceuticalisation has little analytical value beyond what medicalisation already offers. Those advocating pharmaceuticalisation, such as Coveney et al. (2019b), have suggested that pharmaceuticalisation can intertwine with medicalisation in complex ways which should not be conflated or collapsed one into the other. Coveney et al. (2019b) demonstrate this complexity in their study of the medical management of sleeplessness as insomnia where, for example, sleep experts seemed to want to have greater medicalisation of sleeplessness as insomnia without necessarily more pharmaceuticalisation, given the availability of other non-pharmaceutical alternatives.

In sum, since the concept of pharmaceuticalisation was first introduced there have been attempts to extend and elaborate it, alongside critical assessments of its utility. Further research will continue to assess and develop this concept as a means of exploring the dynamic interactions between the pharmaceutical industry, medicines and society, and the shaping of health and illness.

Conclusion

In this chapter, we have charted how pharmaceuticalisation as a concept has developed and evolved. This concept initially developed out of dissatisfaction with medicalisation as a means to understand the considerable increase in the power and influence of the pharmaceutical industry. We outlined and discussed six key dimensions of pharmaceuticalisation (Williams et al., 2011a) that shape and define the concept. Several common features can be identified across these dimensions, including the expansion of drug markets beyond traditional areas to include new medical conditions and new uses in healthy individuals, the increasing significance of state regulatory systems, and attempts to bypass the authority of the medical profession and create more direct relationships between Big Pharma and patients and health consumer groups. We then considered ways in which the concept has been recently extended and elaborated and its utility assessed.

Overall, it is clear that pharmaceuticalisation as a process is distinct from medicalisation in important respects. In particular, pharmaceuticalisation is valuable in drawing attention to the growing power of the pharmaceutical industry and its ability to bypass medical control and reconstruct the role of patients and consumers. As such, it provides a useful analytical framework for empirical research and thereby helps to shift the gaze of scholarship into health and illness.

Note

1 This chapter is based on and extends the argument in a chapter published by the first author in Giarelli et al., 2016.

References

Abraham, J. (1995). *Science, politics and the pharmaceutical industry*. London: University College Press.

Abraham, J. (2007, October). Key socio-political challenges of pharmaceutical development, regulation and public health. Keynote address to the *International Conference of the Social Sciences and Health Research Councils of Canada*, Montreal.

Abraham, J. (2009a). The pharmaceutical industry, the state and the NHS. In J. Gabe & M. Calnan (Eds.), *The new sociology of the health service* (pp. 99–120). London: Routledge.

Abraham, J. (2009b). Sociology of pharmaceuticals development and regulation: A realist empirical research programme. In S. J. Williams, J. Gabe & P. Davis (Eds.), *Pharmaceuticals and society: Critical discourses and debates* (pp. 54–70). Oxford: Blackwell.

Abraham, J. (2010). Pharmaceuticalization of society in context: Theoretical, empirical and health dimensions. *Sociology, 4*, 603–622.

Abraham, J. (2011). Evolving sociological analysis of "pharmaceuticalisation". A reply to Williams, Martin and Gabe. *Sociology of Health & Illness, 33*, 729–730.

Abraham, J., & Davis, C. (2005). Risking public safety: Experts, the medical profession and 'acceptable' drug injury. *Health Risk & Society, 7*, 379–395.

Angell, M. (2005). *The truth about drug companies*. New York: Random House.

Bell, S., & Figert, A. (2012a). Starting to turn sideways to move forward in medicalization and pharmaceuticalization studies: A response to Williams et al. (2012). *Social Science & Medicine, 75*, 2131–2133.

Bell, S., & Figert, A. (2012b). Medicalization and pharmaceuticalization at the intersections: Looking backward, sideways and forward. *Social Science & Medicine, 75*, 775–783.

Brown, N. (2003). Hope against hype: Accountability in bio-pasts, presents and futures. *Science Studies, 16*, 3–21.

Brown, P., Graaf, S., Hillen, M., Smets, E., & van Laarhoven, H. (2015). The interweaving of pharmaceutical and medical expectations as dynamics of micro-pharmaceuticalisation: Advanced-stage cancer patients' hope in medicines alongside trust in professionals. *Social Science & Medicine, 131*, 313–321.

Busfield, J. (2003). Globalization and the pharmaceutical industry revisited. *International Journal of Health Services, 33*, 581–603.

Busfield, J. (2010). "A pill for every ill": Explaining the expansion of medicine use. *Social Science & Medicine, 70*, 931–941.

Busfield, J. (2017). The concept of medicalisation re-assessed. *Sociology of Health & Illness, 39*(5), 759–774.

Chabrolab, F., David, P.-M., & Krikorian, G. (2017). Rationing hepatitis C treatment in the context of austerity policies in France and Cameroon: A transnational perspective on the pharmaceuticalization of healthcare systems. *Social Science & Medicine, 187*, 243–250.

Clarke, A. E., Mamo, L., Fishman, J. R., Shim, J. K., & Fosket, J. R. (2003). Biomedicalization: Technoscientific transformations of health, illness and biomedicine. *American Sociological Review, 68*, 161–194.

Cloatre, E., & Pickersgill, M. (2014). International law, public health, and the meanings of pharmaceuticalisation. *New Genetics & Society, 33*(4). doi: 10.1080/14636778.2014.951994

Conrad, P. (1992). Medicalization and social control. *Annual Review of Sociology, 18*, 209–232.

Conrad, P. (2007). *The medicalization of society*. Baltimore: John Hopkins University.

Conrad, P., & Schneider, J. W. (1980a). *Deviance and medicalization. From badness to sickness*. St Louis: Mosby.

Conrad, P., & Schneider, J. W. (1980b). Looking at levels of medicalization. A comment on Strong's critique of the thesis of medical imperialism. *Social Science & Medicine, 14A*, 75–79.

Coveney, C., Williams, S. J., & Gabe, J. (2019a). Cognitive enhancing drugs: Re-imagining the user in drugs policy. *Drugs: Education, Prevention and Policy, 26*(4), 319–328.

Coveney, C., Williams, S., & Gabe, J. (2019b). Medicalisation, pharmaceuticalisation or both? Exploring the medical management of sleeplessness as insomnia. *Sociology of Health & Illness, 41*(2), 266–284.

Daemmrich, A. (2004). *Pharmacopolitics*. Chapel Hill: University of North Carolina.

Davis, C. (2015). Drugs, cancer and end-of-life care: A case study of pharmaceuticalization? *Social Science & Medicine, 131*, 215–217.

Davis, C., & Abraham, J. (2013). *Unhealthy pharmaceutical regulation*. Basingstoke: Palgrave Macmillan.

Department of Health. (2003). *Our inheritance, our future. Realising the potential of genetics in the NHS*. UK Government White Paper. London: Department of Health.

Elbe, S., Roemer-Mahler, A., & Long, C. (2015). Medical countermeasures for national security: A new government role in the pharmaceuticalization of society. *Social Science and Medicine, 131,* 263–271.

Fox, N. J., & Ward, K. J. (2009). Pharma in the bedroom... and the kitchen. The pharmaceuticalisation of daily life. In S. J. Williams, J. Gabe, & P. Davis (Eds.), *Pharmaceuticals and society: Critical discourses and debates* (pp. 41–53). Oxford: Blackwell.

Fox, N. J., Ward, K. J., & O'Rourke, A. J. (2005). Pro-anorexia, weight loss drugs and the internet: An "anti-recovery" explanatory model of anorexia. *Sociology of Health and Illness, 27,* 944–971.

Gabe, J., & Bury, M. (1996). Risking tranquillizer use: Cultural and lay dimensions. In S. J. Williams, & M. Calnan (Eds.), *Modern medicine: Lay perspectives and experiences* (pp. 74–94). London: University College London Press.

Gabe, J., Chamberlain, K., Norris, P., Dew, K., Madden, H., & Hodgetts, D. (2012). The debate about the funding of Herceptin: A case study of "countervailing powers". *Social Science and Medicine, 75,* 2353–2361.

Gabe, J., & Lipshitz-Phillips, S. (1984). Tranquillisers as social control? *Sociological Review, 32,* 524–546.

Gaudillière, J.-P. (2014). Herbalised Ayurveda? Reformulation, plant management and the "pharmaceuticalisation" of Indian "traditional" medicine. *Asian Medicine, 9*(1–2), 171–205.

Geyer, R. (2011). The politics of EU health policy and the case of direct-to-consumer advertising for prescription drugs. *British Journal of Politics and International Relations, 13,* 586–602.

Giarelli, G., Jacobsen, B., Nielsen, M., & Reinbacher, G. S. (Eds.). (2016). *Future challenges for health and healthcare in Europe.* Aalborg: Aalborg University Press.

Halfmann, D. (2012). Recognizing medicalization and demedicalization: Discourses, practices and identities. *Health, 16,* 186–207.

Hedgecoe, A., & Martin, P. (2003). The drugs don't work: Expectations and the shaping of pharmacogenetics. *Social Studies of Science, 33,* 327–364.

Hendlin, Y. H., Elias, J., & Ling, P. M. (2017). The pharmaceuticalization of the tobacco industry. *Annals of Internal Medicine, 167*(4), 278–280.

Hopkins, M. H., Martin, P. A., Nightingale, P., Kraft, A., et al. (2007). The myth of the biotech revolution: An assessment of technological, clinical and organisational change. *Research Policy, 36,* 566–589.

IMS Institute for Health Informatics. (2014). *Global outlook for medicines through 2018.* Danbury, Connecticut: IMS Institute for Health Informatics.

Jones, K. (2009). In whose interest? Relationships between health consumer groups and the pharmaceutical industry. In S. J. Williams, J. Gabe, & P. Davis (Eds.), *Pharmaceuticals and society: Critical discourses and debates* (pp. 112–125). Oxford: Blackwell.

Law, J. (2006). *The big pharma.* London: Constable and Robinson.

Mamo, M., & Epstein, S. (2014). The pharmaceuticalization of sexual risk: Vaccine development and the new politics of cancer prevention. *Social Science & Medicine, 101,* 155–165.

Morrison, M. (2015). Growth hormone, enhancement and the pharmaceuticalisation of short stature. *Social Science & Medicine, 131,* 305–312.

Moynihan, R. (2002). Disease mongering: How doctors, drug companies and insurers are making you feel sick. *British Medical Journal, 324,* 923.

Moynihan, R., & Henry, D. (2006). The fight against disease mongering: Generating knowledge for action. *Public Library of Science Medicine, 3e,* 191.

Nettleton, S., Burrows, R., & O'Malley, L. (2005). The mundane realities of the everyday lay use of the internet for health, and their consequences for media convergence. *Sociology of Health & Illness, 27,* 972–992.

Nightingale, P., & Martin, P. (2004). The myth of the biotech revolution. *Trends in Biotechnology, 22,* 564–569.

Pollock, A., & Jones, D. S. (2015). Coronary artery disease and the contours of pharmaceuticalisation. *Social Science & Medicine, 131,* 221–227.

Salter, B., & Salter, C. (2018). The politics of ageing: Health consumers, markets and hegemonic challenge. *Sociology of Health & Illness, 40*(6), 1069–1086.

Sariola, S., Ravindran, D., Kumarb, A., & Jeffery, R. (2015). Big-pharmaceuticalisation: Clinical trials and contract research organisations in India. *Social Science & Medicine, 131,* 239–246.

Seale, C. (2002). *Media and health.* London: SAGE.

Shendure, J., Findlay, G., & Snyder, M. (2019). Genomic medicine – Progress, pitfalls, and promise. *Cell, 177*(1), 45–57.

Simpson, B., Khatri, R., Ravindran, D., & Udalagama, T. (2015). Pharmaceuticalisation and ethical review in South Asia: Issues of scope and authority for practitioners and policy makers. *Social Science and Medicine*, *131*, 247–254.

Stevenson, F., Britten, N., Barry, C., Bradley, C., & Barber, N. (2002). Perceptions of legitimacy: The influence on medicine taking and prescribing. *Health*, *6*, 85–104.

Stevenson, F., Leontowitsch, M., & Duggan, C. (2009). Over-the-counter medicines: Professional expertise and consumer discourses. In S. J. Williams, J. Gabe & P. Davis (Eds.), *Pharmaceuticals and society: Critical discourses and debates* (pp. 97–111), Oxford: Blackwell.

Taylor, D., & Bury, M. (2007). Chronic illness, expert patients and care transition. *Sociology of Health & Illness*, *29*, 27–45.

Thomann, M. (2018). "On December 1, 2015, sex changes. Forever": Pre-exposure prophylaxis and the pharmaceuticalisation of the neoliberal sexual subject. *Global Public Health*, *13*(8). doi: 10.1080/17441692.2018.1427275

Time. (1960, March). Tranquil but alert. *Time*, *75*(10), 34.

Towghi, F. (2014). Normalizing off-label experiments and the pharmaceuticalization of homebirths in Pakistan. *Ethnos: Journal of Anthropology*, *79*(1), 108–137. doi: 10.1080/00141844.2013.821511.

Vrecko, S. (2015). Everyday drug diversions: A qualitative study of the illicit exchange and non-medical use of prescription stimulants on a university campus. *Social Science & Medicine*, *131*, 297–304.

Williams, S., Martin, P., & Gabe, J. (2011b). Evolving sociological analysis of "pharmaceuticalisation". A reply to Abraham. *Sociology of Health & Illness*, *33*, 729–730.

Williams, S. J., & Calnan, M. (Eds.). (1996). *Modern medicine: Lay perspectives and experiences*. London: University College London Press.

Williams, S. J., Gabe, J., & Martin, P. (2012). Medicalization and pharmaceuticalization at the intersections: A commentary on Bell and Figert. *Social Science & Medicine*, *75*, 2129–2130.

Williams, S. J., Martin, P., & Gabe, J. (2011a). The pharmaceuticalisation of society? A framework for analysis. *Sociology of Health & Illness*, *33*, 710–725.

5

GOVERNING MEDICAL TECHNOLOGY

Stuart Hogarth and Fiona A. Miller

Introduction

Health technologies really began to blossom in the last of the century, when engineering and medicine became increasingly interdisciplinary, and the human body was more fully recognized as a complex system of electrical fields, fluid and biomechanics, chemistry, and motion – ideal for an engineering approach to many of its problems.

(National Academy of Engineering, 2000, p. 1)

This quote is rich material as a starting point for a critical investigation of medical technology. It offers a typical account of uncomplicated progress in the ability of technology to cure disease and dysfunction, a viewpoint that social scientists have been keen to challenge. It points to the complex interaction of different fields of expertise in biomedical innovation, highlighting another key concern for social scientists – the ways in which technologies are bound up with disciplinary change in the biosciences and in medicine, and, more broadly, how the social and the technical are intertwined. It suggests that technological advance is linked to new ways of thinking about the body, a relationship that critical analysts view as interactive. Technologies may indeed change what we can see, support new perspectives on how the body functions, and foster new conceptions of health and illness, but technologies also reflect and reinforce our expectations about what is worth knowing or acting upon, and how we should do so.

Beyond these classic themes in the critical analysis of medical technologies, this quote is also illustrative of what it does *not* name – notably, the "vast industrial undertakings" that produce these technologies, and the role of the state in promoting and regulating them (Moran, 1995, p. 768). Indeed, the enterprises that create and market the biomedical innovations that play such a vital role in modern healthcare are among the largest and most profitable multi-national industries in the world; their activities are "central to the competitive struggles that lie at the heart of modern capitalist economies" (Ibid.). Thus, as Moran (1995) noted in his classic work, the healthcare state has multiple faces – as a guarantor of the safe and accessible use of biomedical innovations within public healthcare systems that are financially redistributive, while also supporting strategically important industries that compete locally and globally for "market share and profits" (p. 769).

In this chapter, we seek to address both sets of issues, reflecting our ambition to straddle the common divide between analytic and normative work on health technology governance. We begin with what is often termed in policy studies an analysis "of" the policy process – offering a brief review of themes in the critical social scientific study of medical technologies. This review is important for demonstrating how technologies – in their design and deployment – reflect and reproduce the societies in which they have been developed and used. Such work aims at analytic depth and precision but largely eschews policy recommendation. We next move to analysis "in and for" the policy process, adopting an explicitly normative stance to review the nature of the medical technologies industry, the regulatory regime that governs it and the multiple – sometimes conflicting – public policy expectations of its governance.

In doing so, we focus specifically on technologies that, in some settings, are identified simply by what they are not: that is, "non-drug technologies". This focus avoids overlap with the chapter on pharmaceuticals (see Chapter 4, this volume). More importantly, it reflects critical differences between pharmaceutical and medical technologies with respect to the industry, regulatory regime, and epistemic community, even given the marked heterogeneity within the category of medical technology itself.

We characterise our interest using the language of "governance" – how networks of public and private authority co-produce social arrangements and outcomes – with particular attention to regulation (i.e. rulemaking and enforcement), rather than distributive and redistributive forms of governance. In this we follow Keating and Cambrosio's injunction that "to understand biomedicine is to understand its regulation". In this co-constructionist approach, regulation and innovation are intimately entangled: regulation shapes the boundaries of a new technology, stabilising its character, networks, and effects through processes of definition, standardisation, and legitimation. The form that regulation takes is also a work in progress – shaped, in part, by the features of specific sociotechnical systems (Holloway and Miller, 2020). Regulation is also shaped by international politico-economic trends, which for Tombs (2016) should be understood as "a relentless programme of *re*-regulation" that serves private rather than public interests (p. 334, emphasis in original).

Shaping medical technologies

In this first section, we offer a brief review of classic and emerging themes in the critical social scientific study of medical technologies, following the thread of the medicalisation thesis. We first document a shift in analytic focus from classic studies of technology as an exercise of power by single dominant groups to analyses that see technology as a site of contest among multiple groups. We next review classic work on the co-production or "social shaping" of technology, which documents processes of socio-technological emergence. Each brief review highlights the exercise of power, the intersection of interests and the role of commercial and industrial actors – a theme that serves as the focus of our second section.

The power of medical technologies

A classic theme in the critical study of medical technologies concerns their role in the exercise of medical power, often under the auspices of the "medicalisation" thesis. Medicalisation identifies those processes whereby a wide range of issues come to be construed as medical problems, bringing them within the scope of medical authority and intervention. It has been identified as "one of the most potent social transformations of the last half of the twentieth century in the West" (Clarke et al., 2003, p. 161).

Medical technologies have often been seen to bolster the power of medicine relative to patients, and to reproduce broader power relations in society – of men relative to women, for example, or of the Global North relative to the Global South. Over time, this monolithic view of medical power has given way to more nuanced analyses: the growing authority of medical technology may diminish the felt-authority of individual medics, for example, and there is potential for women and communities in the Global South to shift the terms of technology use, and for consumers to increase their power relative to medics. The power of medicalisation, this work suggests, is not only wielded by medics, but also by non-medical actors, including consumers and industry.

From the perspective of classic medicalisation theory, technology has an instrumental role in the ascendancy of medical power. Conrad's (1979) analysis of medicine's institutional function as a mechanism of social control of deviant behaviour is illustrative. Medical and social norms become intertwined and enforced through new forms of technological intervention that target various forms of deviance: lasers and brain implants to treat violent behaviour, genetic testing for eugenic purposes.

The history of diagnostic technologies exemplifies the rise of scientific medicine, changing models of disease and the body, and their association with medical hegemony and the disempowerment of the patient. The history of diagnosis in the last two centuries has been broadly understood by many historians as a shift from the physiological to the ontological, driven by a proliferation of techniques and technologies for eliciting clinical data directly from the bodies of the sick, and with a corresponding diminution in the importance of patients' attempts to render into language their subjective experiences of pain and discomfort. In summary, there are three interlinked historical changes which underpin the contemporary understanding of the normal and the pathological: *localisation*, i.e. a shift in focus from the idea of disease as an imbalance of the individual's system to the definition of disease as a lesion observable at the level of tissue or cell; *generalisation*, i.e. the nosological effort to organise diseases into categories (and subcategories) based on symptoms; and *quantification*, i.e. an increasing reliance on the precise measurement of bodily function *and* statistical measure of the normal and the pathological by reference to healthy and morbid populations. This transformation in understanding was enabled by new diagnostic technologies, from the humble stethoscope to genetic testing, and facilitated medical hegemony both at the level of the clinical encounter by diminishing the importance of dialogue with the patient, and at the level of the population by new forms of surveillance medicine such as screening (see Chapter 7, this volume).

From a feminist perspective, medical technologies raise familiar issues about the nature of male power and the ways in which gender is socially constructed through the control of women's bodies. Early feminist scholarship on reproductive technologies like IVF conceptualised medicine as a system of patriarchal domination that allows male doctors to exercise power over female sexuality and fertility, serving to reinforce essentialised concepts of motherhood based on a pro-natalist ideology that naturalises childbearing as both biological destiny and social obligation (Corea, 1987). Oppression may be immanent in the very design of technology; for instance, why target women's infertility, and not that of men? As reproductive medicine has become a global business, concerns about patriarchal power have intersected with issues of racial inequality. The international trade in commercial surrogacy has been viewed as a regime that exploits women of colour in the Global South (Nelson, 2013).

Alternative perspectives have enriched these insights: drawing on research on the lived experience of patients, many scholars now suggest that new reproductive technologies disrupt established ideologies, reconceptualising the relation of mother and child (Franklin, 2013). Scholarship on the global surrogacy market has taken a similar turn – ethnographic research on the attitudes of the women providing surrogacy services has uncovered the agency of this female labour force, not only its economic exploitation (Parry, 2018). Similarly, Reiser's (1978) humanist critique of the mechanisation of diagnosis suggests that doctors too have become disempowered as they become more reliant on technology, and less confident in their exercise of clinical judgement. For Reiser (1978), mechanical objectivity subverts both the subjective dimensions of the doctor-patient dialogue and that mode of objectivity Foucault described as the clinical gaze.

A less empowered medical workforce is also suggested by those who have identified the emergence of a more consumerist form of healthcare, in which medical technologies are no longer the sole preserve of medical professionals. This argument is weakened, in our view, by the limited historical scholarship on a supposedly less consumerist past. Moreover, consumerisation is not a zero-sum power contest between consumers and medical professionals; it is fostered by, and signals the power of, a third actor: industry. Indeed, Conrad (2005) has updated his classic work to suggest that the growth of consumer medical markets exemplifies "the shifting engines of medicalisation". The growth of new technologies means that medicalisation is now "more driven by commercial and market interests than by professional claims-makers" (p. 3).

Classic views of medical technology as the exercise of power by a single dominant group have given way to views of medical technology as sites of contest among multiple groups, even recognising that not all social groups have equal resources in these contests. Moreover, the growing importance of commercial and market interests means that these contests have normative consequence for public policy, not just analytic significance, as we discuss in in the second part of this chapter. Before doing so, we turn to consider critical social science scholarship on the innovation system for medical technologies.

Theorising medical innovation

The idea of the "construction" or social shaping of technology has been highly influential in science and technology studies and cognate fields. Technology is a social practice and society and technology are mutually constitutive. Rather than technologies simply acting on society – shaping opportunities for certain social groups or social practices – and rather than societies acting on technologies – permitting certain technological solutions to emerge and not others – both should be understood to evolve in tandem. Such analytical approaches stress the indeterminacy of technological change. The eventual design and applied uses of a technology are not immanent in the blueprint; the development of any new technology has no single predetermined endpoint. Rather, the power and interests of competing user groups, their conflicting visions of future applications and their values influence choices made in the design of a technology, in its uses and in the final form, or forms, that it takes (Pinch & Wiebe, 1984). As well, a technology is not just the artefact itself – the device or diagnostic tool. Rather, it is the "sociotechnical ensemble" (Bijker, 1995) or system of artefacts and techniques embodied in people, whose operations are structured by a regime of norms, regulations, and organisational conditions.

Blume's (1992) early and influential account of the development of medical imaging technologies (MRI, ultrasound, CT scanners) in the second half of the 20th century provides an illustrative example of these themes. For Blume, the development of a new medical technology was conceived as occurring through the formation of networks of actors who shape artefacts, techniques, and regimes, according to a shared vision of its future application. Blume (1992) suggested that technology evolves through a series of *problematisations*, whereby groups of actors seek to address features of their environment, a technology, or its usage that they find problematic. Influential actor groups often occupy a position of power over others in the network and such influence is traceable through *inter-organisational links* (e.g. contracts to provide services, grant provision, formal or informal research collaborations). Influence may also be found in explicit statements of intent to the future shaping and application of technology. These *visions* are an important way of enrolling support by appealing to common objectives. The final aspect of Blume's model was the temporal trajectory of development and diffusion – the dynamics of technological innovation can be followed longitudinally using the concept of the *career*, a sequence of four phases (1. exploration, 2. development, 3. diffusion, evaluation, and assessment, and 4. feedback). By the third stage, the new technology becomes established in the clinic, a process that entails "a renegotiation of the hospital's social order," as the division of labour between different professional groups is reorganised to accommodate the new organisational regime.

Blume's interest in "visions" has been renewed in more recent work on the sociology of expectations, which explores how new fields are constituted through future-oriented visions, and how these expectations play a key function in the enrolment of support, the mobilisation of resources and the shaping of technological artefacts (Brown & Kraft, 2006). The sociology of expectation lens has commonly been applied at the broad level of new technoscientific fields, such as nanotechnology. It has also been used to analyse specific technological applications within a given field, where grand visions may prove "fragile" or subject to intense "hype–disappointment dynamics" (Borup, 2006, p. 294). Moreira and Palladino (2005), for example, argue that contemporary biomedicine is "shaped by two, seemingly incommensurable, organisational logics, the 'regime of truth' and 'the regime of hope'" (p. 55). Using experimental treatments for Parkinson's Disease as their case study, they explore the underlying logics of advocates and sceptics contesting the value of new technologies. The regime of hope is characterised by an optimism about the potential of new treatments, a willingness to defer judgement in expectation of good news to come; the regime of truth is focused on the prosaic assessment of present knowledge. Extending the sociology of expectations lens to industry decisions, Hogarth (2017) argues that a bold future-oriented vision of "disruptive innovation" is as important to the interactions between start-up firms and prospective investors in Silicon Valley as a sound business plan, or a management team with a proven track record.

The social environment's constitutive role in technological change is highlighted in these literatures, but rarely explored across jurisdictions. A rare attempt to compare trajectories of development and diffusion across countries is provided by Parthasarathy's (2007) account of genetic testing for breast cancer in the UK and the USA. Previous research has shown that adoption of some molecular diagnostics has proceeded much more rapidly in the USA compared to the UK (Institute for Prospective Technological Studies, 2006), but Parthasarathy goes beyond this to show how the configuration of technologies within clinical care pathways also varies significantly between the two countries. Her conceptual model combines structural factors, such as regulatory regimes, with cultural elements and she uses the concept of "national toolkits", to emphasise the agency of actors in fashioning a "strategy of action" within their local context.

Two common criticisms of the co-constructionist literature warrant mention here. First, by focusing on artefacts and their design, and the processes by which technologies stabilise as "black boxes", later processes of technology refinement are often downplayed. Yet when users configure the technology for practical application in their own institutional context, the "black box" may be reopened and the technology reshaped (Mackay & Gillespie, 1992). As well, the structural dimensions of political and economic power that underpin sociotechnical change are sometimes downplayed in this scholarship (Russell, 1986). For Blume (1992), by contrast, medicine had a "structural dependency" on technological innovation that was bolstered by industry: "medical equipment has become very big business and today physicians, engineers, manufacturers, and patients make common cause in supporting technological advance in medicine" (p. 12). In Blume's account, the professional power of clinicians and the economic power of industry are integrated in a symbiotic relation of co-dependence in which neither party is dominant. Faulkner (2009) has provided an account of how, in recent decades, the state has increasingly sought to steer the direction of this medical-industrial complex through a restructuring of the relationship between the clinic and the laboratory (captured in the concept of "translational research"), and through efforts to restructure regulatory institutions.

Just as Conrad (2005) saw the growth of commercial markets in healthcare as "the shifting engines of medicalisation" in the delivery of care, Clarke and colleagues (2003) identified an industry-assisted shift toward "biomedicalisation", made possible by technoscientific innovation – the linked technological and scientific shifts that have converted medicine into biomedicine. The new era of "biomedicalisation" draws together *inter alia* developments in technoscience from molecularisation to information technology; the corporatisation and commodification of biomedical research and healthcare institutions; and the proliferation of new sites for the production and distribution of medical and health knowledges. This framework is notable for the breadth of its analytic scope although its geographical focus is restricted to describing developments in the USA and its empirical validation is thus far limited to micro-level case studies.

Regulating medical technologies

As these brief reviews make clear, medical technologies are not neutral technical artefacts; their development and deployment reflects and reproduces social and economic power in complex ways. Here, we turn to some of the analytic and normative questions such analyses provoke for the shaping of public policy, with a particular focus on regulation.

Industry and innovation

Any discussion of corporate power in the medical technologies industry must start from an appreciation of the size of the sector and of the structural inequalities within it. Industry estimates suggest that the medical technology market was worth €425 billion in 2017, about a third the size of the pharmaceutical market (MedTech Europe, 2019). This market is not uniformly distributed across the globe, however. The two largest markets, the USA and Europe, account for 43% and 27% of the global market, respectively (Ibid.). In addition to being the largest market, the USA is home to most of the major firms. Measured by 2017 revenues, seven of the ten largest firms are US-based, with the remaining three based in Europe (Evaluate, 2018). Finally, a small number of large firms dominate the market even despite the presence of many small firms – Europe has 27,000 firms and 95% of them are small and medium-sized enterprises (MedTech Europe, 2019). In respect of revenues, the industry is highly concentrated, with the top ten firms accounting for 39% of revenues, and a further 20 firms accounting for 25%. Industrial concentration is even more intense in sub-sectors such as diagnostics – in medical imaging the top ten firms account for 91% of revenues and in the *in vitro* diagnostics sector it is 74%.

The industrial organisation of innovation in the medical technology sector has long relied on a mergers and acquisition model: buying-in technology by acquiring smaller firms (Faulkner, 2009). This is illustrated by the molecular diagnostics sector, where the largest firms (such as Roche, Qiagen, and Illumina) have all grown through acquisitions that have generally provided access to new technologies, rather than simply increasing market share. Historically, however, the medical technology sector differed markedly from the pharmaceutical sector in this respect (Faulker, 2009); until the 1990s, the largest pharmaceutical firms relied on in-house R&D to propel innovation (Rosenbloom and Spencer, 1996). With the growing move to what Tulum and Lazonick (2018) have termed a "downsize and distribute" model of innovation in the pharmaceutical industry, the drug pipeline is increasingly fed through bidding wars to buy-in innovation from biotech SMEs. One might speculate, therefore, that the medical technology industry has served as a negative role model for shifts in the pharmaceutical innovation system.

Regulating medical technologies

The study of regulation is a fruitful avenue for the critical social scientific study of medical technology. Regulatory dynamics expose the sociotechnical contours of technology and technological change, and the significant role of the politico-economic shifts of globalisation in these sociotechnical processes. Two key actors within the regulatory regime for health technology govern the availability and use of medical products by consumers and within collectively financed health systems – market access regulation and reimbursement regulation (e.g. through Health Technology Assessment). Yet, these classic "regulatory state" institutions do not stand apart as independent gatekeepers of established technological entities. Rather, they participate in an array of "formal, informal, and tacit relationships that involve complex configurations of regulatory actors" (Abbott et al., 2017, p. 31).

In the contemporary era, regulation is often "de-centred", with authority exercised by non-majoritarian institutions of elite – technocratic – control (Jasanoff, 1990), rather than under the direct bureaucratic administration of the state (Black, 2001). Regulation is also typically "polycentric" (Black, 2008), exercised by a wide array of "regulators" and an equally wide array of "regulatory intermediaries" – consultancies, credit rating agencies, standard-setting bodies, accounting firms, and civil society groups – which co-produce regulatory objectives, regulatory efforts and the regulated products themselves (Abbott et al., 2017; Meyer and Kearns, 2013; Cambrosio et al., 2017). The multiplicity of these actors, and their often-seamless coordination across public agency, industry, professional association, and civil society group, highlights the extent to which globalisation has engendered re-regulation rather than de-regulation (Tombs, 2015), in ways fundamental to "the continuing expansion, adaptation and transformation of capitalism" (Levi-Faur, 2017, p. 290).

Market access regulation

A first set of regulatory institutions for medical technologies governs industry access to specific geopolitical territories, through classic regulatory state institutions such as the US Food and Drug Administration (FDA), the Chinese FDA and Health Canada. These agencies set the terms of sale within jurisdictional borders for the vast majority of medical products – governing, as Marks (2009) wryly notes, what can be *said* about marketed products more than what can be *done* with them.

In its structural features, the regulatory regime for medical devices mirrors that for pharmaceuticals, though with some important differences. Notably, regulation by bodies like the FDA establishes a far lower bar to market entry for medical devices, diagnostics, and other medical technologies than for pharmaceuticals (Sorenson & Drummond, 2014). As Altenstetter (2013) points out, there is "a double standard for drugs and devices", with "more rigour and strict rules for drug approvals but less rigour and laxer rules for high-risk medical devices". As market access regulation of medical technologies is risk-based, requirements for lower-risk medical technologies (e.g. ventilators, imaging systems) are laxer still.

Market access regulation offers a classic example of the workings of the regulatory state, through extensive rulemaking, monitoring, and enforcement. It thus provokes questions about the capacity of such institutions to defend the public interest, given the state's competing health policy and innovation policy goals (Lehoux et al., 2008). In this regard, literature on the market access regulation of pharmaceuticals has highlighted the challenge of "corporate bias". For example, Davis and Abraham (2013) suggest that even "gold standard" regulators such as the US FDA have become increasingly responsive to industry interests in the neo-liberal era.

Though less studied, non-drug technologies are also illustrative of this dynamic. In Europe, for example, the development of coordinated medical device regulation was first and foremost concerned with opening up internal markets to trade, though that priority has been progressively tempered by the elevation of public health concerns (Altenstetter, 2013). Nonetheless, policy priorities related to a certain form of "economic development" continue to inform market access regulation. In the European Union, for example, uncertainty about the market access regulation of "regenerative medicine" products, which saw member states regulating these technologies variably as devices, drugs, biologics, or a combination of these approaches, has since 2007 been replaced with single approval pathway defined by the EU's centralised pharmaceutical regulatory framework. Exemplifying the dynamic of re-regulation for market growth, this change was driven by industry concerns that wide variations in regulation across member states had created a "heterogeneous and segmented market in Europe" (Hughes-Wilson & Mackay, 2007). The post-2007 EU regulatory framework also demonstrates how technological change is interlinked with broader political shifts, such as the increasing importance of transnational governance.

Market access regulation seems, in some respects, to serve as a gate-keeper – a checkpoint in the progress of a medical product from its developer to its consumer. However, studies of novel technologies suggest otherwise. Regulation in these contexts "does not simply adapt to the development of 'disruptive' innovations, but also participates in their shaping and framing" (Cambrosio, 2017, p. 163). Exploring how molecular biomarkers for cancer can be invoked to suggest new nosologies and therapeutic options, Cambrosio and colleagues (2017) show how these new technologies emerge through processes that collapse, confuse, or confound the orderly sequence of regulatory phases of evidence development, from discovery through a clinical trial to market access approval. Transnational scientific networks link researchers, industry, research funders, and market access regulators in selecting biomarkers, defining thresholds for their detection or relevance, and standardising their measurement. This web of regulatory action encompasses knowledge and evidence production. This process also transforms regulatory agencies: no longer simply adjudicators of the results of biomedical research, they are now active participants in the construction of research activities and the associated standard-setting processes.

Health technology assessment

While market access regulation plays a role in the governance of almost all health technologies in most jurisdictions, a second set of regulatory institutions plays a more partial but increasingly visible role in decisions about reimbursement – which technologies are covered, under what conditions and at what price. Such institutions have particular relevance for collectively financed health systems, whether publicly or privately financed, given the central importance of collective finance for healthcare access within rich countries.

Decisions about reimbursement have traditionally been exercised by clinicians, through "light-touch, peer-controlled" systems of what Moran (2003) has characterised as "club government" (p. 147). The rise of regulatory state institutions has threatened exclusive clinical jurisdiction over such decisions (Moran, 1995, 2003; Salter, 2004), mobilising "evidence-based medicine" and state managerialism as alternate forms of expertise and authority (Harrison and Dowswell, 2002; Salter, 2004).

One formalised instantiation of these efforts is Health Technology Assessment (HTA). HTA agencies have been created in many wealthy countries since the 1980s, adhering to the typical quasi-independent public-agency model of providing "expertise in order to advise decision-makers or make decisions themselves on reimbursement matters" (Löblová, 2016, p. 255). By centralising responsibility for resource allocation within technocratic institutions, HTA purports to render inherently political decisions neutral, transparent, standardised, and rational (Brown, 2011).

Though some HTA agencies are nationally prominent and well resourced, as with the National Institute for Health and Care Excellence in the UK (Williams, 2013), HTA often has a partial role in coverage and pricing; most HTA agencies focus on decisions about initial adoption of novel, expensive technologies; they are more influential for drug than non-drug technologies; as well, they typically offer recommendations rather than exercising decision-making authority (Miller et al., 2020). Despite this, HTA has emerged as an influential epistemic community in resource allocation decisions. And while the founding conception of HTA was quite expansive – extending to the aim of public engagement and social responsibility in the anticipation and shaping of technologies (Guston, 2002; Schot & Rip, 1997) – a more limited and technocratic science has taken root in practice, strongly influenced by the utility-maximising logic of health economics (Williams, 2013).

Even as the community of HTA practitioners and health economists anticipate the necessary ascendance of their rationalist logic, more critical social scientific work has consistently highlighted the limitations of this aspiration – emphasising the context-specific, political, and socially mediated nature of resource allocation institutions and processes (Löblová et al., 2020). Such work includes a body of literature that highlights the variegated meanings of an HTA agency, which have been established in different countries for different reasons, reflecting domestic imperatives, articulated through the efforts of domestic epistemic communities (Löblová, 2016). As well, the HTA agencies that emerge have distinct national styles – with their own "processes, methods and evidential requirements" (Wright et al., 2017, p. 69). Even with a jurisdiction, HTA agencies may have distinct epistemic and organisational styles, operating as separate "regulatory niches" (Hogarth and Löblová, 2020), even within the same sociotechnical field. Finally, the logic of HTA is poorly adapted to the institutional realities of local resource allocation (Williams and Bryan, 2007), including through procurement (Miller, 2020). Despite its declaratory promise, HTA guidance and specifically health economic judgements are little used in localised resource allocation processes, which necessarily "combine altruism, pragmatism and settlement between interest groups" (Williams, 2013, p. 233).

Multiplicity of diffuse regulators

Even while regulatory institutions related to market access and reimbursement have a prominent place – at least rhetorically – in the governance of medical technologies, a wide range of other regulatory institutions play consequential roles. One dimension of this multiplicity is that the "fit" between regulators and the technologies they govern cannot be taken for granted. Just as with regenerative medicine technologies, multiple regulatory frameworks may be applicable to different technologies, depending on the broader socio-political dynamics at stake.

The pap smear offers a useful example. The pap smear is a well-established tool for cervical cancer screening, which first entered routine clinical practice in the USA in the 1960s. Problems with the quality of testing in both the USA and the UK led to new processes of standardisation through quality assurance. In the USA, this proceeded through new statutory regulation governing the country's network of (predominantly commercial) clinical laboratories (Casper &

Clarke,1998). In the UK's public healthcare system, by contrast, the solution was centralisation of screening activity as a national programme (Hogarth & Löblová, 2020).

In addition to the under-determined nature of regulatory fit, the sheer number and diversity of health sector regulators points to the expanding and evolving contours of medical governance. The issue of patient safety, for example, exemplifies how organisational complexity increases as the focus moves from the evaluation of new technologies (the focus of much innovation-centric social science scholarship on medical technologies) to the governance of established (often mundane) technologies in routine use, such as the pap smear. A recent review of patient safety regulations identified 126 organisations (statutory regulators, national agencies, professional and charitable bodies) that exert some regulatory influence on provider organisations in the UK NHS, "from formal regulatory inspections, attempts to promote good practice, to efforts to support and initiate culture improvement" (Oikonomou et al., 2019, p. 2). The infusion pump illustrates the impact of this burgeoning regulatory complex on medical technologies. A ubiquitous presence on hospital wards, delivering medicines, nutrients, and blood or blood products, the technology is clinically important but also risky, in part due to the weakness of market access regulation (Dixon-Woods & Pronovost, 2016). In response a new sociotechnical system of technology governance has emerged, comprising "information systems, reporting procedures, [and] risk managers" (Faulkner, 2009, p. 129).

In these contexts, technologies may themselves be regulatory. The policy preference for single-use devices is, for example, a form of design-based regulation, which uses "technical constraints to stop, or significantly inhibit, action at the moment it is attempted" (Yeung & Dixon-Woods, 2010, p. 503). Such "action-forcing" (Yeung & Dixon-Woods, 2010) may not go uncontested, given varied interpretations of – and values related to – technology cost, quality, availability, infection risk and the importance of professional discretion (Currie et al., 2009). Though less obviously constraining of clinical behaviour, the growing integration of interpretive algorithms within biomarker tests and gene panels suggests that medical diagnostics increasingly "regulate" clinical judgement (Bourret et al., 2011), highlighting once again the extent to which regulation co-produces "the entities it regulates" (Cambrosio et al., 2017, p. 161).

Conclusion

The theme of regulation might be seen as a thread through this overview of social scientific perspectives on medical technology. Medical technologies are implicated in strategies of control, whether as instruments of medicalisation that enhance professional or consumer power and corporate influence, as objects of regulatory governance that constrain the scope and pace of technology diffusion, or deployed as governance devices.

Research on medical technologies spans the mundane and the disruptive, but there is a clear bias towards novel technologies at the expense of established technologies, a preference to study innovation rather than maintenance. One direction for future research is to redress this balance. As to research on innovation, a notable lacuna is the comparative analysis of technological trajectories across countries.

References

Abbott, K.W., Levi-Faur, D., & Snidal, D. (2017). *Introducing regulatory intermediaries*. Los Angeles, CA: SAGE Publications.

Altenstetter, C. (2013). US perspectives on the EU medical devices approval systems and lessons learned from the United States. *European Journal of Risk Regulation, 04*, 443–464.

Bijker, W. E. (1995). *Of bicycles, bakelites, and bulbs: Toward a theory of sociotechnical change*. Cambridge, MA: MIT Press.

Black, J. (2001). Decentring regulation: Understanding the role of regulation and self-regulation in a "post-regulatory" world. *Current Legal Problems, 54*, 103–146.

Black, J. (2008). Constructing and contesting legitimacy and accountability in polycentric regulatory regimes. *Regulation & Governance, 2*(2), 137–164.

Blume, S. (1992). *Insight and industry: On the dynamics of technological change in medicine*. Cambridge, MA: MIT Press.

Borup, M., Brown, N., Konrad, K., & Van Lente, H. (2006). The sociology of expectations in science and technology. *Technology Analysis & Strategic Management, 18*(3–4), 285–298.

Bourret, P., Keating, P., & Cambrosio, A. (2011). Regulating diagnosis in post-genomic medicine: Re-aligning clinical judgment? *Social Science & Medicine, 73*(6), 816–824.

Brown, N., & Kraft, A. (2006). Blood ties: Backing the stem cell promise. *Technology Analysis & Strategic Management, 18*(3–4), 313–327.

Brown, P. R. (2011). The dark side of hope and trust: Constructed expectations and the value-for-money regulation of new medicines. *Health Sociology Review, 20*, 410–422.

Cambrosio, A., Bourret, P., Keating, P., & Nelson, N. (2017). Opening the regulatory black box of clinical cancer research: Transnational expertise networks and "disruptive" technologies. *Minerva, 55*(2), 161–185.

Casper, M., & Clarke, E. (1998). Making the Pap smear into the "right tool" for the job: Cervical cancer screening in the USA, circa 1940–1995. *Social Studies of Science, 28*, 255–290.

Clarke, A. E., Shim, J. K., Mamo, L., Fosket, J. R., & Fishman, J. R. (2003). Biomedicalization: Technoscientific transformations of health, illness, and US biomedicine. *American Sociological Review, 68*(2), 161–194.

Conrad, P. (1979). Types of medical social control. *Sociology of Health and Illness, 1*(1), 1–11.

Conrad, P. (2005). Shifting engines of medicalization. *Journal of Health and Social Behavior, 46*, 3–14.

Corea, G., et al. (Eds.). (1987). *Man-made women: How new reproductive technologies affect women*. Bloomington, IN: Indiana University Press.

Currie, G., Humpreys, M., Waring, J., & Rowley, E. (2009). Narratives of professional regulation and patient safety: The case of medical devices in anaesthetics. *Health Risk Society, 11*, 117–135.

Davis, C., & Abraham, J. (2013). *Unhealthy pharmaceutical regulation: Innovation, politics and promissory science*. Basingstoke, UK: Palgrave Macmillan.

Dixon-Woods, M., & Pronovost, P. J. (2016). Patient safety and the problem of many hands. *BMJ Quality & Safety, 25*(7), 485–488. doi: 10.1136/bmjqs-2016-005232

Evaluate. (2018). *Evaluate MedTech World Preview 2018, Outlook to 2024*. London, UK: Evaluate.

Faulkner, A. (2009). *Medical technology into healthcare and society: A sociology of devices, innovation and governance*. Basingstoke, UK: Palgrave Macmillan, 34.

Franklin, S. (2013). *Biological relatives – IVF, stem cells and the future of kinship*. Durham, NC: Duke University Press.

Guston, D. H., & Sarewitz, D. (2002). Real-time technology assessment. *Technology in society, 24*(1–2), 93–109.

Harrison, S., & Dowswell, G. (2002). Autonomy and bureaucratic accountability in primary care: What English GPs say. *Sociology of Health and Illness, 24*(2): 208–226. doi: 10.1111/1467-9566.00291.

Holloway, K., & Miller, F. A. (2020). The consultant's intermediary role in the regulation of molecular diagnostics in the US. *Social Science & Medicine*, 112929.

Hogarth, S. (2017). Valley of the unicorns: Consumer genomics, venture capital and digital disruption. *New Genetics and Society, 36*(3), 250–272.

Hogarth, S., & Loblova, O. (2020). Regulatory niches: Diagnostic reform as a process of fragmented expansion. Evidence from the UK 1990–2018. *Social Science & Medicine*, 113363.

Hughes-Wilson, W., & Mackay, D. (2007). European approval system for advanced therapies: Good news for patients and innovators alike. *Regenerative Medicine, 2*(1), 5–6.

Institute for Prospective Technological Studies. (2006). *Pharmacogenetics and pharmacogenomics: State of the art and potential socio-economic impact in the EU*. European Communities: Luxembourg.

Jasanoff, S. (1990). *The fifth branch: Science advisers as policymakers*. Cambridge, MA: Harvard University Press.

Lehoux, P., Williams-Jones, B., Miller, F. A., Urbach, D., & Tailliez, S. (2008). What leads to better health care innovation? Arguments for an integrated policy-oriented research agenda. *Journal of Health Services Research & Policy, 13*(4), 251–254.

Levi-Faur, D. (2017). Regulatory capitalism. In Drahos, P. (Ed.), *Regulatory theory: Foundations and applications* (pp. 289–302). Canberra, Australia: ANU Press.

Löblová, O. (2016). Three worlds of health technology assessment: Explaining patterns of diffusion of HTA agencies in Europe. *Health Economics, Policy and Law*, *11*, 253–273.

Löblová, O., Trayanov, T., Csanádi, M., & Ozierański, P. (2020). The emerging social science literature on health technology assessment: A narrative review. *Value in Health*, *23*, 3–9.

Mackay, H., and Gillespie, G. (1992). Extending the social shaping of technology approach: Ideology and appropriation. *Social Studies of Science*, *16*, 621–662.

Marks, H. M. (2009, Unpublished slide manuscript). What does the FDA do? Regulation, Drug Markets and Medical Practice, 1906–2009.

MedTech Europe. (2019). *The European Medical Technology Industry in figures 2019*. Brussels: MedTech Europe.

Meyer, M., & Kearnes, M. (2013). Introduction to special section: Intermediaries between science, policy and the market. *Science and Public Policy*, *40*(4), 423–429.

Moran, M. (1995). Three faces of the health care state. *Journal of Health Policy, Politics and Law*, *20*(3), 767–781.

Moran, M. (2003). *The British regulatory state: High modernism and hyper-innovation*. Oxford, UK: Oxford University Press.

Moreira, T., & Palladino, P. (2005). Between truth and hope: on Parkinson's disease, neurotransplantation and the production of the 'self.' *History of the Human Sciences*, *18*(3), 55–82.

Miller, F. A. (2020). Modes of coordination for health technology adoption: Health Technology Assessment Agencies and Group Procurement Organizations in a Polycentric Regulatory Regime. *Social Science & Medicine*, 113528.

National Academy of Engineering. (2000). *Health technologies: Greatest engineering achievements of the twentieth century, no 16*. Washington, DC: NAE.

Nelson, E. (2013). Global trade and assisted reproductive technologies: Regulatory challenges in international surrogacy. *Journal of Law, Medicine & Ethics*, *41*(1), 240–253.

Oikonomou, E., Carthey, J., Macrae, C., & Vincent, C. (2019). Patient safety regulation in the NHS: Mapping the regulatory landscape of healthcare. *BMJ Open*, *9*(7), e028663.

Parry, B. (2018). Surrogate labour: Exceptional for whom? *Economy and Society*. doi: 10.1080/03085147.2018.1487180

Parthasarty, S. (2007). *Building genetic medicine: Breast cancer, technology and the comparative politics of health care*. Cambridge, MA: MIT Press.

Pinch, T., & Bijker, W. (1984). The social construction of facts and artifacts: Or how the sociology of science and the sociology of technology might benefit each other. *Social Studies of Science*, *14*, 399–441.

Reiser, S. J. (1978). *Medicine and the reign of technology*. Cambridge: Cambridge University Press.

Rosenbloom, R. S., & Spencer, W. J. (Eds.). (1996). *Engines of innovation: U.S. industrial research at the end of an era*. Boston, MA: Harvard Business School Press.

Russell, S. (1986). The social construction of artifacts: A response to Pinch and Bijker. *Social Studies of Science*, *16*, 331–346.

Salter, B. G. (2004). *The new politics of medicine*. Basingstoke, UK: Palgrave Macmillan.

Schot, J., & Rip, A. (1997). The past and future of constructive technology assessment. *Technological Forecasting and Social Change*, *54*(2–3), 251–268.

Tombs, S. (2015). *Social protection after the crisis: Regulation without enforcement*. Bristol, UK: Policy Press.

Tombs, S. (2016). Making better regulation, making regulation better? *Policy Studies*, *37*(4), 332–349.

Tulum, Ö., & Lazonick, W. (2018). Financialized corporations in a national innovation system: The US pharmaceutical industry. *International Journal of Political Economy*, *47*(3–4), 281–316.

Williams, I. (2013). Institutions, cost-effectiveness analysis and healthcare rationing: The example of healthcare coverage in the English National Health Service. *Policy & Politics*, *41*, 223–239.

Williams, I., & Bryan, S. (2007). Cost-effectiveness analysis and formulary decision making in England: Findings from research. *Social Science & Medicine*, *65*, 2116–2129.

Yeung, K., & Dixon-Woods, M. (2010). Design-based regulation and patient safety: A regulatory studies perspective. *Social Science & Medicine*, *71*, 502–509.

6

HEALTH SERVICES AND CARE

Political and affective economies

Rebecca E. Olson

Introduction

Though rarely a direct feature of everyday interactions within hospitals and clinics, health, health services, and care are "inherently political", reflecting a country's and family's political and economic context (Munro & McIntyre, 2016, p. 156). Those countries that lean right, towards neoliberal ideologies, tend to treat healthcare as a professional service – no different to other professional services (such as accounting and law) – exchanged in the free market. Those leaning left, towards the social-democratic, publicly funded pole, position healthcare as a merit good with benefits to a community far surpassing those of the purchaser, and thus deserving of public support (Lin, Smith, & Fawkes, 2014). Some have argued that social-democratic and neoliberal ideologies have converged over the past century across countries with advanced economies (Gauld, 2009), but most would still agree that these political and economic underpinnings continue to shape care delivery. A separate body of scholarship demonstrates how patriarchal and affective economies (Ahmed, 2004) similarly inform questions of who cares, how, and for how much. Antiquated, but nonetheless resilient, gender ideologies that position women as homemakers and men as breadwinners, men as rational and women as emotional, continue to situate (un)paid care work as taken-for-granted lower status women's work. This chapter draws these two bodies of scholarship together.

In this chapter, I offer an exploration of the intersecting political, economic, familial, and emotional relations which work in concert to structure the delivery of both formal healthcare services and informal care. Building on arguments for the inclusion of the family and the private sphere, in addition to the state and market, in analyses of shifting post-industrial political economies (Esping-Andersen, 1999; Folbre, 2012), in this chapter I evaluate the political, economic, affective, and gendered forces underpinning formal health services *and* informal family care. Overall, the chapter draws on existing scholarship to expand the critical discussion on the political and economic organisation of healthcare services and care from a macro-level focus on national policies to a multifocal appreciation of the intersections across policies, ideologies, and emotions.

The chapter begins by situating healthcare services and informal care in economically advanced countries[1] within their historical and political contexts, before examining the neoliberal and social-democratic principles underpinning the organisation of healthcare services and family caregiving. Drawing on examples from the United States of America (USA), United

Kingdom (UK), Costa Rica, Sweden, and Australia, I illustrate the range of offerings: from marketised healthcare services explicitly reliant on family caregiving in neoliberal leaning political economies, to universal healthcare services and care in social-democratic countries where – in theory – reliance on family caregivers is superseded by state support. I then go on to examine the affective economy of care which structures both informal caregiving and formal healthcare services. Specifically, I show how patriarchal framings of emotion and care position women as carers, anchoring them – especially within systems organised following neoliberal principles – in lower status and unpaid care work.

Historical and political contexts of health services and care

Throughout much of human history, food insecurity and infectious disease meant life was short (Kellehear, 2007). By the mid-20th century, improvements in public health, affluence, and farming, along with advances in medicine and surgery, ushered in an era of improved life expectancy (Baum, 2015; Szreter, 2002). And, by the late 20th century and early 21st century, despite increases in chronic and non-communicable diseases along with a renewed concern of fast-spreading infectious diseases (Snowden, 2019), life expectancy has continued to improve. Coupled with low birth rates,[2] extended life expectancy has contributed to an ageing population outside of the formal economy, with many older people involved in providing and receiving informal care (Esping-Andersen, 1999; Olson, 2015). Two decades into the 21st century, life is characterised by health with between three and ten years of illness and disability at the end of life, or intermittent throughout (Kyu et al., 2018).

Supporting recuperation and convalescence during these periods of sickness and disability is the care provided by the family in the community, and by clinicians through formal health services. Historically, families were responsible for providing care during times of illness (Blank & Burau, 2014). By the mid-20th century, the professionalisation of medicine and nursing, along with advances in facilities, infection-control, and technology, saw much care shift from home-based to hospital-based care – especially for serious illnesses (Bella, 2010; Bruhn & Rebach, 2014). This shift was supported by the rise of the welfare state in the decades following World War II, which saw many countries, such as the UK, Canada, and, eventually, Australia, introduce universal healthcare coverage (Bella, 2010; Duckett & Willcox, 2015; Gauld, 2009).

A stronger political hunger for neoliberalism in the late 20th century, along with a growing distaste for institutional care, saw much care shift again from hospital to home, with family carers in many places playing an essential role in allowing patients to remain in the community (Duckett & Willcox, 2015; Olson, 2012). This shift, from home to hospital and back again, was a consequence of an assemblage of ideological, economic, and sentimental forces: an intensifying assessment of institutional care as cold and bureaucratic, a growing critique of paternalism in medical care, a need to contain rising healthcare costs, and a reconceptualisation of individuals – following neoliberal reforms – as autonomous, self-sufficient, and responsible rather than in need of state protection (Olson, 2015). Thus, the organisation of care – who performs what tasks, where, and with what support – is deeply political, reflecting the ideological underpinnings of all social relations. I turn to an examination and evaluation of the political underpinnings of formal and informal care next.

The political organisation of healthcare services

A wide variety of care is offered through formal healthcare services: from general practice and nursing services, through to allied healthcare and specialised surgical and psychiatric care. How these healthcare services are organised varies substantially across the globe, in terms of priorities and financing. Some focus on offering the most technologically advanced diagnostic and treatment services; others prioritise equity in access to basic or primary healthcare. Overall, approaches to healthcare financing and regulation can be placed on a scale, with highly privatised systems relying on market mechanisms positioned at one pole, and publicly funded systems regulated through state intervention at the other pole (Gauld, 2009; Joumard, Hoeller, André, & Nicq, 2010). Although healthcare systems might lean more towards one pole, most offer a complex combination of private and public funding. A comparison of the healthcare systems across three countries – the USA, Costa Rica, and the UK – exemplifies the political underpinnings of the organisation of healthcare, while also illustrating the diversity and complexity of healthcare offered.

The USA's healthcare system leans heavily towards the privatised pole, reflecting its political commitment to free-market principles and distaste for social welfare, cast as interference in the free market (Scribano, 2018). A notoriously neoliberal capitalist country, the USA's healthcare system is often depicted as epitomising a marketised approach (Willis & Parry, 2012). However, veterans, people over 65, and the very poor are eligible for healthcare services through government-funded insurance. Other residents and citizens must rely on private health insurance, often through group plans (called Health Maintenance Organisations) with their employers, to cover the cost of basic and acute healthcare services (Wright & Rogers, 2011). Many, especially those who are unemployed or underemployed, go uninsured and risk incurring the full cost of these services (Wright & Rogers, 2011). Obama's Affordable Care Act prompted a substantial decrease in the number of Americans without health insurance – from 16% in 2010 to 9.1% in 2015 – but a significant number are still uninsured (Obama, 2016). The USA's marketised approach to healthcare is the most costly in the world (Anderson, Hussey, & Petrosyan, 2019). At 17% of gross domestic product (GDP) in 2016, Americans spent well above the global average for health expenditure, around 10% of a country's GDP (World Bank, 2019). In terms of life expectancy, the return on investment is not comparable (Joumard et al., 2010). A child born in the USA in 2016 has a life expectancy of 78.6. years, placing the USA 28th of 44 OECD and partner countries for life expectancy, above the Czech Republic and below Chile (OECD data, 2017).

Costa Rica, in comparison, spends a mere 7.56% of its GDP on healthcare (World Bank, 2019) and has a life expectancy at birth of 79.6%, a full year higher than the USA (OECD data, 2017). Primary healthcare and strategic investment in social services allow for high life expectancies with comparably low health expenditure in Costa Rica, positioning it as a "health without wealth" country (Baum, 2015, p. 315). In terms of its political positioning, Costa Rica leans more to towards the social-democratic, publicly funded pole. Rather than relying on market principles and prioritising cutting-edge technology, equity in access to care drives health and social policy. Costa Rica's social insurance system means the cost of healthcare is shared by the government, employer, and worker. For mothers, children, indigenous people, the elderly, people with disabilities, and those below the poverty line, healthcare is free, covered by the government through taxes raised on luxury, alcoholic, and imported goods (Montenegro Torres, 2013).

Life expectancy in the UK is also substantially higher than in the USA. Children born in the UK in 2016 have a life expectancy of 81.4 years (OECD data, 2017), at the comparatively reasonable cost of 9.76 per cent of their GDP (World Bank, 2019). Despite strong support for neoliberalism, and the dismantling of many aspects of its welfare state following the election of the Thatcher government in 1980s and subsequent governments, the UK has maintained a strong commitment to publicly funded healthcare (Bella, 2010). Indeed, the UK is often used as the primary example of a country with universal healthcare. The UK's National Health Service (NHS) has been in place since the end of World War II, famously offering health services from "cradle to grave" funded by the government through taxes (Blank & Burau, 2014; Givan, 2016, p. 34). However, a minority of UK citizens also take out private health insurance, often through their employers, for acute care and elective surgeries, allowing them access to quicker and more comfortable care (Harley et al., 2011).

These three examples illustrate the intimate, but complex, relationship between the political economy and the organisation of health services, with social-democratic principles underpinning the provision of universal healthcare services and neoliberalism informing privatised healthcare. They also point to the merits of universal, state-funded healthcare, and the drawbacks of marketised approaches. Universal healthcare prioritises equitable access to healthcare services treating health as a merit good: a good that is not just contained within the "consumer", but is conceptualised as a relational good, with benefits to a society far exceeding those to any one individual (Fisman & Laupland, 2009; Lin, Smith, & Fawkes, 2014). Indeed, countries with lower health inequalities tend to have better health on average (Joumard et al., 2010). An emphasis on accessible primary healthcare within universal publicly funded healthcare systems mean fewer people delay treatment because of financial barriers. This translates to better population health outcomes: lower infant mortality rates and longer life expectancy (Baum, 2015). Universal systems, however, are not without drawbacks. In publicly funded healthcare systems, the newest technology will not be made available if analyses suggest the cost outweighs the benefit (Duckett & Willcox, 2015). Waiting times for appointments and treatment – especially for elective procedures – can also be substantially longer (Harley et al., 2011).

In contrast, the USA's marketised approach is often heralded as offering one of the best health services in the world, with a highly skilled workforce and more CT scanners and MRIs than almost any other country (Anderson et al., 2019). However, the perceived benefits of this marketised system – shorter waiting times, easier access to new technology, and elective surgeries – are only available to those who can afford top private health insurance. Furthermore, some of these "benefits" are problematic. First, within a healthcare system regulated by supply and demand, the development of more profitable treatments is regularly prioritised over less profitable (life-saving) interventions and prevention (Wright & Rogers, 2011). As the market responds to consumer demand and not medical need, highly profitable drugs for issues like male-pattern baldness and impotence famously attract more research and development funding than less profitable treatments for life-threatening diseases such as tuberculosis and malaria (Santoro, 2005). Second, because healthcare markets can operate differently to other markets – due to information inequalities and the extraordinary value of the service provided – supply can also precede demand (Bodenheimer & Grumbach, 2005). As Wright and Rogers (2011) explain, if expensive new technology has been purchased by a hospital, then it must be paid for through using that technology and charging insurers. This can lead to overdiagnosis: where more tests and treatments – often with harmful side effects – are ordered than are necessary. Overall, a marketised healthcare system can be described as "a paradox of excess and deprivation" where some "receive too much care that is costly and may be harmful" while others "receive too little care because they are uninsured [or] inadequately insured" (Enthoven & Kronick, 1989; cited by Bodenheimer & Grumbach, 2005, p. 1).

Clearly, the broader political economy is implicated in the organisation of formal healthcare services, with neoliberalism informing marketised approaches and social-democratic principles informing universal approaches to healthcare delivery. Although the political organisation of formal healthcare services is often discussed separately to family life and the private sphere, they are connected. In the next section, following the work of Esping-Andersen (1999) and Folbre (2012), I show the political economy of healthcare to be intimately intertwined with, and in some settings, reliant on, informal care provided by family and friends.

The political organisation of care

Political ideologies underpin the organisation of informal care provided outside of hospitals and GP's clinics, most often by friends and families. During periods of illness and disability, many people experience emotional, physical, and behavioural changes necessitating reliance on an informal carer. By definition, an informal carer (also referred to as a caregiver) provides support to a patient[3] at home in a range of formats, such as emotional support, assistance with mobility and activities of daily living, coordination across medical modalities, and patient advocacy (Blum & Sherman, 2010; Given, Given, & Sherwood, 2012; Olson, 2015). Informal carers provide an important role in providing care which decreases reliance on formal health services, and allows people with a disability or illness to remain in the community (Duckett & Willcox, 2015). Although many carers find fulfilment in the role (Cassidy, 2013; Mutch, 2010), it comes at a cost in the form of a carer's lost wages (Duckett & Willcox, 2015), musculoskeletal injuries from lifting another adult (Evandrou, 1996), exacerbation of pre-existing health problems (Thomas & Morris, 2002), and high rates of mental illness (Li, Mak, & Loke, 2013). The extent to which families are relied on, supported in, or even superseded in providing care varies according to their country's broader political orientation (Glenn, 2010). Comparison of the support offered to informal carers across the USA, Sweden and Australia illustrates the centrality of politics to the organisation of care.

In the USA, the family is responsible for the care provided outside of formal healthcare services. As Glenn (2010, p. 9) explains in her book *Forced to care: Coercion and caregiving in America*, "family members (parents, spouses), are [legally] obligated to provide care for other family members" in the USA. Social programmes are available to help elderly and disabled citizens based in the community with daily activities, though many of these programmes are reliant on charitable donations and provide only supplemental support, leaving many patients dependent on family to meet their everyday needs. Thus, carers in the USA are relied on to care for their ill or disabled family member without state-funded financial support, training, counselling, or respite; only carers of veterans are eligible for these services (Bruhn & Rebach, 2014). Indeed, patients (and families) are typically disqualified from receiving public services when they have identified that a family member is able to provide care (Glenn, 2010). The approach to organising care in the USA is aligned with the country's neoliberal political orientation, where the taxation needed to fund social services is cast in economically conservative political rhetoric as interference in the free market.

In sharp contrast to the USA, the state is responsible for care in Sweden. Citizens pay taxes in return for a range of health and social entitlements (Blank & Burau, 2014). In addition to publicly funded healthcare, patients, the elderly, and people with disabilities can draw on a range of home help services to support everyday activities in the community that they may need assistance with, such as help with shopping, cleaning, and food preparation (Johansson, Long, & Parker, 2011). Unlike the USA, where family are expected to provide care and patients are dependent on family for care, the provision of comprehensive support services in Sweden allows patients, if they so choose, independence from family (Blank & Burau, 2014). If, however, patients prefer to rely on their family for support – and many do – financial and psychosocial support is available to carers. Through the Social Services Act, carers are eligible for respite, counselling, and a financial stipend (Johansson et al., 2011). The conceptualisation of informal care as a social, rather than a family, responsibility reflects Sweden's egalitarian political culture and commitment to social democracy.

Australia's approach to care sits in between the USA and Sweden. Like the USA, family are largely relied on to care for ill or disabled family members in the community. However, financial support is available for carers and has been since the 1990s through a Carer Allowance and Carer Payment. Entitlements, however, are not as comprehensive as the support offered to carers in Sweden. The amount of financial support is low – far below minimum wage – making the Carer Allowance and Carer Payment symbolic recognition for carers rather than full financial support (Blank & Burau, 2014; Olson, 2015). Respite and counselling are also available, but like in the USA, these supplemental services are offered through employers and charities, rather than through government programmes (Olson, 2012). Thus, Australia's conceptualisation of care as a family responsibility deserving of some financial compensation reflects its global political positioning as a neoliberal free-market state, with a continuing, but contracting, commitment to social welfare.

These approaches to organising informal care, underpinned as they are by political ideologies, have been charted by Twigg and Atkin (1994, p. 14) into four different conceptualisations of caregiving: (1) "carers as resources"; (2) "carers as co-workers"; (3) "carers as co-clients"; and (4) "superseded carers". Conceptualisations of care in the USA clearly reflect the first category. With the exception of carers of veterans, family carers are assumed to be an available asset. Policies operate on the presumption that all people in need of care have family able to provide it, without financial or psychosocial support (Olson, 2015). In Australia, conceptualisations of care resonate with Twigg and Atkin's second category: carers as co-workers. Family is relied on to provide care in the community, but offered (tokenistic) financial compensation in return (Duckett & Willcox, 2015). The respite, counselling and financial support made available to all carers in Sweden suggest that the second and third categories of "co-worker" and "co-client" resonate with conceptualisations of care in this social-democratic country. The state commitment to providing care, where patients can choose to rely on government services for help with activities of daily living rather than family, also suggests the relevance of category four, "superseded carers", to Sweden's conceptualisation of care.

Thus, political ideologies underpin both the organisation of formal and informal care. What's more, the organisation of health services is intertwined with the organisation of informal care (Esping-Andersen, 1999; Folbre, 2012), with costly marketised approaches to organising healthcare services in neoliberal countries largely dependent on the availability of family carers. And this dependence is projected to increase, as populations continue to age (Jegermalm & Grassman, 2012). Not all families and not all family members, however, are equally as likely to be called on to care. In the next section, I examine the affective economy undergirding the division of labour within formal and informal care, following intersecting emotional, sexual and class dynamics.

The affective economy of (in)formal care

All care involves emotions. Facing sickness, disability, and life-limiting illness can be frustrating for patients, health professionals and informal carers alike. Giving care involves more than the administration of treatments, assistance with everyday activities, and coordination. For formal and informal carers, care also involves emotional labour:[4] work performed to change one's own and others emotions, in terms of intensity, direction, and duration, to comply with institutional norms (Hochschild, 1983). All carers work to manage their own and the patient's emotions to comply with cultural and organisational expectations and respond to the challenges that come with a diagnosis or disability: grief for unrealised plans, and a revised temporal and emotional orientation to the present and future (Olson, 2011, 2014).

Emotions and emotional labour, however, are far from politically neutral. As Ahmed (2004, p. 119) articulates concisely in her affective economies thesis, "emotions do things". They connect some individuals through social relations, but they also exclude or privilege others, with affect "crucial to the very making of a difference" (Ahmed, 2004, p. 121). In the context of the affective economy of care,[5] patriarchal conceptualisations of emotions serve to position caregiving as lower status women's work. Patriarchal ideologies and debunked mind–body dualist discourses, which situate reasoning and emotion as separate entities, have advanced an understanding of men as rational and women as emotional, while also positioning women as more apt for caregiving and financially devalued emotional labour (Hekman, 1990; James, 1992; Olson & Dadich, 2019). Essentially, because "women are deemed to be emotional … they are [seen to be] the best people to deal with others' emotions" (James, 1992, p. 501). The influence of this affective economy of care, underpinned by a mind–body dualist conceptualisation of emotion and patriarchal ideology, is clearly evident within both formal and informal caregiving.

The emotional dimensions of giving care within formal health services has been the focus of much research. Within nursing especially, it has long been acknowledged that caregiving involves emotional labour, with nurses performing work to listen to, acknowledge, and alter their own emotions, and those of their patients (James, 1992). Although all formal caregiving involves emotions shared with patients, families, and colleagues as well as emotional labour, how much varies across professions, following an affective economy of care, informed by locally articulated gender *and* status dynamics. Those in higher status professions, such as medicine, aligned with reductionist mind–body dualist understandings of emotion (McNaughton, 2013), tend to treat emotions as irrelevant or threats to reasoning (Olson & Dadich, 2019) and delegate emotional labour to lower status, female-dominated professions such as social work and nursing (Dragojlovic & Broom, 2018; James, 1992). In lower status, female-dominated professions, in contrast, emotions are more often treated as central to caregiving, with many adopting a conceptualisation of emotional labour as a skill and an inevitable part of their job (McNaughton, 2013; Olson & Dadich, 2019).

Within and across female-dominated professions, intersecting division lines underpinned by differences in training and status inform the distribution of emotional labour. Physiotherapy offers one example of this; nursing offers another. Despite similarities in training and role overlap across occupational therapy and physiotherapy, the latter has a higher standing. Contributing to this higher status are historical efforts to separate physiotherapy from the emotions and emotional labour performed in other female-dominated professions, and elevate its status as a skilled health profession. In her analysis of physiotherapy's beginnings as a profession in the early 20th century, Linker (2005) suggests that unlike other female-dominated health professions which were supported by women's charity organisations, "leaders of the physiotherapy profession" worked hard to align their profession with medicine, "encouraged distance more than empathy" (p. 114) and "actively avoided rhetoric that even hinted at maternalism" (p. 116). Within contemporary nursing work, an affective economy based on status divisions can also be observed, informing who performs emotional labour. In the USA, for example, many hospitals employ patient care technicians – a role requiring a one-year vocational qualification, dominated by females from working-class, minority and migrant backgrounds. It is common for nurses, who (have afforded and) completed a four-year university degree, to delegate physical and emotional labour to these lower-paid and lower-status workers (DiBenigno & Kellogg, 2014). Thus, formal caregiving is "stratified along class, gender", racial and emotional lines (Willis, 1994, p. 24), as this section shows.

Compared to formal caregiving, informal caregiving is thought to involve more intense emotional experiences. Because informal caregiving typically emerges from an existing relationship, and from the associated feelings of commitment and responsibility for the person in need of care (Bruhn & Rebach, 2014), it is seen to be particularly laden with emotions (James, 1992). Said another way, informal caregiving involves more than caring *for* another human being; it involves caring *about* that person (Glenn, 2010). And, caring for and caring about are strongly implicated in the affective economy of care, influencing who cares and how much.

Patriarchal divisions in informal caregiving are easily observed. Who provides informal care has traditionally followed gendered lines, with women, particularly in more neoliberal countries that rely on families for care, viewed as automatic caregiving assets. Glenn's (2010) historical analysis of the institutional practices and judicial decision-making in the USA throughout the 19th and 20th century illustrates how domestic work and care work came to be seen as a woman's duty. State reform schools to develop skills in cooking and mending for imprisoned women offer one example of the many government-imposed activities which entrenched domestic labour and care work as lower status, women's work. Twentieth-century judicial rulings on family inheritance disputes offer another example. These rulings enforced a woman's duty to care, positioning it as an act of love and not paid labour. People (most often women) who arranged to provide care for an individual at the end of life in exchange for a financial inheritance who then married the care recipient consistently had their reparation claims rejected by the courts (Glenn, 2010).

Illustrating intersections across the political and affective economies of care, contemporary informal caregiving continues to be viewed as women's work (Langer et al., 2015), but the extent to which it follows patriarchal dividing lines is shaped by the political organisation of care. According to recent OECD data (2017), on average 60% of all caregivers across all OECD countries are women. The percentage of women involved in caregiving in the USA and the UK fall above this average, at 64.3% and 62.9%, respectively. Australia falls below this average with women making up 54.5% of carers. Australian Bureau of Statistics (2016) data, however, suggests the importance of looking not just at who cares, but how much time is spent in caring. Caregiving women in Australia spend more time than caregiving men in their caregiving roles, with women representing 68.1% of all primary carers: those carers who provide the most assistance with daily activities such as self-care, mobility, and communication. Sweden goes against the OECD trend with more male carers (54.4%) than female carers (45.6%). However, like the Australian data, Swedish data also suggests that "women spend considerably more time" performing caregiving activities than men (Jegermalm & Grassman, 2012). These data illustrate the connections across the political economies and affective economies of formal and informal care, with marketised approaches to organising health services and care more reliant on a sexual division of unpaid labour, and with patriarchal divisions of labour still present, but less prominent, in social-democratic welfare states.

The relevance of the political economy to the affective economy of care is again apparent in an examination of the gendered and class dimensions of informal care. The extent to which women (and men) are expected to provide informal care is tempered by class. Especially in countries with marketised healthcare services, patients and families with access to greater financial resources can choose not to rely on an informal carer, and instead outsource some or all of their care (Hochschild, 2012). Even in Sweden, where state-funded services are meant to supersede the need for informal carers, cutbacks in formal support disproportionately affect those on a lower income. Jegermalm and Grassman (2012), for example, found that during a period of welfare provision cutbacks in the late 1990s and early 2000s there was a slight increase in the care given by lower-income and blue-collar workers, but not middle-income white-collar workers, presumably because middle-income workers were able to buy these services from the market. Thus, the affective economy of care is clearly underpinned by intersecting patriarchal, emotional, and political ideologies, which see reliance on family to provide care disproportionately affecting women who are less economically advantaged in neoliberal countries.

Conclusion

In this chapter, I have offered a critical examination of the political and affective economies of care. The care offered through formal health services and family carers in the community has historically been conceptualised separately. Others have made important contributions by explicating the political ideologies underpinning the organisation of healthcare services (Gauld, 2009) and the support made (un)available to informal carers (Twigg & Atkin, 1994). Following re-conceptualisations, amid analyses of the changes simultaneously being faced by families and labour markets in post-industrial economies, of public and private spheres as interdependent (Esping-Andersen, 1999; Folbre, 2012), I have shown the political economies of formal and informal care to be interdependent. Especially in market-based medical systems underpinned by neoliberal ideologies, and in shrinking social welfare states seeking to reduce medical spending, families are relied on to provide care at home. Patients are now discharged from hospitals "quicker and sicker" than in previous decades to reduce costs and improve profit margins (Glenn, 2010, p. 154). What's more, the division of caregiving labour follows an affective economy of care. Women are over-represented amongst carers, especially primary carers, because caregiving is emotional work and (lower status) women are seen to be more apt at dealing with emotions and performing emotional labour, echoing the classed, raced, and gendered division of emotional labour within formal healthcare services. This affective economy of care intersects the political organisation of healthcare, with women's overrepresentation amongst carers more prominent in neoliberal settings, and less pronounced in social democracies.

Overall, in this chapter, I offer a call to recognise political and affective economies as intersecting, with real consequences for the gendered, classed, and raced organisation of care within healthcare systems and homes. Specifically, I highlight the impact of patriarchal values and the potential of intersecting political ideologies to exacerbate or ameliorate population health disparities. Furthermore, I draw attention to the power of our current conceptualisations of emotions to anchor women to lower-paid emotional labour and unpaid informal caregiving duties. In sum, health, health services and care are "inherently political" (Munro & McIntyre, 2016, p. 156), and these politics work with gendered ideologies and debunked notions of emotions as inherently feminine to constrain who provides care and how.

Notes

1 In addition to historical and political variation, intersecting cultural (colonial), economic and geographical forces also underpin population health patterns. For brevity, this chapter focuses on the health, health services and caregiving of people in economically advanced, Organisation for Economic Co-Operation and Development (OECD) and partner countries.

2 Esping-Andersen (1999, p. 1) describes this as a "fertility strike", illustrating the intimate connection across markets and families, with lower birth rates attributed to women's greater involvement in the labour market.

3 While acknowledging critiques of the term "patient" as disempowering, this term is used intermittently here for clarity. The term "customer" implies an individualised market relationship. The term "client" can be problematic as carers can also be recipients of formal health service care (Olson, 2015).

4 Some distinguish between "emotional labour" performed for a wage and "emotion work", informed by culturally defined "feeling rules" and performed outside of paid work. Acknowledging the influence of cultural norms on (gendered) institutional feeling rules and the influence of institutional expectations on interpretations of emotions in unpaid roles, such as caregiving (Lois, 2006; Olson & Connor, 2015), the term "emotional labour" is used inclusively here to refer to efforts to alter one's own and others' feelings across contexts of paid and unpaid work.

5 Drawing on Ahmed's (2004) influential work, Dragojlovic and Broom (2018) also use the term affective economy of care. They use the term to emphasise emotions and feelings, such as suffering, as shared across clinicians, informal carers, and patients, rather than located within individuals. Inspired by

the critical capacities of Ahmed's (2004) work, I use the term to denote the embodied and discursive potential of emotions (used interchangeably with affect here) to constitute, coerce and position individuals within ideologically informed and structured social relations.

References

Ahmed, S. (2004). Affective economies. *Social Text, 22*(2), 117–139.

Anderson, G. F., Hussey, P., & Petrosyan, V. (2019). It's still the prices, stupid: Why the US spends so much on health care, and a tribute to Uwe Reinhardt. *Health Affairs, 38*(1), 87–95. doi:10.1377/hlthaff.2018.05144

Australian Bureau of Statistics. (2016). *Disability, ageing and carers, Australia: Summary of findings, 2015, Cat. No. 443.0*. Retrieved from Canberra: http://www.abs.gov.au/ausstats/abs@.nsf/mf/4430.0

Baum, F. (2015). *The new public health* (4th ed.). Melbourne: Oxford University Press.

Bella, L. (2010). In sickness and in health: Public and private responsibility for health care from Bismarck to Obama. In R. Harris, N. Wathen, & S. Wyatt (Eds.), *Configuring health consumers: Health work and the imperative of personal responsibility* (pp. 13–29). New York: Palgrave Macmillan.

Blank, R. H., & Burau, V. (2014). *Comparative health policy* (4th ed.). New York: Palgrave Macmillan.

Blum, K., & Sherman, D. (2010). Understanding the experience of caregivers: A focus on transitions. *Seminars in Oncology Nursing, 26*(4), 243–258.

Bodenheimer, T. S., & Grumbach, K. (2005). *Understanding health policy: A clinical approach* (4th ed.). New York: Lange Medical Books, McGraw-Hill.

Bruhn, J. G., & Rebach, H. M. (2014). *The sociology of caregiving*. New York: Springer.

Cassidy, T. (2013). Benefit finding through caring: The cancer caregiver experience. *Psychology & Health, 28*(3), 250–266. doi:10.1080/08870446.2012.717623

DiBenigno, J., & Kellogg, K. C. (2014). Beyond occupational difference: The importance of cross-cutting demographics and dyadic toolkits for collaboration in a U.S. hospital. *Administrative Science Quarterly, 59*(3), 375–408. doi:10.1177/0001839214538262

Dragojlovic, A., & Broom, A. (2018). *Bodies and suffering: Emotions and relations of care*. London: Routledge.

Duckett, S., & Willcox, S. (2015). *The Australian health care system* (5th ed.). Melbourne: Oxford University Press.

Esping-Andersen, G. (1999). *Social foundations of postindustrial economies*. Oxford: Oxford University Press.

Evandrou, M. (1996). Unpaid work, carers and health. In D. Blane, E. Brunner, & R. Wilkinson (Eds.), *Health and social organization: Towards a health policy for the twenty-first century* (pp. 204–231). New York: Routledge.

Fisman, D. N., & Laupland, K. B. (2009). The sounds of silence: Public goods, externalities, and the value of infectious disease control programs. *Canadian Journal of Infectious Diseases & Medical Microbiology, 20*(2), 39–41.

Folbre, N. (2012). *For love and money: Care provision in the United States*. New York: SAGE.

Gauld, R. (2009). Health and health care in post-industrial society. In J. Powell & J. Hendricks (Eds.), *The welfare state in post-industrial society: A global perspective* (pp. 125–140). Dordrecht: Springer.

Givan, R. K. (2016). *The challenge of change: Reforming health care on the front line in the United States and the United Kingdom*. Ithaca, NY: Cornell University Press.

Given, B., Given, C., & Sherwood, P. (2012). Family and caregiver needs over the course of the cancer trajectory. *Journal of Supportive Oncology, 10*(2), 57–64.

Glenn, E. N. (2010). *Forced to care: Coercion and caregiving in America*. Cambridge, MA: Harvard University Press.

Harley, K., Willis, K., Gabe, J., Short, S. D., Collyer, F., Natalier, K., & Calnan, M. (2011). Constructing health consumers: Private health insurance discourses in Australia and the United Kingdom. *Health Sociology Review, 20*(3), 306–320.

Hekman, S. (1990). *Gender and knowledge: Elements of a postmodern feminism*. Cambridge: Polity Press.

Hochschild, A. R. (1983). *The managed heart*. Berkeley, CA: University of California Press.

Hochschild, A. R. (2012). *The outsourced self: Intimate life in market times*. New York: Metropolitan Books: Henry Holt and Company.

James, N. (1992). Care = organisation + physical labour + emotional labour. *Sociology of Health and Illness, 14*(4), 488–509.

Jegermalm, M., & Grassman, E. J. (2012). Helpful citizens and caring families: Patterns of informal help and caregiving in Sweden in a 17-year perspective. *International Journal of Social Welfare, 21*, 422–432. doi:10.1111/j.1468-2397.2011.00839.x

Johansson, L., Long, H., & Parker, M. G. (2011). Informal caregiving for elders in Sweden: An analysis of current policy developments. *Journal of Aging & Social Policy, 23*(4), 335–353. doi:10.1080/08959420.2011.605630

Joumard, I., Hoeller, P., André, C., & Nicq, C. (2010). *Health care systems: Efficiency and policy settings.* Retrieved from https://read.oecd-ilibrary.org/social-issues-migration-health/health-care-systems_9789264094901-en

Kellehear, A. (2007). *A social history of dying.* Cambridge: Cambridge University Press.

Kyu, H. H., Abate, D., Abate, K. H., Abay, S. M., Abbafati, C., Abbasi, N., … Murray, C. J. (2018). Global, regional, and national disability-adjusted life-years (DALYs) for 359 diseases and injuries and healthy life expectancy (HALE) for 195 countries and territories, 1990–2017: A systematic analysis for the Global Burden of Disease Study 2017. *The Lancet, 392*, 1859–1922. doi:10.1016/S0140-6736(18)32335-3

Langer, A., Meleis, A., Knaul, F. M., Atun, R., Aran, M., Arreola-Ornelas, H., … Frenk, J. (2015). Women and health: The key for sustainable development. *The Lancet, 386*, 1165–1210.

Li, Q. P., Mak, Y. W., & Loke, A. Y. (2013). Spouses' experience of caregiving for cancer patients: A literature review. *International Nursing Review, 60*(2), 178–187. doi:10.1111/inr.12000

Lin, V., Smith, J., & Fawkes, S. (2014). *Public health practice in Australia: The organised effort.* Crows Nest, NSW: Allen & Unwin.

Linker, B. (2005). Strength and science: Gender, physiotherapy, and medicine in the United States, 1918–35. *Journal of Women's History, 17*(3), 106–132. doi:10.1353/jowh.2005.0034

Lois, J. (2006). Role strain, emotion management, and burnout: Homeschooling mothers' adjustment to the teacher role. *Symbolic Interaction, 29*, 507–530.

McNaughton, N. (2013). Discourse(s) of emotion within medical education: The ever-present absence. *Medical Education, 47*, 71–79. doi:10.111/j.1365-2923.2012.04329.x

Montenegro Torres, F. (2013). *Costa Rica case study: Primary health care achievements and challenges within the framework of the Social Health Insurance.* Retrieved from Washington, DC: http://documents.worldbank.org/curated/en/991581468233939710/Costa-Rica-case-study-Primary-health-care-achievements-and-challenges-within-the-framework-of-the-social-health-insurance

Munro, J., & McIntyre, L. (2016). (Not) getting political: Indigenous women and preventing mother-to-child transmission of HIV in West Papua. *Culture, Health and Sexuality, 18*(2), 156–170. doi:10.1080/13691058.2015.1070436

Mutch, K. (2010). In sickness and in health: Experience of caring for a spouse with MS. *British Journal of Nursing, 19*(4), 214–219.

Obama, B. (2016). United States health care reform progress to date and next steps. *Journal of the American Medical Association, 316*(5), 525–532. doi:10.1001/jama.2016.9797

OECD Data. (2017). *Health at a glance 2017: OECD indicators.* Paris: OECD Publishing Retrieved from https://data.oecd.org/healthstat/life-expectancy-at-birth.htm

Olson, R. (2011). Managing hope, denial or temporal anomie? Informal cancer carers' accounts of spouses' cancer diagnoses. *Social Science & Medicine, 73*, 904–911. doi:10.1016/j.socscimed.2010.12.026

Olson, R. (2012). Is cancer care dependant on informal carers? *Australian Health Review, 36*, 254–257. doi:10.1071/AH11086

Olson, R., & Connor, J. (2015). When they don't die: Prognosis ambiguity, role conflict and emotion work in cancer care. *Journal of Sociology, 51*(4), 857–871. doi:10.1177/1440783314544996

Olson, R. E. (2014). Indefinite loss: The experiences of carers of a spouse with cancer. *European Journal of Cancer Care, 23*(4), 553–561. doi:10.1111/ecc.12175

Olson, R. E. (2015). *Towards a sociology of cancer caregiving: Time to feel.* Surrey: Ashgate.

Olson, R. E., & Dadich, A. (2019). Power, (com)passion and trust in interprofessional healthcare. In R. Patulny, A. Bellocchi, R. Olson, S. Khorana, J. McKenzie, & M. Peterie (Eds.), *Emotions in late modernity* (pp. 267–281). London: Routledge.

Santoro, M. (2005). Introduction: Charting a sustainable path for the twenty-first century pharmaceutical industry. In M. Santoro & T. M. Gorrie (Eds.), *Ethics and the pharmaceutical industry* (pp. 1–7). New York: Cambridge University Press.

Scribano, A. (2018). Introduction: The multiple Janus faces of neoliberalism. In A. Scribano, F. T. Lopez, & M. E. Korstanje (Eds.), *Neoliberalism in multi-disciplinary perspective* (pp. 1–20). London: Palgrave Macmillan.

Snowden, F. M. (2019). *Epidemics and society: From the Black Death to the present.* New Haven, CT: Yale University Press.

Szreter, S. (2002). Rethinking McKeown: The relationship between public health and social change. *American Journal of Public Health, 92*(5), 722–725.

Thomas, C., & Morris, S. (2002). Informal carers in cancer contexts. *European Journal of Cancer Care, 11,* 178–182.

Twigg, J., & Atkin, K. (1994). *Carers perceived: Policy and practice in informal care.* Buckingham: Open University Press.

Willis, E. (1994). *Illness and social relations: Issues in the sociology of health care.* St Leonards, NSW: Allen & Unwin.

Willis, E., & Parry, Y. (2012). The Australian health care system. In E. Willis, L. Reynolds, & H. Keleher (Eds.), *Understanding the Australian health care system* (pp. 3–12). Chatswood, NSW: Elsevier.

World Bank. (2019). *Current health expenditure.* Retrieved from https://data.worldbank.org/indicator/SH. XPD.CHEX.PC.CD

Wright, E. O., & Rogers, J. (2011). *American society: How it really works.* New York: W. W. Norton & Company.

7

DIAGNOSIS

A social and political phenomenon

Annemarie Jutel

Diagnosis plays an important part in understanding health, illness, and disease; its critical consideration is important for anyone concerned with health studies. Diagnosis is both a process and a classification tool (Blaxter, 1978). We diagnose (verb) people with diagnoses (noun). Both the action (verb) and the object (noun) deserve careful critical scrutiny. In this chapter, I present diagnosis in both of these capacities, and I expose the social, cultural, and political "content" of diagnosis. I also delineate the difference between diagnosis and disease, and demonstrate how the concealment of this difference creates an ideological and deterministic position that underpins hierarchies of power.

To think critically is to not accept the premises of taken-for-granted truths without an exploration of the assumptions which anchor them. Particularly useful here is to explore the social content of truths, that is to say, the degree to which they are shaped by human agency, as opposed to being the result of some natural arrangement of the world. In relation to diagnosis, the salient point is that to be critical; we must consider the degree to which a particular classification is always inevitably a human agreement about what should be so classified, rather than being a fact of nature.

Once conditions are thought of as diseases, with diagnostic labels, belonging in agreed-upon classification systems, we are inclined to think of them as naturally that way, when, as Zerubavel (1996) reminds us, nature is a continuum that is only divided into categories on the basis of our understanding and conventions. And further, Hacking (2001) points out the risk of seeing classification as natural when he explains that nature can disguise ideology and convey an illusion of neutrality. "No study of classification can escape the obligation to examine the roots of this idea … no study of the word 'natural' can fail to touch on that other great ideological word, 'real'" (p. 7). Hacking's discussion points to the fact that classification is seeking out a picture of an object, a "fixed target", which is true to nature. So, the serious critical scholar will look carefully at what counts as a diagnosable disease to see what assumptions such categories carry with them.

In relation to diagnosis, the first step in the critical analysis is therefore to explore the association between diagnosis and disease. Any one of a number of medical definitions of diagnosis will link it to the material condition of the disease. Diagnosis is, according to the Merriam-Webster definition, the "act of identifying a disease from its signs and symptoms". The *Oxford Concise Medical Dictionary* calls it "the process of determining the nature of a disorder by considering the patient's signs and symptoms, medical background, and – when necessary – results of laboratory

tests and X-ray examinations" (Martin & Oxford University Press Content, 2010). Both definitions fail to note the complex social actions that create the framework that defines what counts
as disease, how disease will be understood, who gets to decide what counts, who can allocate
diagnostic labels, and what social goods and benefits will be associated with the diagnosis. We
will explore these social issues in diagnosis in the following section.

Diseases to diagnoses

To critically understand diagnosis, it is helpful to look back more than a century and a half ago
to the emergence of scientific medicine. This is when diagnosis established its importance in the
practice of medicine. Doctors had indeed been working with diseases, but the introduction of
diagnosis as an organising principle of medicine caused them to reorganise their understanding
of the patient, the condition and their professional practice.

The focus on diagnosis was to anchor the formation of professional medicine (notably the
British and American Medical Associations), and to differentiate medicine from the ever-expand-
ing range of healing practices in vogue. Nineteenth and early 20th-century medical doctors
battled to overcome what Warbasse referred to as the "ruinous competition" (Warbasse, 1912,
in Light, 2004) of myriad competing alternative healers and dispensaries, and used scientific
diagnosis and its study as what distinguished them from non-scientifically qualified practitioners
over whom they were struggling to gain supremacy. More than just the process of naming an
ailment, diagnosis was a rational process that doctors felt they alone had truly mastered.

What scientific medicine claimed as distinguishing it from other forms of healing arts, and
what has since been imprinted upon the practice of medicine today, is the idea that the general
can be discovered in the individual. The symptoms and explanations that the individual patient
brings to the doctor, medicine held, should be classified according to disease models, which
are forms of generalisation. Nineteenth and early twentieth-century medical doctors fought to
draw attention to both the clinical function and social importance of diagnosis (see Chapter 2,
this volume). What distinguished the doctor from non-scientifically qualified practitioners was
diagnosis: a rational and scientific system for classifying disease. Diagnostic skill was lauded as
the mark of a doctor's success (Cathall, 1890), and its absence seen as a "fatal flaw" (Little, 1926).

Diagnostic classification enables the disorder of the individual to be linked to other cases,
and to use the knowledge of other cases to shape and explain the condition, choose the treatment, and predict outcomes. As the introduction to the *Bertillon Classification* (Diverses Autorités
Statistiques, 1909), an early diagnostic nomenclature, made clear: "A statistical nomenclature
… has the more humble but practical goal of enabling statistical organisations to summarise
the thousands of reports that are submitted to them in as truthful and as comparable a way
as possible" (p. 7, my translation). This power of summary, and the knowledge of other cases,
leads to the ability to generalise. Whether it is, as in the Bertillon and subsequently in successive International Classification of Diseases (ICD), an attempt to generalise about the health
of populations, the differences between nations, the progress or advance of disease, or if it is in
relation to the individual case and its link to other cases like it, this summary draws attention
away from the individual case, in favour of collective power. Classifying necessarily obfuscates
difference. Once the individual case is filed under its collective heading, idiosyncrasy disappears
in favour of generalisation.

If we think about diagnosis as classifying individual cases, the social impact of generalisation
becomes more clear. Classifying is not a simple task, because to classify we have to take items (in
this case, diagnoses) that are both similar to, and distinct from, one another. The idea is that the
points of commonality bring a benefit of some kind (in the case of diagnosis, usually to explain,

treat, and predict outcomes). But classifying is not straightforward. Features of a case may fit into several potential categories: pneumonia may be accompanied by the wheeze typical of asthma in one individual, and not in another. So a diagnosis doesn't describe the actual case; it says where the ailment should be most usefully classified.

Classification also presents a predicament, as captured in Ockham's Razor, "*entia non sunt multiplicanda praeter necessitatem*" (Leff, 1997), which posits that one should not split a category/concept/thing any more than is necessary. This axiom attempts to explain that there must be some use to grouping particular conditions with one another rather than seeing them as either independent to one another, or similar to a different condition. Otherwise, we end up concealing important differences which would be better revealed. Pneumonia is a logical way of categorising a case that fits the criteria, because of its acute nature, and because of the benefit that recognition and treatment can bring to the outcome from the person thus diagnosed. However, the focus on pneumonia, and the subsequent administrative identification of the case as being one of pneumonia (in case notes and administrative coding) will effectively subordinate any other potential disease labels.

Contemporary thinkers will be familiar with the expression "lumping or splitting", which underlines the complexity of classification even as it tries to echo Ockham's axiom. Too much emphasis on the group, and we start treating the disease and not the person; splitting until everything is an individual case, on the other hand, prevents any benefit that generalising could have provided, notably in relation to research and epidemiology. Whether to lump or to split is the debate that must be had about units (the patient) in relation to the category (the diagnosis).

The point of classification, as mentioned above, is to make sense of what is really an immense continuum; classification makes islands of meaning (Zerubavel, 1996). It reduces, wrote Richardson (1901) famously (albeit a long time ago), "a disorderly mass to an orderly whole", providing us with ways to communicate about diseases.

We would be hard put to do away with diagnostic classification in relation to diseases and their management. Classification enables epidemiologists to count cases and make generalisations about trends in illness, and points of concern: a point that we have seen well illustrated by the recent COVID-19 pandemic. Diagnosis allows countries to count cases, identify clusters, monitor contagion, and develop treatments. It enables statistical analysis, which is at the heart of today's evidence-based medicine.

We would be hard put to even consider how medicine could achieve its aims in the absence of classification. Therapy would be empirical, without the benefit of understandings developed by previous cases. Disease patterns could not be established, and prediction of outcomes would not be possible. Diagnosis therefore organises medical knowledge on the basis of clusterings and similarity.

Looking at diagnosis with a critical eye requires us to consider how classifications are arrived upon, where power resides in that designation, what interests are served by seeing the similarity in one way as opposed to another, and what the consequences result from the classifications thus created. Even the most physical of disorders requires social negotiations before they can be classified as a disease.

Classification takes place through recognised systems of diagnosis, of which there are many and with each using their own mechanisms for deciding what should be included. These include such nomenclatures as Systematized Nomenclature of Medicine (SNOMED), Diagnosis-related Groups (DRG), International Classification of Diseases, Diagnostic and Statistical Manual of Mental Disorders (DSM), Read Codes and more. Some diseases have additional, more specific diagnostic systems, such as the International Classification of Headaches, the International Classification of Sleep Disorders (ICSD), and the International Classification of Functioning,

Disability, and Health. Different countries will adapt international systems to suit their local contexts, such as national modifications to the DRG or the ICD.

The myriad diagnostic systems may not define diseases in identical ways; different countries and even different states within same countries may apply diagnostic criteria differently. Diagnosis may also be used differently in the clinical setting than in the administrative one. A clinician – or their auxiliary "medical coder" – may note a diagnosis in one way in patient notes, yet may record it in another way for administrative purposes to ensure that the most advantageous treatment plan or reimbursement is enabled. Or, alternatively, they may choose to reduce the potential impact of a diagnosis by choosing a term that is less stigmatising, or less likely to brand the patient with a diagnostic label that could have future social implications. Bowker and Star (1999) described how death certificates often provided socially acceptable diagnoses to explain death to the families of the deceased, with the actual cause of death provided only to the administrations. "In this case", they write, "syphilis can become heart failure, or suicide can become a stroke" (p. 25).

Nevertheless, let us return to the question of diseases and their link to diagnosis. Phil Brown's seminal paper *Naming and Framing* (Brown, 1995) raised the notion that diseases had to be "discovered" before they could be diagnosed, and underlined the social nature of the discovery process. I have further emphasised this in my *Putting a Name to It* (Jutel, 2011). For conditions to be diagnosable, they need to be visible, meaningful, political, and serve particular interests.

To be visible is, although not exclusively, a technological matter. For example, before the advent of microscopy, it would be impossible to distinguish one systematic blood disorder from another. Sickle cell anaemia could only become a disorder when the sickle-shaped red blood cells appeared on glass slides (Feldman & Tauber, in Wailoo, 1997), then distinguishable from other diseases in general and other anaemias in particular. The same holds true for any of a number of disorders, whose aetiologies or profiles become apparent by way of technology. Influenza was explained in the 18th century as the result of the "cold acting on the surface of the body" or "contagious matter mixed with the mass of fluids, and thrown off on particular parts" (Broughton, 1782, p. 7), and was attributed to a bacterium by the late 19th century (Taubenberger, Hultin, & Morens, 2007). While this was actually not correct (influenza is caused by a virus, and not a bacterium), it set science on the right track to recognise the influenza virus (Bresalier, 2012). Similarly, we don't know what diagnoses, hidden today, will become apparent tomorrow as a result of advancing technology, or different ways of explaining disorders.

We can draw, of course, on the example of the 2020 pandemic. China informed the WHO of a pneumonia cluster of unknown origin on 31 December 2019. The "novel virus" was identified on 7 January as 2019-nCoV (World Health Organisation, 2020, 21 January). As it was given diagnostic status (COVID-19) and spread around the world, genetic sequencing revealed variants from Europe to China and elsewhere. These variants begged the questions: Are we still talking about the same disease? How is it helpful to see each variant as different? Clearly one answer was political: demonstrating the prevalence of the European genome in American cases attempted to quell anti-Chinese sentiment (Zimmer, 2020, 8 April).[1] (See also Chapter 5, this volume).

But, as alluded to above, diagnoses are not just a matter of technology. Before we can set our microscopes loose on tissue samples, we also need to have a social will and ability to see a disease that will be diagnosed. The example of Lyme's disease (named for the community in which it was first "seen") is a salient one. A symptom cluster was noticed in a small, affluent community where families talked amongst themselves and compared the symptoms of their children. These educated families were able to recognise the cluster, discuss it with their GPs, who were of a similar social class and inclined to listen, and then to work with the Center for Disease Control to identify the condition as diagnosable, and then to look for the spirochete responsible for the disease (Aronowitz, 1991). One could imagine such clusters might be less conspicuous in other conditions and within other social groups, as with the initial identification of COVID-19. Li Wenliang, the Chinese doctor who first identified the cluster, was forced to apologise for "disrupting the public order" by "spreading false rumours" (Davidson, 2020, 20 March).

Similarly, the problem to be diagnosed must be meaningful. It has to be seen in terms of "problem" or deviant, as well as medical in nature, in order to enter into a diagnostic classification. The example of reading disorders in non-literate societies is a facile example. However, so too might be a gluten intolerance in a society with rice, rather than bread, as its dominant carbohydrate staple. Fadiman's description of epilepsy in a Hmong child illustrates eloquently how culture shapes what conditions might be seen as medical or not (Fadiman, 1997).

Diseases may have to be political in order to "count" as diagnosable. Post-traumatic Stress Disorder (PTSD) and Alzheimer's disease are widely touted examples of how political imperatives were satisfied by diagnostic categories. This is not to say that the material conditions were political creations, rather it is to underline how material conditions come to be recognised as worthy of diagnosis, and the trappings it will bring (more on that to follow). PTSD was a condition recognised in the DSM III after a significant investment by a group of champions using all the tools of the activist – lobbying, coalitions, struggle, and strategic planning – in the propitious context of an American Psychiatric Association needing to reassert its professional dominance amongst the counselling and psychological professions, but also to assert its worthiness in the broader medical edifice (Kirk & Kutchins, 1992; Scott, 1990).

And finally, diseases serve interests. The previous example of politics is a useful starting point for pondering this. The interests of psychiatry were behind the explosion of its little DSM-II pamphlet into the huge manual of today, as were the interests of the Chair of the DSM task force, Robert Spitzer. A researcher and former psychoanalyst, he was committed to removing psychoanalytic influence from the DSM, and saw many issues within the previous edition of the DSM as needing to be addressed. An ambitious man who wanted to leave his mark on the field, Spitzer also felt that a coherent diagnostic index could protect the discipline. This would shape many of the decisions made about what would become diagnosis, and what would be removed (homosexuality, for example) (Kirk & Kutchins, 1992).

Many other interest groups stand to benefit from the belief that particular conditions are diseases and these groups wield significant influence. From overweight to short stature, shyness, or low libido, the number of commercial players who lean on the shaping of diagnostic categories, or their emphasis, is significant (Horwitz & Wakefield, 2007; Jutel, 2010a; Jutel & Mintzes, 2017; Moynihan, 2014, 2016; Moynihan & Cassels, 2005; Tiefer, 2006). The gym, diet, self-help, cosmetic, pharmaceutical, fashion, publishing, and many other industries all have a financial stake in ensuring that particular conditions are seen as diseases rather than as something else (see also Chapter 4, this volume).

We will now turn to diagnosis (v.) or diagnosis-as-process. We will discuss the practice of implementing diagnoses (the labels); to obtain, or to deliver, a diagnosis is a social action that also requires critical scrutiny.

Diagnosis-as-process

The pursuit of a diagnosis starts with some perception of dysfunction, which compels the sick person to see a doctor. That visit triggers a range of social actions, and calls upon a number of social structures, all closely linked to diagnosis, in order to offer the sick person explanation and treatment. While the feeling of dysfunction may very well be a clear, material, physical matter of pathophysiology, it is not a state which comes pre-labelled with some kind of "correct" answer that the doctor can scratch to reveal as a diagnosis; rather, it is a complex decision-making process which is anchored in the social practices of modern science.

The diagnosis also imposes a form of social order, one which defines the roles of clinician and sick person alike. The latter becomes "patient", from the Latin verb *pati* "to suffer" and implying tolerance, perseverance, and passivity in the medical encounter. The former is instilled with the ability to confer a name to the illness. This is a form of power, and the relationship has an imbalance in power because diagnosis is an important means by which social resources are allocated, whether these be the sick note which allows the individual to miss one or another form of social responsibility (work, family duties), the therapy, the insurance payment, or even the ability to discuss a dysfunction in terms that are understandable to one's entourage.

Friedson (1972) has described the power to name disease as:

> the most important foundation upon which the strength of a profession rests, a foundation which establishes and supports the profession's claim to honor, income, and power. Where illness is the ubiquitous label for deviance in an age, the profession that is custodian of the label is ascendant.
>
> *(p. 244)*

Balint's classic work placed the power of diagnosis in its organisational power (Balint, 1964). The most pressing and immediate problem for the patient, he wrote, is "*the request for the name of the illness, for a diagnosis*. It is only in the second instance that the patient asks for therapy" (p. 25, italics in original). Until such time as the doctor presents a diagnosis, the patient is in a state of disarray. The symptoms are not synthesised; they are evidence of disorder. The diagnosis creates order. Mike Kelly (2015) writes more recently that "the provision of a diagnosis by the doctor may form an important turning point in the experience. The diagnostic category provided by the doctor is a potentially very deep well of information" (p. 94).

We can understand how naming the disease creates order, as it provides in shorthand, both a generalisation, and at the same time, a summary. Rather than having to say: "I have a contagious viral infection that has left me weary, with sore joints and a fever, yet with every chance to recover unless I have an untoward complication", one can say, "I have influenza", and in three words, reduce a messy tangle of individual details into an informative sound bite.

Drew Leder made sense of this diagnostic process as interpretive, a hermeneutic process (Leder, 1990). The patient brings, he wrote, an experiential text to the consultation, which is supplemented by the narrative text (the guided history), the physical text (physician examination of the patient) and the instrumental texts (testing and imaging). The division of labour in relationship to who authors which text underlines the cultural authority of medicine and the required submission of the patient. Leder writes:

> That is, diagnostic interpretation leads to treatment and thus to subsequent changes in the person-as-ill. The patient's reaction to treatment then feeds back to refine or transform the original diagnosis. A circular movement unfolds between the medical reading and the responses of a living, changing text.
>
> *(1990, p. 18)*

Yet, the balance of power that is enacted during the diagnostic process may actually transform the text presented by the patient. This is what Arthur Frank calls a *narrative surrender* (Frank, 1995), in which the patient's story is relinquished to the doctor's, told through diagnosis, and "the one against which others are ultimately judged true or false, useful or not" (p. 5–6). However, Kelly (2015) adds that the narrative is broadly one about the future: "a future where a return to the pre-morbid condition can be expected, where a life with chronic illness might be anticipated, or where a trajectory to a decline in health or death might be the end point" (p. 94).

In any case, the point is that there is a transformation – from an individual story to a generic one, from personal tale to medicalised interpretation – and this transformation has stakes (Jutel, 2019). The fact that the diagnosis is linked to explanation and treatment is only part of the story. Yes, the diagnosis (and the power associated with it) is linked to resources, whether those resources be the therapy (without a diagnosis, this is hard to come by), the sick leave, insurance reimbursement, something else, and the like.

But at an individual level, the ability to assign the diagnosis confers power to the doctor, as allocator of scarce resources (De Swaan, 1989), and legitimisation to the patient. By being diagnosed, the patient gains access to the sick role, exempt from certain, otherwise expected, contributions to society, and obliged to a commitment to get better (Parsons, 1958). At the same time as it legitimises, diagnosis can stigmatise. Not all diagnoses are equal, because a diagnosis projects particular social features on the diagnosee: lung cancer presupposes smoking; gout implies gluttony; obesity, sloth. Even the now-common expression "lifestyle" diseases supposed a kind of self-contribution to one's pain. A different lifestyle, a different outcome, regardless of how fatuous the relationship between lifestyle and disease may be for many of these diseases.

Dag Album and his colleagues have commented widely on what they call "disease prestige": a hierarchical valuing of some diagnoses over others by the medical community and others. Although one might wonder whether it matters that there are such preferences, the impact on policy, funding, and research when a disorder is at the bottom, rather than the top, of such a list exposes the importance of highlighting such hidden value systems (Album, Johannessen, & Rasmussen, 2017; Album & Westin, 2008).

That such power is concentrated in medicine, or in its delegates, and is conveyed by the allocation of particular diagnoses, creates a space of potential tension, with laypeople and doctors tussling over what is worthy of diagnosis, and who should be able to make the determination. This is nowhere more apparent than when no diagnosis is arrived upon at the end of a long diagnostic trajectory. Such circumstances are likely to leave the patient bereft, and at a loss to explain their inability to fulfil expected social roles (Dumit, 2006; Nettleton, 2006). Conditions with complex, unexplainable, debilitating symptoms – such as endometriosis, chronic fatigue syndromes, and chronic pain – engender conflict, with competing explanations, frustrations, and interminable testing for what seems an elusive diagnostic label. A frequent medical response is to categorise such disorders as psychosomatic in nature, as a kind of wastebasket diagnosis (Jutel, 2010b).

In turn, the patient reaction to non-diagnosis, and indeed, to diagnosis in general, may be to frequent the web and the many online social media resources available for, and devoted to, the subject of diagnosis. This may be in advance of seeking medical advice, or for evaluation of diagnostic and therapeutic recommendations by doctors. Referred to as the "Doctor Google" phenomenon, it has been widely critiqued in medical circles based on a range of apprehensions: self-diagnosis contributing to misdiagnosis by the physician (Avery, Ghandi, & Keating, 2012; Feke, 2015); disruption of the patient–doctor relationship (Hesse, 2012; Limb, 2014); increased health anxiety, with very rare malignant diseases frequently linked to banal symptoms (Doherty-Torstrick, Walton, & Fallon, 2016; Fergus & Dolan, 2014; Tyrer, Eilenberg, Fink, Hedman, & Tyrer, 2016); and the exploitative actions of industry such as big pharma, big data, and big food (Kim, 2015; Lupton & Jutel, 2015); and more. Not unexpectedly perhaps, this patient incursion into the medical domain has garnered its own diagnostic term: *cyberchondria*, referring to health anxiety resulting from internet use.

In a critical evaluation of diagnosis, one must look beyond the web and social media to understand why diagnosis matters so much to laypeople. I have argued elsewhere that the web is simply a new medium for an activity which people have undertaken for well over a century and against which doctors have ranted for just as long. After all, as early as 1899, Gersuny (1889) wrote words which sound as if they could have been written today: "Sick people who imagine that they know the exact nature of their ailment, or who have read up their complaint in some book, are a great source of trouble to their doctors and themselves". Such caution continued into the next century with Dr Robert Keith (1918) warning that "A patient may give a diagnosis of his own, but you must never accept this without making full examination" (p. 16). Similarly, a few decades later, Dr Albert Krecke lamented "[the patient] has heard so much about all manner of diseases that every time he [sic] feels a little poorly, he imagines the worst" (Krecke, 1934).

So, it's more of the same. What is important to reflect on is why patients would consider diagnosis so important that they would need to explore their problems via sources other than their doctors. I would argue that it is patient conviction of the importance of diagnosis, which leads to this pursuit. This faith in diagnosis is pivotal both to the expansion of medicine's reach, and also to the cultivation of self-diagnosing patients. Believing in medicine's explanatory framework – to locate the individual case in a general category – compels the individual to forge ahead when medicine is at a loss to provide the answer, or when the category provided is at odds with the individual's sense of their condition. This conviction is evidence that medicine has prevailed, but, at the same time, a challenge to the individual clinician.

The complex range of contested diagnoses and medically unexplained symptoms, which preoccupy the social media and the medical profession alike underline the coveted appeal of the diagnosis (Lum, 2018). Here, we might start to recognise where the power of the diagnosis fails. The old adage "You must treat the patient and not the disease" recognises the limitations of the diagnosis to explain all ailments.

Undeland and Malterud (2002) proposed that, by seeing diagnosis as the primary reason goal of a medical consultation, we fail to see many other avenues of succour. The encounter between patient and doctor should be recast, they believe, as a help-seeking interaction rather than a diagnostic endeavour. The doctor–patient dyad may still end up with a diagnosis, but beyond diagnosis, symptoms *sans* diagnosis can still be managed, palliated; and matters which seem to be non-medical in nature can be so identified, and perhaps referred on. This helps remove the inclination to settle on a psychiatric diagnosis when a physical diagnosis cannot be found. Such labels can be particularly offensive to the patients. Stone and his colleagues called for the restoration of the label "functional", which, while value-laden in the medical arena, appears to be acceptable in that of patients. The functional disorder they wrote, provides, "a rationale for pharmacological, behavioural, and psychological treatments aimed at restoring normal functioning … a useful and acceptable diagnosis for physical symptoms unexplained by disease" (Stone et al., 2002).

Conclusion

A critical scholar must consider how diagnosis goes beyond its labelling function. It is far more than a label, rather a social agreement which can allocate prestige, power, and resources. With such power conferred by the diagnosis, it is both a social structure and a social good over which people, professions, and other interested parties squabble. Not only do the patient and the doctor tussle ("negotiate" as Balint (1964) describes it) over what diagnosis should be assigned to what disorder, so to do health professionals over who and what they can diagnose. This negotiation also applies to medical sub-specialities; the health professionals who have wrangled diagnostic rights from medicine (notably nurse practitioners and physiotherapists) have had to fight hard to succeed, and are limited in what they are allowed to diagnose (Keeling, 2015).

Diagnosis plays an important role in how we understand health, illness, and disease, but, as I have discussed above, its social content is remarkable, and under-recognised. Critical reflection must always linger upon such social phenomena, and ponder: to what extent has are such social phenomena infrastructural, providing what looks to be a solid physical foundation to a system which is, in fact, only partially so? The point is not as much to refute a particular organisation of disease, as it is to recognise that there may be other ways for organising it. It is an opening of possibilities.

Note

1 We might also ponder the complexities of even those diseases we think we understand. The influenza virus mutates readily and appears in different forms from year to year, and the ways in which they are diagnosed doesn't always keep up. Readers may be entertained to know that the 2009 (check) H1N1 pandemic commonly referred to as the Swine Flu ended up "coded" or administratively diagnosed as "avian (bird) flu". The instructions from the world health organisations to coders was to use the under-utilised 2005 code, J-09 ("Influenza due to identified *avian* influenza"), to record any deaths by H1N1, but with the addition of the free text entry: "Influenza A H1N1 – confirmed". (WHO, 2010). WHO did recognise the limitation of their coding structure, and the inefficacy of setting up new categories for each and every influenza mutation. They also made a nod towards Ockham, recognising that they had been hasty when they had established J-09 in 2005. It would have been wiser to have been less specific, in order to give space for emerging influenza strains. Reflecting this reality, the code has been changed to read "*certain* identified influenza virus": a more general category (Jutel, 2013).

References

Album, D., Johannessen, L. E., & Rasmussen, E. B. (2017). Stability and change in disease prestige: A comparative analysis of three surveys spanning a quarter of a century. *Social Science and Medicine, 180,* 45–51. doi:10.1016/j.socscimed.2017.03.020

Album, D., & Westin, S. (2008). Do diseases have a prestige hierarchy? A survey among physicians and medical students. *Social Science & Medicine, 66*(1), 182–188. doi:10.1016/j.socscimed.2007.07.003

Aronowitz, R. (1991). Lyme disease: The social construction of a new disease and its social consequences. *Milbank Quarterly, 69*(1), 79–112.

Avery, N., Ghandi, J., & Keating, J. (2012). The "Dr Google" phenomenon – missed appendicitis. *New Zealand Medical Journal, 125*(1367), 135–137.

Balint, M. (1964). *The doctor, his patient and the illness* (2nd ed.). Kent: Pitman Medical.

Blaxter, M. (1978). Diagnosis as category and process: The case of alcoholism. *Social Science and Medicine, 12,* 9–17.

Bowker, G. C., & Star, S. L. (1999). *Sorting things out: Classification and its consequences.* Cambridge, MA: MIT Press.

Bresalier, M. (2012). "A most protean disease": Aligning medical knowledge of modern influenza, 1890–1914. *Medical History, 56*(4), 481–510. doi:10.1017/mdh.2012.29

Broughton, A. (1782). *Observations on the influenza, or epidemic catarrh; as it appeared in Bristol and its environs, during the months of May and June 1782. to Which Is Added, a Meteorological Journal.*

Brown, P. (1995). Naming and framing: The social construction of diagnosis and illness. *Journal of Health and Social Behavior, 35*(extra issue), 34–52.

Davidson, H. (2020, 20 March). Chinese inquiry exonerates coronavirus whistleblower doctors. *The Guardian.* Retrieved from https://www.theguardian.com/world/2020/mar/20/chinese-inquiry-exonerates-coronavirus-whistleblower-doctor-li-wenliang

De Swaan, A. (1989). The reluctant imperialism of the medical profession. *Social Science & Medicine, 28*(11), 1165–1170.

Doherty-Torstrick, E. R., Walton, K. E., & Fallon, B. A. (2016). Cyberchondria: Parsing health anxiety from online behavior. *Psychosomatics, 57*(4), 390–400. doi:10.1016/j.psym.2016.02.002

Dumit, J. (2006). Illnesses you have to fight to get: Facts as forces in uncertain, emergent illnesses. *Social Science & Medicine, 62*(3), 577–590.

Fadiman, A. (1997). *The spirit catches you and you fall down: A Hmong child, her American doctors, and the collision of two cultures* (1st ed.). New York: Farrar, Straus, and Giroux.

Feke, T. (2015). Dr. Google should be sued for malpractice. Here's why. Retrieved from http://www.kevi nmd.com/blog/2015/08/dr-google-should-be-sued-for-malpractice-heres-why.html

Fergus, T. A., & Dolan, S. L. (2014). Problematic internet use and internet searches for medical information: The role of health anxiety. *Cyberpsychology, Behaviour and Social Networking, 17*(12), 761–765. doi:10.1089/cyber.2014.0169

Frank, A. W. (1995). *The wounded storyteller: Body, illness and ethics*. Chicago, IL: University of Chicago Press.

Freidson, E. (1972). *Profession of medicine: A study of the sociology of applied knowledge* (fourth printing ed.). New York: Dodd, Mead & Company.

Gersuny, R. (1889). *Doctor and patient: Hints to both*. Bristol: John Wright & Co.

Hacking, I. (2001). Inaugural lecture: Chair of philosophy and history of scientific concepts at the Collège de France, 16 January 2001. *Economy and Society, 31*(1), 1–14.

Hesse, B. W. (2012). The patient, the physician, and Dr. Google. *Virtual Mentor, 14*(5), 398–402. doi:10.10 01/virtualmentor.2012.14.5.stas1-1205

Horwitz, A. V., & Wakefield, J. C. (2007). *The loss of sadness: How psychiatry transformed normal sorrow into depressive disorder*. New York: Oxford University Press.

Jutel, A. (2010a). Framing disease: The example of female hypoactive sexual desire disorder. *Social Science and Medicine, 70*, 1084–1090. doi: 10.1016/j.socscimed.2009.11.040

Jutel, A. (2010b). Medically unexplained symptoms and the disease label. *Social Theory and Health, 8*, 229–245.

Jutel, A. (2011). *Putting a name to it: Diagnosis in contemporary society*. Baltimore, MD: Johns Hopkins University Press.

Jutel, A. (2013). When pigs could fly: Influenza and the elusive nature of diagnosis. *Perspectives in Biology and Medicine, 56*(4), 513–529. doi:10.1353/pbm.2013.0033

Jutel, A. (2019). *Diagnosis: Truths, and tales*. Toronto, ON: University of Toronto Press.

Jutel, A., & Mintzes, B. (2017). Female sexual dysfunction: Medicalizing desire. In B. Cohen (Ed.), *Routledge international handbook of critical mental health* (pp. 162–168). London: Routledge.

Keeling, A. W. (2015). Historical perspectives on an expanded role for nursing. *Online Journal of Issues in Nursing, 20*(2), 1. Retrieved from http://ojin.nursingworld.org/MainMenuCategories/ANAMarketpla ce/ANAPeriodicals/OJIN/TableofContents/Vol-20-2015/No2-May-2015/Historical-Perspectives -Expanded-Role-Nursing.html

Keith, R. D. (1918). *Clinical case-taking*. London: H.K. Lewis & Co, Ltd.

Kelly, M. P. (2015). Diagnostic categories in autobiographical accounts of illness. *Perspectives in Biology and Medicine, 58*(1), 89–104. doi:10.1353/pbm.2015.0002

Kim, H. (2015). Trouble spots in online direct-to-consumer prescription drug promotion: A content analysis of FDA warning letters. *International Journal of Health Policy Management, 4*(12), 813–821. doi:10.15171/ ijhpm.2015.157

Kirk, S. A., & Kutchins, H. (1992). *The selling of DSM: The rhetoric of science in psychiatry*. New York: A. de Gruyter.

Krecke, A. (1934). *The doctor and his patients*. London: Kogan Paul, Trench, Trubner.

Leder, D. (1990). Clinical interpretation: The hermeneutics of medicine. *Theoretical Medicine, 11*, 9–24.

Leff, W. (1997). William of Ockham. In M. Parry (Ed.), *Chambers biographical dictionary* (pp. 1386). New York: Chambers.

Light, D. W. (2004). Ironies of success: A new history of the American health care "system". *Journal of Health and Social Behavior, 45*(Suppl), 1–24.

Limb, M. (2014). Technology must not replace human contact in drive for self care, conference hears. *BMJ British Medical Journal, 348*, 4278.

Little, E. G. (1926). *Doctors and the public: An address delivered at the opening of the medical session at St. George's Medical School on 1 October, 1926*. Foxton: Burlington Press.

Lum, I. (2018). Between illness and disease: Reflections on managing medically unexplained symptoms. *Canadian Family Physician, 64*(11), 859–860.

Lupton, D., & Jutel, A. (2015). "It's like having a physician in your pocket!" A critical analysis of self-diagnosis smartphone apps. *Social Science and Medicine, 133*, 128–135. doi:10.1016/j.socscimed.2015.04.004

Martin, E. A., & Oxford University Press. (2010). *Concise Medical Dictionary* (8th ed.). Oxford: Oxford University Press.

Moynihan, R. (2014). Evening the score on sex drugs: Feminist movement or marketing masquerade? *British Medical Journal, 349*. doi:10.1136/bmj.g6246

Moynihan, R. (2016). Caution! Diagnosis creep. *Australian Prescriber, 39*(2), 30–31. doi:10.18773/austprescr.2016.021

Moynihan, R., & Cassels, A. (2005). *Selling sickness: How drug companies are turning us all into patients.* Sydney: Allen & Unwin.

Nettleton, S. (2006). "I just want permission to be ill": Towards a sociology of medically unexplained symptoms. *Social Science and Medicine, 62*(5), 1167–1178.

Parsons, T. (1958). Definitions of health and illness in the light of American values and social structure. In E. G. Jaco (Ed.), *Patients, physicians and illness: Behavioral science and medicine* (pp. 165–187). Glencoe, IL: Free Press.

Richardson, E. C. (1901). *Classification.* New York: Charles Scribner's Sons.

Scott, W. J. (1990). PTSD in DSM-III: A case in the politics of diagnosis and disease. *Social Problems, 37*(3), 294–310.

Stone, J., Wojcik, W., Durrance, D., Carson, A., Lewis, S., MacKenzie, L., . . . Sharpe, M. (2002). What should we say to patients with symptoms unexplained by disease? The 'number needed to offend'. *British Medical Journal, 325*(7378), 1449–1450. Retrieved from http://www.ncbi.nlm.nih.gov/entrez/query.fcgi?cmd=Retrieve&db=PubMed&dopt=Citation&list_uids=12493661

Taubenberger, J. K., Hultin, J. V., & Morens, D. M. (2007). Discovery and characterization of the 1918 pandemic influenza virus in historical context. *Antiviral therapy, 12*(4 Pt B), 581–591.

Tiefer, L. (2006). Female sexual dysfunction: A case study of disease mongering and activist resistance. *PLoS Medicine, 3*(4), e178.

Tyrer, P., Eilenberg, T., Fink, P., Hedman, E., & Tyrer, H. (2016). Health anxiety: The silent, disabling epidemic. *British Medical Journal, 353*, i2250. doi:10.1136/bmj.i2250

Undeland, M., & Malterud, K. (2007). The fibromyalgia diagnosis: Hardly helpful for the patients? A qualitative focus group study. *Scandinavian Journal of Primary Health Care, 25*(4), 250–255. doi:10.1080/02813430701706568

Wailoo, K. (1997). *Drawing blood: Technology and disease identity in twentieth-century America.* Baltimore, MD: Johns Hopkins University Press.

World Health Organisation. (2020, 21 January). *Novel virus (2019-ncov) situation report – 1.* Retrieved from Geneva: https://www.who.int/docs/default-source/coronaviruse/situation-reports/20200121-sitrep-1-2019-ncov.pdf?sfvrsn=20a99c10_4

Zerubavel, E. (1996). Lumping and splitting: Notes on social classification. *Sociological Forum, 11*(3), 421–433.

Zimmer, C. (2020, 8 April). Most New York coronavirus cases came from Europe, genomes show. *New York Times.* Retrieved from https://www.nytimes.com/2020/04/08/science/new-york-coronavirus-cases-europe-genomes.html

8

POPULATION-BASED SCREENING FOR DETECTION AND PREVENTION

Natalie Armstrong

Introduction

The focus of this chapter is on population-based screening and its use as a means of detecting and preventing disease. Screening is a public health intervention that aims to improve health outcomes at a population level by identifying pre-disease risk states and intervening to prevent progression or identifying established disease before it becomes symptomatic, thereby enabling earlier treatment. It does this by seeking to identify healthy people who may have an increased chance of a disease or condition and subsequently offering them further investigations and treatment. Screening involves the purposeful application of tests to an asymptomatic population in order to classify people into those who are likely to have or develop a disease (and therefore require further investigation) and those who are not (Raffle, Mackie, & Gray, 2019).

Screening is not without its challenges, though. The crucial distinction from diagnosis means that all screening involves an inescapable risk of false positives and false negatives, in which people are either incorrectly identified as at risk (and therefore subjected to unnecessary further investigation and possibly treatment) or falsely reassured (and therefore not offered the further investigation and treatment they may require) (Armstrong, 2014). As an example of secondary prevention, screening aims to detect a disease in its early stages and enable intervention (Raffle et al., 2019). This creates the distinctive dilemma of not necessarily knowing whether the screening-induced diagnosis brought benefit to the individual patient, or whether the anomalies identified would either have regressed on their own or else progressed so slowly that they would never have caused a problem. Concerns around "overdiagnosis" are covered later in this chapter.

Healthcare systems across the world vary in terms of the range of screening programmes offered, the groups targeted, the frequency of invitation, and the cost to the "consumer" (which is obviously dependent on the country's system of healthcare provision). Costs aside, however, a similar position is taken by many developed countries in terms of currently available and recommended screening programmes. A full account of screening provision across these countries is beyond the scope of this chapter, but England is a useful example. Its current screening programmes include those for cervical cancer; breast cancer; bowel cancer; abdominal aortic aneurism; diabetic retinopathy; and a range of antenatal and newborn screening (including foetal anomalies, infectious diseases in pregnancy, newborn screening, newborn hearing screening, Sickle Cell and Thalassaemia, and the Newborn and Infant Physical Examination Programme).

The potential reach of medical screening is growing and developing; it is now possible to screen for an ever-increasing range of conditions, using ever more advanced and sophisticated technologies and techniques. Screening is far from simply a medical matter, though; rather, it raises fundamental issues and dilemmas that are amenable to and indeed benefit from scrutiny informed by social theory (Armstrong, 2019; Armstrong & Eborall, 2012a, 2012b). These issues are of interest to social scientists because screening gives rise to a range of uncertainties, and the debates and controversies that result are rarely confined to policymakers and health professionals. Contestations about the science underlying screening are common, and frequently enter the public sphere, engaging with wider societal themes and normative questions. Different groups engage, prioritise, and mobilise different forms of knowledge and ways of knowing about screening.

This chapter will provide an overview of social science research on screening to date, identifying key themes and conceptual developments. While social science research is the main focus, the chapter will also touch on other disciplines from time to time as relevant. It will consider current discussions and debates about the potential for harm as well as benefit from screening, including those relating to overdiagnosis and overtreatment, as well as taking a critical look at the increased move to screening participation based on informed choice.

The uncertainties of screening and the change to the doctor–patient relationship

We have already established that screening is importantly different to diagnosis because screening is targeted at individuals who have no symptoms and as such have not sought medical help. In this way, the usual contract between the doctor and patient is reversed. In clinical practice, people present asking for help on the basis of symptoms they are experiencing or other concerns they have, thereby defining themselves as in need of medical advice. Because screening targets apparently healthy people who have not sought the help of health professionals with the offer of an intervention for something they may have never thought about, this relationship is reversed. The very different contract that can then be seen to exist between the doctor and the patient in the two scenarios is summed up very well in the following quote:

> Screening will inevitably turn some people who test "positive" into patients – a transformation not to be undertaken lightly. If a patient asks a medical practitioner for help, the doctor does the best possible. The doctor is not responsible for defects in medical knowledge. If, however, the practitioner initiates screening procedures, the doctor is in a very different situation. The doctor should, in our view, have conclusive evidence that screening can alter the natural history of the disease in a significant proportion of those screened.
>
> *(Cochrane & Holland, 1971)*

Put simply, if a patient seeks medical advice from a doctor, and the doctor ultimately cannot offer any effective treatment or intervention for the condition diagnosed then that is not the doctor's fault – s/he is not responsible for gaps or defects in medical knowledge. If the doctor approaches the patient with the offer of screening, though, it is incumbent upon her/him to be able to help the patient should they test positive and the condition later be diagnosed.

One of the important ways in which screening is different to diagnosis, and an important means through which uncertainty begins to creep in, is that all screening programmes involve an inescapable risk of false positives and false negatives, in which people are either incorrectly identified as at risk (and therefore subjected to unnecessary further investigation and possibly treatment) or are falsely reassured (and therefore not offered the further investigation and treatment they may require). Uncertainty therefore exists about whether people who screen positive really do have the condition and, vice versa, about whether those who screen negative definitely do not. These uncertainties are relevant not only to those individuals being screened but, particularly in the case of false positives, also to those healthcare professionals involved in providing further investigations.

Screening is not definitive; rather, it is a preliminary "sort" – the notion of a sieve is increasingly being used in this context as an explanatory metaphor – of those having been screened into two broad groups based on the probability of them having or developing the condition in question. This element of uncertainty is inescapable as screening is not a definitive diagnosis – that comes later, at least for those who screen positive and who do really have the condition or its precursor (although see later in the chapter for a discussion on the uncertainties posed by potential overdiagnosis). What this means is that a fine balance is needed between having the sieve catch too many people that do not have anything wrong with them (and are therefore false positives) and letting through too many people for whom further investigation is actually warranted (and are therefore false negatives).

A further source of uncertainty, and one which relates more to the level of epidemiological evidence, arises because it is in fact quite challenging to evaluate and assess screening's particular contribution to any observed reduction in mortality and morbidity – several sources of bias are often quoted here (Raffle et al., 2019). One is length-time bias, which refers to the appearance that a person's life expectancy has been increased because the condition has been detected earlier through screening when in fact all that has lengthened is the period of time that they have been aware of the disease. A second is a lead-time bias, in which the kinds of cases that are amenable to and identified through screening are arguably those that are by definition less aggressive or less likely to go on to be a problem for the patient. A third is selection bias, in which people who engage in screening programmes are also likely to be doing other things that are health promoting, such as not smoking, taking exercise, and eating well. These potential biases combine to mean that surfacing the particular contribution that screening is making in any particular case under consideration is not necessarily a straightforward thing to do.

Screening and normative expectations

The 1990s saw a proliferation of work that applied Foucault's ideas on governmentality to public health and health promotion, and argued that individuals were increasingly being constrained to think and act in particular ways in order to maximise their health and be regarded as responsible and moral citizens (Burrows, Nettleton, & Bunton, 1995; Castel, 1991; Lupton, 1995; Nettleton, 1995; Nettleton & Bunton, 1995; Petersen & Lupton, 1996). Focusing broadly on how health status and the means for initially achieving and subsequently ensuring the maintenance of good health has become a predominant concern of modern life, of particular interest within what has been termed the "New Public Health" (Green, 2004) was a well-documented shift towards "promoting" good health and encouraging populations to monitor their own health. Tolerating uncertainty about one's status as either healthy, ill, or "at risk" in some way has arguably become increasingly undesirable.

At the same time, the influential work of David Armstrong (Armstrong, 1983, 1993, 1995) to develop the concept of "surveillance medicine" was influential in using social science theory to examine and problematise the increased observation and surveillance of the population in health terms. The premise of the surveillance medicine concept is that the model of medicine that emerged during the 20th century is concerned with the observation and monitoring of apparently healthy populations, and that asymptomatic individuals are increasingly expected to make their bodies available to health professionals for regular inspection in order to minimise uncertainty by prompt identification of asymptomatic abnormalities. Such observation and monitoring breaks down the traditional distinction between those that are healthy and those that are ill. Medicine is no longer concerned simply with the latter; instead, the whole population comes under surveillance and is potentially "at risk" (Armstrong, 1995).

A significant thread of sociological work on screening has drawn on and developed these ideas, often using cervical screening as a case study – a particularly amenable example as it involves women being invited at regular intervals through much of their adult life, therefore providing a large and easily accessible pool of potential research participants. An important contribution arising from the application of social science theory to what might look more like an issue only of interest to public health specialists is the way in which this enables us to conceptualise engagement with and attendance for screening as a response to normative expectations about what constitutes the most sensible and responsible course of action (Bush, 2000; Howson, 1998, 1999; McKie, 1995). Alexandra Howson's work is notable here for the theoretically sophisticated way in which she problematises women's attendance for cervical cancer screening and links this to wider debates about the exercise of power within society. In her work, Howson argues that attendance for screening can be highly problematic as through the application of social science theory it is possible to understand it not simply as a neutral outcome of public health activity but alternatively "as a response to a particular expression of power or set of normative expectations … a social practice, which is embedded within a moral framework of responsibility and obligation" (Howson, 1999). Attendance at screening may thus be understood as signifying responsible behaviour that demonstrates good citizenship by engaging in forms of health practices that seek to minimise uncertainty and risk – in Howson's terms, screening attendance becomes a form of "moral obligation". This is not to say that individuals are unable to think and behave in ways other than those suggested to them through such powerful discourse, though (Armstrong, 2005, 2007; Armstrong & Murphy, 2012).

Screening as an informed choice?

A second theme on which social scientific scrutiny has been of significant value is whether and how truly "informed consent" for screening can be achieved. The application of social theory has helped to unpick the complex interplay of factors that shape how people make decisions about whether to have screening, and indeed to question whether decisions are being made at all. There has been an increasing focus in recent years on screening based on informed consent rather than on an expectation or assumption of participation; from the invitee's perspective, this has meant that the information leaflets accompanying invitations to participate in screening have begun to include more about the possible harms as well as the potential benefits (Gummersbach et al., 2010; Zapka et al., 2006).

There are important questions about what constitutes both full and accessible information, and when such information may be available. Importantly, the extent to which "the facts" can ever be fully known is questionable; sometimes the very act of screening itself changes what we know about a condition and how we think about it by creating uncertainties in epidemiological understandings. This may be the case because, prior to screening, knowledge about a condition is based almost solely on cases in which it has become symptomatic. A good example of this is work on medium-chain acyl-CoA dehydrogenase deficiency (MCADD) in the context of expanded newborn screening in the US (Timmermans & Buchbinder, 2012). Here, beginning to screen for a condition started to reveal new information that challenged how the condition was understood. From a singular disease it morphed into a condition with several variants, new kinds of patients with different risk factors were identified, the incidence appeared much higher than anticipated, and it seemed to affect a wider range of ethnic groups than had previously been thought. Presenting complex, technical information (which may be incomplete) in ways that are easily accessible necessarily involves selectivity and selection over what is included and how it is explained, which may have implications for how those invited for screening come to understand what it is all about (Armstrong & Murphy, 2008). There are also questions about the quality of information about screened for conditions, in particular the differences between medical descriptions and lived realities (Boardman, 2017).

However, information leaflets are just one part of a bigger, complex picture of the influences on how screening is understood and the decision to participate or not in screening approached. Other pertinent issues include: the technologies or techniques used in screening and their acceptability, particularly when they transgress often strongly felt social taboos (Armstrong, James, & Dixon-Woods, 2012; Chapple, Ziebland, Hewitson, & McPherson, 2008); how individuals think about and understand their own risk of developing a particular condition (Armstrong, 2005; Pfeffer, 2004); the wider contextual and interactional circumstances in which screening offers are made and received (Pilnick, 2008; Pilnick & Zayts, 2012; Todorova, Baban, Balabanova, Panayotova, & Bradley, 2006); and how those invited to participate in particularly sensitive or new types of screening can be understood as acting as "moral pioneers" navigating new and unfamiliar terrains (Markens, Browner, & Mabel Preloran, 2010; Williams et al., 2005).

One response to the increased acknowledgement that screening be considered an informed choice that individuals make on the basis of having had access to good quality information is the increasing development of decision aids. The production and use of decision aids tend to assume that there is a body of stable and agreed on information to be included. The way we communicate with people about screening is, at least in theory, changing (Hersch, Jansen, & McCaffery, 2016), but an informed choice must be based on adequate knowledge, which may or may not be present (Ward, Coffey, & Meyer, 2015). As Stephenson, Mills, and McLeod (2017) argued in the context of antenatal screening, "distinguishing information from choice is underpinned by a questionable fact–value distinction" (Stephenson, Mills, & McLeod, 2017).

Risk and uncertainty

Wider sociological concern with issues of risk and uncertainty has also proved to be fertile ground, and empirical work exploring the experiences and understandings of those for whom screening indicates there may be a problem is plentiful. As examples, Green, Thompson, and Griffiths (2002) explored the role that health technologies such as breast cancer screening may play in the "management" of midlife women's bodies, and the way in which messages about these technologies and their potential are interpreted by women; Griffiths, Green, and Bendelow (2006) used uncertainty as a way of thinking about the issues faced by professionals in balancing individual and population costs and benefits of screening for breast cancer. In the latter example, the focus is on how healthcare professionals understand, talk about, and cope with the tension between the individual and distributive ethic of medicine within the breast screening context – a tension between focusing on what may be beneficial to any individual and attending to health issues for the population as a whole.

In cases where screening has highlighted that there may be a problem, the uncertainty experienced by individuals, and the ways in which they attempt to understand and cope with this, has been a particular area of focus; for example, in relation to cervical abnormalities (Blomberg, Forss, Ternestedt, & Tishelman, 2009; Forss, Tishelman, Widmark, & Sachs, 2004; Kavanagh &

Broom, 1998), antenatal screening (Heyman et al., 2006; Lotto, Armstrong, & Smith, 2016; Lotto, Smith, & Armstrong, 2018), and newborn screening (Grob, 2008). Gillespie's work on risk experience nicely draws out the profound social effects, in addition to the physical and psychological, for those who are screened. By exploring the social implications of screening for those designated as being at risk of potential disease, Gillespie draws attention to the increased medical contact, restructuring of everyday routines, and altered social relationships (Gillespie, 2015). Being "at risk", Gillespie argues, symbolically alters health identities through the "measured vulnerability" some forms of screening have the potential to invoke through their focus on quantification of risk factor (Gillespie, 2012).

A valuable additional focus has been on the work healthcare professionals do in order to attempt to navigate the uncertainties of screening, both in terms of the screening act itself but also the possible follow-ons in terms of diagnosis and prognosis, and the making of decisions about possible interventions. Examination of the interactional work at the "sharp end" of screening has offered important insights into the way in which this form of work gets done and is received (Pilnick, 2008; Pilnick & Zayts, 2012, 2014), including problematising ideals of nondirective counselling on the part of healthcare professionals (Schwennesen & Koch, 2012). As is increasingly being recognised, while there is a wealth of literature on patients' experiences of various forms of screening, research on the everyday work practices of the healthcare professionals working in these situations remains relatively small in comparison (Gale, Thomas, Thwaites, Greenfield, & Brown, 2016; Thomas, 2014).

Governance of screening programmes

In making decisions about whether or not to implement population-based screening programmes, healthcare policymakers typically seek to assess the evidence for and against screening for different conditions. Generally speaking, decisions about screening programmes still draw to a large extent on Wilson and Jungner's classic principles developed for the World Health Organisation over 50 years ago (Sturdy et al., 2020; Wilson & Jungner, 1968). While over five decades old now, Wilson and Jungner's principles are remarkably enduring, with a recent systematic review finding they inform a significant amount of the principles used to govern screening internationally (Dobrow, Hagens, Chafe, Sullivan, & Rabeneck, 2018). The review did highlight, though, that interest in and concern about principles relating to the screening programme or system (rather than, e.g. the test, the condition, or the treatment) are receiving increasing amounts of focus than was present in Wilson and Jungner's original principles.

As discussed at the outset of this chapter, screening involves the making of an offer to asymptomatic populations to assess for the probable presence or absence of disease or its precursors. Because of this, there is a need to be sure that the possible benefits of screening outweigh any potential harms (Gray, 2004). Yet evaluating a screening programme's effectiveness can be challenging, as highlighted earlier, especially in the absence of high-quality trial data. Perhaps the most high profile recent attempt to do this was the review of the NHS Breast Screening Programme in the UK, which ultimately concluded that screening did reduce breast cancer mortality but with the associated cost of overdiagnosis, meaning that some women would be diagnosed with anomalies that would never have troubled them in their lifetime (Marmot et al., 2012). The review placed the figure at about three over-diagnosed cases identified and treated for every one breast cancer death prevented. Echoing the increasing shift towards informed choice already highlighted, the review called for information about the possible costs and benefits of screening to be made clearer and more transparent to women when they were invited to attend for screening and when they were making decisions about treatment options.

Yet, even following the publication of the review's findings, contestations around the newly produced evidence continued, with vocal criticisms of the methods used and the robustness of the conclusions drawn (Thornton, 2012). What is troubling is that many healthcare professionals do not themselves seem to understand these issues – a study in the US showed that clinicians mistakenly interpreted improved survival and increased detection through screening as evidence that screening saves lives (Wegwarth, Schwartz, Woloshin, Gaissmaier, & Gigerenzer, 2012). These complexities combined with the ongoing public and political interest in and enthusiasm for screening mean that arriving at robust decisions about whether or not to implement screening programmes, and communicating these publicly and in policy circles, is not straightforward.

In a recent study of breast and cervical cancer screening in Australia, Pienaar and colleagues argued that screening-related information comes to assume the status of scientific "facts", and that presenting information as neutral and objective in this way obscures the political choices involved in its generation and use (Pienaar, Petersen, & Bowman, 2019). As in other contexts, Pienaar et al. argue the claims about screening's effectiveness presented in the type of policy documents they analyse tend to emphasise the potential benefits and minimise the possible harms. This is a problem, they argue, not least because this then contributes to sustaining expectations of screening that are higher than warranted, meaning that screening becomes further entrenched and more resistant to challenge.

Overdiagnosis and overtreatment

Population-based screening is increasingly being discussed as part of wider debates around over-diagnosis and overtreatment, which are increasingly highlighted as a significant problem in contemporary healthcare. Attention globally is increasingly focused on the harms and avoidable waste of "too much medicine" (BMJ, 2017), with a recent report by the Organisation for Economic Co-operation and Development highlighting wasteful healthcare spending such as tests and interventions which have little or no patient benefit.

While not necessarily straightforward to define (Carter et al., 2015), overdiagnosis and any subsequent overtreatment are terms generally used about instances in which a diagnosis is "correct" according to current standards, but the diagnosis or associated treatment has a low probability of benefitting the patient, and may instead be harmful (Moynihan, Doust, & Henry, 2012). While now extending to a wide range of clinical activities, these types of concerns originated largely in the context of cancer screening (Welch, Schwartz, & Woloshin, 2011).

The potential consequences of overdiagnosis and overtreatment may be significant and include such harms as the psychological and behavioural effects of disease labelling, physical harms and side effects of unnecessary tests or treatments, unnecessary treatment negatively affecting the quality of life, increased financial costs to individuals and wasted resources and opportunity costs to the health system (Heath, 2014; Hicks, 2015; Moynihan et al., 2012). A key theme of psychological research on screening is the psychological impact on individuals, driven by the imperative that screening must not do more harm than good. This has involved investigations into the anxiety associated with receipt of abnormal test results and the requirement to attend for further tests (Brett, Bankhead, Henderson, Watson, & Austoker, 2005; Orbell et al., 2008).

Overdiagnosis is driven by a range of factors, including increasingly sensitive tests that identify indolent, non-progressive, or regressive abnormalities; expanded disease definitions and lowered thresholds; creation of pseudo diseases; public enthusiasm for screening or testing and the desire for reassurance (Chen, Eborall, & Armstrong, 2014); clinicians' fear of missing a diagnosis or of litigation; and financial incentives (Pathirana, Clark, & Moynihan, 2017). The relevance of this to population-based medical screening is that there are increasingly questions about the clinical significance of at least some of the anomalies being identified and treated, in particular whether they would go on to become problematic in a person's lifetime and therefore whether or not intervention to "treat" them is warranted. In this way, uncertainties pertain to the body of epidemiological evidence as well as to how things will work out for any particular individual.

A good fairly recent example of where these issues were played out is the review of the NHS Breast Screening Programme in the UK highlighted above, with the verdict being that screening does reduce breast cancer mortality but with the associated cost of overdiagnosis, meaning that some women will be diagnosed with anomalies that would never have troubled them in their lifetime (Marmot et al., 2012).

Informed choice vs high uptake?

The tension between informed choice and ensuring high uptake of screening has long been recognised (Raffle, 2001). The balance between ensuring informed choice on one hand while also facilitating participation for those that do wish to engage is not straightforward. Screening has received significant attention from health psychology, with the focus primarily upon non-attendance (McCaffery et al., 2001; Neilson & Jones, 1998) and the investigation of factors that may predict screening attendance/non-attendance, including sociodemographic factors (Jepson et al., 2000); variations in invitation type (Norman & Conner, 1992); social cognition models (Bish, Sutton, & Golombok, 2000); educational interventions (Wardle et al., 2003); and variations in information leaflet content, including details about the costs and benefits of screening (Marteau et al., 2010). The interest in establishing the barriers and facilitators to screening participation continues to this day (Priaulx et al. 2020), along with experimental work assessing the effects of different strategies to encourage attendance, such as manipulating normative beliefs about cancer screening uptake rates (von Wagner et al., 2019).

In contrast to this type of health psychology work, a more critical social science perspective may focus instead on the issue of when seeking to facilitate screening participation for those who want to engage could slip into attempted coercion of those that have made an informed decision not to. Earlier in this chapter I drew attention to sociological work on surveillance medicine and in particular work emphasising the perceived moral obligation to engage in preventative interventions such as screening. I also highlighted that individuals are not necessarily without the ability to resist such dominant framings of preventative behaviours (Armstrong & Murphy, 2012).

An interesting question to consider in this context is whether and how we can distinguish between non-participation based on informed choice and that which may be shaped by other, potentially remediable, factors. Scott's work on the sociology of nothing is relevant here (Scott, 2018). In it, Scott draws a distinction between acts of commission, which occur when we choose to avoid doing or being something either through conscious disengagement or disidentification and acts of omission, which occur when we more passively neglect or fail to act, ending up in another position by default rather than conscious intention.

One of the examples Scott uses for acts of commission is the refusal of medical treatment, but we could, of course, extend that to preventative interventions such as screening. The acts of omission are also of relevance here in the context of those who do not take up the offer of screening. As discussed above, given the possible harms and benefits of screening, participation is increasingly positioned as an informed choice based on consideration of the best available evidence. But there are important questions about how we balance seeking to give people every opportunity to attend with respecting that they have thus far opted not to do so. Do we need some display of an act of commission before we stop seeing people as "fair game" for potential behaviour modification?

Conclusion

This chapter has provided an overview of (predominantly) social science research on screening to date, identifying key themes of scholarship in this area and some of the particular conceptual developments and contributions. The chapter has considered how screening brings inherent uncertainties and the different configuration it suggests for the relationship between doctor and patient, given that screening is distinct from patient-initiated help-seeking. The argument that screening is laden with normative expectations and moral judgements has been considered, alongside the experiences of risk and uncertainty for those participating in and those delivering screening programmes and any follow-on further investigation and treatment. The challenges of evidence generation and evidence use in this area of healthcare have also been considered, including the argument that the initiation and continuation of screening programmes may be, at least in part, politically motivated. The chapter has also considered more recent and ongoing discussions and debates about the potential for harm as well as benefit from screening, including those relating to overdiagnosis and overtreatment, and taken a critical look at the increased emphasis on understanding screening participation as an individual decision based on informed choice, but one that is likely to be in tension with a desire for high rates of screening uptake.

The tension between individual informed choice about screening participation and the ongoing interest in how behavioural science strategies and techniques can be used to encourage people to engage, and therefore increase uptake, is one that perhaps warrants further consideration both in terms of future research but also the implications for policy and practice. Concerns about inequalities in screening uptake are well-founded. Evidence from a number of countries shows that there are disparities in the uptake of different kinds of screening. For example, work from New Zealand on prostate cancer testing of asymptomatic men shows that Māori men had significantly lower rates of screening (Matti, Lyndon, & Zargar-Shoshtari), while a systematic review of uptake of colorectal cancer screening showed that men were less likely to participate in screening and that attendance was higher in the least deprived areas (Mosquera et al., 2020). Given these inequalities in uptake, efforts to make screening more accessible and convenient for those that do want to engage are helpful. However, the question of when facilitating and encouraging participation slips into coercion of those who have made a decision not to participate is an important one. The tension between informed choice and high uptake will no doubt persist while uptake remains a key metric through which the quality of screening is assessed. Consideration of other possible options for assessing quality may be valuable, such as the receipt of offers, individuals' satisfaction with their decision making, or the extent to which decisions made about attendance or non-attendance are congruent with an individual's preferences and values.

References

Armstrong, D. (1983). *Political anatomy of the body*. Cambridge: Cambridge University Press.
Armstrong, D. (1993). Public health spaces and the fabrication of identity. *Sociology, 27*(3), 393–410.
Armstrong, D. (1995). The rise of surveillance medicine. *Sociology of Health and Illness, 17*(3), 393–404.
Armstrong, N. (2005). Resistance through risk: Women and cervical cancer screening. *Health, Risk and Society, 7*(2), 161–176.
Armstrong, N. (2007). Discourse and the individual in cervical cancer screening. *Health: An Interdisciplinary Journal for the Social Study of Health, Illness and Medicine, 11*(1), 69–85.

Armstrong, N. (2014). Screening for disease: Challenges. In William C. Cockerham, Robert Dingwall, and Stella R. Quah (Eds.), *The Wiley-Blackwell encyclopedia of health, illness, behavior, and society*. Wiley Blackwell.

Armstrong, N. (2019). Navigating the uncertainties of screening. *Social Theory and Health*, 17(2), 158–171.

Armstrong, N., & Eborall, H. (2012a). *The sociology of medical screening: Critical perspectives, new directions*. Chichester: Wiley Blackwell.

Armstrong, N., & Eborall, H. (2012b). The sociology of medical screening: Past, present and future. *Sociology of Health and Illness*, 34(2), 161–176. doi:10.1111/j.1467-9566.2011.01441.x

Armstrong, N., James, V., & Dixon-Woods, M. (2012). The role of primary care professionals in women's experiences of cervical cancer screening: A qualitative study. *Family Practice*, 29(4), 462–466. doi:10.1093/fampra/cmr105

Armstrong, N., & Murphy, E. (2008). Weaving meaning? An exploration of the interplay between lay and professional understandings of cervical cancer risk. *Social Science and Medicine*, 67(7), 1074–1082. doi:10.1016/j.socscimed.2008.06.022

Armstrong, N., & Murphy, E. (2012). Conceptualizing resistance. *Health*, 16(3), 314–326. doi:10.1177/1363459311416832

Bish, A., Sutton, S., & Golombok, S. (2000). Predicting uptake of a routine cervical smear test: A comparison of the health belief model and the theory of planned behaviour. *Psychology and Health*, 15(1), 35–50.

Blomberg, K., Forss, A., Ternestedt, B. M., & Tishelman, C. (2009). From "silent" to "heard": Professional mediation, manipulation and women's experiences of their body after an abnormal Pap smear. *Social Science and Medicine*, 68(3), 479–486. doi:10.1016/j.socscimed.2008.11.007

BMJ. (2017). Too much medicine. http://www.bmj.com/too-much-medicine.

Boardman, F. K. (2017). Experience as knowledge: Disability, distillation and (reprogenetic) decision-making. *Social Science & Medicine*, 191, 186–193.

Brett, J., Bankhead, C., Henderson, B., Watson, E., & Austoker, J. (2005). The psychological impact of mammographic screening. A systematic review. *Psycho-Oncology*, 14(11), 917–938. doi:10.1002/pon.904

Burrows, R., Nettleton, S., & Bunton, R. (1995). Sociology and health promotion: Health, risk and consumption under late modernism. *The Sociology of Health Promotion: Critical Analyses of Consumption, Lifestyle and Risk*, 1–9.

Bush, J. (2000). "It's just part of being a woman": Cervical screening, the body and femininity. *Social Science & Medicine*, 50(3), 429–444.

Carter, S. M., Rogers, W., Heath, I., Degeling, C., Doust, J., & Barratt, A. (2015). The challenge of overdiagnosis begins with its definition. *BMJ British Medical Journal*, 350. doi:10.1136/bmj.h869

Castel, R. (1991). From dangerousness to risk. In G. Burchell, C. Gordon, & P. Miller (Eds.), *The Foucault effect* (pp. 281–298). London: Harvester Wheatsheaf.

Chapple, A., Ziebland, S., Hewitson, P., & McPherson, A. (2008). What affects the uptake of screening for bowel cancer using a faecal occult blood test (FOBt): A qualitative study. *Social Science and Medicine*, 66(12), 2425–2435. doi:10.1016/j.socscimed.2008.02.009

Chen, J. Y., Eborall, H., & Armstrong, N. (2014). Stakeholders' positions in the breast screening debate, and media coverage of the debate: A qualitative study. *Critical Public Health*, 24(1), 62–72. doi:10.1080/09581596.2013.788787

Cochrane, A. L., & Holland, W. W. (1971). Validation of screening procedures. *British Medical Bulletin*, 27(1), 3–8. Retrieved from https://www.scopus.com/inward/record.uri?eid=2-s2.0-0014976153&partnerID=40&md5=642cb67676847748f2645d0e79fa8556

Dobrow, M. J., Hagens, V., Chafe, R., Sullivan, T., & Rabeneck, L. (2018). Consolidated principles for screening based on a systematic review and consensus process. *Cmaj*, 190(14), E422–e429. doi:10.1503/cmaj.171154

Forss, A., Tishelman, C., Widmark, C., & Sachs, L. (2004). Women's experiences of cervical cellular changes: An unintentional transition from health to liminality? *Sociology of Health and Illness*, 26(3), 306–325. doi:10.1111/j.1467-9566.2004.00392.x

Gale, N. K., Thomas, G. M., Thwaites, R., Greenfield, S., & Brown, P. (2016). Towards a sociology of risk work: A narrative review and synthesis. *Sociology Compass*, 10(11), 1046–1071. doi:10.1111/soc4.12416

Gillespie, C. (2012). The experience of risk as "measured vulnerability": Health screening and lay uses of numerical risk. *Sociology of Health and Illness*, 34(2), 194–207. doi:10.1111/j.1467-9566.2011.01381.x

Gillespie, C. (2015). The risk experience: The social effects of health screening and the emergence of a proto-illness. *Sociology of Health and Illness*, 37(7), 973–987. doi:10.1111/1467-9566.12257

Gray, J. M. (2004). New concepts in screening. *British Journal of General Practice*, 54(501), 292–298.

Green, E. E., Thompson, D., & Griffiths, F. (2002). Narratives of risk: Women at midlife, medical "experts" and health technologies. *Health, Risk and Society, 4*(3), 273–286. doi:10.1080/1369857021000016632

Green, J. (2004). The new public health. In J. Gabe, M. Bury, & M. A. Elston (Eds.), *Key concepts in medical sociology* (pp. 233–237). London: SAGE.

Griffiths, F., Green, E., & Bendelow, G. (2006). Health professionals, their medical interventions and uncertainty: A study focusing on women at midlife. *Social Science and Medicine, 62*(5), 1078–1090. doi:10.1016/j.socscimed.2005.07.027

Grob, R. (2008). Is my sick child healthy? Is my healthy child sick?: Changing parental experiences of cystic fibrosis in the age of expanded newborn screening. *Social Science and Medicine, 67*(7), 1056–1064. doi:10.1016/j.socscimed.2008.06.003

Gummersbach, E., Piccoliori, G., Oriol Zerbe, C., Altiner, A., Othman, C., Rose, C., & Abholz, H. H. (2010). Are women getting relevant information about mammography screening for an informed consent: A critical appraisal of information brochures used for screening invitation in Germany, Italy, Spain and France. *European Journal of Public Health, 20*(4), 409–414. doi:10.1093/eurpub/ckp174

Heath, I. (2014). Role of fear in overdiagnosis and overtreatment-an essay by Iona Heath. *BMJ (Online), 349*. doi:10.1136/bmj.g6123

Hersch, J., Jansen, J., & McCaffery, K. (2016). Informed and shared decision making in breast screening. In *Breast cancer screening: An examination of scientific evidence* (pp. 403–420).

Heyman, B., Hundt, G., Sandall, J., Spencer, K., Williams, C., Grellier, R., & Pitson, L. (2006). On being at higher risk: A qualitative study of prenatal screening for chromosomal anomalies. *Social Science and Medicine, 62*(10), 2360–2372. doi:10.1016/j.socscimed.2005.10.018

Hicks, L. K. (2015). Reframing overuse in health care: Time to focus on the harms. *Journal of Oncology Practice, 11*(3), 168–170. doi:10.1200/jop.2015.004283

Howson, A. (1998). Surveillance, knowledge and risk: The embodied experience of cervical screening. *Health, 2*(2), 195–215.

Howson, A. (1999). Cervical screening, compliance and moral obligation. *Sociology of Health and Illness, 21*(4), 401–425.

Jepson, R., Clegg, A., Forbes, C., Lewis, R., Sowden, A., & Kleijnen, J. (2000). The determinants of screening uptake and interventions for increasing uptake: A systematic review. *Health Technology Assessment, 4*(14), i–vii+1–123

Kavanagh, A. M., & Broom, D. H. (1998). Embodied risk: My body, myself? *Social Science and Medicine, 46*(3), 437–444.

Lotto, R., Armstrong, N., & Smith, L. K. (2016). Care provision during termination of pregnancy following diagnosis of a severe congenital anomaly – A qualitative study of what is important to parents. *Midwifery, 43*, 14–20. doi:10.1016/j.midw.2016.10.003

Lotto, R., Smith, L. K., & Armstrong, N. (2018). Diagnosis of a severe congenital anomaly: A qualitative analysis of parental decision-making and the implications for healthcare encounters. *Health Expectations, 21*, 678–684.

Lupton, D. (1995). *The imperative of health*. London: SAGE.

Markens, S., Browner, C. H., & Mabel Preloran, H. (2010). Interrogating the dynamics between power, knowledge and pregnant bodies in amniocentesis decision making. *Sociology of Health and Illness, 32*(1), 37–56. doi:10.1111/j.1467-9566.2009.01197.x

Marmot, M., Altman, D. G., Cameron, D. A., Dewar, J. A., Thompson, S. G., & Wilcox, M. (2012). The benefits and harms of breast cancer screening: An independent review. *The Lancet, 380*(9855), 1778–1786. doi:10.1016/S0140-6736(12)61611-0

Marteau, T. M., Mann, E., Toby Prevost, A., Vasconcelos, J. C., Kellar, I., Sanderson, S., … Kinmonth, A. L. (2010). Impact of an informed choice invitation on uptake of screening for diabetes in primary care (DICISION): Randomised trial. *BMJ (Online), 340*(7757), 1176. doi:10.1136/bmj.c2138

Matti, B., Lyndon, M., & Zargar-Shoshtari, K. Ethnic and socio-economic disparities in prostate cancer screening: Lessons from New Zealand. *BJU International*. doi:https://doi.org/10.1111/bju.15155

McCaffery, K., Borril, J., Williamson, S., Taylor, T., Sutton, S., Atkin, W., & Wardle, J. (2001). Declining the offer of flexible sigmoidoscopy screening for bowel cancer: A qualitative investigation of the decision-making process. *Social Science and Medicine, 53*(5), 679–691. doi:10.1016/S0277-9536(00)00375-0

McKie, L. (1995). The art of surveillance or reasonable prevention? The case of cervical screening. *Sociology of Health and Illness, 17*(4), 441–457.

Mosquera, I., Mendizabal, N., Martín, U., Bacigalupe, A., Aldasoro, E., Portillo, I., & Group, f. t. D. (2020). Inequalities in participation in colorectal cancer screening programmes: A systematic review. *European Journal of Public Health, 30*(3), 558–567. doi:10.1093/eurpub/ckz236

Moynihan, R., Doust, J., & Henry, D. (2012). Preventing overdiagnosis: How to stop harming the healthy. *BMJ British Medical Journal, 344.* doi:10.1136/bmj.e3502

Neilson, A., & Jones, R. K. (1998). Women's lay knowledge of cervical cancer/cervical screening: Accounting for non-attendance at cervical screening clinics. *Journal of Advanced Nursing, 28*(3), 571–575.

Nettleton, S. (1995). *The sociology of health and illness.* Cambridge: Polity Press.

Nettleton, S., & Bunton, R. (1995). Sociological critiques of health promotion. *The Sociology of Health Promotion,* 41–59.

Norman, P., & Conner, M. (1992). Health checks in general practice: The patient's response. *Family Practice, 9*(4), 481–487. doi:10.1093/fampra/9.4.481

Orbell, S., 'Sullivan, I., Parker, R., Steele, B., Campbell, C., & Weller, D. (2008). Illness representations and coping following an abnormal colorectal cancer screening result. *Social Science and Medicine, 67*(9), 1465–1474. doi:10.1016/j.socscimed.2008.06.039

Pathirana, T., Clark, J., & Moynihan, R. (2017). Mapping the drivers of overdiagnosis to potential solutions. *BMJ, 358,* j3879. doi:10.1136/bmj.j3879

Petersen, A., & Lupton, D. (1996). The new public health: Health and self in the age of risk. *The New Public Health: Health and Self in the Age of Risk.*

Pfeffer, N. (2004). Screening for breast cancer: Candidacy and compliance. *Social Science & Medicine, 58,* 151–160.

Pienaar, K., Petersen, A., & Bowman, D. M. (2019). Matters of fact and politics: Generating expectations of cancer screening. *Social Science & Medicine, 232,* 408–416. doi:10.1016/j.socscimed.2019.05.020

Pilnick, A. (2008). "It's something for you both to think about": Choice and decision making in nuchal translucency screening for Down's syndrome. *Sociology of Health and Illness, 30*(4), 511–530. doi:10.1111/j.1467-9566.2007.01071.x

Pilnick, A., & Zayts, O. (2012). "Let's have it tested first": Choice and circumstances in decision-making following positive antenatal screening in Hong Kong. *Sociology of Health and Illness, 34*(2), 266–282. doi:10.1111/j.1467-9566.2011.01425.x

Pilnick, A., & Zayts, O. (2014). "It's just a likelihood": Uncertainty as topic and resource in conveying "positive" results in an antenatal screening clinic. *Symbolic Interaction, 37*(2), 187–208. doi:10.1002/symb.99

Priaulx, J., Turnbull, E., Heijnsdijk, E., Csanádi, M., Senore, C., de Koning, H. J., & McKee, M. (2020). The influence of health systems on breast, cervical and colorectal cancer screening: An overview of systematic reviews using health systems and implementation research frameworks. *Journal of Health Services Research & Policy,* 1355819619842314. doi:10.1177/1355819619842314

Raffle, A. E. (2001). Information about screening – Is it to achieve high uptake or to ensure informed choice? *Health Expectations, 4*(2), 92–98.

Raffle, A. E., Mackie, A., & Gray, J. A. M. (2019). *Screening: Evidence and Practice.* Oxford: Oxford University Press.

Schwennesen, N., & Koch, L. (2012). Representing and intervening: "doing" good care in first trimester prenatal knowledge production and decision-making. *Sociology of Health & Illness, 34*(2), 283–298. doi:10.1111/j.1467-9566.2011.01414.x

Scott, S. (2018). A sociology of nothing: Understanding the unmarked. *Sociology, 52*(1), 3–19. doi:10.1177/0038038517690681

Stephenson, N., Mills, C., & McLeod, K. (2017). "Simply providing information": Negotiating the ethical dilemmas of obstetric ultrasound, prenatal testing and selective termination of pregnancy. *Feminism and Psychology, 27*(1), 72–91. doi:10.1177/0959353516679688

Sturdy, S., Miller, F., Hogarth, S., Armstrong, N., Chakraborty, P., Cressman, C., … Zappa, M. (2020). Half a century of Wilson & Jungner: Reflections on the governance of population screening [version 2; peer review: 3 approved]. *Wellcome Open Research, 5*(158). doi:10.12688/wellcomeopenres.16057.2

Thomas, G. M. (2014). Prenatal screening for Down's syndrome: Parent and healthcare practitioner experiences. *Sociology Compass, 8*(6), 837–850. doi:10.1111/soc4.12185

Thornton, H. (2012). Re: Breast screening is beneficial, panel concludes, but women need to know about harms (rapid response). *British Medical Journal, 345.*

Timmermans, S., & Buchbinder, M. (2012). Expanded newborn screening: Articulating the ontology of diseases with bridging work in the clinic. *Sociology of Health and Illness, 34*(2), 208–220. doi:10.1111/j.1467-9566.2011.01398.x

Todorova, I. L. G., Baban, A., Balabanova, D., Panayotova, Y., & Bradley, J. (2006). Providers' constructions of the role of women in cervical cancer screening in Bulgaria and Romania. *Social Science and Medicine, 63*(3), 776–787. doi:10.1016/j.socscimed.2006.01.032

von Wagner, C., Hirst, Y., Waller, J., Ghanouni, A., McGregor, L. M., Kerrison, R. S., … Stoffel, S. T. (2019). The impact of descriptive norms on motivation to participate in cancer screening – Evidence from online experiments. *Patient Education and Counseling, 102*(9), 1621–1628. doi:10.1016/j.pec.2019.04.001

Ward, P. R., Coffey, C., & Meyer, S. (2015). Trust, choice and obligation: A qualitative study of enablers of colorectal cancer screening in South Australia. *Sociology of Health and Illness, 37*(7), 988–1006. doi:10.1111/1467-9566.12280

Wardle, J., Williamson, S., McCaffery, K., Sutton, S., Taylor, T., Edwards, R., & Atkin, W. (2003). Increasing attendance at colorectal cancer screening: Testing the efficacy of a mailed, psychoeducational intervention in a community sample of older adults. *Health Psychology, 22*(1), 99–105. doi:10.1037/0278-6133.22.1.99

Wegwarth, O., Schwartz, L. M., Woloshin, S., Gaissmaier, W., & Gigerenzer, G. (2012). Do physicians understand cancer screening statistics? A national survey of primary care physicians in the United States. *Annals of Internal Medicine, 156*(5), 340–349. Retrieved from https://www.scopus.com/inward/record.uri?eid=2-s2.0-84857724590&partnerID=40&md5=4f44f8265c0ad4c7976577ff0616457b

Welch, H. G., Schwartz, L. M., & Woloshin, S. (2011). *Overdiagnosed: Making people sick in the pursuit of health.* Boston: Beacon Press.

Williams, C., Sandall, J., Lewando-Hundt, G., Heyman, B., Spencer, K., & Grellier, R. (2005). Women as moral pioneers? Experiences of first trimester antenatal screening. *Social Science and Medicine, 61*(9), 1983–1992. doi:10.1016/j.socscimed.2005.04.004

Wilson, J. M. G., & Jungner, G. (1968). Principles and practice of screening for disease. *Public Health Papers 34*. Geneva: World Health Organization.

Zapka, J. G., Geller, B. M., Bulliard, J. L., Fracheboud, J., Sancho-Garnier, H., & Ballard-Barbash, R. (2006). Print information to inform decisions about mammography screening participation in 16 countries with population-based programs. *Patient Education and Counseling, 63*(1–2), 126–137. doi:10.1016/j.pec.2005.09.012

9

PERSONALISED MEDICINE

Michael Morrison and Susan Kelly

Introduction

Personalised medicine can be understood as a concept, a label or brand, and a set of promissory, future-orientated visions of how technologies might transform medical practice. The exact meaning of "personalised medicine" varies over time and in different contexts. It has been associated with a range of different technologies from genetic testing, to whole-genome sequencing, "big data", and even stem cell science. It is discussed in policy documents, peer-reviewed articles in the scientific and medical literature, at conferences, and in the popular press, where it has been accompanied by a range of related, parallel labels, including pharmacogenetics, stratified medicine, and precision medicine (Hedgecoe, 2004; Erikainnen & Chan, 2019). Personalised, and latterly "precision", medicine appears in the branding and mission statements of commercial companies and cancer care centres alike, is the stated topic and purpose of scientific consortia, major infrastructure building initiatives, national innovation policies, and increasingly of partnerships between public and private sector organisations to deliver healthcare.

The purpose of promissory discourse about science, technology, or medicine is to stimulate and coordinate collective action in the present by providing an account of a desirable future and a "roadmap" for how to get there. Although intended to drive investment of time, capital, and labour in new technologies and research endeavours, these visions are typically bigger than any specific technology. At its core, the contemporary notion of personalised medicine is one of ever more finely grained stratification of "messy" heterogeneous patient populations into small, tightly defined groups – or at the extreme perhaps even individuals – whose prognosis and response to a range of available treatments can be predicted with increasing accuracy. The "personal" here does not refer to an individual's situated socioeconomic and cultural needs, but to the quantified "person" defined in terms of biological and digital data. Much of the promissory force of personalised medicine lies in the cultural authority granted to quantitative data and mechanical calculation, but its attraction lies in its appeal to the interests of different groups.

Promissory visions like personalised medicine tend to be ambiguous and interpretively flexible, allowing them to promise different things to different people, the better to promote collective action (Tarkkala, Helén, & Snell, 2019; Hoyer, 2019). For industry, the value of prediction is orientated to drug discovery and development, promising more efficient, better-targeted, and therefore less expensive research and development processes and improved profitability. For clinicians there is the promise of more accurate diagnosis and treatment with fewer side effects, based on the idea that more data means more objective classification, a notion alluded to in the term "precision medicine" (Erikainen & Chan, 2019). Policymakers and healthcare funders hope that a more predictive medicine will reduce healthcare costs by enabling more people to stay healthy and avoiding the expense of managing chronic diseases. Universities, companies, and national governments alike aspire to establish international leadership and competitive advantage in a new and emerging marketplace for personalised medicine products and services.

For patients and the public, there is the somewhat nebulous promise of "better medicine" with the corollary that "personalised medicine" can evoke, albeit spuriously, more patient-centred, holistic forms of medical practice (Budin-Ljosne & Harris, 2016; Tutton, 2014). At the same time, discourses of personalised medicine also require a particular moral orientation of individuals. The responsible person – and often in national projects the "good citizen" – is obliged to make data about themselves knowable and accessible to researchers and to act upon the recommendations made in light of this information to improve, protect and sustain their health.

The idea of personalised medicine is thus a force for scientific, social, organisational, and economic change. Attempting to realise the promise of personalised care requires new infrastructures, professional roles, data collection and curation practices, invokes new moral and social responsibilities, obligations, ideas of care, personhood, and ways of living. Enthusiasm for personalised medicine initiatives runs the usual risk of hype triumphing over hope, of significant, often public sector, expenditure for limited genuine public benefit, but there are other concerns too. The data-intensive nature of much current personalised or precision medicine raises the spectre of new forms of surveillance, inequality, discrimination, exploitation, and a loss of accountability. This chapter traces the origins of the contemporary notion of personalisation, the technologies, and practices now associated with the labels and explores the underlying contradictions and dangers.

History of personalisation

Among the many systems or "cosmologies" of medical knowledge preceding clinical biomedicine (see Chapter 1, this volume), "personalisation" is most closely identifiable with what Jewson (1976) describes as "bedside medicine". Here, disease was understood as encompassing physiological, mental, and environmental aspects of the individual patient. Treatment rested as much on the personal rapport between physician and patient as on material intervention. By contrast, the medicine of the clinic, and increasingly the laboratory, which emerged in the 18th and 19th centuries, viewed diseases as discrete entities existing independently of any particular manifestation in the body of an individual patient (Foucault, 1973). Diagnosis operationalised this by classifying patients into disease categories (see Chapter 7, this volume). To fit individuals into groups, the assessment needed to focus more on what was the same about each patient, not on what was unique. Individuals' self-reported symptoms were supplanted by standardised measurements and categorisations such as age, height, race, gender, or physical signs of disease.

Standardisation renders individuals comparable, but also allows for differentiation on the basis of categories, or "types" of person. Here, medicine was in step with wider state projects of a bureaucratic management of populations. This is especially clear in public health (and the insurance industry), where the application of statistics used detailed bureaucratic records of the present to make probabilistic calculations about the future. In essence, knowing how many individuals belonging to the category "A" have been diagnosed with disease "B" allows calculation of how likely an individual assigned to category "A" is to be diagnosed with disease "B" in future. The "personal" was reconfigured as the assignment of individuals to a set of standardised bureaucratic categories and associated calculations of disease risk. As this version of medicine became institutionalised in hospitals and the apparatus of public health during the 19th and 20th centuries, there were occasional counter-movements, pushing for a return to more holistic notions of medicine, which charged that ever more rationalised, technology-orientated health-care was resulting in an "impersonalised medicine", with limited scope for relations of interpersonal care between doctors and their patients (Tutton, 2014).

The reification of broad disease categories also paved the way for mass production of pharmaceuticals targeted at the standardised "typical patient" (Tutton, 2014, and see also Chapter 4, this volume). This model of mass-produced "blockbuster" drugs was very successful, despite the reality that many drugs designed for the "average" patient often do not work for all patients in a given disease category, and in some cases actually produce harms. Towards the end of the 20th century, falling numbers of innovative new drugs coming to market and threats to the profitability of the pharmaceutical industry gave rise to new currents of "personalisation" (Hedgecoe, 2004). Dumit (2012) reported that pharmaceutical marketing increasingly encouraged individual consumers to internalise disease risk calculations, such as "high" cholesterol levels or blood pressure, as personal moral responsibilities, to be discharged by buying products and services to prevent future ill health.

Elsewhere, advances in genetics, especially the Human Genome Project (1990–2003), gave rise to the idea that patients might be stratified into groups of "good responders" and "poor responders" to drugs on the basis of genetic markers (Hedgecoe, 2004). Drugs at risk of being taken off the market, or of failing to get regulatory approval, because of a high incidence of adverse responses might be "rescued" if they could be found to work well in a genetically-defined subset of patients, while new drugs in development might be targeted at patient populations defined by genetic markers indicating a positive response, even if these new ways to define the target population cut across existing disease categories. A variety of terms was used to describe and promote this new model. "Pharmacogenetics" a term first coined in the 1950s, was popularised, and was also rebranded "pharmacogenomics", both abbreviated as "PGx" (Hedgecoe, 2003) Other terms included stratified medicine, tailor-made medicine, "getting the right drug to the right person", and most notably "personalised medicine" (Tutton, 2014).

Since then, a number of PGx tests have been developed, mainly, though not exclusively, for existing drugs. Verbelen, Weale, and Lewis (2017) report that the US Food and Drug Administration (FDA) lists 137 associations between genetic variants and drugs that have so far been incorporated into the prescribing advice labels issued with FDA-approved pharmaceuticals. However, the wider "pharmacogenomic revolution" predicted by some commentators has largely failed to materialise. There are a number of reasons for this. Many gene-drug associations relied on genetic studies done in primarily white, Western cohorts, so their results are not always valid in other populations. Only some variation in response to pharmaceuticals is due to simple genetic variants, and many variants only explain some proportion of observed variability in drug response, reducing their clinical utility. The economic case for PGx tests has also been patchy; Verbelen, Weale, and Lewis (2017) found that some PGx tests had several published cost–benefit analyses, although these were not always in agreement, while others had not been evaluated at all. There were also questions about whether physicians actually read the PGx advice on drug labels and whether pharmaceutical companies would risk fragmenting the market for a potential new "blockbuster" drug by introducing a PGx test, or whether testing would be reserved for "failing" products (Martin & Morrison, 2006).

In addition, PGx tests stratify users into a limited number of groups, usually "normal" and "poor" responders. In terms of "tailoring" medical treatment to individuals this, as Hedgecoe has remarked, "is more a case of buying a small, medium or large T-shirt from the Gap than being fitted for a Saville row suit" (2004, p. 5). This exposes some of the discrepancies between the promise of personalisation, which evokes a lost ideal of holistic personal care, and the reality of PGx as an additional or alternative measure for assigning people to groups in the course of medical treatment.

Nonetheless, the concept or "brand" of personalisation was sufficiently attractive that it was adopted and adapted for other technologies and practices, even as the limitations of pharmacogenetic testing gradually became apparent. BiDil, a treatment for congestive heart failure, was often described as a "personalised medicine" because its FDA approval controversially limited the drug's use to African American patients. Although there was no genetic test associated with BiDil, it was associated with PGx because "scientific and popular accounts … implicated genetic explanations for the efficacy of the drug in African Americans" (Tutton et al., 2008, p. 465), providing an early example of the recurring concern that the new genetics, and later genomics, might give renewed credibility to ideas of a biological basis for racial differences.

Another practice marketed as a "personalised therapy" was the collection and storage of umbilical cord blood. Cord blood contains stem cells similar to those in bone marrow, and parents were encouraged to pay for the collection and storage of this material on the grounds that it might one day be a source of immune-compatible material for cell therapies for their new-born child. Here "personalisation" combines biological differentiation on the basis of immunology (Brown, Machin, & McLeod, 2011) with the "personal" domain of private transactions between individuals and cord blood banking companies, operating in clear distinction to the ethos of donation for *public* benefit evident in some public cord blood banks and national blood donation programmes (Dickenson, 2013).

Technologies of personalised medicine

Biomedical technologies have been deeply implicated in the notion of personalised medicine, from genomics to stem cell therapies, "big data" driven algorithms, and systems biology. As with historic examples, from the stethoscope to X-rays, the novel capacities offered by technologies do not mandate any particular organisation of medical care, nor do they determine relationships between physicians and patients, but they do provide an impetus and a focal point for projects of reorganisation and reordering. Medical technology, with its links to the underlying idea of technological progress, is deeply linked to the political economy of hope that drives and sustains so much societal activity and investment in contemporary biomedicine (Delvecchio-Good, 2001). As novel technologies like genomics, and research fields like big data or systems medicine, develop they become enrolled in particular promissory narratives, which in turn shape further processes of development. In this way medical technologies do not determine the future of healthcare, but rather have particular futures, and the values that inform them, scripted into the technologies and research fields.

The human genome is the map of one's DNA, the double helix that contains all of one's genes. Genomics signals the movement away from single-gene testing and the identification of relatively simple gene-phenotype associations to studies of the whole genome, including how sections of the genome interact, are silenced, and are expressed. Genomics is driven by increasing understanding of the human genome and by technology; that is, by the increasing ability to understand how the genome is put together and by the increasing ability to study it quickly and cheaply. In many ways, "genomics" is a successor to pharmacogenomics, in that it aims to overcome the limitations of gene-association studies by using bigger and more complex data sets. That means, of course, drawing more and more people into the research enterprise to accomplish large-scale genome-wide association studies, and the integration of other "omics" into our knowledge of the human genome and its variations.

These other "omic" technologies (proteomics, metabolomics, transcriptomics, proteomics, microbiomics, epigenomics, etc.) further increase the scope and scale of biological data to be correlated with physiological (and sometimes social and behavioural) outcomes by measuring additional molecules such as proteins, or ribonucleic acids (RNA), other entities such as micro-organisms that live in the human gut, and modifications to DNA that activate or "silence" some genes (known as "epigenetics"). In terms of "precision medicine", the integration of multiple "omics" into our understanding of the individual has so far largely been through the promises of systems biology, or systems medicine. In a similar fashion, stem cell technology is also giving a new lease of promissory life to the idea of PGx screening. Induced pluripotent stem cell technology creates stem cells from ordinary blood or skin samples. These can produce an array of tissue types, from heart muscle to liver cells, and even three-dimensional tissue clusters called "organoids", all with the original donor's DNA. It is hoped that using "personal" cells and tissues to test for adverse responses to drugs will have greater predictive power than the single-gene markers of earlier PGx (Shi et al., 2016).

A growing number of large-scale "big science" (Davies, Frow, & Leonelli, 2013) projects in different countries are attempting to support – and drive – the development and clinical application of "personalised" or "precision" medicine technologies. Examples include the 100,000 Genomes project in the UK, the Precision Medicine Initiative in the USA, the Tohoku Medical Megabank in Japan, and the European Bank for induced pluripotent Stem Cells (Minari et al., 2018). Genomics is clearly central to these visions of personalisation, but many projects also collect multiple information types, building large integrated data sets for future personalised medicine systems (Green, Carusi, & Hoyer, 2019).

In addition, small scale "personalisation" in the form of commercial digitally-available individual genomes, whether purchased for health (Harris, Kelly, & Wyatt 2016), ancestry, love, or other reasons (Phillips, 2016) mean that millions of individuals have their "own" genetic code at their fingertips. This genomic data in particular is often presented as "raw" data, giving unmediated and thus unbiased access to the (genetic) truth of identity and risk status. However, the very idea of "raw" data is a misnomer, as all information is the product of methodologies, practices of collection, organisation, and interpretation, and of ontological assumptions about what it is that is even capable of being captured as "data" in the first place (Gitelman, 2013). The obfuscation of the produced nature of data lends a compelling but flawed appeal to personalised genomic data as a means to "know oneself". There exist on the internet ways of mining these individual genomes for "personal" information, from Promethease to DNA Land to Nutrahacker, providing individual reports based on the data submitted, and, in some cases, surveys relating to individual behaviours. Most of these require some technical know-how in order to gain knowledge of one's personal results. Providing reports may not be the only business model being followed by these companies; the databases of customers containing both DNA and survey results have been sold for large sums (Harris, Kelly, & Wyatt, 2016).

One challenge, where genomics echoes the previous limitations of PGx, is that much of the research on "human genomics" has been done on Western, largely white, populations (Currie et al., 2006). This has the effect of limiting our knowledge to that of genomic variation in the referent population, leaving other groups under-represented and limiting the usefulness of the data produced. In short, if we take seriously the origin of much of our knowledge of the frequency and effects of genomic variation identified through whole-genome sequencing, we know more about the population to whose genomes we have access to than we do about the "human genome". This matters when we "personalise" medicine.

Significant political investment in personalised medicine by regional and national govern-ments is underpinned by the multi-faceted promise that such endeavours will bring patient benefit, reduce long-term health expenditure, transform organisational arrangements and build infrastructure, and provide opportunities for industrial and economic development (Samuel & Farsides, 2017; Hoyer, 2019; Tarkkala, Helén, & Snell, 2019). This includes the aspiration to stimulate the growth of new genomics and big data companies at the local and national level, and the hope that building large, high-quality data resources will attract investment from major multinational pharmaceutical and IT firms who will pay for access. It is therefore unsurprising that many personalised or precision medicine programmes involve partnerships between public sector healthcare organisations and private companies, including the 100k Genomes project, the European Bank for induced pluripotent Stem Cells, and the Wellcome Trust collaboration with AstraZeneca to collect and analyse genomic data and health records from 2 million research participants.

In addition to the aspirations of states to promote economic growth, private sector organi-sations are increasingly seen as the only actors with sufficient expertise to process and develop machine-learning tools for the mass of public sector data. Not only traditional pharmaceutical and medical device firms, but increasingly "big tech" players like IBM, Google, Apple, and Amazon are entering the health sphere to provide personalised medicine services (Powles & Hodson, 2017; Sharon, 2018; Zwart, 2016). This move represents a convergence with broader trends of large-scale processing of data by algorithms and machine-learning processes in sec-tors beyond healthcare. Ideas of "personalisation" and data-driven profiling that surface in the tailored (i.e. correlation-based) recommendations made to Amazon shoppers, targeted online advertisements, or the selection of news stories presented to individual social media users, have infused medical and healthcare contexts through the existing discourses of per-sonalised and precision medicine. This has raised fears about privacy, confidentiality of sen-sitive medical information, private enclosure of health data through intellectual property rights, profiling of patients as customers through "shadow health records" to enable targeted advertising, and potential bias and lack of accountability in algorithms developed for medical decision-making (Powles & Hodson, 2017; Sharon, 2018). "Shadow health records" are health information, including profiles of individuals, derived from sources not covered by traditional legal protections for health data, such as information derived from fitness trackers or social media posts, and de-identified health data combined with other, identifying, information from non-protected datasets. Nonetheless, the political impetus behind various personalised medicine programmes has meant that these concerns have been given limited credence from state actors to date.

Areas of application

In contrast to some of the rhetoric, applications of personalised medicine are not evenly dis-tributed. Personalisation of one form or another is most evident in the clinical areas of cancer, rare disease, cardiology, and public health. Most of the "big science" genomics projects described above incorporate cancer and rare disease cohorts. Rare disease is a collective label for a wide range of mainly genetic, usually childhood-onset, conditions that each only occur very infre-quently in the population. Symptoms are often non-specific, such as developmental delay or learning difficulties, while their scarcity means most rare diseases are unfamiliar to physicians. Here the main benefit of genome sequencing is diagnostic, allowing clinicians to finally "put a name" to the condition and end the "diagnostic odyssey" of patients and their families (see Chapter 7). Projects such as the 100,000 genomes study frequently report instances of successful diagnoses of a rare paediatric disease as "good news stories", to illustrate and promote the benefits of clinical whole-genome sequencing. At the same time, extrapolating from rare disease populations can mask a lack of robust evidence for the clinical, economic and personal benefits of expanding the routine provision of whole-genome sequencing to broader populations. The UK House of Commons Science and Technology Committee report "Genomics and genome editing in the NHS" noted that:

> Despite the apparent importance of the 100,000 Genomes Project as a source of evidence on the clinical and cost-effectiveness of whole-genome sequencing, [the NHS England representative] could not say whether there were plans for a formal evaluation of the 100,000 Genomes Project.
>
> *(Science and Technology Committee, 2018, p. 18)*

Despite the committee's recommendations that a formal evaluation is carried out, there has, to date, been no publicly available evidence of the projects clinical or cost-benefit utility.

Cancer and cardiac disease, by contrast are major causes of morbidity and mortality among most populations, and a significant economic burden on healthcare systems. Cancer is in many ways the prototype condition for personalised medicine. It is well established as a disease produced by genetic defects, and studied, diagnosed and treated at the molecular level (Fujimura, 1988). In cancer care, the tumour, as much as the patient, was already the object of stratification; by location (breast, colon, prostate, etc.), size, spread, appearance, and other factors (Hedgecoe, 2004; Day et al., 2017). Many of the PGx tests developed to date target cancer. The best known is probably the use of human epidermal growth factor receptor 2 (HER2) levels to determine the suitability of the drug trastuzumab (trade name Herceptin) for breast cancer patients. Tumours with a high level of HER2 respond well to Herceptin, while those with low HER2 levels do not, meaning patients with a HER2 negative tumour are not eligible for the drug. However, as Kimmelman and Tannock (2018) note, Herceptin was approved for women with HER2 positive breast cancers in 1998, but accumulating enough evidence that women with HER2 negative cancers did not receive any significant benefit took a further 20 years of work. This, they argue, illustrates a persistent problem with both PGx and later genomic and data-driven forms of personalisation in cancer care. The stratification into ever smaller patient populations makes it easier to get the evidence of effectiveness needed to get new cancer drugs or decision-making algorithms accepted, but actively disincentivises doing larger, more rigorous follow-up studies to confirm the utility of the approved treatment or tool. In some cases, personalised medicine can actually promote greater uncertainty and a lower quality of evidence for clinical decision-making (Kimmelman & Tannock, 2018).

Nonetheless, the potential of genetic and genomic characterisation and stratification of tumours is well established in clinical care. Ethnographic studies of cancer genetics have illustrated how implementation into routine practice changes both how the technology is understood and operated, and the organisation of clinical care itself (Beaudevin, Peerbaye, & Bourgain, 2019; Day et al., 2017). Moreover, Day et al. (2017) have suggested that personalised medicine strategies can be a catalyst for *other kinds of stratification* of healthcare, as different steps of the cancer care pathway are increasingly parcelled out to different technically-orientated specialisms, which may, in turn be provided through competing public or private service organisations. As further projects aim to implement whole-genome sequencing in routine care, further reorganisation and restructuring can be anticipated.

Whole-genome sequencing has also been proposed as a tool for screening in a public health context. Unlike diagnosis, screening involves systematically testing asymptomatic individuals with the aim of detecting conditions or increased risk of disease in individuals, who can then be followed up with further confirmatory diagnosis and treatment. Genomics-based screening has been proposed for new-born populations, as a prenatal test, using circulating DNA detected in maternal blood, and in adult cancer surveillance programmes, through the technique of polygenic risk-stratified screening. To date these public health technologies have been tested in research settings with limited populations, but are not yet implemented into routine care. As Kerr et al. (2019) note in relation to cancer screening, the proposed changes envisage new roles and responsibilities for both lay participants and professionals, in relation to collecting data, making it available, responding to risk with appropriate behaviours, and accommodating new practices and routines. As with Dumit's (2012) observation on pharmaceutical drug marketing, adopting a moral frame of personal duty, individual responsibility for self-care and maintenance of good health is an important part of this vision.

Similar messages have been reported in other personalised aspects of public health, such as self-monitoring devices and wearable biosensors. A huge variety of self-monitoring tools are available through smartphones and smartwatches (Lupton, 2013), but cardiac care is particularly prominent, through wearable digital devices that monitor everything from amount and extent of exercise, pulse, blood pressure, heart rhythm, and even electrocardiogram readouts. These devices not only move personalised medicine from the clinic into the home, but are also part of the growing market for products whose marketing strongly echoes public health messages of self-surveillance and responsible behaviour (Williams et al., 2020). Direct-to-consumer (DTC) provision of genetic and genomic testing services does something similar for DNA (Saukko, 2018). One of the highest-profile consumer genomics companies is US-based firm 23&Me, whose CEO Anne Wojcicki has been an outspoken advocate of market-based direct provision of healthcare and individual responsibility as the best method to prevent, rather than treat, disease (Hogarth, 2017).

Globally there is a large, though fluctuating, number of DTC genomics companies, providing services ranging from PGx and detecting variants associated with disease risk to nutrition and wellbeing advice, profiling genetic ancestry, detecting genetic relatedness (including paternity testing), assessing athletic, musical and intellectual ability, and even matchmaking (Phillips, 2016). Concerns have been expressed about the quality and scientific validity of many of the DTC genomics services being provided. The US Food and Drug Administration was involved in a much-publicised dispute with 23&Me over regulation of its disease-relevant findings (Hogarth, 2017), and that agency has also taken action against DTC companies providing PGx services (FDA, 2019). However, firms providing "edutainment" genomic services such as ancestry tracing are exempt from the oversight of healthcare regulatory agencies.

There has also been debate about whether the direct provision of information about disease risk would create a "flood" of worried customers turning to doctors and genetic counsellors for advice and reassurance not provided by the companies (Dickenson, 2013). This has not, to any great extent, materialised, perhaps because lay DTC genomics users draw on their existing range of health beliefs and knowledge to interpret the plausibility of DTC results (Harris, Kelly, & Wyatt, 2016), or because many tests are ordered by users who already have some medical or genetic expertise with which to evaluate the credibility of reported findings (Finlay, 2017). However, it does suggest that a divergence between companies' framing of personal responsibility as empowerment and choice, and public health professionals' advocacy of individual responsibility coupled with an appeal to a certain kind of common good, as for example, individuals identified through polygenic risk-stratified screening as being at lower risk are encouraged to accept a lower level of follow-up surveillance and monitoring to free up resources for those with greater need (higher risk) (Kerr et al., 2019).

Imaginaries of personalised medicine

The stated goals of personalised medicine are to use data-driven technologies to develop and drive new approaches to diagnosis, prevention and treatment of disease that take into account individual biological variation. Each step, from pharmacogenomics, to whole-genome sequencing, multi-"omics", and big data-driven medicine, attempts to compensate for the limitations of previous efforts by invoking the power of ever bigger and more complex data sets. Ultimately, the "personal" in personal medicine relates not to the holistic notion of a socio-culturally-situated actor, but the quantified "person" defined in terms of biological and digital data. Personalised medicine in this sense is not a rupture with the disciplinary, measurement-based, object-orientated medicine of the clinic; it is an extension and an intensification of it (Foucault, 1973). Both draw on the cultural authority of quantified measurement and perceived mechanical objectivity; the idea that data expressed in numbers and measurements and calculations made by impersonal rule-following machines capture underlying reality and render the "messy" experienced world amenable to rational calculation and planning (Espesland, 1997; Zwart, 2016).

The aim, whether the data is genomic, proteomic, electronic healthcare records, records of self-surveillance through wearable devices, online shopping habits, or the fusion of all these elements, is to move from the particular (the data given off by individuals) to the general (the pooled set of heterogeneous data on large cohorts and populations) and back to a new formulation of "the individual" as a particular pattern or correlation in this data set, defined by multiple points of measurement and comparison. This quantified, transparent, "data self" is envisaged as the locus for neoliberal "projects of the self"; hence the intense emphasis on "responsibilisation" in personalised and precision medicine discourses. As Zwart (2016, p. 72) observes, "[b]y combining 'static' data (on individualized genome sequences) with 'dynamic' data (on the impact of lifestyle, diet and other characteristics, framed as changeable by individuals), personalized medicine *summons us to invest in self-optimization*". This echoes, and amplifies, the other meaning of personalisation previously noted by Dumit (2012), the assumption of "personal" moral responsibility for managing risk to be undertaken by the informed person or citizen.

As the "datafication" of populations, and the associated subjectivities this is anticipated to create, proliferates, new markets for targeted health products and services are expected to arise. Ultimately, it is through this self-governance that the interconnected promises of personalised medicine for generating "health and wealth" are to be realised.

Challenges, critiques, and responses to personalised medicine

We are concerned with the following challenges to, and critiques of, personalised medicine. Conceptually, we have pointed to personalised medicine's combination of big data and biology as potentially reifying two of the most prevalent modernist essentialisms. The combined cultural authority of mechanical computation and of "the gene" threaten to present the categories and predictions of personalised medicine as unassailable, incontestable truths. This obscures that data collection and correlation requires work, incorporates judgements, and holds potentially hidden biases. There are also concerns about what counts as a valid test and who decides, introducing biases and raising questions of power and voice. As previously discussed, the meaning of many genetic, and later genomic, variants is calculated from reference populations, but these are mainly white Caucasian. This is detrimental to other ethnicities in terms of access and fairness, but also gives a perverse value to collecting "racial" genome sequences, raising the spectre of a scientific re-inscription of race. Racialising trends have been seen even where genetic data was not directly implicated, as with BiDil, and have a particular, disturbing manifestation in the use of genomic ancestry tests to mediate racial ancestry claims (Panofsky & Donovan, 2019).

Combined with the discourse of personal moral responsibility to give away one's data, the power relations and predictive categories produced by personalised medicine have the potential to open up novel currents of surveillance:

> Rather than opening up practices of the Self, allowing individuals to refashion their own lives, the Big Data repositories which provide reference data (i.e. standards for normality) can easily become a ubiquitous electronic panopticon: a molecularized version of the super-ego, the "voice of conscience" of the terabyte age. On a daily basis, computer "monitors" will be telling individuals that they better change their lives in order to optimize somatic functioning, and to live up to health and normalcy standards, and/or to postpone the impacts of unhealthy lifestyles and ageing.
>
> *(Zwart, 2016, pp. 84–85)*

The economic counterpart of this injunction to "know yourself" is to buy new products and services to repair the deficiencies made visible by this surveillance (Dumit, 2012). We have already seen the discourse of "empowered choice" used to promote products from pharmaceutical marketing to cord blood banking and genomic "edutainment" tests of dubious provenance and merit. Beyond simply dubious marketing practices, there is a social cost to the individual responsibilisation for health: we see that it ignores social determinants of health, is harmful to marginalised or vulnerable groups, and requires the ability to "be healthy", which is linked to the ability to act which comes from wealth and social status.

Second, we are concerned with the privatisation of risk. This entails a loss of the power to "choose not to choose" (Kelly, 2009); that is, to choose not to accept a risk label and the biotechnological options that go along with it. We are concerned that risk is becoming politicised as a moral imperative to act, and we have seen how the means to respond to that imperative are not evenly distributed. We are also concerned that personalised medicine reduces social cohesion and promotes the individual above all else; it seems to entail "me medicine" over "we medicine" (Dickenson, 2013). Relatedly, the idea of personalised medicine does not address or make room for "relational autonomy" (Dove et al., 2017). Relational autonomy is a reformulation of the idea of "autonomy" that locates personal identity as constituted (though not determined) through interpersonal relationships and situated in particular cultural and economic contexts (Brahim, 2019). Although the rational, self-determining model of the individual still dominates in many medical and legal accounts of agency and responsibility, calls have been made to adopt a more relational approach in clinical care and medical research (Dove et al., 2017; Brahim, 2019)

Third, we are concerned with issues around privacy, data sharing, discrimination, the private ownership of public data, and so on, which the "big data" era surrounding personalised medicine entails. Many versions of personalised or precision medicine depend on a growing interpenetration of the public and private sectors. It is not coincidental that the responsibilised, quantified citizen of personalised medicine bears many similarities to the rational, self-serving information-rich *homo economicus* of economic theory. Prainsack is among those who have called for a "solidarity" model of bioethics as an alternative to the individualised approach upon which "personalisation" depends (Prainsack & Buyx, 2012). Like "relational autonomy", the notion of solidarity draws on ideas of connectedness and situatedness, signifying "shared practices reflecting a collective commitment to carry 'costs' (financial, social, emotional, or otherwise) to assist others" (Prainsack & Buyx, 2012, p. 346).

Conclusions

The ambition of personalized medicine to ensure a dynamic revision of disease tax-onomies is at odds with requirements for continuity of data, to ensure the preservation and support of existing health systems but also to generate the data sources personal-ized medicine needs. Personalization is dependent on the ability to identify similar patients, which presupposes continuity in the (historical) health records and across sites. Yet, the aim of a highly dynamic taxonomy risks undermining existing practices of data generation and validation, and thereby the very data that personalized diag-nostics need.

(Green, Carusi, & Hoyer, 2019, p. 7)

This quote shows that the requirements of personalisation are at odds with the requirements of health systems, as well as the reliance of personalisation on technological and organisational change. There is an inherent paradox in the idea of a perpetually fluid, updating classification of disease that incorporates a variety of novel types of data, but which is founded on correla-tions with historic data sets that use stable classifications of disease derived from standardised practices of measurement and assessment, which is rarely addressed. In simplified form, if you collect genomic data from people with diabetes and use that information to produce a new way of defining the category of diabetes, some of the people, and the data, collected under the old definition may no longer meet the criteria of the new definition, thus undermining the basis on which the calculation was made in the first place. While governmental policies and editorials in life sciences journals espouse the "big picture" promise of personalised or precision medicine, implementing new technologies and practices of personalisation must play out in heterogene-ous, local contexts, where the outcomes can be hard to predict.

Empirical evidence from the implementation of personalised medicine shows that "person-alisation" is highly complex (Beaudevin et al., 2019; Day et al., 2017), with results more like the lumping, splitting, and reordering of classifications previously seen with the introduction of clinical genetic testing (Featherstone & Atkinson, 2011; Green et al., 2019). These in turn have implications for other aspects of healthcare systems, distant from the clinic, such as reimburse-ment or epidemiology, which are often poorly accounted for in visions of personalised medicine (Green et al., 2019). Further, the political pressure to implement personalisation projects and schemes can limit the capacity of healthcare practitioners themselves to point out the limita-tions of personalised or precision medicine in local practices (Samuel & Farsides, 2017). As has been discussed, we are missing robust evidence of a favourable cost-benefit assessment for many aspects of personalised medicine. Finally, personalisation introduces new uncertainties and can actually lower the quality of evidence for clinical decision-making by disincentivising the col-lection of robust clinical evidence to supplement and verify calculations made on small, often preclinical, data sets (Kimmelman & Tannock, 2018). Nonetheless, these local sites of person-alisation can also be spaces of resistance, co-option, and subversion of the doctrines of person-alised medicine, for example, by actions that support solidarity, recognise relational rather than individual autonomy, or that provide evidence for the limitations of projects of personalisation.

Further sociological research into these specific manifestations of personalised medicine is warranted; the infrastructure building projects, practices of collecting, curating, mobilising, and evaluating the data on which personalisation and precision depend, the lived realities, relation-ships, obligations, and moral and social responsibilities evoked, and of the ideas of personhood and of care that are supported or suppressed by personalised medicine.

Acknowledgements

MM would like to thank Chris Goldsworthy (InSiS, Oxford) for helpful discussions and documents relating to the 100,000 Genomes project.

References

Beaudevin, C., Peerbaye, A., & Bourgain, C. (2019). "It has to become true genetics" Tumour genetics and the division of diagnostic labour in the clinic. *Sociology of Health and Illness, 41*(4), 643–657.

Brahim, O. L. (2019). Reconsidering the "self" in self-management of chronic illness: Lessons from relational autonomy. *Nursing Enquiry, 26*(3), e12292

Brown, N., Machin, L., & McLeod, D. (2011). Immunitary bioeconomy: The economisation of life in the international cord blood market. *Social Science and Medicine, 72*(7), 1115–1122.

Budin-Ljøsne, I., & Harris, J. R. (2016). Patient and interest organizations' views on personalized medicine: A qualitative study. *BMC Medical Ethics*, 17, 28. doi:10.1186/s12910-016-0111-7

Currie, G. P., Lee, D. K., & Liworth, B. J. (2006). Long-acting β_2-agonists in asthma. *Drug Safety, 29*(8), 647–656.

Davies, G., Frow, E., & Leonelli, S. (2013). Bigger, faster, better? Rhetorics and practices of large-scale research in contemporary bioscience. *BioSocieties, 8*(4), 386–396.

Day, S., Coombes, R. C., McGrath-Lone, L., Schoenborn, C., & Ward, H. (2017). Stratified, precision or personalised medicine? Cancer services in the "real world" of a London hospital. *Sociology of Health and Illness, 39*(1), 143–158.

Delvecchio Good, M.-J. (2001). The biotechnical embrace. *Culture, Medicine and Psychiatry, 25*, 395–410.

Dickenson, D. (2013). *Me medicine vs we medicine: Reclaiming biotechnology for the common good.* New York: Columbia University Press.

Dove, E. S., Kelly S. E., Lucivero, F., Machirori, M., Dheensa, S., & Prainsack, B. (2017). Beyond individualism: Is there a place for relational autonomy in clinical practice and research? *Clinical Ethics, 12*(3), 150–165.

Dumit, J. (2012). *Drugs for life: How pharmaceutical companies define our health.* Durham, NC: Duke University Press.

Erikainen, S., & Chan, S. (2019). Contested futures: Envisioning "personalized," "stratified," and "precision" medicine, *New Genetics and Society, 38*(3), 308–330.

Espeland, W. N. (1997). Authority by the numbers: Porter on quantification, discretion, and the legitimation of expertise. *Law & Social Inquiry, 22*, 1107–1133.

Featherstone, K., & Atkinson, P. (2011). *Creating conditions: The making and remaking of a genetic syndrome.* London: Routledge.

Finlay, T. (2017). Testing the NHS: The tensions between personalized and collective medicine produced by personal genomics in the UK, *New Genetics and Society, 36*(3), 227–249.

Foucault, M. (1973). *The birth of the clinic: An archaeology of medical perception.* London: Routledge.

FDA. (2019). FDA issues warning letter to genomics lab for illegally marketing genetic test that claims to predict patients' responses to specific medications. *US Food and Drug Administration News Release*, 4 April 2019, available from https://www.fda.gov/news-events/press-announcements/fda-issues-warning-letter-genomics-lab-illegally-marketing-genetic-test-claims-predict-patients

Fujimura, J. H. (1998). The molecular biological bandwagon in cancer research: Where social worlds meet. *Social Problems,* 35(3), 261–283

Gitelman, L. (Ed.). (2013). *"Raw data" is an oxymoron.* Cambridge, MA: MIT Press.

Green, S., Carusi, A., & Hoyer, K. (2019). Plastic diagnostics: The remaking of disease and evidence in personalised medicine. *Social Science and Medicine* (e-pub ahead of print) *Social Science & Medicine*. https://doi.org/10.1016/j.socscimed.2019.05.023

Harris, A., Kelly, S., & Wyatt, S. (2016). *Cybergenetics: Health genetics and new media.* Abingdon: Routledge.

Hedgecoe, A. (2004). *The politics of personalised medicine: Pharmacogenetics in the clinic.* Cambridge: Cambridge University Press.

Hedgecoe, A. M. (2003). Terminology and the construction of scientific disciplines: The case of pharmacogenomics. *Science, Technology and Human Values, 28*(4), 513–537.

Hogarth, S. (2017). Valley of the unicorns: Consumer genomics, venture capital and digital disruption. *New Genetics and Society, 36*(3), 250–272.

House of Commons Science and Technology Committee. (2018). *Genomics and genome editing in the NHS*. London: House of Commons.

Hoyer, K. (2019). Data as promise: Reconfiguring Danish public health through personalized medicine. *Social Studies of Science, 49*(4), 531–555.

Jewson, N. D. (1976). The disappearance of the sick-man from medical cosmology, 1770–1870. *Sociology, 10*(2), 225–244.

Kelly, S. E. (2009). "Choosing not to choose": Reproductive responses of parents of children with genetic conditions or impairments. *Sociology of Health and Illness, 31*(1), 81–97.

Kerr, A., Broer, T., Ross, E., & Cunningham-Burley, S. (2019). Polygenic risk-stratified screening for cancer: Responsibilization in public health genomics. *Social Studies of Science, 49*(4), 605–626.

Kimmelman, J., & Tannok, I. (2018). Comment: The paradox of precision medicine *Nature Reviews. Clinical Oncology, 15*, 341–342.

Lupton, D. (2013). Quantifying the body: Monitoring and measuring health in the age of mHealth technologies. *Critical Public Health, 23*(4), 393–403.

Martin, P., & Morrison, M. (2006). *Realising the potential of genomic medicine*. London: Royal Pharmaceutical Society of Great Britain.

Minari, J., Brothers, K. B., & Morrison, M. (2018). Tensions in ethics and policy created by National Precision Medicine Programs. *Human Genomics, 12*, 22. doi:10.1186/s40246-018-0151-9.

Panofsky, A., & Donovan, J. (2019). Genetic ancestry testing among white nationalists: From identity repair to citizen science. *Social Studies of Science, 49*(5), 653–681.

Phillips, A. (2016). Only a click away – DTC genetics for ancestry, health, love…and more: A view of the business and regulatory landscape. *Applied & Translational Genomics, 8*, 16–22.

Powles, J., & Hodson, H. (2017). Google DeepMind and healthcare in an age of algorithms. *Health Technology, 7*, 351–367.

Prainsack, B., & Buyx, A. (2012). Solidarity in contemporary Bioethics: Towards a new approach. *Bioethics, 26*(7), 343–350.

Samuel, G. N., & Farsides, B. (2017). The UK's 100,000 Genomes Project: Manifesting policymakers' expectations. *New Genetics and Society, 36*(4), 336–353.

Saukko, P. (2018). Digital health – A new medical cosmology? The case of 23andMe online genetic testing platform. *Sociology of Health and Illness, 40*(8), 1312–1326.

Sharon, T. (2018). When digital health meets digital capitalism, how many common goods are at stake? *Big Data and Society, 5*(2). doi:10.1177%2F2053951718819032

Shi, Y., Inoue, H., Wu, J. C., & Yamanaka, S. (2016). Induced pluripotent stem cell technology: A decade of progress. *Nature Reviews. Drug Discovery, 16*(Feb), 115–130.

Tarkkala, H., Helén, I., & Snell, K. (2019). From health to wealth: The future of personalized medicine in the making. *Futures, 109*, 142–152.

Tutton, R. (2014). *Genomics and the reimagining of personalised medicine*. Farnham: Ashgate.

Tutton, R., Smart, A., Martin, P. A., Ashcroft, R., & Ellison, G. (2008). Genotyping the future: Scientists' expectations about race/ethnicity after BiDil. *Journal of Law, Medicine and Ethics, 36*(3), 464–470.

Verbelen, M., Weale, M. E., & Lewis, C. M. (2017) Cost-effectiveness of pharmacogenetic-guided treatment: Are we there yet? *Pharmacogenomics Journal, 17*, 395–402.

Williams, R., Weiner, K., Henwood, F., & Will, C. (2020). Constituting practices, shaping markets: Remaking healthy living through commercial promotion of blood pressure monitors and scales. *Critical Public Health, 30*(1), 28–40.

Zwart, H. A. E. (2016). The obliteration of life: Depersonalization and disembodiment in the terabyte era. *New Genetics and Society, 35*(1), 69–89.

10

COMPLEMENTARY AND ALTERNATIVE MEDICINE

Kevin Dew and Supuni Liyanagunawardena

Introduction

Complementary and alternative therapeutic approaches have elicited great interest from social scientists. In this chapter we consider the opposing forces of marginalisation and popularisation of Complementary and Alternative Medicine (CAM), and possibilities for integrating CAM and biomedicine. We show how these different forces shaping CAM practices play out in similar and different ways in the West and in non-Western countries, with a focus on South Asia. CAM practices and utilisation are shaped by multiple forces, including scientific and economic drivers, gender issues, nationalism, and colonialism, and also by relations between people and between organisations offering different therapeutic services. Social science interest in CAM has had a focus on processes that have marginalised CAM in relation to biomedicine (Saks, 1995; Starr, 1982; Willis, 1983) and patient and practitioner experiences of CAM use (Sharma, 1992). There is, however, little that looks at the complex interactions between patients, practitioners, organisations, and the state. By exploring the dynamics of CAM practice, we suggest that, in addition to considerations about political manoeuvrings at state level and between different professional bodies, it is the general population, individuals in homes, villages, and cities, who decide how and when to use CAM.

The concept of alternative medicine could only emerge once a reasonably stable form of orthodox medicine was established, and this took place from the 19th century in Europe (Bivins, 2007). As such, alternative medicine can be defined as therapeutic practices that are not part of contemporary orthodox practices. We can consider orthodox medicine as those approaches that state-sanctioned medical doctors are trained to use, and that we find in use in hospitals and the clinics of general practitioners and family physicians, often referred to in the social science literature as biomedicine. This might seem straightforward enough, but such a definition does get messy on closer examination. Some medical practitioners, for example, use therapies that were not part of their medical education, such as acupuncture, naturopathy or homeopathy (Dew, 2001). In some countries medical training may include approaches that are seen as unorthodox in other countries – such as osteopathy in the USA.

Varying definitions of CAM are used by different organisations, such as the World Health Organization, The Cochrane Collaboration, and the US National Center for Complementary and Alternative Medicine (Gale & Mchale, 2015). These definitions position CAM as approaches that are not fully integrated into, or operate outside of, conventional or state-funded medicine, and can include well-established therapeutic systems developed in the Western world, such as osteopathy, chiropractic, and homeopathy, non-Western traditions that have been developed over hundreds or even thousands of years, such as Chinese medicine and Ayurveda, through to folk healing practices passed down through communities, such as spiritual healing. What is considered CAM will vary across different jurisdictions. However CAM is defined, research on its use shows significant increases in its popularity throughout Europe, North America, and Australasia since the 1970s, whether that is measured by consumption of CAM products or consultations with CAM practitioners (Sointu, 2012).

The marginalisation of CAM

As CAM operates in a marginal position outside of state-funded medicine it does not have the status or prestige of biomedicine. Historically the marginal position of CAM has been seen as an outcome of political processes. To summarise and simplify this process (as there is variation in how this played out throughout the world), the medical profession became united in the middle of the 19th century and a whole range of levers were then used to empower the profession in relation to the state and disempower therapeutic regimes and organisations that could challenge it. In the UK, this process of marginalising CAM was given major impetus when the state handed the regulation of the medical profession over to a General Medical Council in 1858. The Council could then determine who was in and who was out of the medical profession. General practitioners and surgeons were in, bone-setters, herbalists, and others were out (Larkin, 1983). In the USA, the subordination of alternative therapeutic practices was strongly influenced by changes in education practices, particularly for homeopathy. Funding support for medical education institutes became based on German education models, with laboratories grounding understandings of disease processes and treatments in anatomy and physiology (Breslaw, 2012). This supported orthodox or conventional approaches to medicine, but not unorthodox ones. In some jurisdictions, alternative practices met a slow and drawn-out death. In the state of Victoria in Australia, legislation was passed in 1908 designed to eliminate competition from trained homoeopathic practitioners, with only one new homoeopathic practitioner allowed per year, effectively undermining the capacity to staff homoeopathic hospitals in that state (Willis, 1983).

In more contemporary times, the subordination of alternative practices has been achieved through additional means. One particularly powerful mechanism has been through the development and impact of the evidence-based medicine movement. The idea of basing medicine on evidence would seem to be common sense; however, sitting at the top of the hierarchy of evidence-based medicine is the evaluation procedure of the randomised double-blind, placebo-controlled trial. This particular type of trial was designed to assess the efficacy of medications, the first trial in 1946 evaluating the use of streptomycin in the treatment of pulmonary tuberculosis (Porter, 2006). Following the fallout from the thalidomide tragedy in the 1950s and 1960s, there was an increased impetus to put in place rigorous procedures for the assessment of potentially toxic pharmaceuticals by clinical trials (Light, 2010). This effort to prevent lethal and dangerous drugs from entering the market was transformed from a test of these drugs to a standard that all therapeutic interventions were expected to meet – even though many therapeutic interventions do not work like drugs and are not as easy to assess as drugs. For example, in the double-blind trial, the person performing the therapeutic act is not supposed to know whether they are giving the patient the real treatment or a placebo treatment. For a surgeon, or for someone who uses spinal manipulation, or for an acupuncturist inserting needles – these all require some level of expertise and technical proficiency, so the person administering the treatment will know if it is the real treatment or some fake version of it. However, something given as a pill can look exactly the same, whether it is an inert substance or a potential remedy. As a consequence of placing this form of trial at the top of the evidential hierarchy, medications based on standard pharmacology are almost the only form of therapeutic intervention that can successfully become evidence-based.

Some alternative therapeutic approaches may have treatments based on something in pill form, such as homeopathy. However, homeopathy's philosophy of diagnosing and prescribing is not the same as that used by orthodox practitioners. Orthodox medical practitioners diagnose a condition, say a migraine, and prescribe a medication that would be the same for all those who have the same condition. As such, it is easy to do a trial on all migraine patients because they would all get the same medication. Homoeopaths diagnose and prescribe on the basis of finding a single remedy that is right for that particular person, not the condition. So, two people with migraine might get different remedies prescribed. This makes it more difficult to conduct a randomised controlled trial because many remedies may be used, not just the one. This does not mean randomised controlled trials are impossible to do; it just makes them much more complicated.

An issue related to this is that conducting randomised controlled trials is a very expensive process and requires the backing of corporations who will look forward to large returns on their investment, which is based on being able to patent pharmaceuticals. Rewards for homoeopathic remedies would not return that investment.

The popularity of CAM

To this point, we have noted some of the reasons – professional, political, methodological, and economic – for the marginalisation of some therapeutic practices that are labelled CAM. There are a range of other influences that promote some of these CAM practices. There has been a growing popularity of alternative therapies since the 1960s, particularly in Anglophone countries (Saks, 2001). A common reason put forward for this rise in popularity of CAM is dissatisfaction with orthodox medicine (Sharma, 1992), particularly in relation to the treatment of chronic conditions (Kelner & Wellman, 1997). To simplify the argument here, there has been something of a shift in disease profiles over the last century or so, from a primary concern with acute infectious diseases to a focus on chronic conditions. This shift is known as the epidemiological transition. Orthodox medicine, particularly with the development of antibiotics, has been particularly good at treating acute infectious disease. However, the very word "chronic" suggests something that is not so easily treated – it is something that is on-going. Therefore, by definition, chronic diseases are diseases that orthodox medicine has not been able to "cure". The different kinds of arthritis and other musculoskeletal problems (sore backs, shoulders, etc.), respiratory conditions like asthma, and intestinal problems ranging from chronic indigestion to Crohn's disease, are just some of the conditions that orthodox medicine struggles with. The argument here is that many people then turn to something else to try to deal with their on-going problems. This does not necessarily mean that orthodox medicine is rejected, but that it might be added to, with research suggesting that where the use of CAM has increased there has been no decline in the use of orthodox medicine (Northcott & Bachynsky, 1993).

The idea of the empowered patient and health consumerism have been suggested as reasons for the increase in the popularity of CAM (Sointu, 2006). The argument here is that shifts in the role of the state from caring for populations to a view that people are responsible for their own health choices and outcomes means that people are more likely to seek out alternatives to conventional medicine (Sointu, 2012). Although a critical analysis of the changes in the rhetoric around state responsibility for its citizens is warranted, this should be considered in relation to the significant proportion of state budgets that are spent on healthcare and the increasing levels of the medicalisation of populations. In other words, the state retains a strong focus on caring for the population, seen in the financial support provided for medical and health services.

Some researchers suggest that there are more philosophical reasons for the use of CAM, such as the rejection of scientific and professional authority (Siahpush, 1998). However, most people who use CAM do not start using it because they believe in the alternative principles of that approach. It seems that most people with chronic conditions take a more pragmatic approach, trying to find something that works. If they find something they perceive to be helpful and continue with that treatment, then they may start to consider the underpinnings of the approach and come to sympathise with those ideas (Sharma, 1992). Or CAM users may find other aspects of the treatment of value, such as the therapist providing positive outcomes beyond symptom relief, taking more time, or providing a sense of "balance" and wellbeing (Jakes & Kirk, 2015). This is captured by one of Kim McLeod's research participants, all of whom were seeing a general practitioner and on antidepressants, stating that after seeing a kinesiologist, she experienced a "massive increase in understanding on every level" (McLeod, 2017, p. 91).

The term medicalisation has been used by sociologists to describe a process in which medicine increasingly dominates our lives under the oversight, or as a result of the influence of, the medical profession and allied institutions (Conrad, 2007; Chapter 3, this volume). The expansion of conditions that are deemed amenable to medical intervention makes it more likely that a proportion of the population will seek out alternative approaches to deal with these conditions. The terms proto-disease and pre-disease, for example, have been coined to describe one aspect of medicalisation. Proto-diseases are new "disorders" that are based on risk profiles where the disease is not present, and symptoms are not felt (Greene, 2005). Proto-diseases can be identified in an ever-growing proportion of the population – as our cholesterol, blood pressure, and glucose levels need to be brought into line. Having high cholesterol may mean you will be prescribed cholesterol-lowering drugs, and now, with a new identity as a person who might suffer future heart disease, you might embark on other therapeutic approaches to reduce your cholesterol, such as consulting a naturopath and changing your diet.

Other trends that promote the use of CAM relate more to the operations of capitalism. Historically CAM practitioners have operated as small businesses with little in the way of state interference. However, by the end of the 20th century, a trend was apparent of CAM practitioners becoming employees of larger companies with, for example, naturopaths being employed by supplement and vitamin companies or even by pharmaceutical companies in Australia (Collyer, 2004). Pharmaceutical companies also distribute CAM products. The expansion of CAM products into supermarkets and pharmacies is a further manifestation of these developments in the corporatisation of CAM.

Capitalist modes of production and distribution also impact on therapeutic practices in non-Western countries. In China, market reforms introduced in the post-Mao period impacted upon the provision of Tibetan medicine. Tibetan medical practices could be provided at a low cost, with many medications produced from locally available materials. The scientific valuation of Tibetan medicine from a biomedical perspective was replaced by an assessment of Tibetan medicine based on its "authenticity"; and its capacity to support economic development goals (Janes, 2002). However, this support of Tibetan medicine reshaped it with the mass manufacture of medicine requiring standardised approaches to diagnosis and treatment. Standardised approaches are in friction with Tibetan healing principles – these have a basis in the principles of karma, with the physician assessing the particular body types of patients that are determined at conception and an outcome of karmic deeds from past lives (Janes, 2002). These global economic imperatives work to reshape Tibetan medicine to a more de-personalised form of treatment (Janes, 2002).

The increasing movement of peoples between countries as colonisers, migrants, refugees, and tourists can also lead to the promotion of CAM, although the CAM practices may also change as a result of these flows of people and ideas (see Chapters 22 and 23, this volume). The expansionary goals and imperialism of European states in the 16th to 18th centuries led to encounters with other healing systems, introducing the possibilities of seeking out forms of treatment that were not available to orthodox medical practitioners (although we need to be cautious about the whole concept of orthodoxy at that time). Some therapeutic offerings aligned well with the use of remedies and preparations based on plant material, a conventional medical approach up until the 20th century. An example is the use of cinchona bark in the treatment of malaria (cinchona bark being a rich source of quinine). Others were more challenging, such as the use of acupuncture (Bivins, 2007). There was no obvious explanation for the effect of acupuncture that would align with 18th-century Western systems of thought.

We have noted how Tibetan medicine has changed in its native land because of neo-liberal economics, but Tibetan medicine has also spread to other parts of the world has taken on other forms. Tibetan medicine was taken to the West by Tibetan migrants, including physicians trained in Tibetan medicine. In the West, Tibetan medicine has the aura of spirituality, but in a context of middle-class ageing populations with chronic conditions desiring ways to sustain health and wellbeing (Janes, 2002). We can then see a contrast in how Tibetan medicine is transformed and used in its place of origin and as it has been exported to new territory. In Tibet, it has become a cheaper option, particularly for the rural poor who have difficulty accessing biomedically focused hospitals and clinics, and in the West it is "principally a privilege of the urban elite" (Janes, 2002, p. 284).

Integrating therapeutic approaches

Orthodox medical practitioners also have an interest in CAM. Conventional medical practitioners, particularly in general practice, refer patients on to complementary therapists, and this appears to be becoming more common (Poynton, Dowell, Dew, & Egan, 2006), and some studies show that nearly half of all nurses use complementary therapies in clinical practice (Shorofi & Arbon, 2010). There has also been the development of what has been termed integrative medicine, where conventional and alternative medical practices may be available through the one clinical practice or even the one clinical practitioner. However, integrative medicine tends to be based on the terms of conventional medicine where, for example, CAM may be added into hospital-based programmes, or CAM can be claimed by conventional medicine if it is shown to pass the rigours of the conventional evidence-based medicine hierarchy (Coulter, 2004). Some medical practitioners claim that CAM practices can be reconfigured in orthodox medical terms and so be legitimately used in medical practice. For example, the needling used in acupuncture is thought, in CAM terms to act on entities like chi and meridians according to Traditional Chinese Medicine, but Western medical acupuncturists can claim that needling acts through conventional physiological mechanisms by, for example, releasing endorphins (Dew, 2000). This Western explanation became available from the late 20th century when endorphins were identified.

People who seek out therapeutic help for conditions they identify as needing care from others have their own ways of integrating orthodox and alternative medicines. Research on household use of medications shows how people mix and match different therapies, try out different approaches, take advice from many sources, including family, friends, work colleagues, as well as health practitioners both orthodox and unorthodox. Through this process people may establish regimes that suit their own sense of what is beneficial and that align with their own values and assumptions (Chamberlain, Madden, Gabe, Dew, & Norris, 2011; Dew et al., 2014). That is, users of medications take a pragmatic approach, mixing different health approaches, particularly in the face of chronic conditions. This mixing and matching also happens in cultures with indigenous healing practices. For example, Tibetans will draw on Tibetan medicine particularly for chronic conditions but also use biomedical approaches (Janes, 2002). In the next section, we discuss how CAM is positioned in the non-Western world.

CAM/traditional medicine in South Asia

In the Global South, or the non-Western world more broadly, the term "medical pluralism" has been used to describe the situation where Western medicine and local or indigenous medical systems co-exist (Leslie, 1976). There, Western medicine is a more recent introduction and often a vestige of colonialism, whereas local/indigenous medicine tends to be deep-rooted in national cultures that shape people's health-related knowledge and beliefs (Obeyesekere, 1976). Due to the vast heterogeneity of the therapeutic landscape in the Global South, this section focuses on the South Asian subcontinent to illustrate the position and dynamics of CAM within the non-Western world.

The term "medical pluralism" has been criticised for glossing over the political dimensions involved in therapeutic practices in the non-Western world (Gale, 2014; Khan, 2006). In many "pluralist" settings there is a commonly a clear hierarchy of medical systems, with Western biomedicine often being the dominant system, favoured and privileged over the others. Consequently, local and indigenous medicines exist as an alternative or complement to the orthodox system represented by Western biomedicine. This is similar to the position of CAM in the global north, though the term CAM is hardly used to refer to the local or indigenous medicines in non-Western settings. Rather, they continue to be referred to as "traditional medicine" (TM), evoking their historical and cultural associations with particular communities.

The history of TM in Asia dates back several millennia. Charles Leslie's seminal work *Asian Medical Systems* (1976) placed them on the research agenda. Leslie focused on three "great tradition medicines" in Asia, namely, Ayurveda, Unani, and Traditional Chinese Medicine. These had disparate origins (in South Asia, in the Mediterranean, and in China, respectively) from where they spread to other regions. Further, they had all achieved professionalisation within the millennium from the 5th century BC to the 5th century AD (Leslie, 1976). By then, they featured a wealth of written texts, established professional and ethical codes of conduct, and formalised pathways to become a practitioner, which often involved years of education and practice.

In conjunction with those institutionalised TMs, there have always been "folk medicines" or other less well-established forms of TM. These include a variety of therapeutics ranging from specialised treatment for specific conditions (e.g. bone setting, snakebite treatment), midwifery, religious or spiritual healing, and ritualistic practices. These were generally neither institutionalised nor professionalised, with the relevant knowledge and skills often passed down through successive generations. They would likely have been complementary to the then orthodox system represented by the "great tradition medicines" such as Ayurveda, as well as offering a popular and less expensive alternative available for the masses (Leslie, 1976). Today, with the "great tradition medicines" themselves being displaced by Western medicine, "folk" healing practices have been relegated further to the periphery of the medical scene and have become "subaltern therapeutics" (Hardiman & Mukharji, 2012).

However, the different TMs and "folk" therapeutic practices within a specific community are often closely intertwined with, and at times hardly distinguishable from, each other. This is illustrated by Nordstrom (1988) in her study of TM practitioners from a single town in Sri Lanka. None of her practitioners fit the statutory definition of a TM practitioner as a provider of "empirical, herbal-based medical services" due to the eclecticism of their practices. For instance, Nordstrom gives examples of a government-registered Ayurvedic practitioner whose services included writing "was kavi" (powerful poems to bring malediction on someone), an exorcist who dispensed indigenous medicines where necessary, and a Buddhist priest who treated drug addiction using religious teachings, herbal medicine, and counselling. Therefore, Nordstrom argues against the identification of Ayurvedic medicine as being a system separate from other popular therapeutic practices in the country, since they all form different faces of the same pluralistic traditional medical system (Nordstrom, 1988).

The popularity of TM

The sparse reports on the uptake of TMs in South Asia impede cross-regional comparisons, though they indicate certain trends. Nearly 80% of the rural populations of Bangladesh and Pakistan are said to rely on TMs (Haque, Chowdhury, Shahjahan, & Harun, 2018; Sher, Bussmann, Hart, & de Boer, 2016); while in Sri Lanka, there appears to be a general decline in demand even in rural regions (Weerasinghe & Fernando, 2011). In India, around 7% of the population are reported as users of TM, with significant usage differences between different states (Chowdhury & Kundu, 2018; Rudra, Kalra, Kumar, & Joe, 2017).

The high demand for TM in South Asian villages is partially linked to the substandard development of infrastructure in those rural regions. Most healthcare facilities are located in urban centres, and a lack of good transport infrastructure to reach those urban centres, as well as a shortage of medical staff and medical supplies in regional hospitals are common issues faced by rural populations. In Bangladesh, for example, only 20–25% of people can access any modern healthcare facilities (Haque et al., 2018). In this context, the services of traditional practitioners and "folk" healers – often based in the neighbourhood – present a more convenient alternative (Albert, Porter, & Green, 2019; Haque et al., 2018; Weerasinghe & Fernando, 2011). Further, such healers usually provide their services either free or for a low fee, which makes them highly sought after by the local community.

Preference for TM treatment can be condition-specific. Sri Lankans are said to opt for a traditional home remedy for minor illnesses and seek TM treatment for conditions such as snakebite, fractures, rheumatism, asthma, and paralysis (Liyanage, 2000; Weerasinghe & Fernando, 2011; Wolffers, 1988). There may also be conditions that cannot be clearly mapped onto a biomedical framework, such as the "*niangsophet*" (a problem of infancy that could be represented by a range of signs and symptoms) among Meghalayan tribals in India (Albert et al., 2019), and so biomedical treatments are viewed as inappropriate. Further, the popular view of TM as being "natural therefore benign" (as opposed to Western medicine, which is "artificial, therefore harmful to the body") could be a strong motive for choosing the former where long-term treatment is required.

Many people turn to TM in the hope of a cure when Western medicine fails, such as for cancer (Broom, Wijewardena, Sibbritt, Adams, & Nayar, 2010). Associated with this is the belief that TM provides definitive treatment addressing the root cause of the illness, whereas Western medicine offers merely temporary relief. This also relates to the discourse of spiritual and mystical power associated with TM. As on-going fieldwork in Sri Lanka by one of the authors indicates, there are healers who are reported to perform miraculous cures based on their specialised knowledge or psychic powers, thus inspiring pilgrimages of hopeful patients from near and far.

Marginalised groups in TM

The history of TM clearly reflects the power dynamics in the cultures where they originated. The gender and caste-based segregation in Ayurvedic medicine, for example, stems from the hierarchical social structure in ancient India. In reviewing Ayurvedic texts, Shah (2006) notes a complete erasure of women's health and sexuality apart from where it may affect their ability to bear children, which was of paramount importance for men in terms of preserving their lineage. Ayurveda was considered sacred knowledge in ancient India, and hence was largely dominated by men of high caste. In any case, the rigorous education and training required to become an Ayurvedic practitioner proved an effective barrier that excluded all socially marginalised groups.

However, "folk" medicines or "subaltern therapeutics" presented some contrast to orthodox medicine in this regard. These forms did not involve formal education or scholarship, and people from underprivileged social groups who perform ritualistic, spiritual, and folk healing practices can be found in many communities. Midwifery, for example, was performed almost exclusively by women. The "dai" tradition (midwifery) in India is founded on thousands of years of experience, mainly of women, of assisting childbirth (Sadgopal, 2012). Further, as certain aspects of childbirth (such as the cutting of the umbilical cord) were considered "sinful" and unsuitable to be performed by anybody of high caste, there was always a demand for "dai" of low-caste.

Regardless of their importance to their community, the position of such "folk" practitioners can remain unlegitimised. Nordstrom (1988) identifies one set of TM practitioners in Sri Lanka who treat common general ailments, as "local-level healers". These are mostly women who work from home on an as-needed basis but are not recognised as medical practitioners, even by those who seek their help: the community links their success as healers to their feminine nature and to their being accessible at the house throughout the day (unlike men). In India, Sadgopal (2012) points out that over one-third of all childbirths are attended by a "dai" (midwife), making theirs the most widely accessed maternity service in the country. However, the contribution of the "dai" remains unacknowledged, or even negated, within the state maternity services. Such erasure of certain "folk" healers can arguably be traced to their challenge to the dominant power structures and ideologies involving gender, social class, caste, medicalisation, and/or commercialisation within their community or in the work setting (Nordstrom, 1988; Sadgopal, 2012).

Colonialism and nationalism

As we have argued, the positioning of CAM and TM practices in relation to biomedicine can be distinctly different in the Global South. It can take on a more overt political hue in contexts where biomedicine is conflated with colonialism and empire, giving rise to "medicinal politics" (Whyte, Van der Geest, & Hardon, 2002).

The colonial history of medicine in Sri Lanka is a case in point. The country had a thriving indigenous medical tradition, with one of the world's first hospitals established by the 4th century BC (Uragoda, 1987). During the colonial era in the 18th–19th century, the British enforced a comprehensive medical system into the local medical scene, which was in disarray at that time. TM no longer had a place in the colonial state-funded healthcare sector and was pushed to the periphery of legitimacy. The Western-educated local elite favoured "modern" Western medicine over the traditional, sealing the fate of the latter (Arseculeratne, 2002). When

Sri Lanka became an independent sovereign state in the mid-20th century, it was with a fully functional and comprehensive Western medical system in place (Uragoda, 1987). Successive governments have continued that system without significant change. The patronage of Western medicine by post-colonial governments, as Khan (2006) argues in the case of India, possibly had a more detrimental effect on TM and therapeutics than the centuries of colonial rule. Though recognised as part of the state health system, TM in Sri Lanka remains subordinated to Western biomedicine in the medical hierarchy as well as in social status (Arseculeratne, 2002; Jones & Liyanage, 2018; Leslie, 1976).

TMs are imbued with indigenous culture, evoking a strong sense of the local and the historical. When juxtaposed against Western medicine, TMs can become symbols of the nation itself and may feature strongly in nationalist discourses. In colonial India, the iconic national leader Mahatma Gandhi was a major critic of Western medical hegemony. As Khan (2006) analyses, Gandhi's rejection of Western culture underpinned his critique of Western medicine. As an alternative he advocated greater emphasis on the prevention of illness through self-control and spiritual awareness, reflecting Ayurvedic teachings. In post-colonial Sri Lanka, a nationalist political movement that called for the reinstatement of Sinhalese as the sole official language of the country came into power in 1956. The development of TM was a priority in the political agenda of this movement. Waxler (1984) notes that TM practitioners, who had been marginalised under the then pro-Western government, were one of the main interest groups that propelled the nationalist movement to victory. The status and state support of TM thus continue to ebb and flow in line with political trends of colonialism, modernisation, and a nationalist revival.

Regulating and modernising TM

The World Health Organization, in its *Traditional Medical Strategy 2014–2023*, encourages regulating TMs and including them in the country's healthcare system to complement Western medicine (World Health Organization, 2013). One such instance of this approach is reported from India. Since the late 1990s, India has taken steps to mainstream several of its TMs, namely, Ayurveda, Yoga and Neuropathy, Unani, Siddha, Homeopathy, and Sowa Rigpa (known by the acronym AYUSH). This culminated in establishing the Ministry of AYUSH in 2014. Integrating TMs into the healthcare system is primarily expected to overcome the severe shortage of biomedical professionals in the country and to strengthen the healthcare system as a whole (Shrivastava, Shrivastava, & Ramasamy, 2015). The Ministry also aims for greater state funding and resources for the development of these medicines and professionalising of their practitioners.

A key aspect of developing, revitalising, or legitimising TMs involves "modernising" them to meet the accepted norms of Western science. With Western medicine being the undisputed orthodox system in most parts of the Global South, "modernising" TMs often means adapting them into a similar framework. Such adaptation, however, may undermine the whole idea of promoting TM. The process of redefining and reconfiguring TMs in India has led to them losing many of their unique features and practices (Hardiman & Mukharji, 2012). As a result, what is legitimised within the AYUSH framework today is not the Ayurveda or the Unani that has been practised in the region for centuries: it is a "syndicated Ayurveda" and a "syndicated Unani" consisting only of elements that are acceptable under a Western scientific framework. The "disowned" elements may not disappear from use entirely, as they will continue to be used by "subaltern" practitioners functioning beyond the sanctioned national framework (Hardiman & Mukharji, 2012).

Hybridisation of TM and biomedicine

In Sri Lanka, Waxler (1984) identifies a "behavioural convergence" of Western and Ayurvedic medicines, which can be understood as a blurring of borders between the two systems at the patient level. Where practitioners are concerned, such border crossing can be useful and even essential at times. For instance, there are traditional practitioners who follow Western diagnostic techniques and prescribe Western pharmaceuticals based on patients' wishes (Waxler, 1984; Wolffers, 1988). On the other hand, Western medical practitioners may instruct patients based on Ayurvedic teachings such as bathing patterns and avoiding excessively hot/cold food (Waxler, 1984), or explain illnesses by resorting to traditional local idioms of demons being exorcised from the body (on-going fieldwork observation by author).

For the general public, Western and TMs may be constitutive of one hybrid system of healing, which they understand broadly in terms of Ayurvedic teachings that are entrenched in Sri Lankan culture. This explains why, for example, people feel the need to balance the "heat" of Western pharmaceuticals with a "cooling" substance (Nichter, 1987). With such merging of the Western and the traditional, seamless movement between different healing practices can occur. As Amarasingham (1980) demonstrates, a mentally-ill patient seeks treatment (sequentially as well as simultaneously) from exorcists, astrologers, Buddhist priests, Ayurvedic, and Western medical practitioners. At each engagement, the patient and her family are able to define and interpret the condition anew according to the treatment being prescribed, locating each explanation within a broadly Ayurvedic framework. Such pragmatic hybridising – by patients and practitioners – illustrate the complexities of health-seeking practices undertaken every day within the pluralistic medical landscapes in the non-Western world.

Concluding comments

For all its diversity we can see some similar influences and trends related to CAM occurring across the globe. Economic drivers can expand CAM use, but for different reasons. In the West, the corporatisation of CAM as a profitable industry is one driver. In South Asia, access to therapeutic help in poor rural areas can drive CAM, or rather, TM use. Standardisation processes can also be discerned that reshape CAM therapeutic practices, processes that intersect with both economic and scientific credibility concerns. The demands of the evidence-based medicine hierarchy or authority can limit the type and form of practices that gain credibility, and the standardisation of medications harmonises with corporate concerns, creating more uniform forms of therapeutics that may significantly shift away from the original philosophy of the CAM practice.

Intertwined with these processes of standardisation are a complex range of other concerns, such as nationalism, colonialism, globalisation, power differentials by gender and class, and professionalisation strategies of different occupations, that shape and reshape CAM practices in diverse social, political, and cultural milieux.

Counterposed to these forces of standardisation and assimilation of CAM to the epistemic standards of biomedicine are people's practices. People make their own decisions about what therapeutic regime to engage in and how they will mix and match different regimes. Issues of cost, relations with others, relations to tradition and politics, sense of empowerment or responsibility, and so on all come into play when decisions are made about the use of CAM, what type of CAM to use, and what else might be used besides CAM. People themselves integrate the diversity of practices into their own frameworks and many practitioners and patients take a pragmatic approach to the use of CAM around the globe.

References

Albert, S., Porter, J., & Green, J. (2019). Doktor Kot, Doktor Sla – book doctors, plant doctors and the segmentation of the medical market place in Meghalaya, northeast India. *Anthropology & Medicine*, *26*(2), 159–176. doi:10.1080/13648470.2017.1368830

Amarasingham, L. (1980). Movement among healers in Sri Lanka: A case study of a Sinhalese patient. *Culture, Medicine & Psychiatry*, *4*(1), 71–92.

Arseculeratne, S. N. (2002). Interactions between traditional medicine and "western" medicine in Sri Lanka. *Social Scientist*, *30*(5/6), 4–17. doi:10.2307/3517999

Bivins, R. (2007). *Alternative medicine: A history*. Oxford: Oxford University Press.

Breslaw, E. (2012). *Lotions, potions, pills, and magic: Health care in early America*. New York: New York University Press.

Broom, A., Wijewardena, K., Sibbritt, D., Adams, J., & Nayar, K. R. (2010). The use of traditional, complementary and alternative medicine in Sri Lankan cancer care: Results from a survey of 500 cancer patients. *Public Health*, *124*(4), 232–237. doi:10.1016/j.puhe.2010.02.012

Chamberlain, K., Madden, H., Gabe, J., Dew, K., & Norris, P. (2011). Forms of resistance to medication within New Zealand households. *Medische Anthroplogie*, *23*(2), 299–308.

Chowdhury, S., & Kundu, P. (2018). Alternate systems of medicine in India – How pervasive and why? *Journal of Health Management*, *20*(2), 178–189. doi:10.1177/0972063418763653

Collyer, F. (2004). The corporatisation and commercialisation of CAM. In P. Tovey, G. Easthope, & J. Adams (Eds.), *The mainstreaming of complementary and alternative medicine: Studies in social context* (pp. 81–99). London: Routledge.

Conrad, P. (2007). *The medicalization of society: On the transformation of human conditions into treatable disorders*. Baltimore, MD: Johns Hopkins University Press.

Coulter, I. (2004). Integration and paradigm clash: The practical difficulties of integrative medicine. In P. Tovey, G. Easthope, & J. Adams (Eds.), *The mainstreaming of complementary and alternative medicine: Studies in social context* (pp. 103–122). London: Routledge.

Dew, K. (2000). Deviant insiders: Medical acupuncturists in New Zealand. *Social Science & Medicine*, *50*(12), 1785–1795.

Dew, K. (2001). Modes of practice and models of science in medicine. *Health: An Interdisciplinary Journal for the Study of Health, Illness and Medicine*, *5*(1), 93–111.

Dew, K., Chamberlain, K., Hodgetts, D., Norris, P., Radley, A., & Gabe, J. (2014). Home as a hybrid centre of medication practice. *Sociology of Health & Illness*, *36*(1), 28–43.

Gale, N. (2014). The sociology of traditional, complementary and alternative medicine. *Sociology Compass*, *8*(6), 805–822. doi:10.1111/soc4.12182

Gale, N., & Mchale, J. (2015). Introduction: Understanding CAM in the 21st century – the importance and challenge of multi-disciplinary perspectives. In N. Gale & J. Mchale (Eds.), *Routledge handbook of complementary and alternative medicine* (pp. 1–9). London: Routledge.

Greene, J. (2005). Releasing the flood waters: Diuril and the reshaping of hypertension. *Bulletin of the History of Medicine*, *79*(4), 749–794.

Haque, M. I., Chowdhury, A. B. M. A., Shahjahan, M., & Harun, M. G. D. (2018). Traditional healing practices in rural Bangladesh: A qualitative investigation. *BMC Complementary and Alternative Medicine*, *18*(1), 62–62. doi:10.1186/s12906-018-2129-5

Hardiman, D., & Mukharji, P. B. (Eds.). (2012). *Medical marginality in South Asia: Situating subaltern therapeutics*. London: Routledge.

Jakes, D., & Kirk, R. (2015). How and why patients use acupuncture: An interpretive phenomenological study. *Journal of Primary Health Care*, *7*(2), 124–129.

Janes, C. (2002). Buddhism, science, and market: The globalisation of Tibetan medicine. *Anthropology & Medicine*, *9*(3), 267–289.

Jones, M., & Liyanage, C. (2018). Traditional medicine and primary health care in Sri Lanka: Policy, perceptions, and practice. *Asian Review of World Histories*, *6*(1), 157–184. doi:10.1163/22879811-12340029

Kelner, M., & Wellman, B. (1997). Health care and consumer choice: Medical and alternative therapies. *Social Science & Medicine*, *45*(2), 203–212.

Khan, S. (2006). Systems of medicine and nationalist discourse in India: Towards "new horizons" in medical anthropology and history. *Social Science & Medicine*, *62*(11), 2786–2797.

Larkin, G. (1983). *Occupational monopoly and modern medicine*. London: Tavistock Publications.

Leslie, C. (Ed.). (1976). *Asian medical systems: A comparative study*. Berkeley, CA: University of California Press.

Light, D. (2010). The Food and Drug Administration: Inadequate protection from serious risks. In D. Light (Ed.), *The risks of prescription drugs* (pp. 40–68). New York: Columbia University Press.

Liyanage, J. H. C. (2000). *"Rogi charyawa" (Illness behavior: A sociological analysis)* Mullariyawa: Wijesuriya Publishers.

McLeod, K. (2017). *Wellbeing machine: How health emerges from the assemblages of everyday life*. Durham, NC: Carolina Academic Press.

Nichter, M. (1987). Cultural dimensions of hot, cold and sema in Sinhalese health culture. *Social Science & Medicine*, *25*(4), 377–387.

Nordstrom, C. R. (1988). Exploring pluralism – The many faces of Ayurveda. *Social Science & Medicine*, *27*(5), 479–489. doi:10.1016/0277-9536(88)90371-1

Northcott, H., & Bachynsky, J. (1993). Concurrent utilization of chiropractic, prescription medicines, non-prescription medicine and alternative health care. *Social Science & Medicine*, *37*(3), 431–435.

Obeyesekere, G. (1976). The impact of Āyurvedic ideas on the culture and the individual in Sri Lanka. In C. Leslie (Ed.), *Asian medical systems: A comparative study* (pp. 201–226). Berkeley, CA: University of California Press.

Porter, R. (2006). Medical science. In R. Porter (Ed.), *The Cambridge history of medicine* (pp. 136–175). Cambridge: Cambridge University Press.

Poynton, L., Dowell, A., Dew, K., & Egan, T. (2006). General practitioners' attitudes toward (and use of) complementary and alternative medicine: A New Zealand nationwide survey. *New Zealand Medical Journal*, *119*(1247).

Rudra, S., Kalra, A., Kumar, A., & Joe, W. (2017). Utilization of alternative systems of medicine as health care services in India: Evidence on AYUSH care from NSS 2014. *PloS one*, *12*(5), e0176916.

Sadgopal, M. (2012). Strengthening childbirth care: Can the maternity services open up to indigenous traditions of midwifery? In V. A. Sujatha (Ed.), *Medical pluralism in contemporary India* (pp. 211–231). Hyderabad: Orient Blackswan.

Saks, M. (1995). *Professions and the public interest: Medical power, altruism and alternative medicine*. London: Routledge.

Saks, M. (2001). Alternative medicine and the health care division of labour: Present trends and future prospects. *Current Sociology*, *49*(3), 119–134.

Shah, S. (2006). Representation of female sexuality in the ayurvedic discourse of the early medieval period. *Studies in History*, *22*(1), 45–58.

Sharma, S. (1992). *Complementary medicine today: Practitioners and patients*. London: Routledge.

Sher, H., Bussmann, R. W., Hart, R., & de Boer, H. J. (2016). Traditional use of medicinal plants among Kalasha, Ismaeli and Sunni groups in Chitral District, Khyber Pakhtunkhwa province, Pakistan. *Journal of Ethnopharmacology*, *188*, 57–69. doi:10.1016/j.jep.2016.04.059

Shorofi, S. A., & Arbon, P. (2010). Nurses' knowledge, attitude and professional use of complementary and alternative medicine (CAM): A survey of five metropolitan hospitals in Adelaide. *Complementary Therapies in Clinical Practice*, *16*(4), 229–234.

Shrivastava, S. R., Shrivastava, P. S., & Ramasamy, J. (2015). Mainstreaming of Ayurveda, Yoga, Naturopathy, Unani, Siddha, and Homeopathy with the health care delivery system in India. *Journal of Traditional and Complementary Medicine*, *5*(2), 116–118. doi:10.1016/j.jtcme.2014.11.002

Siahpush, M. (1998). Postmodern values, dissatisfaction with conventional medicine and popularity of alternative therapies. *Journal of Sociology*, *34*, 58–70.

Sointu, E. (2006). The search for wellbeing in alternative and complementary health practices. *Sociology of Health & Illness*, *28*, 330–349.

Sointu, E. (2012). *Theorizing complementary and alternative medicines: Wellbeing, self, gender, class*. Basingstoke: Palgrave.

Starr, P. (1982). *The social transformation of American medicine*. New York: Basic Books.

Uragoda, C. G. (1987). *A history of medicine in Sri Lanka from the earliest times to 1948*. Colombo: Sri Lanka Medical Association.

Waxler, N. E. (1984). Behavioral convergence and institutional separation: An analysis of plural medicine in Sri Lanka. *Culture, Medicine and Psychiatry*, *8*(2), 187–205.

Weerasinghe, M. C., & Fernando, D. N. (2011). Paradox in treatment seeking: An experience from rural Sri Lanka. *Qualitative Health Research*, *21*(3), 365–372. doi:10.1177/1049732310385009

Whyte, S. R., Van der Geest, S., & Hardon, A. (2002). *Social lives of medicines*. New York: Cambridge University Press.

Willis, E. (1983). *Medical dominance: The division of labour in Australian healthcare*. Sydney, NSW: George Allen & Unwin.

Wolffers, I. (1988). Illness behaviour in Sri Lanka: Results of a survey in two Sinhalese communities. *Social Science & Medicine, 27*(5), 545–552.

World Health Organization. (2013). *WHO traditional medicine strategy 2014–2023*. Retrieved from https ://apps.who.int/iris/bitstream/handle/10665/92455/9789241506090_eng.pdf;jsessionid=21742BE E9CB95BD807EB2CD91C7686E2?sequence=1

PART II

Life contexts

11

HEALTH INEQUALITY

Dennis Raphael and Toba Bryant

"Social injustice is killing people on a grand scale"

Introduction

Profound differences in health outcomes exist between nations. There are also significant differences in health outcomes amongst members within these same nations. The World Health Organization reports a child born in Sierra Leone can expect to live 50 years versus 84 years for a child born in Japan, a gap of 34 years (World Health Organization, 2017). In the USA, there is a 27-year gap in life expectancy between people living in different parts of the Washington DC area. Those in the Northwest DC neighbourhood of Georgetown can expect to live 94 years versus a 67-year life expectancy for those in Anacostia in Southeast DC (World Health Organization, 2008). Similar gaps are omnipresent between and within other nations.

These gaps result from differences in living and working conditions and access to healthcare (Whitehead, 1985). These health gaps can be dispassionately described as "health disparities" with little said about their sources. They can also be described as "health inequalities" with attention paid to how these differences manifest amongst nations as a function of level of development, existing political and economic structures, and ideological convictions of governing political parties, and within nations as a function of one's social locations of class, race, ethnicity, or gender. Finally, when described as "health inequities", it is made explicit that since most of these health differences are avoidable, they are therefore unfair and morally unjust (Kawachi, Subramanian, & Almeida-Filho, 2002). This is the position taken by the World Health Organization's Commission on Social Determinants of Health that stated, "Social injustice is killing people on a grand scale" (World Health Organization, 2008).

Since most health inequalities are avoidable, in this chapter we use the more common term "health inequality" to refer to these avoidable, unfair, and unjust health outcomes. These differences in life circumstances and health outcomes are not natural, but rather the result of what the World Health Organization calls, "A toxic combination of poor social policies and programmes, unfair economic arrangements and bad politics" (World Health Organization, 2008). This approach directs attention to how public policy, shaped by historical traditions, societal structures, and power dynamics across and within nations distribute the economic, political, and social conditions necessary for health. The shorthand for these conditions has come to be known as the social determinants of health (Raphael, 2016b).

Addressing health inequalities through action on the social determinants of health has become an important public policy focus among many governing authorities around the world (Donkin, Goldblatt, Allen, Nathanson, & Marmot, 2018). These inequalities include differences in life expectancy, death rates from various diseases and injuries, and incidence of these diseases and injuries. The best means of tackling these health inequalities is to "level-up" the health of those experiencing adverse health outcomes closer to those with the best health outcomes (Dahlgren & Whitehead, 2006; Whitehead & Dahlgren, 2006). How to go about doing so is the source of much debate.

This chapter begins with an overview of the nature of health inequalities and how these are defined and measured. It then provides various means by which the causes of these health inequalities can be conceptualised. These conceptualisations shape thinking of how health inequalities come about and how to reduce them. The chapter concludes with an examination of the moral imperatives involved in identifying and tackling health inequalities as well as the barriers to such action.

Defining health and social inequality

Health inequalities are differences in health outcomes among nations and groups of individuals within these nations (Kawachi et al., 2002). There are striking differences between developed and developing nations in life expectancy, with those born in Switzerland expecting to live 83.5 years, in Norway, 82.3 years, and in Ireland, 81.6 years, while corresponding figures are 52.9 years in the Central African Republic, 53.2 years in Chad, and 54.1 years in the Ivory Coast (United Nations Development Program, 2018). There are also significant differences amongst nations similar in level of development, with one example being 72.8 years of expected life in Bangladesh while only 66.6 years in Pakistan and another being life expectancy of 79.5 years in the USA versus 82.6 years in Sweden (United Nations Development Program, 2018).

Within nations, health inequalities result from differences in life circumstances, and the term social inequality describes these differences (Grabb, 2007). In Canada, the overall life expectancy is 81.0 years, but for persons of Indigenous ancestry it is much lower (75.1 years for First Nations, 77.0 years for Metis (mixed ancestry), and 68.5 years for Inuit (Statistics Canada, 2017). In relation to income, Canadian men in the highest quintile of earnings can expect to live 83 years, while those in the lowest quintile live eight years less, at 75 years (Milligan & Schirle, 2018). For women, these income-related differences are three years, 86 years for the top 20% versus 83 years for the bottom 20%.

Unfortunately, the link between social and health inequalities is frequently ignored with attention diverted to biomedical, behavioural, and cultural risk factors, which though relevant, makes action to reduce the bulk of health inequalities between and within nations difficult (Raphael, 2011a). This is the case as the neglect of how social inequality creates health inequalities separates the problem of health inequalities from the societal structures and processes that drive them, thereby normalising their presence (Hofrichter, 2003).

There are, of course, health inequalities that are "natural" in the sense that they result from biological characteristics such as genetically-determined diseases like Huntington's chorea, a choice to engage in a high-risk recreational activity such as automobile racing, ageing, or just plain bad luck (Whitehead, 1985). But the overwhelming proportion of health inequalities between specific groups, communities, and nations are not natural and result from adverse living circumstances created through public policies that threaten health (World Health Organization,

2017). Since most health inequalities are preventable through governmental action, the failure to address them is unfair and unjust (Braveman & Gruskin, 2003).

Identifying health inequalities

Three tasks must be undertaken prior to identifying and reducing health inequalities. The first is to identify which health indicators to use. These usually include measures of life expectancy and infant mortality rates and, especially in the case of developing nations, maternal mortality. Other indicators include morbidity and mortality rates for various physical, mental, and social health problems such as cardiovascular disease, depression and suicide, and delinquency and crime. Choosing health indicators is a relatively easy task.

Second, it is necessary to formulate the basis upon which health inequalities are defined (Braveman & Gruskin, 2003). As noted, health inequalities exist at the group and national levels. But on what basis of comparison is a health inequality identified? Inquiry is not made into whether health inequalities exist between persons with blue versus brown eyes. Nor do we look for health inequalities between people who play board games versus those in solitary play.

This second task is more difficult as it requires the researcher or health advocate to have recourse to each of the following: a) a theory of justice; b) a theory of society; and c) a theory of the genesis of these health inequalities (Kawachi et al., 2002). These theories direct attention to what is relevant and important. Without such normative frameworks, justifying one basis for comparison over others is problematic (Wemrell, Merlo, Mulinari, & Hornborg, 2016).

Most theory-driven inquiry into health inequalities consider between-nation differences in terms of stage of development, form of their welfare state, approaches to public policymaking, and other structural factors. Within societies, the focus is upon how individuals occupying social locations related to social class, gender, and race come to experience differing health outcomes (Garthwaite, Smith, Bambra, & Pearce, 2016). There are many others, such as being employed versus unemployed, low versus middle versus high income, disabled versus able, Indigenous versus non-Indigenous, and urban versus rural, among others (Canadian Institute for Health Information, 2018; Public Health Agency of Canada, 2018; Smith, Bambra, & Hill, 2015).

As it turns out, many of the factors that are used to identify – and also explain – health inequalities between nations are useful for identifying and explaining health inequalities within nations. As one such example, Wilkinson and Pickett have argued that the extent of income inequality within a nation explains their overall health profile, with nations such as the UK and USA having worse health profiles as compared to more equalitarian nations such as Norway and Sweden (Wilkinson & Pickett, 2009). But income inequality is also a key factor in health inequalities within a nation as those with higher income experience better health outcomes than those with less income. The same can be said for other factors as well: they both identify and explain health inequalities between as well as within nations.

The Organisation for Economic Cooperation and Development (OECD) provides national data profiles for many health indicators as well as classification variables that allow for the identification of health inequalities. National statistics agencies such as Statistics Canada provide these indicators by groups differing in income, education, and other markers (Organisation for Economic Cooperation and Development, 2018; Statistics Canada, 2018). While the great majority of health inequalities inquiries to date have been from high-income nations (Cash-Gibson, Rojas-Gualdrón, Pericàs, & Benach, 2018), the growing availability of high-quality data in the developing world should change this (Global Health Observatory, 2018).

One broad category upon which health inequalities both between and within nations can be examined is that of developed versus developing nations (Gordon, 2010). Health inequalities and the social inequalities that drive them are actually greater within developing nations than in developed nations (Khazaei, Ayubi, Nematollahi, S., & Khazaei, 2016; Simson, 2018). Another is the form of the welfare state, a concept that represents the basket of public policies developed to ensure citizen economic and social security (Bambra, 2013). Related to welfare state concepts, analysis has been made of how having the state versus the market distributing resources to meet the needs of societal members shapes the extent of health inequalities, finding the state has an indispensable role in managing these inequalities (Bryant & Raphael, 2018, 2020). Finally, analyses have focused on amount of public spending on programmes and benefits, and how degree of stratification and decommodification within a society leads to health inequalities. Table 11.1 provides a summary of some of the concepts that have been applied towards understanding the extent of health inequalities between and within nations.

Concerning health inequalities within nations, an especially useful concept which identifies dimensions upon which group health inequalities exist is that of social location(s): "An individual's social locations consists of her ascribed social identities (gender, race, sexual orientation, ethnicity, caste, kinship status, etc.) and social roles and relationships (occupation, political party membership, etc.)" (Anderson, 2011). As it turns out, significant health inequalities are present among people who differ in these and other social locations such as social class, income, gender, and race (Smith et al., 2015). In developing nations, there is a focus on tribe, caste, and other specific identities (Wood & Gough, 2006). The concept of intersectionality considers

Table 11.1 Concepts applied to understandings health inequalities between and within nations

Concept	Definition
Stage of development	Nations are usually defined in terms of low, middle, and high income, representing progress towards economic development.
National wealth	Nations differ in terms of their overall wealth.
Form of welfare state	Nations differ in their general approaches towards the provision of economic and social security to their members.
Political ideology	Governing authorities differ in their approach towards the provision of economic and social security along a socialism-liberalism dimension.
Legitimacy	Nations differ in the extent to which their rulers are accountable to the governed via democratic processes.
Competency	Nations differ in their abilities to accomplish their goals.
State role in providing social security	Nations may identify the state, market, or family as the primary arbiters of resource distribution and provision of economic and social security.
Public spending	Nations differ in the extent to which they spend on programmes and supports to members.
Stratification	Nations differ in the extent to which differences exist amongst society members in terms of wealth and income, education and power and influence.
Decommodification	Nations differ in the extent to which members can have a decent quality of life independent of involvement in the labour force.
Income inequality	Nations differ in their extent of skewed distributions of income.

Source: Bryant, T. & Raphael, D. (2018). Welfare states, public health and health inequalities. Oxford: Oxford University Press. Retrieved 15 February 2019, from http://www.oxfordbibliographies.com/view/document/obo-9780199756797/obo-9780199756797-0178.xml.

how those occupying numerous social locations come to experience specific health outcomes (Kapilashrami, Hill, & Meer, 2015).

Explaining health inequalities

The third task is to formulate the mechanisms by which national characteristics and membership in specific groups leads to health inequalities. The very influential UK *Black report* and *Health divide* volumes considered two primary mechanisms for understanding this process with emphasis on occupational grade – a variant of social class: cultural/behavioural and materialist/structuralist (Townsend, Davidson, & Whitehead, 1992). These reports took as a given that access to healthcare is important for health, but also recognised that healthcare in developed nations such as the UK usually responds to the presence of illness rather than being responsible for illness in the first place. Of course, this is not the case in many developing nations where lack of access to healthcare is a key contributor to adverse health outcomes (Gordon, 2010).

The cultural/behavioural explanation was that individuals' behavioural choices (e.g. tobacco and alcohol use, diet, physical activity, etc.) are shaped by their attitudes and values (i.e. culture) were responsible for their developing and dying from a variety of diseases. The materialist/structuralist explanation emphasised the material conditions under which people live, such as the availability of resources to access the amenities of life, working conditions, and quality of available food and housing, among others. Both the *Black report* and the *Health divide* accepted the materialist/structuralist explanation and showed that in addition to the direct health effects of living conditions, the risk behaviours associated with the cultural/behavioural explanation were themselves heavily structured by one's material conditions of life.

Since then, research has shown that behavioural risk factors account for a relatively small proportion of variation in the incidence and death from various diseases in developed nations and developing nations (Davey Smith, 2003; Raphael, 2011d; Raphael, Chaufan, et al., 2019; Scott-Samuel & Smith, 2015). Additional models have added nuance to these two basic models: psychosocial (identifying how material factors lead to stress and risk behaviours), lifecourse (how exposures to living and working conditions accumulate benefit and risk across the lifecourse), and macro-social (the examination of the effects of broader societal factors and public policymaking) (Bartley, 2016).

In Table 11.2 we illustrate these approaches through an overview of how various models both explain health inequalities and suggest means of reducing them. Approach 1 focuses on access to healthcare, and such access certainly contributes to health inequalities, especially in the developing world (Gordon, 2010; McGibbon, 2016). The Commonwealth Fund provides ongoing analyses of access to care in selected developed nations, identifying shortfalls in numerous cases (Osborn, Squires, Doty, Sarnak, & Schneider, 2016; Schneider, Sarnak, Squires, & Shah, 2017) while the World Health Organization does so for all member nations (World Health Organization, 2018). Clearly, universal healthcare systems funded through general revenues are the most effective in preventing and responding to disease and illness. This applies to both the developed and developing worlds (Giedion, Andrés Alfonso, & Díaz, 2013; Savedoff, de Ferranti, Smith, & Fan, 2012).

In developed and even developing nations, however, sole focus on healthcare can divert attention from the living and working conditions that are primary determinants of health (Stoddart & Evans, 2017). It can also take attention away from the broader systems in which healthcare systems are embedded and may lay the blame for shortcomings in health on the healthcare system that cannot solve the pressing social problems that produce adverse health outcomes.

Table 11.2 Various framework and their implications for explaining and reducing health inequalities

Health inequalities interpretation	Key health promotion concept	Health promotion practice approach	Practical implications of the approach
1. Health inequalities result from differences in access and quality of health and social services.	Health inequalities can be reduced by strengthening healthcare and social services.	Create "health-promoting" hospitals, clinics, and social service agencies.	Focus is limited to promoting the health of those already experiencing health inequalities.
2. Health inequalities result from differences in important modifiable medical and behavioural risk factors.	Health inequalities can be reduced by enabling people to make "healthy choices" and adopt "healthy lifestyles".	Develop and evaluate healthy living and behaviour modification programmes and protocols.	Healthy lifestyle programming may ignore the material basis of health inequalities and widen existing health inequalities.
3. Health inequalities result from differences in material living conditions.	Health inequalities can be reduced by improving material living conditions.	Ensure that community development and participatory research enable people to gain control over their health.	There is the assumption that governmental authorities are receptive to and will act upon community voices and research findings.
4. Health inequalities result from differences in material living conditions that are a function of group membership.	Health inequalities can be reduced by improving the material living conditions of particularly disadvantaged groups.	Targeted development and research activities among disadvantaged groups improve their material living conditions.	There is the assumption that governmental authorities are receptive to such activities and anticipated outcomes.
5. Health inequalities result from differences in material living conditions shaped by public policy.	Health inequalities can be reduced by advocating for healthy public policy that reduces disadvantage.	Analyse how public policy decisions impact health (i.e. health impact analysis).	There is the assumption that governments will create public policy on the basis of its effects upon health.
6. Health inequalities result from differences in material living conditions that are shaped by economic and political structures and their justifying ideologies.	Health inequalities can be reduced by influencing the societal structures that create and justify health inequalities.	Analysing how the political economy of a nation creates inequalities identifies avenues for social and political action.	Requires health promotion to engage in building social and political movements that will reduce health inequalities.

(Continued)

Table 11.2 Continued

Health inequalities interpretation	Key health promotion concept	Health promotion practice approach	Practical implications of the approach
7. Health inequalities result from the power and influence of those who create and benefit from health and social inequalities.	Health inequalities can be reduced by increasing the power and influence of those who experience these inequalities.	Critical analysis empowers the disadvantaged to gain an understanding of, and a means of increasing, their influence and power.	Require health promotion to engage in building social and political movements that increase the power of the disadvantaged.

Source: Adapted from Raphael, D. (2017). Implications of inequities in health for health promotion practice, Table 8.2, p. 153. In I. Rootman, S. Dupéré, A. Pederson, and O'Neill, M. (Eds.). *Health promotion in Canada: New perspectives on theory, practice, policy, and research* (4th ed, pp. 146–166). Toronto: Canadian Scholars' Press.

Approach 2 is certainly the dominant approach in many developed nations, and this is especially the case in nations identified as liberal welfare states (see Approach 6) where individual responsibility for health is consistent with market approaches to resource distribution (Raphael, 2011b, 2011c). It is also common in developing nations (Ferrari, 2018). An extensive literature has established that the effects of these risk behaviours pale beside risks posed by living and working conditions. Analyses are also available on how this focus on behavioural risk factors is consistent with the general underlying ideologies of the liberal welfare state (Chaufan & Saliba, 2019; Raphael et al., 2019; Scott-Samuel & Smith, 2015).

Approach 3 recognises the importance of living and working conditions and Approach 4 directs attention to those most likely to experience these problematic living circumstances. These are certainly advances over the concern with risk behaviours. Approach 5 makes explicit that these differences in living conditions are a result of public policies that determine the quality and distribution of the social determinants of health. This is the view taken by the WHO Commission on Social Determinants of Health (Commission on Social Determinants of Health, 2008). However, these models say little about the societal structures and processes that lead to these public policy decisions.

Approaches 6 and 7 constitute political economy approaches, with the latter taking on a critical materialist stance on the health inequalities problem. Both consider how the economic and political systems shape the making of public policy that distributes the resources necessary for health. The critical materialist political economy approach (Approach 7) incorporates the roles played by power and influence and how some sectors possess more power than others with resultant effects upon health and health inequalities (Chernomas & Hudson, 2007; Navarro, 2009; Olsen, 2010; Raphael, 2015).

We suggest that the most useful models for explaining and responding to health inequalities are Approaches 5 to 7. The focus of these higher-level models – public policy, societal structures, and processes, and the forces shaping these structures and processes – are themselves determinants of the factors identified in the lower-level approaches. In addition, the effectiveness of these lower-level approaches for reducing health inequalities is scant (Nettleton, 1997; Popay, Whitehead, & Hunter, 2010; Scott-Samuel & Smith, 2015). Nevertheless, Approaches 1 and 2 can dominate governmental approaches and public understandings and do so in market-oriented societies such as Canada, the UK, and the USA (Conference Board of Canada,

2012; Scott-Samuel & Smith, 2015). In the following section, we provide a comprehensive model that draws upon the latest theorisations and findings concerning the sources of health inequalities to identify the means by which health inequalities come about as well as means for reducing them.

Critical materialist analyses of the sources of health inequalities

The approach we take towards explaining and responding to health inequalities is a critical materialist political economy approach that considers how the structures and processes of political and economic systems distribute economic and social resources amongst their populations (Coburn, 2010). As such it draws from Approaches 5 to 7 depicted in Table 11.2. The approach directs attention to how these differences in access to these resources lead to health inequalities between nations and between groups of individuals within nations (Bambra, 2009). Key to understanding these differences in access to resources are the concepts of power and influence (Scott, 2014).

Power and influence of societal sectors

Three key sectors influence the entire public policy process in a nation. The business and corporate sector is centrally placed as it has the greatest potential power and influence in capitalist societies – and virtually all developed and developing nations are capitalist – to shape aspects of economic and political systems, public policymaking, and the quality and distribution of the factors that shape health.

The business and corporate sector include the owners and managers of corporations and other large businesses and of smaller businesses who believe their interests are aligned with the larger corporate sector (Carroll & Sapinski, 2018). The goal of this sector is to maximise the returns of the owners and investors in companies. It possesses various levers of power – primarily its ability to move and invest money – that shape how governments develop and implement public policies that distribute economic and social resources that shape health (Langille, 2016). In regard to these public policies, the business and corporate sector usually favour less governmental provision of social and economic security, and advocates for weakened government management of employment practices and fewer support programmes and benefits, all of which result in less redistribution of income and wealth, all important determinants of health (Langille, 2016; Leys, 2001; Macarov, 2003).

The organised labour sector includes labour unions and their members. This sector usually supports greater redistribution of income and wealth from the wealthy to others through higher taxation on the business and corporate sector and the wealthy, greater government management of the workplace, and wider provision by governing authorities of supports and benefits (Peters, 2012). It gains power and influence through the percentage of the population that belong to trade unions and through alliances with governing parties of the left (Brady, 2009; Bryant, 2016; Swank, 2010)

When the labour sector has more influence, public policies are created that equalise the power imbalances between employers and employees (Navarro et al., 2006). This happens at the macro-level where governments are pressured to create equity-related public policies such as more progressive income taxes, and mandate that workplaces provide fairer wages and greater benefits. When the labour sector has less power and influence, public policies that enhance economic and social security become less likely, and workplaces and employment become more precarious with lower wages and benefits (Olsen, 2008).

The civil society sector consists of the agencies, groups, and organisations that try to shape public policy for various causes such as the environment, reducing poverty, providing child care and other programmes and services. It includes citizens who desire that the government operate in certain ways, such as providing fairer taxation policies or helping to provide employment training and other opportunities to members of society. It gains power and influence from its ability to influence public opinion and shape public policy through networks of agencies, organisations and other non-governmental institutions (Brady, 2009). And of course, the citizenry itself has influence through its ability to elect representatives to governments.

Another especially important sector, not explicitly shown in Figure 11.1, are international financial institutions such as the International Monetary Fund and the World Bank who have a profound influence upon the public policy practices of nations that are indebted (Cerami, 2013; Labonté & Schrecker, 2006; Ruckert & Labonté, 2012). In many cases, these institutions have come under strong criticism for their demanding the weakening of public institutions and public services in developing nations and invoking austerity measures that threaten health (De Vogli, 2011; Labonté & Stuckler, 2016; Stubbs, Kentikelenis, Stuckler, McKee, & King, 2017).

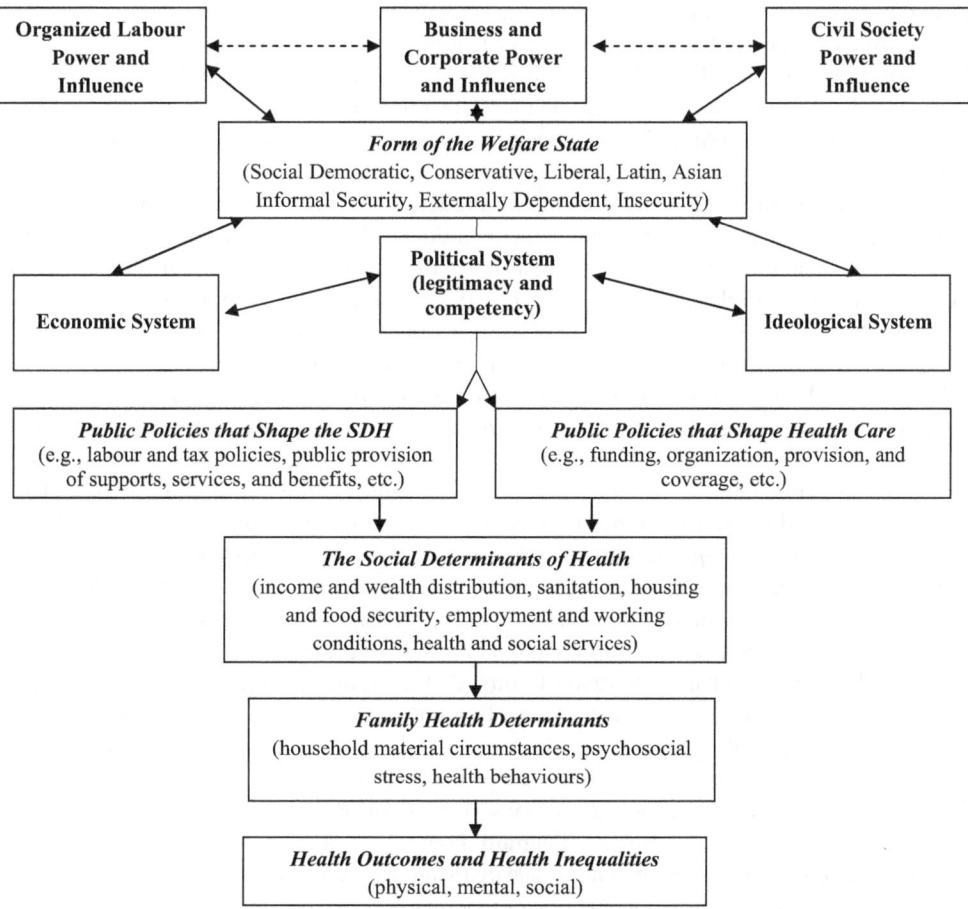

Figure 11.1   Provides a model for making sense of health inequalities between and within nations. Further details concerning this model are available elsewhere (Raphael & Bryant, 2015).

The balance of power among sectors differs among nations, with resulting impacts on the distribution of the factors that shape health and the nature of the healthcare system (Raphael, 2013b). This analysis helps explain why in some nations, citizens are provided with comprehensive healthcare that covers prescription medicines, rehabilitation, and dental care for children (Olsen, 2010). These same nations are likely to provide universal and affordable childcare, free or very low tuition at postsecondary institutions, and employment for most that provide well-above-poverty-line wages and numerous benefits. And if employment is lost, they provide support and job retraining until employment is gained (Raphael, 2011a). This package of benefits and supports by which a nation provides economic and social security to its citizens has been termed the welfare state (Briggs, 1961; Teeple, 2000).

The welfare state and its different forms

Nations differ widely as to the extent that they meet the essential needs of their citizenry. These result from differences in the balance of power between the business and corporate, labour, and the civil society sectors (Esping-Andersen, 1990, 1999). In developing nations, it may also reflect the power of the military and the influence of financial organisations such as the International Monetary Fund and the World Bank (Cerami, 2013; Wood & Gough, 2006).

Five forms of the welfare state have been identified in developed nations. These are social democratic, conservative, Latin, liberal, and Asian (Karim, Eikemo, & Bambra, 2010). In the developing world four have been identified: welfare, informal security, and externally dependent (Wood & Gough, 2006), and a permanent emergency welfare regime in Sub-Saharan Africa (Cerami, 2013).

Welfare state models are political economy models as they conceive ideas, institutions and public policy evolve from societal arrangements influenced by historical traditions and power relations. The central features of welfare regimes are their extent of social stratification, decommodification, and the relative role of the state, market, and family in providing economic and social security to the population (Eikemo & Bambra, 2008). The literature on developing nations includes these concepts but adds legitimacy and competency of governing authorities (Wood & Gough, 2006). These latter concepts have also been applied to developed nations and this is especially the case in regard to liberal welfare states (Raphael, Komakech, Bryant, & Torrence, 2019).

The social-democratic welfare state (e.g. Denmark, Finland, Norway, and Sweden) has been strongly influenced by social-democratic ideology, politics, and governance (Esping-Andersen, 1990). Its concern with *equality* outlines a key role for the state in addressing inequality and providing the population with various forms of economic and social security (Saint-Arnaud & Bernard, 2003). Its provision of programmes and supports on a universal basis is consistent with its goal of reducing social stratification and decommodifying the necessities of life. In essence, the social-democratic welfare state strives to provide the means by which one can live a decent life independent of employment market involvement. They do so by emphasising universal welfare rights and provide generous benefits and entitlements. The healthcare systems are comprehensive and run by governments. They cover pharmaceuticals and children's dental care in addition to primary and secondary healthcare services (Côté & Raynauilt, 2015).

The conservative welfare state (e.g. Belgium, France, Germany, and Netherlands) is distinguished by its concern with maintaining *stability* (Saint-Arnaud & Bernard, 2003). Historically, governance is by Christian Democratic parties that maintain many aspects of social stratification, a moderate degree of decommodification of societal resources, and an important role for the family in providing economic and social support (Esping-Andersen, 1990). The Church played a significant role in its development. An underdeveloped form of the conservative welfare state – the Latin (e.g. Greece, Italy, Portugal, and Spain) – has been added to Esping-Anderson's three regimes by Saint-Arnaud and Bernard (2003).

Conservative welfare states also offer generous benefits but provide these based on social insurance plans associated with employment status with primary emphasis on male wage earners (Esping-Andersen, 1990). They support citizens but maintain status differences and promote adherence to authority. These tendencies sometimes manifest in corporatist approaches (e.g. Germany), where business interests have major influence or in *Statist* approaches (e.g. France), where the state plays a key role in the provision of citizen security (Pontusson, 2005).

In these nations, the corporate and business sector acts in collaboration with the labour sector and the state to maintain levels of income and social programmes that maintain human dignity and well-being. In practicalities, the conservative welfare state looks very similar to the social-democratic welfare state in terms of quality of life and overall health (Pontusson, 2005). Their healthcare systems are also comprehensive, although they may be financed and delivered through non-profit private organisations and insurance agencies.

The emphasis of the Liberal welfare state (e.g. Australia, Canada, the United Kingdom, and the United States) is on *Liberty* and is dominated by the market and ruled by generally pro-business political parties (Saint-Arnaud & Bernard, 2003). Little attempt is made to reduce social stratification, and its degree of decommodification is the lowest (Esping-Andersen, 1990, 1999). There is little State intervention in the operation of the economic system.

Liberal welfare states provide modest benefits, and the State usually steps in with assistance only when the market fails to meet citizens' most basic needs. Their political and social history is one of dominance by business interests that has led the population to give its loyalty to the economic system rather than the state as a means of providing economic and social security. These liberal welfare states are the least developed in terms of the provision of citizen economic and social security. A key feature is their use of means-tested benefits that are targeted only to the least well-off. Their healthcare systems are likely to be two-tiered, offering both public and private systems alongside each other and cover less than the social-democratic and conservative welfare states. Liberal welfare states' healthcare systems are more subject to privatisation and profit-making as well.

In addition, liberal welfare states' political systems follow the Westminster model, and all are federal states. Much research shows that federalism reinforces inequalities in part because it fosters distrust of government (Banting & Corbett, 2002). Their electoral systems are first-past-the-post that favours dominant political parties that support less government intervention in the economy. It also makes it difficult for smaller left parties to influence the political process. Social-democratic and conservative welfare states work under proportional representation. This type of electoral system makes them more open to influence by political parties of the left, and to favour greater state intervention in the provision of social and economic security for citizens.

Stratification, decommodification, and the role of the state, family, and market

Three keys differences among these forms of the welfare states are the extent of stratification, decommodification, and the role of the state in providing societal members with economic and social resources. Generally, the social-democratic welfare state provides the most equitable profile regarding these factors, and the liberal welfare state provides the least.

Stratification refers to institutionalised differences amongst society members and is usually defined in terms of wealth and income, education, and in the political economy literature, power, and influence (Scott, 2014). Welfare states are both a result of levels of stratification as well as means of maintaining these status differences. Provision of universal services that decommodify the necessities for health – most common in social-democratic and least common in liberal welfare states – is another means for managing stratification (Menahem, 2010).

Stratification leads to social inequality, which are differences that are "consequential for the lives they lead, most particularly for the rights or opportunities they exercise and the rewards or privileges they enjoy" (Grabb, 2007, p. 1). One social inequality, income difference, is an important theme in health inequalities research.

Decommodification refers to the ability of people to have a decent quality of life independent of involvement in the paid employment market or what Esping-Andersen (1990, 1999) terms the "cash nexus". In addition to replacement income associated with retirement, sickness and disability, and unemployment, important aspects of daily life that can be commodified or decommodified are child care, employment training, elementary, secondary and postsecondary education, dental care, and health and social services, among others (Menahem, 2010).

Roles of the state, family, and market in providing economic and social security differ between the types of welfare state (Saint-Arnaud & Bernard, 2003). The social-democratic welfare state sees a strong State role, the conservative provides *family-directed* benefits based on earnings, and the liberal emphasises *market* involvement. State involvement is most effective for the provision of economic and social security and more equitable distribution of the social determinants of health. These differences help explain differences in what their economic, political, and ideological systems look like.

Economic, political, and ideological systems

The political economy approach directs attention to the structures and processes of economic and political systems and the ideas that societal members have about these systems and the nature of society. The economic system both creates and distributes economic resources amongst the population. Since all economic systems in wealthy developed nations are capitalist, market principles – of which profit-making is paramount – have the potential to drive their operations (Coburn, 2010). Some of the main features associated with market processes that impact health are wage structures, benefits available through work, working conditions, and vacation time, among others (Jackson & Thomas, 2017).

It has long been recognised, however, that without state intervention in the operation of the market economy, the distribution of economic resources becomes skewed in favour of the wealthy and powerful (Macarov, 2003). In addition, some structures and processes necessary for societal functioning may not be made available at all by the economic system. The welfare state arose because the economic system itself is not capable of dealing with the provision of basic societal resources such as education, healthcare, housing, and other programmes and services that provide citizens with resources necessary for wellbeing (Teeple, 2000).

The business and corporate sector has many economic levers, such as its ability to move and invest capital (Brooks & Miljan, 2003). The organised labour sector's levers are the ability to require employment security, benefits, and labour input decision making through collective bargaining and the threat of labour disruption, i.e. strikes. The levers available to the civil society sector is mobilising public opinion through its networks of agencies, organisations, and other non-governmental institutions (Brady, 2009).

The political system consists of the organisation of the state and its collection of laws and regulations. The political structure can intervene in the operation of the economic system by enacting laws and regulations that affect employment practices and by having governments provide supports and services to the citizenry through programmes and benefits. These supports, benefits, and services come from the enactment of corporate and personal taxes, the latter of which are especially progressive in social-democratic welfare states and rather less so in liberal welfare states (Bryant & Raphael, 2020). Usually progressive in that greater proportions of taxes accrue from those with higher incomes.

There are many specific areas where state activity impacts upon the social determinants of health. Working through the making of public policy, these areas include income and income distribution, employment and job insecurity, working conditions, housing and food security, and the availability of health and social services, among others (Raphael, 2016a). These social determinants of health indirectly affect the living conditions – and health – of individuals.

Finally, the means by which economic and political systems distribute resources are usually justified by dominant discourses on the nature of society and the different roles that the state, economic marketplace, and family should play in providing economic and social security. More recently, the analysis had been made of the impact of neo-liberalism as a societal doctrine that shapes the distribution of resources. Neo-liberalism is an ideology that believes that governments should withdraw from managing the economy thereby ceding more power and influence to the business and corporate sector (Schrecker & Bambra, 2015). This has been seen as leading to the skewing of the distribution of the social determinants of health and threatening the health of citizens in general and children in particular. The ideological system is especially important because it shapes the means by which the population comes to understand these issues. If the general public is convinced of the validity of neo-liberal arguments about the primacy of the marketplace over the state, then little can be expected to come from public policies that will manage the economy in the service of promoting equitable distributions of economic and social resources.

Public policy: The factors that shape health and healthcare are affected by a wide range of public policies that include labour and employment, revenue, and tax policies, among others. These policies determine how economic and social resources are distributed among the population. Governments influence this distribution by establishing taxation levels, the nature and quality of benefits, whether benefits are universal or targeted, and how employment agreements are negotiated. Governments are also responsible for establishing housing policies, maintaining transportation systems, enacting labour regulations and laws, and providing training related to employment and education. Profound differences between forms of the welfare state are apparent (Olsen, 2002, 2010).

Social determinants of health: Social determinants of health are the specific economic and social conditions that shape the health of individuals, communities, and nations (World Health Organization, 2009). Numerous sets of such determinants have been developed and Box 11.1 provides one developed by Canadian researchers (Raphael, 2016b). Most are concerned with living and working conditions and how they are distributed between and amongst nations. Others are aspects of individuals' social locations and how these make them vulnerable to public policy that threatens health. Their quality and distribution have been related to public policy and the forms of the welfare states that drive them (Bambra, 2013; Bryant & Raphael, 2018; Schrecker & Bambra, 2015). Social-democratic and conservative welfare states are clearly superior in providing these conditions for health than are the liberal and Latin welfare states (Raphael, 2011b, 2011c).

Familial health determinants: Families' living and working conditions differ within and across jurisdictions. The most obvious manifestations of these differences – important because they predict health outcomes – are familial material circumstances, psychosocial factors including stress experienced by families and coping mechanisms, and health-related behaviours (Benzeval, Dilnot, Judge, & Taylor, 2001).

Material circumstances refer to the concrete exposures to health strengthening and health-threatening conditions that are associated with income and wealth. In response to these material circumstances, families experience differences in a number of psychosocial variables such as stress, sense of efficacy and control, and self-identity. These come to shape parents' and children's health in both the present and the future (Lynch, Kaplan, & Salonen, 1997). The third aspect is how the experience of varying circumstances and the levels of stress associated with these circumstances lead to the adoption of health-supporting or health-threatening behaviours. In the latter case, these behaviours can be seen as coping responses to adverse life circumstances.

Health and health inequalities: Health outcomes are strongly shaped by the components presented in Figure 11.1. Differences in infant mortality rates among nations grouped by form of the welfare state differ profoundly, with liberal welfare states showing the worse outcomes and the greatest inequalities in absolute rates of infant mortality (Raphael & Bryant, 2019). There is greater variation in life expectancy and children's health outcomes within liberal as compared to the other welfare types (Raphael, 2012). Research on health inequalities in developing nations as a form of welfare state are only just beginning.

Box 11. 1 Social determinants of health

Early Life	Immigrant Status
Education	Income and Its Distribution
Disability	Indigenous Ancestry
Employment and Working Conditions	Race
Food Security	Social Safety Net
Gender	Social Exclusion
Geography	Unemployment and Employment
Healthcare Services	Security
Housing	

Source: Raphael, D. (Ed.). (2016c). *Social determinants of health: Canadian perspectives* (3rd ed.). Toronto: Canadian Scholars' Press.

The moral imperative of tackling health inequalities

Why reduce health inequalities? Usually, researchers and advocates answer this question on empirical grounds by showing how the majority of health inequalities are avoidable and taking such action would reduce human misery. These arguments include economic arguments concerning the extra costs to society of the presence of health inequalities and the adverse living conditions that create them. But perhaps a more compelling argument is that governing authorities are obliged to tackle health inequalities because health is a basic human right enshrined in numerous international covenants (Office of the United Nations High Commissioner for Human Rights & World Health Organisation, 2008). Box 11.2 presents some of these covenants to which virtually all nations have committed.

Box 11.2 Selected International Instruments Incorporating a Right to Health

Universal Declaration of Human Rights *(1948)*

Article 25 (1): "Everyone has a right to a standard of living adequate for the health of himself and his family, including food, clothing, housing and medical care and necessary social services".

International Convention on the Elimination of All Forms of Racial Discrimination *(1963)*

Article 5 (e) (iv): States undertake to prohibit and eliminate racial discrimination and equality before the law, in respect to "The right to public health, medical care, social security, and social services".

International Covenant on Economic, Social and Cultural Rights *(1966)*

Article 12(1): States Parties recognise "the rights of everyone to the enjoyment of the highest attainable standard of physical and mental health".

Article 12(2): Illustrates the breadth of areas that needed to be addressed and other human rights that have to be addressed "to achieve the full realization of this right".

Convention on the Elimination of All Forms of Discrimination against Women *(1979)*

Article 12 (1): "States Parties shall take all appropriate measures to eliminate discrimination against women in the field of health care in order to ensure, on a basis of equality of men and women, access to health care in order to ensure, on a basis of equality of men and women, access to health care services, including those related to family planning".

Convention on the Right of the Child *(1989)*

Article 24 (1): "States Parties recognize the right of the child to the enjoyment of the highest attainable standard of health and to facilitate for the treatment of illness and rehabilitation of health. States Parties shall strive to ensure that no child is deprived of his or her right to access to such health care services".

United Nations Declaration on the Rights of Indigenous Peoples *(2007)*

Article 21.1. "Indigenous peoples have the right, without discrimination, to the improvement of their economic and social conditions, including, inter alia, in the areas of education, employment, vocational training and retraining, housing, sanitation, health and social security".

Article 24.2. "Indigenous individuals have an equal right to the enjoyment of the highest attainable standard of physical and mental health. States shall take the necessary steps with a view to achieving progressively the full realization of this right".

> Article 29.3. "States shall also take effective measures to ensure, as needed, that programmes for monitoring, maintaining and restoring the health of indigenous peoples, as developed and implemented by the peoples affected by such materials, are duly implemented".
>
> Source: Abstracted from Rioux, M. (2019). The right to health: Human rights approaches to health. In Bryant, T., Raphael, D. and Rioux, M. (Eds.). *Staying alive: Critical perspectives on health, illness, and health*. Care (3rd ed. pp. 84–112. Toronto: Canadian Scholars' Press).

These commitments provide moral and ethical justifications for addressing health inequalities. They draw attention to making public policy that will enhance health rather than create unnecessary misery and suffering. Such moral imperatives provide the context against which progress in promoting health can be justified.

Conclusion

This chapter has identified various approaches towards understanding and reducing health inequalities between and among members of nations. We argue that the critical materialist political economy approach offers the most useful explanation for the presence of health inequalities and the best path towards reducing them. Since societal structures and processes produce health inequalities, these must be reformed. And since health inequalities occur as a result of the balance of power between various societal sectors, such imbalances must be addressed. The means of doing so is through the building of political and social movements that will promote public policymaking in the service of the many and not the few.

In many cases, this will not be an easy task as powerful economic and political forces may oppose the progressive public policies that will redistribute the economic and political resources necessary for health (Banting & Myles, 2013; Raphael, 2015). Numerous means of accomplishing this have been outlined in the literature on social change as well as in the health inequalities literatures (Carroll & Sapinski, 2018; Langille, 2016; Navarro et al., 2006; Raphael, 2009). Directions for action focus on growing left institutional political power (Brady, 2009), strengthening the labour movement (Navarro & Shi, 2002), and mobilising the public through explications of the means by which health inequalities and the social inequalities that drive them, come about (Langille, 2016).

The literature on social movements offers many avenues for concerted action (Castells, 2015; Della Porta & Diani, 2015; Roggeband & Klandermans, 2017). The UK's Politics of Health Group and Canada's Upstream are two health-related social movements in developed nations (The Politics of Health Group, 2018; Upstream, 2013). The People's Health Movement is a global network bringing together grassroots health activists, civil society organisations and academic institutions from around the world, particularly from low- and middle-income countries (People's Health Movement, 2018). Organisations such as these can help develop the social and political movements that can force governing authorities to promote the quality and equitable distribution of the social determinants of health through public policy action. Only then may we see reductions in the health inequalities that are the source of so much unnecessary suffering.

References

Anderson, E. (2011). Feminist epistemology and philosophy of science. *The Stanford Encyclopedia of Philosophy*. Stanford: Metaphysics Research Lab. Retrieved from http://plato.stanford.edu/archives/spr2011/entries/feminism-epistemology/

Bambra, C. (2009). Welfare state regimes and the political economy of health. *Humanity and Society*, *33*(1–2), 99–117.

Bambra, C. (2013). States of health: Welfare regimes, health, and healthcare. In B. Greve (Ed.), *The Routledge handbook of the welfare state* (pp. 260–273). New York: Routledge.

Banting, K., & Corbett, A. M. (2002). Health policy and federalism: An introduction. In K. Banting & A. M. Corbett (Eds.), *Health policy and federalism: A comparative perspective on multi-level governance* (pp. 1–39). Kingston: Queen's University Press.

Banting, K., & Myles, J. (Eds.). (2013). *Inequality and the fading of redistributive politics*. Vancouver: UBC Press.

Bartley, M. (2016). *Health inequality: An introduction to theories, concepts, and methods* (2nd ed.). Cambridge: Polity Press.

Benzeval, M., Dilnot, A., Judge, K., & Taylor, J. (2001). Income and health over the lifecourse: Evidence and policy implications. In H. Graham (Ed.), *Understanding health inequalities* (pp. 96–112). Buckingham: Open University Press.

Brady, D. (2009). *Rich democracies, poor people: How politics explain poverty*. New York: Oxford University Press.

Braveman, P., & Gruskin, S. (2003). Defining equity in health. *Journal of Epidemiology and Community Health*, *57*, 254–258.

Briggs, A. (1961). The welfare state in historical perspective. *European Journal of Sociology*, *2*, 251–259.

Brooks, S., & Miljan, L. (2003). Theories of public policy. In S. Brooks & L. Miljan (Eds.), *Public policy in Canada: An introduction*. (pp. 22–49). Toronto: Oxford University Press.

Bryant, T. (2016). *Health policy in Canada* (2nd ed.). Toronto: Canadian Scholars' Press.

Bryant, T., & Raphael, D. (2018). *Welfare states, public health and health inequalities*. Oxford: Oxford University Press. Retrieved from http://www.oxfordbibliographies.com/view/document/obo-9780199756797/obo-9780199756797-0178.xml

Bryant, T., & Raphael, D. (2020). *The politics of health in the Canadian welfare state*. Toronto: Canadian Scholars' Press.

Canadian Institute for Health Information. (2018). *Health inequalities*. Ottawa: Author. Retrieved from https://www.cihi.ca/en/health-inequalities

Carroll, W. K., & Sapinski, J. P. (2018). *Organizing the 1%: How corporate power works*. Halifax: Fernwood Publishing.

Cash-Gibson, L., Rojas-Gualdrón, D. F., Pericàs, J. M., & Benach, J. (2018). Inequalities in global health inequalities research: A 50-year bibliometric analysis (1966-2015). *PloS one*, *13*(1), e0191901.

Castells, M. (2015). *Networks of outrage and hope: Social movements in the Internet age*: New York: John Wiley & Sons.

Cerami, A. (2013). *Permanent emergency welfare regimes in sub-saharan Africa: The exclusive origins of dictatorship and democracy*. London: Palgrave MacMillan.

Chaufan, C., & Saliba, D. (2019). The global diabetes epidemic and the nonprofit state corporate complex: Equity implications of discourses, research agendas, and policy recommendations of diabetes nonprofit organizations. *Social Science & Medicine*, *223*, 77–88.

Chernomas, R., & Hudson, I. (2007). *Social murder and other shortcomings of conservative economics*. Winnipeg: Arbeiter Ring Publishing.

Coburn, D. (2010). Health and health care: A political economy perspective. In T. Bryant, D. Raphael, & M. Rioux (Eds.), *Staying alive: Critical perspectives on health, illness, and health care*. (2nd ed., pp. 65–92). Toronto: Canadian Scholars' Press.

Conference Board of Canada. (2012). *Canadians see their own behaviour and lifestyle as the key to their health, not socio-economic factors*. Ottawa: Author. Retrieved from http://www.conferenceboard.ca/press/news release/12-10-16/Canadians_see_their_own_Behaviour_and_Lifestyle_as_the_Key_to_their_Health_not_Socio-Economic_Factors.aspx

Côté, D., & Raynauilt, M.-F. (2015). *Scandinavian common sense: Policies to tackle social inequalities in health*. Montreal: Baraka Books.

Dahlgren, G., & Whitehead, M. (2006). *Levelling up (part 2): A discussion paper on European strategies for tackling social inequities in health*. Copenhagen: World Health Organization, European Office. Retrieved from https://apps.who.int/iris/handle/10665/107791

Davey Smith, G. (Ed.). (2003). *Inequalities in health: Life course perspectives*. Bristol: Policy Press.

De Vogli, R. (2011). Neoliberal globalisation and health in a time of economic crisis. *Social Theory & Health*, *9*(4), 311–325.

Della Porta, D., & Diani, M. (2015). *The Oxford handbook of social movements*. Oxford: Oxford University Press.

Donkin, A., Goldblatt, P., Allen, J., Nathanson, V., & Marmot, M. (2018). Global action on the social determinants of health. *BMJ Global Health, 3*(Suppl 1), e000603.

Eikemo, T. A., & Bambra, C. (2008). The welfare state: A glossary for public health. *Journal of Epidemiology and Community Health, 62*(1), 3–6.

Esping-Andersen, G. (1990). *The three worlds of welfare capitalism.* Princeton: Princeton University Press.

Esping-Andersen, G. (1999). *Social foundations of post-industrial economies.* New York: Oxford University Press.

Ferrari, C. K. (2018). Implementation of public health policies for healthy lifestyles promotion: What Brazil should tell us? *Health Promotion Perspectives, 8*(3), 243.

Garthwaite, K., Smith, K. E., Bambra, C., & Pearce, J. (2016). Desperately seeking reductions in health inequalities: Perspectives of UK researchers on past, present and future directions in health inequalities research. *Sociology of Health & Illness, 38*(3), 459–478.

Giedion, U., Andrés Alfonso, E., & Díaz, Y. (2013). *The impact of universal coverage schemes in the developing world: A review of the existing evidence.* Washington, DC: World Bank. Retrieved from https://openkno wledge.worldbank.org/bitstream/handle/10986/13302/75326.pdf?sequence=1&isAllowed=y

Global Health Observatory. (2018). *Health equity assessment toolkit.* Geneva: Author. Retrieved from http:// www.who.int/gho/health_equity/assessment_toolkit/en/

Gordon, D. (2010). Health inequalities in developing nations. *Social Alternatives, 29*(2), 28–33.

Grabb, E. (2007). *Theories of social inequality* (5th ed.). Toronto: Harcourt Canada.

Hofrichter, R. (2003). The politics of health inequities: Contested terrain. In R. Hofrichter (Ed.), *Health and social justice: A reader on ideology, and inequity in the distribution of disease* (pp. 1–56). San Francisco: Jossey Bass.

Jackson, A., & Thomas, P. (2017). *Work and labour in Canada: Critical Issues* (3rd ed.). Toronto: Canadian Scholars' Press.

Kapilashrami, A., Hill, S., & Meer, N. (2015). What can health inequalities researchers learn from an intersectionality perspective? Understanding social dynamics with an inter-categorical approach? *Social Theory & Health, 13*(3/4), 288–307.

Karim, S. A., Eikemo, T. A., & Bambra, C. (2010). Welfare state regimes and population health: Integrating the East Asian welfare states. *Health Policy, 94*(1), 45–53.

Khazaei, S., Ayubi, E., Nematollahi, S., & Khazaei, S. (2016). Variations of infant and under-five child mortality rates around the world, the role of human development index (HDI). *International Journal of Pediatrics, 4*(5), 1671–1677.

Kawachi, I., Subramanian, S. V., & Almeida-Filho, N. (2002). A glossary for health inequalities. *Journal of Epidemiology and Community Health, 56*(9), 647–652.

Labonte, R., & Schrecker, T. (2006). The G8 and global health. *Canadian Journal of Public Health, 97*(1), 35–38.

Labonté, R., & Stuckler, D. (2016). The rise of neoliberalism: How bad economics imperils health and what to do about it. *Journal of Epidemiology and Community Health, 70*(3), 312–318.

Langille, D. (2016). Follow the money: How business and politics define our health. In D. Raphael (Ed.), *Social determinants of health: Canadian perspectives* (3rd ed., pp. 470–490). Toronto: Canadian Scholars' Press.

Leys, C. (2001). *Market-Driven politics.* London, UK: Verso.

Lynch, J., Kaplan, G., & Salonen, J. (1997). Why do poor people behave poorly? Variation in adult health behaviours and psychosocial characteristics by stages of the socioeconomic lifecourse. *Social Science and Medicine, 44*(6), 809–819.

Macarov, D. (2003). *What the market does to people: Privatization, globalization, and poverty.* Atlanta: Clarity Press.

McGibbon, E. (2016). Oppressions and access to health care: Deepening the conversation. In D. Raphael (Ed.), *Social determinants of health: Canadian perspectives.* (3rd ed., pp. 491–520). Toronto: Canadian Scholars' Press.

Menahem, G. (2010). *How can the decommodified security ratio assess social protection systems? LIS Working Paper No. 529.* Sysracuse: Luxembourg Income Study. Retrieved from http://www.lisdatacenter.org/wps/li swps/529.pdf

Milligan, K., & Schirle, T. (2018). *Rich man, poor man: The policy implications of Canadians living longer.* Toronto: C.D. Howe Institute. Retrieved from https://www.cdhowe.org/sites/default/files/attachments/resea rch_papers/mixed/Rich%20Man,%20Poor%20Man%20-%20The%20Policy%20Implications%20of %20Canadians%20Living%20Longer.pdf

Navarro, V. (2009). What we mean by social determinants of health. *Global Health Promotion, 16*(1), 5–16.

Navarro, V., Muntaner, C., Borrell, C., Benach, J., Quiroga, A., Rodríguez-Sanz, M., … Pasarín, M. (2006). Politics and health outcomes. *The Lancet, 368*, 1033–1037.

Navarro, V., & Shi, L. (2002). The political context of social inequalities and health. In V. Navarro (Ed.), *The political economy of social inequalities: Consequences for health and quality of life* (pp. 403–418). Amityville: Baywood.

Nettleton, S. (1997). Surveillance, health promotion and the formation of a risk identity. In M. Sidell, L. Jones, J. Katz, & A. Peberdy (Eds.), *Debates and dilemmas in promoting health* (pp. 314–324). London: Open University Press.

Office of the United Nations High Commissioner for Human Rights, & World Health Organization. (2008). *The right to health, fact sheet no. 31*. New York: Author. Retrieved from http://www.ohchr.org/Documents/Publications/Factsheet31.pdf

Olsen, G. (2002). *The politics of the welfare state*. Don Mills: Oxford University Press.

Olsen, G. (2008). Labour market policy in the United States, Canada and Sweden: Addressing the issue of convergence. *Social Policy & Administration, 42*(4), 323–341.

Olsen, G. (2010). *Power and inequality: A comparative introduction*. Toronto: Oxford University Press.

Organisation for Economic Cooperation and Development. (2018). *OECD health statistics 2018*. Paris: Author. Retrieved from http://www.oecd.org/els/health-systems/health-data.htm

Osborn, R., Squires, D., Doty, M. M., Sarnak, D. O., & Schneider, E. C. (2016). In new survey of eleven countries, US adults still struggle with access to and affordability of health care. *Health Affairs, 35*(12), 2327–2336.

People's Health Movement. (2018). *Health for all now!* Capetown: Author. Retrieved from https://phmovement.org/

Peters, J. (2012). *Free markets and the decline of unions and good jobs*. In: *Boom, bust and crisis: Labour, corporate power and politics in Canada* (pp. 16–54). Halifax: Fernwood Publishers.

Pontusson, J. (2005). *Inequality and prosperity: Social Europe versus liberal America*. Ithaca: Cornell University Press.

Popay, J., Whitehead, M., & Hunter, D. J. (2010). Injustice is killing people on a large scale – but what is to be done about it? *Journal of Public Health, 32*(2), 148–149.

Public Health Agency of Canada. (2018). *Understanding the report on key health inequalities in Canada*. Ottawa: Author. Retrieved from https://www.canada.ca/en/public-health/services/publications/science-research-data/understanding-report-key-health-inequalities-canada.html

Raphael, D. (2009). Reducing social and health inequalities requires building social and political movements. *Humanity & Society, 33*(1–2), 145–165.

Raphael, D. (2011a). A discourse analysis of the social determinants of health. *Critical Public Health, 21*(2), 221–236.

Raphael, D. (2011b). The political economy of health promotion: Part 1, national commitments to provision of the prerequisites of health. *Health Promotion International, 28*(1), 95–111.

Raphael, D. (2011c). The political economy of health promotion: Part 2, national provision of the prerequisites of health. *Health Promotion International, 28*(1), 112–132.

Raphael, D. (2011d). Poverty in childhood and adverse health outcomes in adulthood. *Maturitas, 69*, 22–26.

Raphael, D. (2012). An analysis of international experiences in tackling health inequalities. In D. Raphael (Ed.), *Tackling Health Inequalities: Lessons from International Experiences* (pp. 229–264). Toronto, Canada: Canadian Scholars' Press.

Raphael, D. (2015). Beyond policy analysis: The raw politics behind opposition to healthy public policy. *Health Promotion International, 30*(2), 380–396.

Raphael, D. (2016a). Social structure, living conditions, and health. In D. Raphael (Ed.), *Social determinants of health* (3rd ed., pp. 32–56). Toronto: Canadian Scholars' Press.

Raphael, D. (Ed.). (2016b). *Social determinants of health: Canadian perspectives* (3rd ed.). Toronto: Canadian Scholars' Press.

Raphael, D. (2017). Implications of inequities in health for health promotion practice. In I. Rootman, S. Dupéré, A. Pederson, & O'Neill, M. (Eds.). *Health promotion in Canada: New perspectives on theory, practice, policy, and research* (4th ed., pp. 146–166). Toronto: Canadian Scholars' Press.

Raphael, D., & Bryant, T. (2015). Power, intersectionality and the life course: Identifying the political and economic structures of welfare states that support or threaten health. *Social Theory & Health, 13*(3–4), 245–266.

Raphael, D., & Bryant, T. (2019). Political economy perspectives on health and health care in T. Bryant, D. Raphael, & M. Rioux (Eds.), *Staying alive: Critical perspectives on health, illness, and health care* (3rd ed.). Toronto: Canadian Scholars' Press.

Raphael, D., Chaufan, C., Bryant, T., Bakhsh, M., Bindra, J., Puran, A., & Saliba, D. (2019). The cultural hegemony of chronic disease association discourse in Canada. *Social Theory & Health*, 17, 172–191.

Raphael, D., Komakech, M., Bryant, T., & Torrence, R. (2019). Governmental illegitimacy and incompetency in Canada and other liberal nations: Implications for health. *International Journal of Health Services*, *49*(1), 17–36.

Roggeband, C., & Klandermans, B. (2017). *Handbook of social movements across disciplines*. New York: Springer.

Ruckert, A., & Labonté, R. (2012). The financial crisis and global health: The International Monetary Fund's (IMF) policy response. *Health Promotion International*, *28*(3), 357–366.

Saint-Arnaud, S., & Bernard, P. (2003). Convergence or resilience? A hierarchical cluster analysis of the welfare regimes in advanced countries. *Current Sociology*, *51*(5), 499–527.

Savedoff, W. D., de Ferranti, D., Smith, A. L., & Fan, V. (2012). Political and economic aspects of the transition to universal health coverage. *The Lancet*, *380*(9845), 924–932.

Schneider, E. C., Sarnak, D. O., Squires, D., & Shah, A. (2017). *Mirror, mirror 2017: International comparison reflects flaws and opportunities for better us health care*. Washington: The Commonwealth Fund. Retrieved 1 March 2020, from https://www.commonwealthfund.org/publications/fund-reports/2017/jul/mirror-mirror-2017-international-comparison-reflects-flaws-and

Schrecker, T., & Bambra, C. (2015). *How politics makes us sick: Neoliberal epidemics*. Houndsmill, Basingstoke: Palgrave Macmillan.

Scott, J. (2014). *Stratification and power: Structures of class, status and command*. New York: John Wiley & Sons.

Scott-Samuel, A., & Smith, K. E. (2015). Fantasy paradigms of health inequalities: Utopian thinking? *Social Theory & Health*, *13*(3–4), 418–436.

Simson, R. (2018). *Mapping recent inequality trends in developing countries*. Working Paper 24. London: International Inequalities Institute, London School of Economics and Political Science.

Smith, K., Bambra, C., & Hill, S. (Eds.). (2015). *Health inequalities: Critical perspectives*. Oxford: Oxford University Press.

Statistics Canada. (2017). Gap in life expectancy projected to decrease between Aboriginal people and the total Canadian population. Ottawa: Author. Retrieved from https://www150.statcan.gc.ca/n1/pub/89-645-x/2010001/life-expectancy-esperance-vie-eng.htm

Statistics Canada. (2018). *Health inequalities data tool*. Ottawa: Author. Retrieved from https://infobase.phac-aspc.gc.ca/health-inequalities/

Stoddart, G., & Evans, R. (2017). *Producing health, consuming health care. Why are some people healthy and others not?* (pp. 27–64): New York: Routledge.

Stubbs, T., Kentikelenis, A., Stuckler, D., McKee, M., & King, L. (2017). The impact of IMF conditionality on government health expenditure: A cross-national analysis of 16 West African nations. *Social Science & Medicine*, *174*, 220–227.

Swank, D. (2010). Globalization. In F. G. Castles, S. Leibfried, J. Lewis, H. Obinger, & C. Pierson (Eds.), *The Oxford handbook of the welfare state*. Oxford: Oxford University Press.

Teeple, G. (2000). *Globalization and the decline of social reform: Into the twenty first century*. Aurora: Garamond Press.

The Politics of Health Group. (2018). *Speaking out on the health impact of politics*. Liverpool: Author. Retrieved from http://www.pohg.org.uk/

Townsend, P., Davidson, N., & Whitehead, M. (Eds.). (1992). *Inequalities in health: The Black report and the health divide*. New York: Penguin.

United Nations Development Program. (2018). *Human development reports*. New York: Author. Retrieved from http://hdr.undp.org/en/2018-update

Upstream. (2013). *Upstream is a movement to create a healthy society through evidence-based, people-centred ideas*. Saskatoon: Author. Retrieved from http://www.thinkupstream.net/

Wemrell, M., Merlo, J., Mulinari, S., & Hornborg, A. C. (2016). Contemporary epidemiology: A review of critical discussions within the discipline and a call for further dialogue with social theory. *Sociology Compass*, *10*(2), 153–171.

Whitehead, M. (1985). *The concepts and principles of equity and health*. Copenhagen: World Health Organization, European Office. Retrieved from http://citeseerx.ist.psu.edu/viewdoc/download?doi=10.1.1.196.7167&rep=rep1&type=pdf

Whitehead, M., & Dahlgren, G. (2006). *Concepts and principles for tackling social inequities in health: Levelling up Part 1*. Copenhagen: World Health Organization, European Office. Retrieved from http://www.euro.who.int/__data/assets/pdf_file/0010/74737/E89383.pdf

Wilkinson, R. G., & Pickett, K. (2009). *The spirit level – Why more equal societies almost always do better.* London: Allen Lane.

Wood, G., & Gough, I. (2006). A comparative welfare regime approach to global social policy. *World Development, 34*(10), 1696–1712.

World Health Organization. (2008). *Closing the gap in a generation: Health equity through action on the social determinants of health.* Geneva: Author. Retrieved from https://www.who.int/social_determinants/final _report/csdh_finalreport_2008.pdf

World Health Organization. (2009). *Social determinants of health.* Geneva: Author. Retrieved from http:// www.who.int/social_determinants/en/

World Health Organization. (2017). *10 facts on health inequities and their causes.* Geneva: Author. Retrieved from https://www.who.int/features/factfiles/health_inequities/en/

World Health Organization. (2018). *World health statistics 2018: Monitoring health for the SDGs, sustainable development goals.* Geneva: Author. Retrieved from https://apps.who.int/iris/bitstream/handle/10665/2 72596/9789241565585-eng.pdf?ua=1

12

BEYOND BINARY CATEGORIES

A contemporary gender studies perspective on health and illness

Lisa Jean Moore and Jonathan N. Torres

Operationalising gender and sexuality studies for health and illness research

This chapter uses some of the contributions of gender and sexuality studies to investigate contemporary research in gender, health, and illness studies. We begin with a primer on terminology that is relevant to gender and health and illness. Next, we turn to a literature review of recent, innovative interventions into the overlapping fields of gender and health and illness. In particular, we highlight recent studies that use emergent methods and theories to understand the limits of binary categorisation as well as the material consequences of sexist practices. Exciting and significant work continues to demonstrate the expansive ways individuals express and experience their sex and gender with respect to age, health, and caregiving. One other area of innovative work in gendered health wrestles with the consequences of public health campaigns and climate change for individual and communities in postcolonial environments. We conclude with a summation and recommendations for new areas of research and identify global gender health priorities.

While many epidemiological studies use the category of gender as a primary social determinant of health status and outcomes, health, and illness researchers are not always adequately educated regarding the theories, methods, and concepts that include a gender analysis. Gender and sexuality studies, also sometimes called gender and women's studies or feminist studies, is the interdisciplinary study of sex, sexuality, and gender, particularly how and with what consequence people are categorised and stratified into the binary categories of "female" and "male". Gender and sexuality studies are committed to investigating how the dual meanings of "sex" – as a classification system and as intimate action – reverberate to put gender and sexuality in very close proximity to each other. The field examines, among other topics, how biological characteristics are used as a basis for social organisation. That is to say, biological attributes that differentiate male and female individuals have been used to produce and in certain cases justify inequalities between genders. While we acknowledge that there is a gender continuum beyond the binary, we must acknowledge that gender also means the legal status of woman or man usually based on sex assigned at birth; there is assumed congruence between sex and gender, although actual biological evidence is often limited to laypeople (Lorber & Moore, 2011). Included in gender studies are investigations of gender representation, gender roles, the social construction of gender and sex, sexuality and its expressions, gender in social institutions, politics and policy, transnational feminisms, LGBTQ identities, and various social processes in their gendered dynamics such as socialisation, reproduction, education, psychoanalysis, migration, and employment.

Many (but not all) scholars of gender and sexuality studies consider themselves to be feminist and/or anti-racist and anti-imperialist in their political and intellectual orientation. The field has been greatly influenced by the growth of queer theory since the 1980s (Jagose, 1996). Queer theory is an interdisciplinary approach to cultural studies that disrupts normative definitions of sex, gender, and sexuality. By the 1990s, a burgeoning body of trans historical and cross-cultural literary, documentary, performance, political, and anthropological work had developed into the new field of transgender studies (see, for example, Currah, Juang, & Minter, 2006; Stryker & Whittle, 2006). Transgender studies, a deeply interdisciplinary field of research, theory, and pedagogy, influences and is influenced by gender and sexuality studies, LGBT activism, and queer theory. This new field linked insights and analyses drawn from the experience or study of transgender experiences with the central disciplinary concerns of contemporary humanities and social science research.

Key terminology in gender studies

Typically, we use the term *sex* to refer to common biological criteria for classification as female or male: chromosomes (XX for female, XY for male), hormones (oestrogen for female, testosterone for male), genitalia (clitoris, vagina, and uterus for female; penis and scrotum for male), procreative organs (ovaries and uterus for female, testes for male), gametes (ova for females, sperm for males). These biological criteria, however, are not as objective as they appear based on phenotypic markers, threshold measurements, and cultural beliefs (Kessler, 1998; Fausto-Sterling, 2000). In other words, using phenotypic markers of anatomical parts such as penises, body hair, and breasts, threshold measurements such as length of clitoris or sex hormone levels, or cultural beliefs about the size of the penis, people make a decision about an individual's gender. Many individuals do not fit into these dichotomous categories. The term *intersex* is an umbrella term to refer to people born with procreative or sexual anatomy that doesn't fit the typical chromosomal, hormonal, or gonadal definitions of female or male – appearing genitally female but having mostly male-typical anatomy internally, or a person born with XX chromosomes, a "large" clitoris or lacking a vaginal opening, or a person born with XY chromosomes, a "small" penis or with a divided scrotum resembling female labia, or a person born with mosaic genetics, so that some cells have XX chromosomes and some have XY. Intersex characteristics may not show up until puberty, or at attempts to conceive.

Gender is the social, cultural, and legal status as a woman or man, usually based on sex assigned at birth, but may be legally changed. Gender status produces patterns of social expectations for bodies, behaviour, emotions, family, and work roles. Gendered expectations can change over time both on individual and social levels. There is an assumed congruence between sex and gender, although the actual biological evidence of sex is often limited. Rather, we assume that when we know someone's gender (their embodied behaviour and presentation), we also know their sex (their physiological and biological status). *Gender expression* is the presentation of self as a gendered person through the use of markers and symbols, such as clothing, hairstyles, and jewellery. Our interaction with others relies on gender display to structure the ways we speak, behave, and socialise with one another.

Transgender is a word that has shifted significantly in meaning since it first began appearing in cross-dresser community publications in the late 1960s. Political theorist Paisley Currah suggests that since the early 1990s, *transgender* has become most commonly used to describe people in the United States whose gender identity or gender expression does not conform to social expectations for their birth sex (Currah, 2006). *Cisgender* is an adjective describing a person whose gender corresponds to the gender they were assigned at birth. The term "cisgender" was first used by biologist Dana Leland Defosse in 1994 "in a Web-based call for research on campus climate and transgender subjectivities" (Enke, 2013, pp. 234–235).

Gender nonconforming is a term that describes people who do not conform to the socially expected gender display of their sex assigned at birth. *Gender nonconforming* can be used for intersex, cisgender, or transgender people. Often these individuals are challenging the idea of the gender binary and can also identify as *non-binary* or *genderqueer*, meaning they do not identify with male or female or exclusively as male or female, and often use they/them pronouns. GNC people can be heterosexual, bisexual, homosexual, or pansexual.

These terms do not have absolute meaning. They are used differently in different parts of the world. While we have tried to define the key terminology above, linguistic and discursive labels are unable to contain all the permutations of the meaning of gender difference between nations and regions of the globe. We have cautiously adopted the terms Global North and Global South to indicate socioeconomic and political divisions and hierarchies across the geographic region while we acknowledge there are other ways to identify geopolitical differences such as high-income countries, or emerging markets, see, for example, Silver (2015). The Global North typically includes North America, Europe, Australia, and "more developed" parts of Asia, for example, Japan and South Korea, whereas the Global South refers to Africa, South and Central America, and "less developed" parts of Asia, for example, Cambodia or Myanmar. Taking our lead from DAWN (Development Alternatives with Women for a New Era), the term "south" is a political and ideological location-position that describes poor and marginalised people's experiences. Thus, we prefer this terminology to the language of "development", which carries with it meanings of value, attainment, and hierarchy.

Health consequences, for the most part, remain tied to normative understandings that construct a notion of active and passive citizens with respect to individual wellbeing (Simon-Kumar et al., 2018). As the literature suggests, people in the Global North are seen as active agents of their wellbeing and as environmentally conscious, whereas people in the Global South are seen as passive recipients of environmental degradation with poor health linked to toxicity or natural disasters. Postcolonial scholars urge for a perspective of interconnectedness that seeks to recognise that health and gender intersections are not solely contained within the immediate social environment but rather are influenced by conditions, both material and ideological, that are global in breadth and that influence the ways in which women, communities, and populations (and their health) are linked to natural environments (Simon-Kumar et al., 2018).

Recent scholarship on sex, gender, and health: complicating causal explanations of gender and health

While the causal link between "sex" and "gender" is often thought to flow automatically from biological to social difference, recent research has forcefully demonstrated that the influence operates in the other direction (Springer et al., 2012). One explanation of how social influences affect health is the gender feedback loop. Through the social policing and surveillance of gender, everyday confirmations reaffirm messages surrounding sex categories, ideas regarding self, and material practices that reaffirm one's gendered body. Through the gender feedback loop (including the surveillance and accountability of gendered behaviour), gendered messages develop gendered consequences (Crawley et al., 2008).

The classic epidemiology phrase "women are sicker, but men die quicker" illustrates this paradox. Researchers have brought attention to this gender and health paradox. Research demonstrates that women have longer life expectancies and higher morbidity (illness) rates than men. Men experience more life-threatening chronic diseases and die younger, whereas women live longer but have more nonfatal acute and chronic conditions and disability (Rieker & Bird, 2005). Often due to *gender socialisation*, men have greater exposure to toxins and risky occupational hazards as well as greater rates of suicide. Medical sociologist Patricia P. Rieker and women's health scholar Chloe E. Bird's (2005) gerontological research explains the gender and health paradox and the need to incorporate social and biological perspectives to solve gender differences in population health.

Two frameworks that include social and biological factors in health differences are sex/gender entanglement and interconnectedness. A collaborative team, including the medical sociologist Kristen Springer, public health scholar Jeanne Stellman, and gender studies scholar Rebecca Jordan Young (2012), introduces the concept of entanglement to provide alternative perspectives for health research. They utilise ideas from quantum physics to describe health research where no individual element can fully describe a quantum mechanical state without the incorporation of other elements, and any attempt to measure a single factor inevitably perturbs the remaining system, rendering results inaccurate (Springer et al., 2012). A quantum explanation breaks components down to their most fundamental unit and then defines these components as part of an interrelated system, as such sex and gender are deconstructed and revealed to be deeply dependent upon one another to define each. Thus, borrowing from the quantum physics field, sex and gender can be viewed as two entangled factors (much like energy and matter) that function together, impacting one's life experience and physical/mental wellbeing.

Additionally, gender and health scholars Rachel Simon-Kumar, Sara Macbride-Stewart, Susan Baker, and Lopamudra Patnaik Saxena develop an interconnectedness framework in theorising gender differences. Simon-Kumar et al. (2018) focus on the shared experiences of women in the Global North and South, and analyses the relationships between gender, environment, and health. Their extensive literature review of these three fields of scholarship led them to conclude the need for additional frameworks beyond simple dualisms such as male/female, North/South, and nature/culture. Furthermore, Ann Öhman et al. (2015) calls for further research into work-related health, which is one of the leading ill-causes of health in the world. Unpaid work is heavily gendered, with women having more responsibilities in terms of childcare, elderly care, and household duties. Öhman et al. (2015) further call for climate change research to focus on global warming's effect on gender, and the need for postcolonial perspectives in the fields of gender and health. The need for a theoretical integration of such perspectives is immense, and would highlight inequalities, disparities, and tensions between the Global South and Global North in terms of public health policy and international declarations (Öhman et al., 2015). Thus, by drawing on the theoretical frameworks featured in Springer et al. (2012), Simon-Kumar et al. (2018), and Öhman et al. (2015) we can further account for sociocultural influences on gender and health.

Trans, GNC, and cis gender differences

A person's relationship to prevailing gender roles, and the social expectations that come with them, may shape social opportunities and present constraints influencing health in ways that are not primarily associated with one's sex assignment at birth (Lagos, 2018). Sociologist Danya Lagos, whose research focuses on gender and social determinants of population health, analysed data from the US' Behavioral Risk Factor Surveillance System in their 2018 study to examine disparities in self-reported health among trans, gender nonconforming, and cisgender individuals. Analyses using survey data from across the United States to compare cis and gender-nonconforming individuals frequently do not account for individuals who may be gender nonconforming as well as transgender. A gender-nonconforming identity can intersect with various expressions of cisgender or transgender identity (Miller & Grollman, 2015). Lagos (2018) found that gender-nonconforming respondents are the only non-cisgender group with a consistently significant health disadvantage compared with both cisgender men and cisgender women. Gender-nonconforming individuals may face discriminatory attitudes in work and/ or clinical spaces. Past research conducted on trans/gender-nonconforming discrimination has focused primarily on the workplace. There is currently a lack of research focusing on gender nonconformity as a factor impacting health.

Sociologists Lisa R. Miller and Eric A. Grollman have helped to fill this gap by focusing on gender nonconformity as a form of "stigma visibility", which is defined as a known, visible, conspicuous, and discredited stigmatised status (Miller & Grollman, 2015). Miller and Grollman specialise in examining the consequences faced by LGBTQ+ individuals due to prejudice and discrimination, using the concept of stigma visibility to demonstrate how these consequences impact wellbeing. Using cross-sectional data from the US National Center for Transgender Equality's Discrimination Survey, Miller and Grollman (2015) used stigma visibility and the minority stress model to analyse the differences in self-reported health. Similar to Lagos (2018), their measures include socioeconomic status, race/ethnicity, marital status, and smoking, as well as health-harming behaviours such as smoking, drug/alcohol abuse, and attempted suicide. They found that trans people who were frequently read by others as trans and gender-nonconforming faced major and everyday events of discrimination and were more likely to engage in health-harming behaviours compared to gender-conforming or "passing" trans individuals. Those who belonged to multiple disadvantaged groups (people of colour, lower-income) faced additional stressors and engaged in higher rates of health-harming behaviours.

Particularly, the constant threat of anti-transgender violence, or the threat of violence against transgender and gender-nonconforming individuals, is one health stressor that should be acknowledged in health and illness frameworks. Researchers Jeremy D. Kidd, who specialises in public health and LGBTQ+ psychiatry, and Tarynn M. Witten, who specialises in biomedical simulation and modelling, reviewed this topic in a 2007 review. Using data on hate crimes from the TranScience Longitudinal Aging Research Study, these researchers state that the most common forms of violence experienced are physical, emotional, or sexually based. Additionally, Kidd and Witten (2007) state that anti-transgender violence is a pandemic that spans the globe. In Argentina, a report identified over 400 transgender deaths in the Buenos Aires metropolitan region between 2000 and 2006; 62% of these deaths were due to people dying of AIDS while 17% were due to people being murdered. In Nepal, police began to jail transwoman, or *metis*. This "sexual cleansing" of the population led to the jailing of HIV outreach workers, thereby threatening public health. In the United States, the Trump Administration has roll backed policies that ban gender identity discrimination, and has barred transgender individuals to serve in the military. This widely prevalent hate violence not only threatens the safety of transgender people, but also detrimentally affects the greater pursuit of universal civil liberties, public health, and democratic governance (Kidd & Witten, 2007). Furthermore, both anti-transgender and violence against cis women go unreported systematically. Under-reporting of gender-based violence is due to numerous social, economic, and personal factors.

Gender-based violence is defined as violence directed at a person because of their gender, and in addition to physical, emotional, or verbal abuse, it can include the denial of resources or access to services. Public health effects of gender-based violence include exposure to sexually transmitted diseases and infections, unwanted pregnancy, and substance abuse. UNICEF Social Policy Specialists Tia Palermo and Amber Peterman, and Jennifer Bleck, who specialise in community and family health, explore the under-reporting of gender-based violence in the Global South. Barriers to reporting or seeking care from formal sources include shame and stigma, financial barriers, lack of awareness of available services, and discriminatory attitudes towards victims in courts and law enforcement settings (Palermo et al., 2014). The researchers used cross-sectional data from Demographic and Health Surveys from Central Asia and Eastern Europe, Latin America, India and East Asia, and Africa. They found that the average woman who did not formally report gender-based violence was typically younger, never or currently married, and living in a rural community. Regional differences in recording reflected important cultural, political, and religious differences as well. Significantly, the highest rates of formal reporting were found in Latin America, whereas the lowest rates were reported in Asia. Reasons described for not reporting suggest that policy initiatives should address the impunity of perpetrators; ensure that gender-based violence, particularly within marriage, is a prosecutable crime; and provide subsidies for gender-based violence-related health costs (Palermo et al., 2014). Furthermore, implementation and enforcement of policies that target gender-based violence use a small sample of data that does not account for the larger population of women who experience such violence. Estimates indicate that rates of physical or sexual gender-based violence in the population may be 7–44 times the number of incidents formally reported (Palermo et al., 2014). Analysing social factors such as caregiving, marriage, and ageing could provide further insight into the different contexts involved in the prevalence of gender-based violence, as discussed below.

The demands of informal caregiving are likely to rise as life expectancies increase globally. According to the National Alliance for Caregiving, a caregiver or informal caregiver, is an unpaid individual who assists someone in daily and or medical tasks. About 43.5 million Americans fulfilled the role of caregiver at home. Caregiving is gendered, and therefore there are gendered implications of caregiving across the globe. In the Global North (where we have the most rigorously collected data), a majority (75%) of caregivers are cis women, who typically spend about 50% more time providing care than cis men. The Alliance for Caregiving also mentions that women caregivers are more likely than men to make alternate work arrangements thereby changing women's economic stability and fiscal security. These challenges of gender norms, caregiving expectations, and work opportunities lead to women pursuing fewer demanding jobs, giving up work entirely, and losing job-related benefits (National Alliance for Caregiving and AARP, 2009).

In terms of marriage, gender, and health, sociologists Umberson and Kroeger (2016) focused on the marital dynamics between married, different-sex, and same-sex couples to explore differences in health outcomes, as well as provide a framework to better understand caregiving among these two populations. Compared to those who are unmarried and or live without a partner, couples who live together reported better self-assessed health, lower rates of chronic illness, were less likely to be institutionalised in old age, more likely to survive heart attacks, and live longer (Umberson & Kroeger, 2016). However, these benefits have changed over time and the legalisation of gay marriage in June of 2015 in the USA has provided a new arena in which to analyse how marriage affects health. Specifically, men and women bring contemporary sociocultural ideas and experiences of gender into their relationships. These cultural ideas include emotional work and support women provide for men.

Using a gender-as-relational perspective, Umberson and Kroeger interviewed 15 gay male couples, 15 lesbian couples, and 15 heterosexual couples. They found that both men and women who are married to women reduce the amount of emotion work they do when their partner is under a lot of stress. Emotion work, outlined by Arlie Hochschild (1979), is the affective work an individual accomplishes to bring the appropriate emotional reaction to a given situation, such as being compassionate when someone is ill.

This finding is consistent with past research that shows men typically give time and space to their wives if they notice stressed attitudes or feelings. Additionally, findings suggest that the emotion work provided by women in same-sex relationships is affected by both their own stress level as well as the spouse's stress level, whereas the emotion work provided by men in same-sex relationships is reduced only when the emotion work provider is under stress. The receipt of emotion work was found to be positive for the health of men, but not women. Furthermore, the provision of emotion work was found to be positively related to the health of same-sex couples, but not significantly related to the health of different-sex couples. The health stressors LGBT people face may influence their decision to marry, and this benefits both partners' long-term health, respectively. The health effects of marital dynamics among same-sex and different-sex couples can further contribute to research regarding both ageing and marriage.

Nine per cent of LGBT people are caregivers, and about 3 million LGBT US citizens are 55 and older, a number that is expected to double in the next two decades. Health stressors such as concern over financial stability, loneliness in old age, and declining physical health affect this population more than non-LGBT individuals. Past research that examines marriage and health has solely focused on heterosexual men and women. The findings outlined above provide a micro-level analysis of trans, gender-nonconforming, and cisgender differences in health. However, the data featured in Lagos (2018), Miller and Grollman (2015), and Umberson and Kroeger (2016), utilised small sample sizes from the US, which can't fully reflect the full variation of differences between and among these populations. Furthermore, Rieker and Bird (2005) state that in order to create a framework fully encompassing of gendered health differences, it needs to incorporate contextual effects at the level of the family, community, and social policy in ways that extend beyond models of gender inequality and inequity. Factors such as globalisation and climate change can be useful in expanding frameworks that analyse gender differences in health.

Postcoloniality and the climate crisis

Health differences among trans, GNC, and cis individuals are also shaped by a globalising world. Using a postcolonial perspective has proven useful to more fully understand health inequality in both the Global North and South. Postcoloniality, or postcolonialism, is a field of study exploring the cultural legacy of colonialism and imperialism. The exploitation and extraction of labour and resources from the Global South by the Global North and the North's imposition of norms and values reverberate well past indigenous liberation movements. Gendered effects of international migration are another issue of importance for future global health research on gender and health (Öhman et al., 2015). Anthropologist Ramah McKay, who specialises in healthcare and policy, conducted a study in Maputo, Mozambique, in 2018 to examine how global health interventions articulate with urban economies, colonial legacies, and gendered relations. Following independence, public health services were nationalised in the country and hospitals used by the former colonial elite became public. However, most medical services were still based in urban centres. Postcolonial medicine thus reinforced colonial health structures (McKay, 2018). During the late 1980s and early 1990s, global health organisations played a large role in providing medical services to Maputo residents, but critics have shown that these processes may fragment and stratify public health systems (McKay, 2018). Simon-Kumar et al. (2018) mention that since this time period, medicine has been transformed by a set of interrelated processes of modernisation, scientisation, technical innovation, and neoliberal economics. This transformation of medicine and medical care directly influences gendered relations. Understanding how colonialism and migration still impact health inequities across populations could lead to better access to care, improved quality of care, and advocacy for the most marginalised groups. For example, McKay (2018) explains how mobility in Maputo is seen as both a risk and resource.

Migratory labour across country lines is seen as a masculine mode of caregiving in that men can provide income through their migrant work; thus, global health organisations targeted men in their campaigns, encouraging these men to get tested for HIV. However, women also use their mobility as a resource to create livelihoods even in the face of restricting gender social norms. Instead of recognising the social and economic benefits of migrant labour for women, global health organisations are pathologising what a "healthy" labourer looks like.

Furthermore, women in McKay's study, such as a participant named Glória, only seek medical treatment based upon the relations they have with both family and clinical spaces. To be a good patient and a good mother also required her to accommodate familial expectations even as they contravened clinic norms (McKay, 2018). Global health organisations may therefore be reinforcing colonial ways of seeking medical care. In order to disrupt this, healthcare interventions will need to be based upon knowledge of local culture and practices in order to deliver meaningful and efficacious response to local issues (Cox & Webb, 2015).

Climate change also presents new gendered challenges in theorising health frameworks for those living in the Global North and Global South. Climate change is the longitudinal change in temperature and normal weather patterns across the globe attributed to global warming. Global warming is due to human activity producing more greenhouse gases which has led to sea-level rise, prolonged droughts, and increased wildfires. According to the Center for Disease Control's National Climate Assessment (2014) climate change is expected to increase the number of respiratory and cardiovascular diseases, injuries and premature deaths due to natural disasters, the prevalence of food and waterborne illnesses, and threats to mental health. Research on the impact climate change will have on public health is still largely unaddressed and developing a framework to support those at risk is crucial as the situation worsens.

Ecofeminist writer and activist Greta Gaard addresses this in their essay regarding ecofeminism and climate change. Gaard suggests a queer feminist climate justice perspective is needed to transform the solutions for climate change. The United States, China, Russia, and India are the leading countries contributing to emissions in the atmosphere. However,

Between 75–80% of the effects of climate change will be felt by the Global South (Gaard, 2015). These effects will exacerbate health-related issues such as air quality, food security and water accessibility. The United Nations' *Women Watch* fact sheet on gender and climate change states women constitute the majority of the world's poor and are more dependent for their livelihood on natural resources being threatened by climate change. Women also make up a majority of victims of natural disasters. Gender inequalities mean that women and children are 14 times more likely to die in ecological disasters than men (Gaard, 2015). The dramatic effects of this statistic play out in disasters within the past 20 years.

Gaard's (2015) research reveals that 75% of those who died in the 2004 Indian Ocean tsunami were women, more women than men died in the 2003 European heatwave, while after Hurricane Katrina in the USA in 2005, African American women faced the most obstacles to survival. In attempts to mitigate the issue, organisations such as the WorldWatch Institute have advocated for population reduction through the advancement of women's rights. However, this strategy is inherently problematic as those targeted for "family planning" are women in the Global South. This area accounts for 80% of the world's population, but only generates about 20% of greenhouse gases. Thus, none of these strategies suggests reducing the North/First World's alarming overconsumption of the planet's resources, or seriously restricting its 80% contribution to greenhouses gases (Gaard, 2015).

Research conducted on climate change and climate justice excludes most queer, gender-nonconforming, and trans individuals. In statements of climate justice to date, there is no mention of the integral need for queer climate justice – although our climates are both gendered and sexualised, simultaneously material, cultural, and ecological (Gaard, 2015). Climate change affects the most marginalised communities first. For example, Hurricane Katrina exacerbated a pre-existing socio-ecological disaster (Haskell, 2014). LGBTQ+ communities in Louisiana, Alabama, and Mississippi were discriminated against by faith-based relief organisations, which refused these populations the aid they required. In regard to health issues after the storm, same-sex partnerships were not granted visitation rights in hospitals, nor any consideration in deciding medical care. Health services provided after the storm failed to treat those living with HIV. These individuals experienced difficulty obtaining antiretrovirals, and often emergency relief doctors had no expertise in handling HIV patients (Haskell, 2014). Furthermore, as a global phenomenon, homophobia infiltrates climate change discourse, distorting our analysis of climate change causes and climate justice solutions, placing a wedge between international activists (Gaard, 2015). As climate change continues to advance towards crisis levels, the health of women and girls, queer, gender-nonconforming, and trans individuals becomes endangered by discriminatory practices and policies.

Climate change has been most widely discussed as a scientific problem requiring technological and scientific solutions without substantially transforming ideologies and economies of domination, exploitation, and colonialism (Gaard, 2015). Using research from both McKay (2018) and Gaard (2015), health differences across gender and sexuality may only be solved by including postcolonial and ecofeminist perspectives. This perspective is utilised in the 27 Bali Principles of Climate Justice (2002), based upon climate justice principles created by the first National People of Color Environmental Summit in 1993. The work of the Summit falls within the interconnectedness framework of Simon-Kumar et al. (2018), which in turn can expand climate policies that are inclusive of vulnerable populations. When examining health and illness between the Global North and Global South, it is important to consider the impact a warming planet has on already vulnerable communities. These communities become diasporic, wandering the planet in search of food, clean water, safety, and shelter and existing gendered stratifications may become exacerbated, leading to intractable social and health problems.

Whither gender binaries: Areas for growth

In the space that remains, we suggest areas for continued development in health and illness research with respect to gender, sex and sexuality. Clearly problematising the taken-for-granted gender and sex binary must be assiduously pursued by researchers as to not reify dichotomous categories as biologically rigid and determinative. It is true that sex and gender exist and have real and material effects on people's health and wellbeing. But as this chapter shows, the ways in which researchers define and operationalise the categories of "sex" and "gender" and how scholars then measure the effects of "sex" and "gender" on health is deeply consequential to the findings of the research. In other words, if we aim to find sex and gender differences between only men and women, we might "find" differences, but this will only tell part of the story. Furthermore, since individuals live self-determined lives that do not neatly fall within gender binaries, health research must consider broadening the available categories of identification.

Research shows that the number of transgender individuals has increased over the decade in the United States (Meerwijk & Sevelius, 2017), and it is likely that the number of individuals identifying as gender-nonconforming, transgender, or non-binary will continue to grow. Therefore, it is critical that researchers and policymakers accurately measure health outcomes for all people as well as create health advocacy that addresses human needs. This inclusion of all humans requires methodological intervention in qualitative and quantitative health research. Specifically, there needs to be a conscious turn toward studying the health outcomes of those with the greatest social and economic disparity.

Simultaneous to generating research that accurately reflects gender diversity, it is crucial that research integrate an understanding of how global social power is deeply gendered into their work. We want to be extremely clear that in reconsidering the gender binary for health research, we do think that sexism exists and structures health and wellbeing in both the Global North and South. Deeply important to all research is the imperative to include an analysis that foregrounds a critique of the overwhelmingly paternalistic, male-dominated, misogynistic global terrain that structures human life. While there may be differences in health outcomes for people based on sex or gender, there absolutely are differences in exposures, risks, quality of care, violence, resources, and labour based on stratification of the sex and gender binary. In other words, bodies are treated differently because of their sex categorisation, and this in turn creates sex differences.

International organisations such as the World Health Organization (WHO), a specialised agency of the United Nations, work to steer global priorities for health care access, delivery, and prevention. In early 2019, WHO released a news report illustrating a worldwide lack of women (and presumably trans and gender-nonconforming people) in leadership positions in healthcare administration and delivery. The report suggests that meeting gender equity goals are severely hampered due to chronic bias, discrimination, and salary gaps; statistics reveal that 69% of global health organisations have male leadership, and 80% of board chairs are male (World Health Organization, 2019). Thus, a priority for gender equity in health care research and delivery is greater gender representation achieved through policies and practices that repair the structural barriers to women and gender-nonconforming people's participation in the health care work-force at the leadership level.

One thing is certain – public health crises such as climate change, gender-based violence, labour shortages, and global pandemics will continue to emerge, possibly with even more rapidity and severity than has been seen to date. But the way we analyse, approach, and prepare for these eventualities can be improved by incorporating a gender studies approach. With a critical perspective on health and illness agenda informed by gender studies, all people can be considered when attempting to address burgeoning health threats as well as acute and chronic health problems.

References

Climate Change and Public Health – Climate Effects on Health | CDC. (n.d.). Retrieved from https://www.cdc.gov/climateandhealth/effects/default.htm

Cox, F., Newsham, K. K., Bol, R., Dungait, J. A., & Robinson, C. H. (2016). Not poles apart: Antarctic soil fungal communities show similarities to those of the distant Arctic. *Ecology Letters, 19*, 528–536.

Crawley, S. L., Foley, L. J., & Shehan, C. L. (2008). *Gendering bodies*. Lanham, MD: Rowman & Littlefield Publishing Group.

Currah, P. (2006). Gender pluralisms under the transgender umbrella. In Paisley Currah, Richard M. Juang, & Shannon Price Minter (Eds.), *Transgender rights*. Minneapolis, MN: University of Minnesota Press.

Currah, P., Juang, R. M., & Minter, S. P. (Eds.). (2006). *Transgender rights*. Minneapolis, MN: University of Minnesota Press.

Enke, A. F. (2013). The education of little cis: Cisgender and the discipline of opposing bodies. In Susan Stryker and Aren Z. Aizura (Eds.), *The transgender studies reader 2* (pp. 234–247). New York: Routledge.

Fausto-Sterling, A. (2000). *Sexing the body*. New York: Basic Books.

Gaard, G. (2015). Ecofeminism and climate change. *Women's Studies International Forum, 49*, 20–33.

Haskell, B. (2014). Sexuality and natural disaster: Challenges of LGBT communities facing hurricane Katrina (10 May 2014). Available at SSRN: https://ssrn.com/abstract=2513650

Hochschild, A. (1979). Emotion work, feeling rules, and social structure. *American Journal of Sociology*, *85*(3), 551–575.

Jagose, A. (1996). *Queer theory: An introduction*. New York: New York University Press.

Kessler, S. (1998). *Lessons from the intersexed*. New Brunswick, NJ: Rutgers University Press.

Kidd, J. D., & Witten, T. M. (2007). Transgender and trans sexual identities: The next strange fruit-hate crimes, violence and genocide against the global trans-communities. *Journal of Hate Studies*, *6*(1), 31–63.

Lagos, D. (2018). Looking at population health beyond "male" and "female": Implications of transgender identity and gender nonconformity for population health. *Demography*, *55*(6), 2097–2117.

Lorber, J., & Moore, L. J. (2011). *Gendered bodies: Feminist perspectives*. Oxford: Oxford University Press.

McKay, R. (2018). Conditions of life in the city: Medicine and gendered relations in Maputo, Mozambique. *Journal of the Royal Anthropological Institute*, *24*(3), 532–549.

Meerwijk, E., & Sevelius, J. (2017). Transgender population size in the United States: A meta-regression of population-based probability samples. *American Journal of Public Health*, *107*(2), 1–8.

Miller, L. R., & Grollman, E. A. (2015). The social costs of gender nonconformity for transgender adults: Implications for discrimination and health. *Social Forum*, *30*, 809–831.

Öhman, A., Eriksson, M., & Goicolea, I. (2015). Gender and health – Aspects of importance for understanding health and illness in the world. *Global Health Action*, *8*(1), 26908.

Palermo, T., Bleck, J., & Peterman, A. (2014). Tip of the Iceberg: Reporting and gender-based violence in developing countries. *American Journal of Epidemiology*, *179*(5), 602–661.

Rieker, P., & Bird, C. (2005). Rethinking gender differences in health: Why we need to integrate social and biological perspectives. *Journals of Gerontology: Series B*, *60*(2), S40–S47.

Silver, M. (2015). If you shouldn't call it the third world, what should you call it? *NPR*, 4 January. www.npr.org/sections/goatsandsoda/2015/01/04/372684438/if-you-shouldnt-call-it-the-third-world-what-should-you-call-it accessed on 30 November 2020.

Simon-Kumar, R., MacBride-Stewart, S., Baker, S., & Saxena, L. P. (2018). Towards North-South interconnectedness: A critique of gender dualities in sustainable development, the environment and women's health. *Gender, Work & Organization*, *25*, 246–263.

Springer, K. W., Stellman, J. M., & Jordan-Young, R. M. (2012). Beyond a catalogue of differences: A theoretical frame and good practice guidelines for researching sex/gender in human health. *Social Science & Medicine*, *74*(11), 1817–1824.

Stryker, S., & Whittle, S. (Eds.). (2006). *The transgender studies reader*. New York: Routledge.

Umberson, D., & Kroeger, R. (2016). Gender, marriage, and health for same-sex and different-sex couples: The future keeps arriving. In McHale S., King V., Van Hook J., & Booth A. (Eds.), *Gender and couple relationships*. *National symposium on family issues*, vol 6. Springer, Switzerland.

World Health Organization. (2019). 10 key issues in ensuring gender equity in the global health workforce. https://www.who.int/news-room/feature-stories/detail/10-key-issues-in-ensuring-gender-equity-in -the-global-health-workforce accessed on 24 May 2019.

13

SEXUAL ORIENTATION AND GENDER IDENTITY AS DETERMINANTS OF HEALTH AND ILLNESS

Alex Müller

Introduction

Over the past two decades, research on sexual and gender minority health (the health of LGBTQ – lesbian, gay, bisexual, transgender, and queer – people) has highlighted substantial health disparities based on sexual orientation and gender identity. Despite increasing legal recognition and social acceptance in many parts of the world, research shows that sexual and gender minority people remain at increased risk of harassment and victimisation, and have higher rates of depression, suicide, smoking, and alcohol use than their heterosexual counterparts, as well as a higher risk for obesity, cardiovascular disease, and malignancies (Mayer et al., 2008). This is not because identifying as lesbian, gay, bisexual, or transgender is a pathology or is physiologically hazardous, but because social stigma, marginalisation, and discrimination confer risk factors for sexual and gender minority people's health. In brief, sexual orientation and gender identity are social determinants of health (Logie, 2012; Pega & Veale, 2015).

In this chapter, I provide an overview of health disparities related to sexual orientation and gender identity and summarise the current theoretical frameworks to explain these. First of all, however, I place the relationship between sexual orientation, gender identity, and health in a historical and global context, to highlight the significant changes across the world and over time.

Lesbian, gay, bisexual, transgender, and queer (LGBTQ) people are not a homogenous population, nor is the acronym exhaustive of the diversity of sexual orientations and gender identities. What individuals grouped together under the acronym share are similar experiences of discriminatory treatment in society because of their sexual orientation, gender identity, and/or gender expression. Whilst such a grouping can be useful for analysing the consequences of marginalisation, it is important not to assume that individuals under this umbrella acronym necessarily have similar experiences or needs. In fact, individual experiences differ greatly across the populations covered under the acronym. Thus, the populations represented by each individual letter in the acronym are complex and heterogeneous, and oppressions and vulnerabilities based on race, age, ability, religion, culture, socioeconomic class, and geographic location often intersect, exacerbate, and amplify the effects of homo- and transphobia. In order to keep the focus on the shared causes of oppression, discrimination and marginalisation, I will refer to individuals whose sexual orientations and/or gender identities do not fit society's norms as sexual and gender minorities. That is, I use the term sexual and gender minorities deliberately because it frames individuals in relation to the dominant majority (heterosexual and cisgender individuals in heteronormative societies, see below), and thus emphasises shared experiences of minority status.

Identifying as lesbian, gay, bisexual, transgender, or queer is not genetically or biologically hazardous, nor is it an inherent pathology. The social stigma related to sexual orientations or gender identities that are regarded not to be the norm, however, leads to marginalisation and discrimination, and can confer risk factors for sexual and gender minority people's health. These phenomena are born out of heteronormativity and homo- and transphobia. Heteronormativity is a social construct that simplifies human sexuality and gender identity by assuming that heterosexual identities, attractions, and relationships are the idealised normality (therefore also "normativity") – that there exist only two, opposite sexes, and each should be attracted to the other. Heteronormativity is part of many societies' ideologies across the world and informs various religious beliefs and political stances. Homo- and transphobia, the irrational fear and hatred of people who are attracted to the same sex (lesbian, gay, and bisexual people) and people whose gender identity is not aligned to the sex assigned to them at birth (transgender people), result from heteronormativity. They lead to social exclusion, experiences of discrimination and stigma, and in the worst-case violence directed against people whose real or perceived sexual orientation or gender identity does not fit the narrowly defined heterosexual norms (Mayer et al., 2008).

Increasingly, awareness about and criticism of heteronormativity has pointed out how this worldwide existing phenomenon makes sexual and gender minorities invisible in all facets of social life, including in healthcare and health-related research. Through its pervasive normative influence, healthcare providers often assume that every patient is heterosexual and either a man or a woman with a respective male or female natal sex (so called "cisgender" as the opposite of transgender). As a result, in many places, sexual and gender minority people's diverse health needs are not recognised, documented, or researched (Logie, 2012). For example, in most clinical records sexual orientation and gender identity are not recorded as part of the patient characteristics. This makes it near impossible to analyse sexual orientation- or gender identity-related health disparities at the population level (Cahill & Makadon, 2014).

Sexuality, gender identity, and health in context
Pathologisation of homosexuality and gender diversity

Medicine itself has, for many years, supported the perception that sexual orientations and gender identities that deviate from the narrow heteronormative norm are pathological (Drescher, 2010). Until 1973, homosexuality was a defined diagnosis in the American Psychiatric Association's *Diagnostic and Statistical Manual of Mental Disorders* (DSM), indicating the consensus of psychiatry at the time: that sexual and romantic attraction to somebody of the same sex or gender was unnatural, pathological, and could be cured through psychotherapy or electro-shock aversion therapy (Smith, 2004). The World Health Organization's International Classification of Diseases (ICD) included a diagnosis of "homosexuality" as a mental disorder until its revision to ICD-10 in 1992. Diagnoses related to gender identity persist in both DSM and ICD, with the ongoing controversy over their contribution to the pathologisation of non-normative gender identities (Drescher, 2010). Gender variance or gender diversity (formerly called non-conforming gender identity), unlike same-sex sexual orientation, remains classified as a mental illness by the American Psychiatric Association, under the diagnosis of "gender dysphoria". Many argue that this is for the same reasons that same-sex sexual orientation was once classified as a mental illness (Drescher, 2015). In the process of revising the ICD, the World Health Organisation has renamed the diagnosis "gender incongruence", and moved it from the list of mental health conditions to the list of conditions related to sexual health (World Health Organization, 2018). There is ongoing controversy about whether gender diversity should be classified under a diagnosis at all – on the one hand, many have pointed out that diversity in and of itself is not a pathology (Suess Schwend, Winter, Chiam, Smiley, & Cabral Grinspan, 2018). On the other hand, others are concerned that losing a classification in the DSM and ICD might jeopardise access to gender-affirming healthcare for people who wish to modify their body in line with their gender identity.

Today, we know that what is considered a mental illness depends on what society and scientists at a certain time and in a certain context agree to be "abnormal" behaviours, cognitions, and emotions (Gergen, 2001). International medical and health organisations, such as the World Psychiatry Association have clearly stated that same-sex orientation, attraction, and behaviour are not mental illnesses, and that attempts to "treat" same-sex sexual orientation are harmful and without evidence of success (Bhugra, Eckstrand, Levounis, Kar, & Javate, 2016). The South African Society of Psychiatrists, for example, agrees that "there is no scientific evidence that reparative or conversion therapy is effective in changing a person's sexual orientation. There is, however, evidence that this type of therapy can be destructive" (Victor, Nel, Lynch, & Mbatha, 2014).

Out of this harmful history, particular vulnerabilities for sexual and gender minority people have occurred in healthcare and health research, but also particular moral-ethical obligations for the health sciences (Martin & Meezan, 2003). The World Health Organization (2013) has called for more research evidence on the impact of sexual orientation and gender identity on health. This is particularly important in countries where state and public attitudes are flagrantly homo- and transphobic and are supported by national laws that criminalise same-sex activity and public gender expressions that transgress heteronormativity. Identifying health risks and vulnerabilities and hopefully improving health services related to sexual orientation and gender identity is therefore a strong need for future research and an important aspect of social justice.

From pathology to concepts of minority stress

After (mostly) shedding the notion that non-heteronormative sexual orientations and gender identities are pathological per se, health research could begin to look into the health and wellbeing of sexual and gender minority individuals in their own right. Over and over again, studies showed that compared to cisgender, heterosexual peers, sexual and gender minority populations suffer from more mental health concerns, such as substance use (including alcohol, tobacco, and illegal drug use), affective disorders (for example, depression and anxiety disorders) and suicide (Meyer, 2003; Hendricks & Testa, 2012). The reason for these disparities in mental health outcomes is that stigma (widespread disapproval held by many people in a society), prejudice, and discrimination lead to stressful social environments for sexual and gender minorities. This is called minority stress.

Minority stress adds to the general stress that all people experience. It is chronic because it is linked to underlying social and cultural norms (and stigma) that are relatively stable and only change slowly, if at all. Minority stress is based in social processes, institutions, and structures (for example, laws that criminalise consensual same-sex activity), and not in individual events (such as a change in financial circumstances, or the death of a loved one). Minority stress linked to a person's sexual orientation or gender identity intersects with and is exacerbated by other factors that determine social in- and exclusion, such as race, age, ability, and geographical location. Meyer (2003) suggests that there are four different processes that contribute to minority stress and mental health concerns among sexual minorities. First, chronic and acute events or social circumstances that might add to stress. This can include experiences of discrimination in education or healthcare facilities, or experiences of insults and harassment in public or private. Second, expecting such stressful events, and guarding oneself against them, also leads to stress, regardless of whether or not the discriminatory encounter actually happens. Third, hearing negative, discriminatory attitudes contributes to an internalisation of the notion that one has less value. And fourth, hiding one's sexual orientation, in anticipation of discriminatory events, in and of itself contributes to further stress.

Building on Meyer's model (which he conceptualised for sexual orientation-related minority stress), Hendricks and Testa (2012) explain how minority stress also affects gender minority people and argue that the same factors shape minority stress based on gender identity. That is, as with same-sex sexual orientation, it is not gender diversity itself that is a mental illness, but "hostile and stressful social environments" (p. 462) that lead to an increase in mental health concerns among gender minority people.

The new understanding of sexual orientation- and gender identity-based minority stress was a fundamental shift. It signifies the current consensus that stigma against same-sex orientation and gender variance is one of the key factors that underlie sexual orientation and gender identity-related health disparities. Thus, while many of the health disparities are ostensibly rooted in individual behaviour (such as alcohol use or suicidality), they are significantly impacted by societal stigmas that devalue non-normative sexual orientations and gender identities (Bogart, Revenson, Whitfield, & France, 2014). A recent report by the Executive Board Secretariat of the World Health Organization summarises this view by pointing out that one of the main challenges to improving the health and wellbeing of sexual minority people is "institutional prejudice, social stress, social exclusion (even within families) and anti-homosexual hatred and violence ..." (World Health Organization, 2013).

Sexual orientation, gender identity, and structural stigma

A number of recent studies have built on the sexual orientation- and gender identity-related minority stress models developed by Meyer (2003) and Hendricks and Testa (2012) and have examined the impact of a specific kind of stigma on the health and wellbeing of sexual and gender minority people. The specific stigma these studies were interested in is structural stigma, defined as social prejudice against lesbian, bisexual and gay people at the community level, or social stigma that is institutionalised or made into law (such as laws that criminalise consensual same-sex behaviour).

A landmark study, conducted in the United States, showed that sexual minority people who lived in areas with high levels of structural stigma died 12 years sooner than sexual minority people living in areas with low structural stigma (Hatzenbuehler et al., 2014). Further, sexual minority individuals who lived in areas with high structural stigma were three times more likely to die from homicide and violence-related deaths, compared to sexual minority individuals living in areas with low structural stigma. The study also showed that sexual minorities in high-stigma areas were more likely to die from suicide. Additionally, those who died from suicide in high-stigma areas were on average 18 years younger than those who died from suicide in low-stigma areas. These findings confirmed an earlier study, which showed that lesbian, gay and bisexual youth in areas with high anti-gay prejudice were more likely to attempt suicide (Hatzenbuehler, 2011). Similarly, another study from the United States showed that transgender adults who lived in areas with lesser structural stigma were less likely to attempt suicide (Perez-Brumer, Day, Russell, & Hatzenbuehler, 2017).

There are thus clear links between the legal status of people with non-normative sexual orientations and gender identities and their health and wellbeing. Further studies from the United States confirm this, and show, for example, that sexual orientation-related discriminatory laws and policies – laws and policies that deprive sexual minorities of certain rights (for example, the right to marry) – contribute to higher levels of mental health concerns among sexual minority populations (Hatzenbuehler, McLaughlin, Keyes, & Hasin, 2010).

This is an important finding in the global context, where, as I will show in the following section, many countries have retained laws that criminalise consensual same-sex activity, and where countries, especially in Eastern Europe, increasingly implement legislation aimed at curtailing expressions of non-conforming sexual orientation or gender identity (International Lesbian, Gay, Bisexual, Trans and Intersex Association: Lucas Ramon Mendos, 2019).

Laws governing sexual orientation and gender identity across the world

The current state of laws pertaining to sexual orientation and gender identity is vastly different in different parts of the world. Whilst in some countries same-sex couples enjoy full civic and political rights, including protection from discrimination based on sexual orientation and/or gender identity, other countries maintain legislation that criminalises private consensual sexual acts between adults of the same sex, as well as diverse gender expressions (International Lesbian, Gay, Bisexual, Trans and Intersex Association: Lucas Ramon Mendos, 2019). Figure 13.1 shows an overview of sexual orientation- and gender identity-related laws, taken from the annual report by the International Lesbian, Gay, Bisexual, Trans, and Intersex Association.

The majority of the countries that criminalise same-sex activity and public gender expressions that transgress heteronormativity are in the Global South (International Lesbian, Gay, Bisexual, Trans and Intersex Association: Lucas Ramon Mendos, 2019). In most of these countries, the laws are remnants of British colonial penal codes. Whilst laws and implementation vary across countries, the penalties for same-sex activity can include arrest, forced medical examination, and imprisonment. For example, in Malawi, as in 30 other African countries, same-sex activity between two men or two women is criminalised and punishable by up to 14 years in prison; in Zambia, police arrested two men on suspicion of "homosexuality" in August 2018; and until March 2019, men who were suspected of having sex with other men in Kenya were forced to medical examinations of their anuses to "prove" their homosexuality, a practice that the UN Special Rapporteur on Torture has strongly condemned as unethical and harmful. Further, the social climate of criminalisation means that people are often in danger of harassment and violence. In Zimbabwe, for example, police arrested over 40 people at a Christmas party of an organisation advocating for the rights of sexual and gender minorities, allegedly under the law that criminalised same-sex activity.

In many countries, gender minority people are also affected by laws that criminalise same-sex sexuality because their non-normative gender identity is read as non-normative sexual orientation. Additionally, gender minority people are vulnerable to interactions with the law and legal system when their identity documents, which form the basis of their legal identity, are based on the sex assigned to them at birth and do not reflect their gender identity. Whilst legal gender recognition – being able to hold identity documents and administrative records that correctly list one's gender identity – is increasingly accessible in Europe and South America, in many countries around the world states do not offer legal or administrative procedures to change one's name or gender marker on official documents.

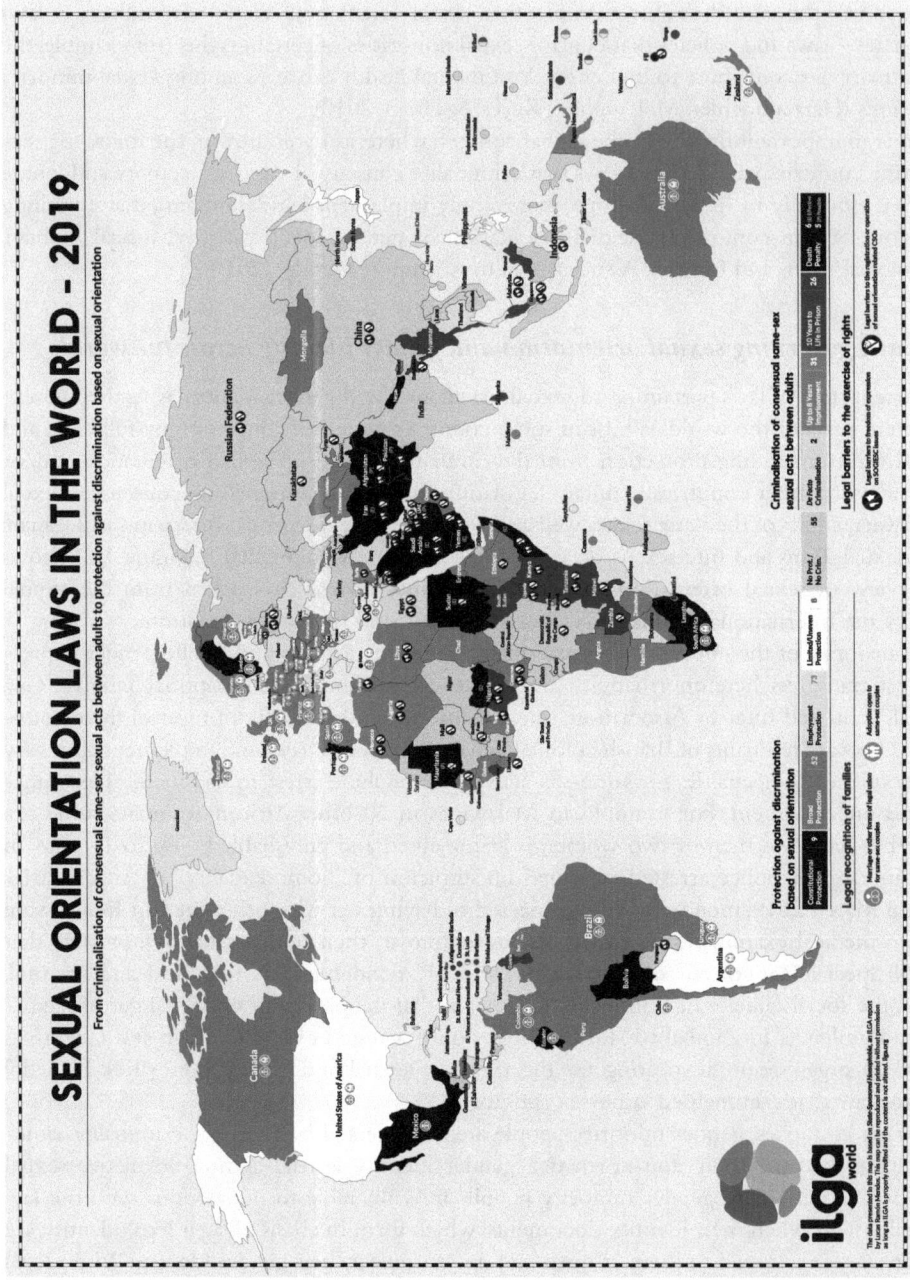

Figure 13.1 Sexual orientation laws across the world. Credit: International Lesbian, Gay, Bisexual, Trans and Intersex Association

Not only do discriminatory and criminalising laws have negative consequences for the health and wellbeing of sexual and gender minority individuals (as I have outlined in the previous section on structural stigma), but they can also impede healthcare provision for sexual and gender individuals. For example, sexual and gender minority individuals who have a health concern directly linked to their sexual orientation and/or gender identity (such as a sexual health concern, for example), often fear being reported to law enforcement and might delay seeking healthcare. This could be seen, for example, after the Nigerian government passed a new law that expressly criminalised marriage between people of the same sex or gender, the Same Sex Marriage Prohibition Act. Schwartz and colleagues, who were conducting a study on the feasibility and effectiveness of engagement of men who have sex with men in HIV prevention and treatment services at the time the law was passed, could show that the passing of the law directly and negatively impacted HIV prevention efforts (Schwartz et al., 2015). After the law was passed, significantly more of the men who had sex with men who were enrolled in their study said that they were afraid to seek healthcare, and that they avoided going to health facilities. This obviously impedes efforts to prevent and treat HIV (when individuals miss their scheduled clinic visits out of fear of being reported), and has detrimental effects on people's health in the long term. Another example are government health services that refuse to provide HIV prevention services aimed at gay men and other men who have sex with men in countries that criminalise same-sex activity, as recently seen in Tanzania. Both these examples highlight how the legal framework, even whilst ostensibly "only" criminalising sexual acts, can justify and further sexual orientation-based discrimination and hinder access to healthcare.

Gender minority people who do not have identity documents with their correct gender identity are often unable to access healthcare when an identity document is required to register as a patient or to enter a healthcare facility. An identity document that does not match a person's gender identity immediately discloses trans and gender diverse identities, which in turn can increase the risk of discrimination or denial of care, or can lead to gender minority people being accused of fraud.

Health disparities

Sexual and gender minority individuals have the same health needs as everyone else. In addition, however, they face unique health concerns that are brought about by sexual orientation- and gender identity-related stigma and discrimination, as I have outlined in the previous sections. Over the past decades, many studies have documented these sexual orientation- and gender identity-related disparities in health and healthcare (Logie, 2012; Pega & Veale, 2015; Plöderl & Tremblay, 2015). Compared to heterosexual and cisgender peers, sexual and gender minority people experience higher levels of depression, suicidality and suicidal ideation, anxiety, and substance use (Mayer et al., 2008). A recent systematic review showed that compared to the general population, transgender women across the world are 49 times more likely to be living with HIV (Baral et al., 2013). Other research shows that lesbian women have increased risks for chronic cardiovascular disease (Eliason, 2014), cervical cancer (Brown, McNair, Szalacha, Livingston, & Hughes, 2015), and obesity (Mason & Lewis, 2015)

As I have shown in the previous sections, we must not assume that these health concerns are inherent to being a sexual or gender minority person (Cochran et al., 2014). Rather, these and other health disparities are the likely result of stigma, marginalisation, and invisibility; stress associated with hiding one's sexuality; and/or the impact of enduring verbal, emotional, physical, and sexual abuse from intolerant peers, family, and community members (Meyer, 2003). In fact, as I have shown, structural stigma, particularly in communities with high anti-gay prejudice, increases the risk of premature mortality or mental health concerns for sexual and gender minority individuals (Hatzenbuehler et al., 2014; Perez-Brumer et al., 2017). Social exclusion due to sexual orientation or gender identity limits access to education, economic opportunities, and public services, including healthcare, and thus considerably reduces sexual and gender minority individuals' educational, economic, and social capital. This in turn impacts health status, health-seeking behaviour and access to healthcare for these individuals (Logie, 2012; Pega & Veale, 2015). In the following sections, I will investigate two specific health concerns (violence and mental health) in more detail.

Violence

Violence against sexual and gender minority individuals is increasingly recognised as a key public health and human rights concern. The UN Human Rights Council passed several resolutions to express concern about violence and discrimination against individuals motivated by their sexual orientation and/or gender identity (Discrimination and violence against individuals based on their sexual orientation and gender identity. HRC/29/23, 2015; Discriminatory laws and practices and acts of violence against individuals based on their sexual orientation and gender identity. HRC/19/41, 2011; Human rights, sexual orientation and gender identity. HRC/RES/17/19, 2011; Human rights, sexual orientation and gender identity. HRC/RES/27/32, 2014). In 2016, the UN Human Rights Council appointed the first *UN Independent Expert on Violence based on Sexual Orientation and Gender Identity* (Protection against violence and discrimination based on sexual orientation and gender identity. HRC/RES/32/2, 2016), who, in a recent report (Report of the Independent Expert on protection against violence and discrimination based on sexual orientation and gender identity), noted that:

> [Violence and discrimination against sexual and gender minorities] are committed in all corners of the world, and victims are presumed to be in the millions, every year. These acts extend from daily exclusion and discrimination to the most heinous acts, including torture and arbitrary killings. At their root lie the intent to punish the non-conformity of victims with preconceived notions of what should be their sexual orientation or gender identity.

A recent systematic review shows that up to 25% of sexual and gender minority people have experienced physical violence because of their sexual orientation or gender identity, and that up to 12% have experienced sexual violence (Blondeel et al., 2018). Among gender minority people specifically, up to 68% have experienced physical violence, and up to 49% sexual violence (ibid.). The systematic review mostly included data from Europe and North America. The SEARCH study, a recent study from Southern and East Africa, suggests that the violence experienced by sexual and gender minority individuals in African countries might be even higher. In this study, between 40% and 63% of sexual and gender minority people had experienced physical violence, and between 36% and 56% had experienced sexual violence (Müller, Daskilewicz, & Southern and East African Research Collective on Health, 2019a).

These studies tell us two important things: First, that the levels of violence, and thus the health consequences of violence, are high; and second, that gender minority people, who may more often visibly defy ideals of heteronormative gender identity and expression, are at an even more increased risk of violence.

The health consequences of violence are manifold: the immediate consequences are physical injuries, and, in the case of sexual violence, increased vulnerability to HIV, other sexually transmitted infections, and pregnancy. But the health consequences of violence often go far beyond the immediate: many survivors of violence experience post-traumatic stress or have long-term physical restrictions (Krug, Mercy, Dahlberg, & Zwi, 2002). For example, among South African sexual and gender minority individuals who had experienced violence, almost half showed signs of post-traumatic stress (Müller, Daskilewicz, & Southern and East African Research Collective on Health, 2019c).

Increasingly, studies are also showing that not all sexual and gender minority individuals are at the same risk for experiencing violence. More often than not, it is individuals who visibly defy heteronormative gender identity and expression who experience sexual and other forms of violence (Logie & Gibson, 2013). This means that what is considered "homophobic violence" may often be motivated by non-conforming gender expression – which the perpetrator(s) *assume* to signify a non-conforming sexual orientation (Nath, 2011). It is also important to recognise the intersectional vulnerabilities that sexual and gender minority people face: sexual and gender minority people of colour, sexual and gender minority people who are poor, and sexual and gender minority people who are homeless are often at greater risk of experiencing violence. Many of the different life contexts, such as the ones described in Part II of this handbook, intersect with sexual orientation and gender identity to affect health and wellbeing.

Mental health

The premises of the minority stress and structural stigma models – that sexual orientation – and gender identity-related stigma and discrimination negatively impact mental health – have, by now, broad empirical support. Many studies show that compared to cisgender and heterosexual people, sexual and gender minority individuals have higher levels of depression, anxiety and suicidality, and also higher levels of substance use (Plöderl & Tremblay, 2015). For example, a representative study from California in the United States showed that compared to cisgender youth, transgender youth were three times more likely to have considered suicide in the past year (Perez-Brumer et al., 2017). Similarly, a recent systematic review and meta-analysis of studies on depression or anxiety showed that lesbian, gay, and bisexual people consistently had higher rates of depression and anxiety than heterosexual people (Ross et al., 2018).

There are differences in the level of mental health concerns between the various sexual orientation and gender identity subgroups. As a recent systematic review of mental health outcomes among sexual minority populations showed, bisexual women tended to have the highest levels of depression and anxiety, whereas sexual minority men (gay men and other men who have sex with men) showed the highest levels of suicidal ideation and attempts (Plöderl & Tremblay, 2015). Transgender and gender diverse individuals often experience even more mental health concerns when compared with sexual minority individuals. For example, the SEARCH study showed that in a sample of almost 4,000 sexual and gender minority individuals in Southern and East Africa, mental health concerns were highest among transgender women and people who identified as gender non-conforming (Müller et al., 2019a).

Sexual orientation and/or gender identity alone of course are not the only factors that influence people's mental health and wellbeing – it is well established that many individual, community, and societal factors act as social determinants of health and thus influence health and wellbeing. These include, for example, one's race, class, including income and social status, employment, education levels, and physical environments. Here, a recent study from the United States is illustrative. The study compared depression among Black sexual minority women to depression among White sexual minority women and Black sexual minority men. It showed that Black sexual minority women, whose social status is triply marginalised based on their race, gender, and sexual orientation, experienced poorer mental health compared to the other two groups, who each only experienced double marginalisation (Calabrese, Meyer, Overstreet, Haile, & Hansen, 2015). This suggests that other determinants of health intersect with sexual orientation and/or gender identity and can exacerbate the mental health risk of, for example, sexual and gender minority people of colour, of poor sexual and gender minority people or of sexual and gender minority people who live with a disability.

Sexuality and gender identity and access to healthcare

Sexual and gender minority individuals often face barriers to accessing appropriate healthcare (Alencar Albuquerque et al., 2016). These barriers are due to a lack of provider education and knowledge, provider-initiated discrimination and a lack of services offering care that addresses the specific needs of sexual and gender minorities (Müller, 2017).

Lack of provider education and knowledge

With few exceptions, sexual orientation and gender identity-related health concerns and topics are not included in most healthcare education. Studies have documented the lack of comprehensive education for health professionals in many countries (see, for example, these studies from the United States and South Africa: Müller, 2013; Obedin-Maliver et al., 2011). This means that most health sciences students are given little opportunity to challenge their heteronormative assumptions, and to learn about sexual orientation- and gender identity-specific health concerns and vulnerabilities. As a result, health sciences students, who go on to become healthcare providers, can feel unprepared and uncomfortable when treating patients who identify as sexual or gender minorities (White et al., 2015).

More importantly, perhaps, health sciences students and healthcare providers often lack the knowledge that is needed to provide appropriate comprehensive healthcare for sexual orientation- and gender identity-related health concerns. This is reflected in the myriad of experiences made by sexual and gender minority patients, which speak to this lack of knowledge. For example, where healthcare providers fail to understand queer women's sexual health and sexual behaviours, they cannot provide adequate information about sexually transmitted infections and how to protect oneself from them (Meer & Müller, 2017).

Provider-initiated discrimination

Experiences made by sexual and gender minority individuals in healthcare contexts are also often shaped by discriminatory and judgemental attitudes by healthcare providers. Despite their ethical obligations to provide non-judgemental care to all patients, some healthcare providers cannot, or do not want to, apply these ethical principles to sexual and gender minority patients. Especially in contexts where non-conforming sexual orientations and gender identities are heavily stigmatised or criminalised, the discriminatory attitudes that exist in wider society also exist among healthcare providers. As a result, sexual and gender minority individuals may experience intrusive questions, name-calling, or even denial of care (Meer & Müller, 2017). As a consequence, sexual and gender minority individuals may delay seeking care, feel forced to seek care elsewhere (often further away, or at a greater inconvenience), or decide to not seek care at all (Müller, 2016). For example, the recent SEARCH study illustrates how widespread sexual orientation- and gender identity-related discrimination is in healthcare in Southern and East Africa: of 813 sexual and gender minority South Africans, 54% said that they had been treated with less respect in a health facility because of their sexual orientation or gender identity; 31% said that they had been insulted or called names; and 22% had been denied care (Müller et al., 2019c). In Kenya, half of the surveyed 976 sexual and gender minority Kenyans said that they had been treated with less respect in a health facility, one third said that they had been insulted or called names, and another third had been denied care (Müller, Daskilewicz, & Southern and East African Research Collective on Health, 2019b).

Lack of health services for specific needs

Because sexual orientation and gender identity-related health concerns are often not recognised, some health systems do not provide treatment guidelines or resources, or specific treatments or interventions may not be covered by health insurance. Perhaps the most prominent example for this is the lack of access to gender-affirming healthcare for transgender and gender diverse people who wish to modify their body to match their gender identity. Gender-affirming care encompasses hormone therapy, and/or surgical interventions, to modify the body. Even though it is recognised as a medical necessity, and even though its benefits to people's wellbeing and safety have been empirically proven, in many countries of the world it is not available in state-funded public health systems, and healthcare providers have not received the training or the clinical guidelines to provide it (Spencer, Meer, & Müller, 2017; Winter et al., 2016). In countries where gender-affirming care is more available and accessible, its cost is often not covered by health insurance, thus making it prohibitively expensive for most transgender and gender diverse people (Winter et al., 2016). Whilst this exclusion is being challenged, and gender-affirming care is increasingly being provided according to international guidelines, especially in the Global South many transgender and gender diverse people remain without access. For example, in Southern and East Africa only one in three transgender individuals has access to hormone therapy, and only one in four has access to surgical gender affirmation (Müller et al., 2019a). Similarly, in Vietnam, a recent study concluded that the healthcare system is under-prepared to meet the complex health needs of transgender individuals, due to numerous gaps at the policy and organisational level combined with discriminatory attitudes and lack of knowledge among healthcare providers (Do & Nguyen, 2020).

Conclusion

Sexual orientation and gender identity are important social determinants of health. In heteronormative societies, they influence the health of and the healthcare for people who identify as lesbian, gay, bisexual, transgender, or queer. Empirical research evidences the health disparities between populations who identify as heterosexual and cisgender, and populations who identify as sexual and gender minorities; the models of minority stress and structural stigma explain how the structural forces of stigma and marginalisation related to sexual orientation and gender identity negatively influence individual health and wellbeing.

Whilst this is increasingly being recognised by international agencies and national government departments and non-governmental organisations, important gaps remain, especially in healthcare provider education and health policy. In order to reduce sexual orientation and gender identity-related health disparities and to ensure equal access to healthcare for all, regardless of sexual orientation or gender identity, healthcare, including healthcare provider education and health policy needs to carefully interrogate its own heteronormative assumptions and actively incorporate the healthcare needs of sexual and gender minority individuals. At the same time, the causes of sexual orientation- and gender identity-related stigma and discrimination, rooted in heteronormativity and homo- and transphobia, need to be addressed through efforts for full legal, political, and social inclusion of sexual and gender minority individuals. This includes legislative efforts to abolish laws that criminalise same-sex activity, and to pass and implement anti-discrimination legislation.

References

Alencar Albuquerque, G., de Lima Garcia, C., da Silva Quirino, G., Alves, M. J. H., Belém, J. M., Dos Santos Figueiredo, F. W., ... Adami, F. (2016). Access to health services by lesbian, gay, bisexual, and transgender persons: Systematic literature review. *BMC International Health and Human Rights, 16*(1), 2. doi:10.1186/s12914-015-0072-9

Baral, S. D., Poteat, T., Strömdahl, S., Wirtz, A. L., Guadamuz, T. E., & Beyrer, C. (2013). Worldwide burden of HIV in transgender women: A systematic review and meta-analysis. *The Lancet Infectious Diseases, 13*(3), 214–222. doi:10.1016/S1473-3099(12)70315-8

Bhugra, D., Eckstrand, K., Levounis, P., Kar, A., & Javate, K. R. (2016). WPA position statement on gender identity and same-sex orientation, attraction and behaviours. *World Psychiatry, 15*(3), 299–300. doi:10.1002/wps.20340

Blondeel, K., de Vasconcelos, S., García-Moreno, C., Stephenson, R., Temmerman, M., & Toskin, I. (2018). Violence motivated by perception of sexual orientation and gender identity: A systematic review. *Bulletin of the World Health Organization, 96*(1), 29–41L. doi:10.2471/BLT.17.197251

Bogart, L. M., Revenson, T. A., Whitfield, K. E., & France, C. R. (2014). Introduction to the special section on lesbian, gay, bisexual, and transgender (LGBT) health disparities: Where we are and where we're going. *Annals of Behavioral Medicine: A Publication of the Society of Behavioural Medicine, 47*(1), 1–4. doi:10.1007/s12160-013-9574-7

Brown, R., McNair, R., Szalacha, L., Livingston, P. M., & Hughes, T. (2015). Cancer risk factors, diagnosis and sexual identity in the Australian longitudinal study of women's health. *Women's Health Issues*. doi:10.1016/j.whi.2015.04.001

Cahill, S., & Makadon, H. (2014). Sexual orientation and gender identity data collection in clinical settings and in electronic health records: A key to ending LGBT health disparities. *LGBT Health, 1*(1), 34–41. doi:10.1089/lgbt.2013.0001

Calabrese, S. K., Meyer, I. H., Overstreet, N. M., Haile, R., & Hansen, N. B. (2015). Exploring discrimination and mental health disparities faced by black sexual minority women using a minority stress framework. *Psychology of Women Quarterly, 39*(3), 287–304. doi:10.1177/0361684314560730

Cochran, S. D., Drescher, J., Kismödi, E., Giami, A., García-Moreno, C., Atalla, E., ... Reed, G. M. (2014). Proposed declassification of disease categories related to sexual orientation in the International Statistical Classification of Diseases and Related Health Problems (ICD-11). *Bulletin of the World Health Organization, 92*(9), 672–679. doi:10.2471/BLT.14.135541

Discrimination and violence against individuals based on their sexual orientation and gender identity. HRC/29/23. (2015). Geneva: United Nations Human Rights Council.

Discriminatory laws and practices and acts of violence against individuals based on their sexual orientation and gender identity. HRC/19/41. (2011). Geneva: United Nations Human Rights Council.

Do, T. T., & Van Nguyen, A. T. (2020). "They know better than we doctors do": Providers' preparedness for transgender healthcare in Vietnam. *Health Sociology Review, 29*(1), 92–107. doi:10.1080/14461242.2020.1715814

Drescher, J. (2010). Queer diagnoses: Parallels and contrasts in the history of homosexuality, gender variance, and the diagnostic and statistical manual. *Archives of Sexual Behavior, 39*(2), 427–460. doi:10.1007/s10508-009-9531-5

Drescher, J. (2015). Queer diagnoses revisited: The past and future of homosexuality and gender diagnoses in DSM and ICD. *International Review of Psychiatry, 27*(5), 386–395. doi:10.3109/09540261.2015.1053847

Eliason, M. J. (2014). Chronic physical health problems in sexual minority women: Review of the literature. *LGBT Health, 1*(4), 259–268. doi:10.1089/lgbt.2014.0026

Gergen, K. J. (2001). Psychological science in a postmodern context. *American Psychologist, 56*(10), 803–813. doi:10.1037//0003-066X.56.10.803

Hatzenbuehler, M. L. (2011). The social environment and suicide attempts in lesbian, gay, and bisexual youth. *Pediatrics, 127*(5), 896–903. doi:10.1542/peds.2010-3020

Hatzenbuehler, M. L., Bellatorre, A., Lee, Y., Finch, B. K., Muennig, P., & Fiscella, K. (2014). Structural stigma and all-cause mortality in sexual minority populations. *Social Science and Medicine*, *103*, 33–41. doi:10.1016/j.socscimed.2013.06.005

Hatzenbuehler, M. L., McLaughlin, K. A., Keyes, K. M., & Hasin, D. S. (2010). The impact of institutional discrimination on psychiatric disorders in lesbian, gay, and bisexual populations: A prospective study. *American Journal of Public Health*, *100*(3), 452–459. doi:10.2105/AJPH.2009.168815

Hendricks, M. L., & Testa, R. J. (2012). A conceptual framework for clinical work with transgender and gender nonconforming clients: An adaptation of the Minority Stress Model. *Professional Psychology: Research and Practice, 43*(5), 460–467. https://doi.org/10.1037/a0029597

Human rights, sexual orientation and gender identity. HRC/RES/17/19. (2011). Geneva: United Nations Human Rights Council.

Human rights, sexual orientation and gender identity. HRC/RES/27/32. (2014). Geneva: United Nations Human Rights Council.

International Lesbian, Gay, Bisexual, Trans and Intersex Association: Lucas Ramon Mendos, V. (2019). *State-sponsored homophobia 2019*. Geneva.

Krug, E. E. G., Mercy, J. A., Dahlberg, L. L., & Zwi, A. B. (2002). *The world report on violence and health*. Geneva: World Health Organization. doi:10.1136/ip.9.1.93

Logie, C. (2012). The case for the World Health Organization's Commission on the Social Determinants of Health to address sexual orientation. *American Journal of Public Health*, *102*(7), 1243–1246. doi:10.2105/AJPH.2011.300599

Logie, C., & Gibson, M. F. (2013). A mark that is no mark? Queer women and violence in HIV discourse. *Culture, Health & Sexuality*, *15*(1), 29–43. doi:10.1080/13691058.2012.738430

Martin, J. I., & Meezan, W. (2003). Applying ethical standards to research and evaluations involving lesbian gay bisexual and transgender populations. *Journal of Gay & Lesbian Social Services*, *15*(1–2), 181–201. doi:10.1300/ J041v15n01_12

Mason, T. B., & Lewis, R. J. (2015). Minority stress, depression, relationship quality, and alcohol use: Associations with overweight and obesity among partnered young adult lesbians. *LGBT Health*, *2*(4), 333–340. doi:10.1089/lgbt.2014.0053

Mayer, K. H., Bradford, J. B., Makadon, H. J., Stall, R., Goldhammer, H., & Landers, S. (2008). Sexual and gender minority health: What we know and what needs to be done. *American Journal of Public Health*, *98*(6), 989–995. doi:10.2105/AJPH.2007.127811

Meer, T., & Müller, A. (2017). "They treat us like we're not there": Queer bodies and the social production of healthcare spaces. *Health & Place*, *45*, 92–98. doi:10.1016/j.healthplace.2017.03.010

Meyer, I. H. (2003). Prejudice, social stress, and mental health in lesbian, gay, and bisexual populations: Conceptual issues and research evidence. *Psychological Bulletin*, *129*(5), 674–697. doi:10.1037/0033-2909.129.5.674

Müller, A. (2013). Teaching lesbian, gay, bisexual and transgender health in a South African health sciences faculty: Addressing the gap. *BMC Medical Education*, *13*, 174. doi:10.1186/1472-6920-13-174

Müller, A. (2016). Health for all? Sexual orientation, gender identity, and the implementation of the right to access to health care in South Africa. *Health & Human Rights: An International Journal*, *18*(2), 195–208. Retrieved from http://search.ebscohost.com/login.aspx?direct=true&db=sih&AN=120294738&site=ehost-live

Müller, A. (2017). Scrambling for access: Availability, accessibility, acceptability and quality of healthcare for lesbian, gay, bisexual and transgender people in South Africa. *BMC International Health and Human Rights*, *17*(1), 16. doi:10.1186/s12914-017-0124-4

Müller, A., Daskilewicz, K., & Southern and East African Research Collective on Health. (2019a). *Are we doing alright? Realities of violence, mental health, and access to healthcare related to sexual orientation and gender identity and expression in East and Southern Africa: Research report based on a community-led study in nine countries*. Amsterdam, Netherlands: COC.

Müller, A., Daskilewicz, K., & Southern and East African Research Collective on Health. (2019b). *Are we doing alright? Realities of violence, mental health, and access to healthcare related to sexual orientation and gender identity and expression in Kenya: Research report based on a community-led study in nine countries*. Amsterdam.

Müller, A., Daskilewicz, K., & Southern and East African Research Collective on Health. (2019c). *Are we doing alright? Realities of violence, mental health, and access to healthcare related to sexual orientation and gender identity and expression in South Africa: Research report based on a community-led study in nine countries*. Amsterdam.

Nath, D. (2011). *"We'll show you you're a woman" – Violence and discrimination against black lesbians and transgender men in South Africa.* New York, NY: Human Rights Watch.

Obedin-Maliver, J., Goldsmith, E. S., Stewart, L., White, W., Tran, E., Brenman, S., … Lunn, M. R. (2011). Lesbian, gay, bisexual, and transgender–related content in undergraduate medical education. *JAMA: The Journal of the American Medical Association, 306*(9), 971–977. doi:10.1001/jama.2011.1255

Pega, F., & Veale, J. F. (2015). The case for the World Health Organization's Commission on social determinants of health to address gender identity. *American Journal of Public Health, 105*(3), e58–e62. doi:10.2105/AJPH.2014.302373

Perez-Brumer, A., Day, J. K., Russell, S. T., & Hatzenbuehler, M. L. (2017). Prevalence and correlates of suicidal ideation among transgender youth in California: Findings from a representative, population-based sample of high school students. *Journal of the American Academy of Child & Adolescent Psychiatry, 56*(9), 739–746. doi:10.1016/j.jaac.2017.06.010

Plöderl, M., & Tremblay, P. (2015). Mental health of sexual minorities. A systematic review. *International Review of Psychiatry, 27*(5), 367–385. doi:10.3109/09540261.2015.1083949

Protection against violence and discrimination based on sexual orientation and gender identity. HRC/RES/32/2. (2016). Geneva: United Nations Human Rights Council.

Report of the Independent Expert on protection against violence and discrimination based on sexual orientation and gender identity. A/HRC/38/43. (2018). Geneva: United Nations Human Rights Council.

Ross, L. E., Salway, T., Tarasoff, L. A., MacKay, J. M., Hawkins, B. W., & Fehr, C. P. (2018). Prevalence of depression and anxiety among bisexual people compared to gay, lesbian, and heterosexual individuals: A systematic review and meta-analysis. *Journal of Sex Research, 55*(4–5), 435–456. doi:10.1080/00224499.2017.1387755

Schwartz, S. R., Nowak, R. G., Orazulike, I., Keshinro, B., Spring, S., Ake, J., … Kennedy, S. (2015). The immediate effect of the Same-Sex Marriage Prohibition Act on stigma, discrimination, and engagement on HIV prevention and treatment services in men who have sex with men in Nigeria: Analysis of prospective data from the TRUST cohort. *Lancet HIV, 2*(7), e299–e306. doi:10.1016/S2352-3018(15)00078-8

Smith, G. (2004). Treatments of homosexuality in Britain since the 1950s – an oral history: The experience of patients. *BMJ, 328*(7437), 427–430. doi:10.1136/bmj.37984.442419.EE

Spencer, S., Meer, T., & Müller, A. (2017). "The care is the best you can give at the time": Health care professionals' experiences in providing gender affirming care in South Africa. *PloS One, 12*(7), e0181132. doi: 10.1371/journal. pone.0181132.

Suess Schwend, A., Winter, S., Chiam, Z., Smiley, A., & Cabral Grinspan, M. (2018). Depathologising gender diversity in childhood in the process of ICD revision and reform. *Global Public Health*, 1–14. doi:10.1080/17441692.2018.1427274

Victor, C. J., Nel, J. A., Lynch, I., & Mbatha, K. (2014). The psychological society of South Africa sexual and gender diversity position statement: Contributing towards a just society. *South African Journal of Psychology, 44*, 292–302. doi:10.1177/0081246314533635

White, W., Brenman, S., Paradis, E., Goldsmith, E. S., Lunn, M. R., Obedin-Maliver, J., … Garcia, G. (2015). Lesbian, gay, bisexual, and transgender patient care: Medical students' preparedness and comfort. *Teaching and Learning in Medicine, 27*(3), 254–263. doi:10.1080/10401334.2015.1044656

Winter, S., Diamond, M., Green, J., Karasic, D., Reed, T., Whittle, S., & Wylie, K. (2016). Transgender people: Health at the margins of society. *The Lancet, 388*(10042), 390–400. doi:10.1016/S0140-6736(16)00683-8

World Health Organization. (2013). *Improving the health and wellbeing of lesbian, gay, bisexual and transgender persons.* Geneva.

World Health Organization. (2018). *WHO ICD-11 beta draft.* Retrieved from https://icd.who.int/dev11/l-m/en

14

REPRODUCTIVE JUSTICE
Revitalising critical reproductive health research

Tracy Morison

We generally think of reproductive matters as deeply personal and private, subject to our personal desires and choices alone. Yet, this impression is belied by the many debates and controversies surrounding reproductive issues, such as the ongoing clash over abortion, disputes over how to curb "teen pregnancy", or more latterly discussions about "test-tube babies". In reality, reproductive issues are profoundly a matter of public concern, perhaps unlike many other areas of health. Reproduction is charged with moral, religious, symbolic, ideological, and political meaning, which spark debate and contention (Joffe & Reich, 2015). Questions of who may reproduce with whom, when, and under what conditions – and, of course, who should be prevented from procreating – entwine with slippery notions of "real" families, nation-state, ethnic identity, class pedigree, racial purity, divine or legal rights, and more. Disputes over these issues arise from deep-rooted beliefs and ideals about belonging and, indeed, our very humanness. It is unsurprising then that reproductive matters – and the area that we have now come to call reproductive health – have always been highly contested and subject to considerable regulation, despite our feeling that it is a personal matter.

Critical approaches to studying reproductive health commonly seek to highlight this fraught socio-political backdrop, situating issues in context and, importantly, trying to tease apart the webs of surrounding power relations that shape people's reproductive lives. Such work spans diverse disciplines – anthropology, history, sociology, psychology – and approaches, covering a vast array of topics. (For contemporary overviews of the range of topics covered in critical reproductive health scholarship, see: Joffe & Reich, 2015; Ussher et al., 2020.) It is impossible to do justice to such a rich and complex terrain in a single chapter. My aim, therefore, is to focus on reproductive politics more broadly, both as they have shaped the field and been interrogated by critical reproductive health researchers. In this chapter I focus on an approach that offers a particularly effective lens for doing such nuanced, critical work across disciplines and topic areas, namely, the reproductive justice framework, a radical cross-disciplinary feminist framework that has been increasingly taken up by critical scholars.

To begin, I provide a background discussion of the global politics that birthed "reproductive health" as its own discreet area and generated important international approaches to policymaking, intervention, and, importantly, scholarship. I trace the emergence of the reproductive justice framework from among the global perspectives on reproductive health, showing how these perspectives are themselves shaped by their socio-political contexts. I then go on to provide some exemplars of critical reproductive health research that uses a reproductive justice lens. Rather than attempting to paint a comprehensive picture of this body of scholarship, my aim is to provide a sense of the ways that the reproductive justice framework can be used and what it can bring to reproductive health research. I close with a discussion of some unresolved issues, oversights, and areas for future work.

Background: the socio-political context of reproductive health

The socio-political contexts within which knowledge is generated invariably shape the questions researchers ask and the ways that they try to answer them. The same is true of reproductive health; in fact, the very notion of "reproductive health" is a relatively recent one. In this section, I discuss how reproductive health came to be its own discreet area of health. I trace its emergence out of global shifts in how reproduction and its attendant social issues were understood, framed, studied, and responded to, beginning with the rise of the reproductive health and rights paradigm and the subsequent push for a more radical reproductive justice approach. I highlight the role played by feminist thinking in these global movements, showing how it has helped to shift the gaze ever more toward the political and toward questions of social justice.

The rise of the reproductive health and rights paradigm

"Reproductive health" as a concept demarcating a distinct health area was officially introduced into the global lexicon relatively recently, at the 1994 International Conference on Population and Development (ICPD). The conference declaration – known as the Cairo Declaration on Population and Development – advocates "an approach that places family planning in the broader framework of reproductive health care" (United Nations Population Fund, 1994a). This was the first and most comprehensive international document officially recognising the new concept of reproductive health, along with the notion of "reproductive rights" (Eager, 2017). This new way of framing reproductive issues, the reproductive health and rights paradigm, was intended to replace the narrow, instrumentalist focus that had dominated until then: the family planning perspective. This older perspective was rooted in a population control agenda and often intertwined with eugenicist thinking (Ross et al., 2017).

Responding to these deeply problematic population control tactics, women's rights and health activists resoundingly criticised the family planning perspective's targeting of women and its reductionist view of reproduction as primarily a biological phenomenon, almost entirely neglecting cultural and socio-political aspects (Morison & Macleod, 2015). In this regard, the new reproductive health and rights paradigm intended to locate reproduction as a gendered phenomenon. Accordingly, women's rights advocates argued that "giving women the ability to make informed choices about their fertility is a key step for their own health and empowerment, but it's also a vital step towards fairer communities and societies" (Ghebreyesus & Kanem, 2018, p. 2585). As such, reproductive health and rights were viewed both as a driver toward, and a fundamental part of, gender equality. While some feminist groups – such as the SisterSong Women of Colour Reproductive Health Collective – did argue that race- and class-based dimensions needed consideration alongside gender, the critique at that time (the early 1990s) was largely articulated in the voice of mainstream (White) feminism and centred on gender (Ross et al., 2017; SisterSong, 2007; see the discussion of feminist politics below).

An important aspect of the women's movement critique – and the hallmark of the new reproductive health and rights paradigm – was the mobilisation of human rights discourse. Framing reproductive rights as human rights offered a powerful defence of these rights, as well as the associated goals of women's empowerment and gender equity (Rebouché, 2017). With human rights already protected under international law, their linkage to reproduction offered a authoritative framework for ensuring that all people – women and men alike – have the ability to make decisions about their reproductive lives and to exercise their reproductive rights. Human rights discourse also allowed for stronger, more positive claims for the full human rights of women, far beyond what was possible within the constraints of national legal frameworks regulating sexuality and reproduction (Ross, 2017a). Importantly, human rights arguments helped reshape abortion access into an issue of transnational significance, rather than simply a local or personal concern (Rebouché, 2017).

The introduction of reproductive rights was a crucial step in reproductive health globally. Yet, the radical possibilities of this discourse, in terms of its social justice and transformative potential, was diluted by the dominant Western ethos of liberal individualism, which focuses on personal freedom, choice, and empowerment. Accordingly, it envisages an empowered, autonomous subject who actively claims individual rights (Rebouché, 2017). Consequently, in the reproductive health and rights paradigm arguments tend to emphasise individual autonomy, neglecting the *contexts* in which pregnancy termination and other reproductive decisions are made (Rebouché, 2017). Reproductive health was therefore largely defined in the rhetoric of individual choice. The International Conference on Population Development's 1994 Programme of Action, for example, asserts that "reproductive health ... implies that people are able to have a satisfying and safe sex life and that they have the capability to reproduce and *the freedom to decide* if, when and how often to do so" (United Nations Population Fund, 1994b, emphasis added). This emphasis on personal freedom and choice has been taken up in advocacy and scholarship for women's reproductive rights, most markedly expressed in the notion of "the right to choose" that strongly undergirds struggles for contraceptive and abortion access.

Moving toward reproductive justice

The reproductive rights paradigm became the globally dominant framework for working with reproductive issues in policy, programming, and scholarship. However, some of its limitations were raised early in the 1990s by Black and women of colour feminists in the USA, who expressed concerns about the emphasis on pro-choice politics in the reproductive rights paradigm. The mainstream women's and human rights movement was largely focused on access to contraception and abortion, under the well-known "pro-choice" rubric, with its slogans of "my body, my choice" and "a woman's right to choose". While this struggle was important, it was articulated within the language of mainstream (White) feminism, which envisaged women as a single homogenous group with more or less common concerns. The reproductive health and rights paradigm thus failed to consider the differences *among* women; how the "choices" available to women differed based on their social location (Luna & Luker, 2013).

Unlike White, middle-class women, women of colour and poor women were more frequently faced with the denial of their right to have and to raise children, along with those who were in other ways deemed potentially "unfit mothers", such as women: with mental or physical disabilities or illnesses, who were unmarried, considered "too young", or were not heterosexual. This was articulated by one of the founding coalitions, SisterSong Women of Colour Reproductive Health Collective, as follows:

> One of the key problems addressed by reproductive justice is the isolation of abortion
> from other social justice issues that concern communities of color: issues of economic
> justice, the environment, immigrants' rights, disability rights, discrimination based on

race and sexual orientation, and a host of other community-centered concerns. These issues directly affect an individual woman's decision-making process. By shifting the focus to reproductive oppression – the control and exploitation of women, girls, and individuals through our bodies, sexuality, labor, and reproduction – rather than a narrow focus on protecting the legal right to abortion, [we are] developing a more inclusive vision of how to build a new movement.

(SisterSong, 2007, p. 4)

As part of this "more inclusive vision", reproductive justice advocates highlighted that the notion of choice favours predominantly White middle-class women who are *able* to choose from reproductive options, while disadvantaging those unavailable to do so, largely poor and low-income women, and especially women of colour (Ross et al., 2017). The social context mediates access to power and resources: the power to make informed choices about one's sexual activity, fertility, pregnancy, and reproductive health and the resources to act on these choices (Thompson, 2017). As an alternative framework to the Reproductive health and Rights paradigm, reproductive justice seeks to locate rights inside a social framework (Gilliam et al., 2009) and so foreground the inter-connection of reproductive issues and wider social justice concerns.

An important aspect of this alternative framework is the illumination of the gendered, classed, raced, and other power relations surrounding reproductive issues. Such a view is enabled by the application of intersectionality theory (Crenshaw, 1989), an integral component of the reproductive justice framework, which draws attention to "the matrix of domination" (Collins, 1991) – or the web of power relations – within which people's ability to exercise their sexual and reproductive rights is enabled or restricted. This matrix comprises: (i) structural and systemic dynamics; (ii) social relations shaped by gender, ethnicity/race, class, and other social categorisations; and (iii) sociocultural discourses and practices (Chiweshe et al., 2017). Thus, while encompassing several reproductive issues and topics, "reproductive justice is essentially a framework about power" (Ross & Solinger, 2017).

In line with the original impetus to go beyond pro-choice politics based upon liberal, individualised notions of rights, the reproductive justice framework is grounded in international human rights discourse, which links the realisation of human rights to the achievement of social justice (Rebouché, 2017). The focus is on structural and systemic changes that can support rights (Luna & Luker, 2013). Reproductive Justice is therefore "based in the human right to make personal decisions about one's life, *and* the obligation of government and society to ensure that the conditions are suitable for implementing one's decisions" (Ross, 2017a, p. 174).

The women's movement and feminist perspectives on reproduction

From the preceding discussion, its plain to see that feminists have played a central role in the development of the field of reproductive health. The second wave of the women's liberation movement, emerging in the 1970s, was central to the ways that reproductive issues have been framed. At the same time, feminist thinking was being taken up in critical scholarship in a range of disciplines, providing new lenses with which to study reproductive issues. Prior to this, a biomedical or public health approach had dominated explorations of fertility, pregnancy, and childbearing, with social scientists considering the impact of social conditions on these narrow areas (Joffe & Reich, 2015). Accordingly, issues such as contraceptive uptake and usage and unintended pregnancy dominated scholarship (Macleod & Morison, 2020; Morison & Macleod, 2015).

This limited population focus was driven by the preoccupation in the Global North with population control as countries turned their attention to economic "development" and prosperity in the aftermath of World War II. Rapid population growth – framed as an impending "global population crisis" – was deemed detrimental to economic growth and "development", and this crisis narrative formed the justification for regulating population size and composition. To forestall that "population crisis", governments around the world were encouraged to control their nation's fertility and family size. Contraceptive uptake and usage, (unintended) pregnancy rates, and rates of maternal and infant mortality therefore became key priorities and focal areas in policy, programming, and research (Macleod & Morison, 2020).

Population control measures zoomed in on women as the most pragmatic and efficient means of fertility regulation. Under the sway of eugenic and colonialist discourses, population control interventions sought in particular to curb the fertility of women deemed to be less desirable members of the population: those deemed "feeble-minded" or unfit to reproduce (Wanhalla, 2007). Women were thus coerced, subtly and forcibly, down specific reproductive paths – towards or away from motherhood – on the basis of their "fitness" to reproduce, determined according to race, class, ability, and moral standing (Eager, 2017). (For further discussion of "stratified reproduction" see Mamo & Alston-Stepnitz, 2015.)

However, the rise of second-wave feminism in the 1970s brought with it an awareness of the social and gendered dimensions of reproduction. This view was founded upon the well-known catchphrase 'the personal is political, and encouraged the application of a critical lens to matters that may previously have been overlooked as simply natural parts of life and as deeply private. Scholars from a range of disciplines began to use a feminist lens to question the taken for granted, considering issues such as the sociocultural meanings attached to infertility and "childlessness", motherhood identities, or the politics surrounding contraceptive and abortion access (Joffe & Reich, 2015; Ussher et al., 2020).

The surge of feminist-inspired scholarship initiated during this time has continued to grow, generating an abundance of critical research using a feminist lens and often (but not exclusively) qualitative research designs to unpack the politics and dynamics around a wide range of reproductive issues, like reproductive technologies, obstetric violence, menopause, and so on (Macleod & Morison, 2020). Indeed, Joffe and Reich (2015) assert that feminist perspectives on reproduction have generated much of the current and strongest scholarship in the field of reproduction. Notably, the work of feminists and the women's movement was also influential in drawing attention to the need to move beyond an emphasis on "family planning" described above, which largely amounted to control of women's fertility and sexuality, and helping to usher in a new approach now known as the reproductive health and rights paradigm (Eager, 2017).

The value of a reproductive justice approach in knowledge production

Having traced the global shifts in how the reproductive justice framework has been taken up more generally, in this section I concentrate on scholarship that has made use of a reproductive justice approach. Originally conceptualised as a framework for activism by Black feminists, reproductive justice has gained popularity among feminist activists and more broadly in reproductive health (Ross, 2017b). While it has long been successfully utilised in reproductive health advocacy and programming, the framework has gained traction somewhat more slowly in scholarship (Luna & Luker, 2013). As an *analytic lens* for research the concept has only recently begun receiving scholarly attention, but its uptake has rapidly increased to the extent that some of the founders have even exclaimed that reproductive justice has "gone viral" (Ross et al., 2017).

As an emerging feminist theory, reproductive justice has the potential to revitalise international reproductive health scholarship by widening the conceptual focus, foregrounding marginalised accounts, and offering ways to apply knowledge for constructive social change (Luna & Luker, 2013). In order to demonstrate these valuable aspects of the theoretical framework, in the following section I discuss research that has used a reproductive justice lens to explore two especially knotty and contentious areas: (i) abortion decision-making in the case of potential foetal anomalies, and (ii) the use of assisted reproductive technologies.

Expanding research on abortion and reproductive decision-making

Although reproductive justice advocates have criticised the reproductive health and rights paradigm for its over-emphasis on abortion, there has been research on abortion that uses a reproductive justice lens to illuminate the more complex intersectional politics surrounding abortion care. A good example is the recent research on the Zika virus infection during pregnancy, which carries the risk of causing foetal anomalies. This research highlights a tension at the intersection of reproductive rights and disability: the right to terminate a pregnancy that one is unable to support, on the one hand, and concerns around eugenic approaches to disabilities, on the other. As Mohapatra (2019) notes, this is an especially tense conflict in reproductive theorising, especially considering that both disability and abortion bear social stigma.

Two studies have focused on the professional guidance available to clinicians for counselling on pregnancy decision-making in cases of Zika infection, analysing guidance papers, frameworks, and practice: Mohapatra (2019), using international and US documents, and Rabionet et al. (2018), using Puerto Rican documents. The outcomes of both studies highlight the need for clinicians to use comprehensive, intersectional counselling approaches. From a reproductive justice perspective, the researchers advocate responses that guarantee access to safe pregnancy termination *as well as* to pregnancy continuation without coercion. They argue that counselling should be comprehensive, advising thoroughly on a range of options (e.g. pregnancy continuation, termination of pregnancy, and adoption) and offering complete information about potential risks (Mohapatra, 2019; Rabionet et al., 2018). Rabionet et al. (2018) further suggest that such counselling should incorporate measures such as destigmatising reproductive choices; acknowledging cultural, religious, and traditional views; and eliminating coercion toward specific decisions. Alongside such non-directive, patient-centred counselling, decision-making should be supported by the provision of information about available medical and social support services and should link patients with these services (Mohapatra, 2019; Rabionet et al., 2018).

These studies illustrate how a reproductive justice lens allows for a holistic approach to reproductive decision-making that allows the right *not* to have children to sit alongside the right to have children, granting both rights equal legitimacy and enhancing patients' agency to make a decision based on their own circumstances, needs, and preferences. Doing so requires cognisance of the differing social locations that people may occupy, which means that reproductive politics are brought to bear in different ways. They also show how competing sets of rights can be considered and potentially reconciled.

Attending to complexity and nuance in research on assisted reproduction

The application of a reproductive justice lens to the issue of assisted reproduction highlights how reproductive technologies can be simultaneously empowering and oppressive. Scholarship interrogating contemporary commercial surrogacy using a reproductive justice lens highlights how "gestational surrogacy resides at the nexus of complex and pressing feminist concerns regarding technology, globalization, flows of capital and labor, reproductive 'choice', and justice" (Fixmer-Oraiz, 2013, p. 126). Furthermore, as Fixmer-Oraiz (2013) argues, attention to reproductive justice makes social and economic injustices visible and open to intervention.

A significant concern related to transnational gestational surrogacy is that the least advantaged women often act as surrogates for the most advantaged (Mohapatra, 2012). Surrogates occupy relatively less powerful positions for negotiation in surrogacy contracts. They take on significant risks (e.g. injury, infertility, death) for a fraction of total profits and, after surrogacy arrangements, are often left with limited access to a sustainable income or healthcare. It has been argued, therefore, that transnational surrogacy practices are a form of reproductive injustice: that a "motherhood market" allows the socioeconomic oppression of poor women who act as surrogates for intending parents from affluent contexts, further entrenching global inequalities (Saravanan, 2016).

This assessment is borne out by Fixmer-Oraiz's (2013) analysis of popular narratives of gestational surrogacy in contemporary US media. Her findings show how the dominant construction of transnational gestational surrogacy as altruistic works alongside choice rhetoric to mask the structural conditions underpinning the "choices" and experiences of women who act as surrogates. Rather than seeing surrogacy as a "choice", Mohaptra (2012) argues that it should be construed as a form of labour, which could serve as a beginning point for achieving reproductive justice for all parties in the surrogacy market.

Alongside this reconceptualisation, Mohaptra (2012) asserts, is the importance of applying an intersectional analysis of race, gender, and class to determine how reproductive justice may be achieved. In this regard, it is also important to consider *who* makes use of assisted reproduction services and why. For instance, we might consider the nature and extent to which single or LGBTQ+ people use assisted reproductive technologies and how their appropriation of these services aligns with or diverges from that of infertile heterosexual couples' practices (Fixmer-Oraiz, 2013). Transnational surrogacy may make pathways to biological parenthood possible for those living in countries with discriminatory laws about who is permitted to commission surrogacy. The use of assisted reproduction by those otherwise barred from (biological) parenthood may be seen as challenging reproductive injustice resulting from the hetero-patriarchal regulation of reproduction and family formation, and may subvert heteronormativity and repronormativity (Mohapatra, 2012).

In this vein, recent research drawing together trans★ and reproductive justice scholarship and advocacy identifies the obstacles to genetic pathways to parenthood encountered globally by trans individuals (Honkasalo, 2018; Nixon, 2013). Assisted reproductive technologies (ARTs) are not only financially costly but also legally regulated and may exclude those on the reproductive margins (e.g. unmarried couples, unpartnered individuals, sexual/gender minorities) who do not live up to normative parenthood ideals. For instance, pioneering research by Riggs and Bartholomaeus (2019) in Australia seeks to investigate how cisnormativity regulates transgender or non-binary people's pathways to parenthood. The researchers interviewed healthcare professionals, transgender and non-binary adults, and parents of transgender and non-binary children about their views on, and experiences with, fertility preservation. Their work shows that trans reproductive justice relies not only on the availability of fertility preservation, but also on the challenging wider social discourses and prohibitions that regulate trans and non-binary people's reproductive lives.

The research reviewed in this section perhaps raises more questions than answers. Yet, this is precisely the value of such work. It questions race- and class-based assumptions about the nuclear family, delving into the associated structural and discursive circumstances that disadvantage some women, families, and communities, and, in so doing, asks us to reconsider the terms upon which family and belonging are legitimised (Fixmer-Oraiz, 2013).

Issues and oversights

As a relatively new framework for critical scholarship, there are still many areas that need attention in reproductive justice scholarship, both in terms of the questions that researchers might ask as well as where research is conducted. Currently, as this section explores further, knowledge production drawing on a reproductive justice frame (i) remains focused on women, (ii) has only just begun to engage fully in issues of sexual justice, and (iii) is largely concentrated in the Global North. I discuss each of these issues in turn below.

The "man question" in reproductive health

Reading the above, one would be forgiven for thinking that reproductive health and justice is almost entirely about women. Certainly, at the turn of the century, the conflation of reproductive health with women's health was questioned as new thinking about gender and gender politics emerged in feminism and beyond. Alongside shifts in theorising gender were global shifts that brought men's role in reproduction into the limelight. The notion of "reproductive rights", ushered in by the reproductive health and rights paradigm, facilitated a growing emphasis on men's concerns and needs. Most notably, the HIV/AIDS pandemic highlighted men's roles in sex and reproduction. It was consequently widely accepted that to deal with these issues meant including men in research and interventions. Initially, the need for reproductive research to turn its attention to men as well as women was spurred by concerns about the integral, but sometimes restrictive, role that men play in women's reproductive health (Morison & Macleod, 2015).

The push to include men in reproductive health research and programming sat uneasily with many feminists and women's health advocates, who feared that women's hard-won gains would be eroded as attention and funding was diverted to men's causes (Cornwall & Esplen, 2010). Indeed, the possibility of men acting as potential allies in the battle for gender justice was met with hesitation, uncertainty, and often hostility (Cornwall & Esplen, 2010). Some raised concerns about problem-focused views of men as wholly negative influences on women's health. The man question, therefore, concerned how best to include men in constructive ways, that did not eclipse women's needs or detract from the aim of women's empowerment, the original impetus for adopting a fuller, gendered perspective in the first place.

Various approaches have emerged to respond to this question. These approaches retain the overarching goal of women's empowerment to varying degrees. The "male equity" approach aims to redress the oversight of men and to take a broader view of men's roles than a problem-oriented approach allows. The intention is to focus on men beyond their roles as women's partners and "in their own right". Including men in reproductive health research and the broader reproductive health and rights arena is seen as a "win–win", beneficial to men themselves, their female partners, their children, and the larger community (Alan Guttmacher Institute, 2003). On the other hand, the "men as partners" framework is founded on an explicit commitment to gender equity and women's empowerment. This framework focuses on including men as women's partners and as allies in working toward gender equity. Men are viewed as potential agents of positive change and this tack is taken in many sexual and reproductive health programmes and interventions (Stern et al., 2009).

Finally, a middle-ground position is found in the gendered and relational approach to studying men's practices. This power-based framework moves beyond the consideration of men's participation in the sexual and reproductive health *of women*, to a view of men as co-actors with women as well as having their own sexual and reproductive health needs (Figueroa-Pera, 2003). This alternative framework recognises the reciprocal and interdependent nature of sexual and reproductive partnerships (Figueroa-Pera, 2003). The value of this approach is that its focus on gender power relations prevents researchers and practitioners from losing sight of the larger hetero-patriarchal context within which sex and reproduction occur.

Of course, the frameworks above are located within the mainstream reproductive health and rights paradigm that is generally used for research and implementation. The shift to reproductive justice necessitates renewed thinking about including men in research and praxis. The obvious focus of reproductive justice is on women in disadvantaged circumstances, and much of the literature centres on women (Morison & Macleod, 2015) – the socio-historical reasons for which have already been detailed. This is not to say that there is no place for men in the reproductive justice movement and framework. To the contrary, proponents of this approach explicitly state that reproductive justice applies to all, not only to women of colour (Ross et al., 2017).

Advocates of reproductive justice argued early on that the focus on women is both necessary and appropriate given the much more direct and profound impact of reproductive issues on women than men (SisterSong, 2007). This is indeed true, given that men *as a group* are certainly in a less precarious position than women *as a group*. However, the intersectional lens of reproductive justice requires more nuanced thinking. Attention still needs to be given to the question of how reproductive justice is relational in nature. In this respect, Morison and Macleod (2015) argue for the importance of recognising men as reproductive beings invested in specific ways of understanding sexuality, reproduction, and parenthood. They contend that the application of the reproductive justice framework, in practice or policy work, needs to attend to the gendered relational discursive frameworks and material realities that maintain inequitable gendered relations around reproduction. To (once more) neglect men as part of the gendered matrix surrounding reproduction would be a serious oversight and further thinking in this avenue is to be welcomed.

Queering reproductive justice

Much of the reproductive justice literature centres, perhaps unsurprisingly given its origins, on *reproductive* freedoms and oppressions, and to a much lesser extent on *sexual* autonomy and freedom. Nonetheless, the framework has always acknowledged the interdependence of sexual *and* reproductive freedoms (Ross & Solinger, 2017). Indeed, the SisterSong coalition affirmed this in their original primer on reproductive justice, asking: "What is reproductive justice without the ability to fully express, control and affirm one's sexuality? Incomplete, at best" (SisterSong, 2007, p. 37). To acknowledge this interlinkage, some writers adopt the term "sexual and reproductive justice".

To date, the issues of sexual autonomy and justice have been taken up in a limited way, for instance, restricted to work related to sexual coercion and violence against women and human trafficking (Asian Communities for Reproductive Justice, 2005). Until recently, far less attention has been devoted to sexual and gender diversity, and the scholarship has by and large not explicitly moved beyond a heterocentric focus on cisgender women. Work that has been done in this area remains largely limited to activism and sexual and reproductive health programmes and interventions. Consequently, attention has turned to the question of "queering reproductive justice" (Price, 2019).

There is undoubtedly scope for work on sexual and gender diversity within the reproductive justice movement and framework, with reproductive justice described as "a natural home" (Nixon, 2013, p. 79) for such efforts. Certainly, lesbian, gay, bisexual, transgender, and queer persons have been a part of reproductive justice and sexual liberation movements for as long as these have existed (Flores et al., 2011). It has only been more recently, however, that queer and reproductive justice movements have consciously and explicitly aligned themselves, foregrounding common concepts and causes across movements, such as bodily integrity and autonomy (Price, 2010; The LGBT Community Center, n.d.). For instance, African American and queer people may share the common cause of the right to have and parent children safely and free from state intrusion despite disparate social policies of injustice enacted against the two groups (Mamo & Alston-Stepnitz, 2015). This alliance-building across what some feminist health psychologists have called "chains of equivalence" (Macleod, 2012) has led to an expansion of what reproductive justice means and represents.

Accordingly, as one commentator explains, "reproductive justice is not just about one's ability to reproduce. It's about autonomy, it's about respect, it's about shared principles based in the human right to health and a desire for real social change" (Perez, 2007, p. 1). In addition to attending to who is able to realise their reproductive and parental rights, reproductive justice includes the human right to engage in sexual activity without state intervention, free from fears of violence, disease, or unwanted pregnancy (Ross & Solinger, 2017). This more comprehensive definition could be further expanded by engagement with feminist and queer scholarship on sexual citizenship, which according to Richardson (2000), encompasses the right to: (i) sexual practice in intimate relationships, including rights to sexual pleasure and to self-determination (e.g. the right to have children); (ii) self-identity and self-definition (e.g. the right to name the kind of sexual person one is); and (iii) institutional recognition and public validation of a variety of sexual relationships (e.g. choice and public recognition of partnerships).

There is clearly much room for scholarly engagement between feminists, queer theorists, and reproductive justice scholars. As intimated above, feminist work around sexual and reproductive citizenship holds promise, as evidenced, for example, in recent work on "queer kinship" (Morison et al., 2019; Morison & Lynch, 2019) or trans reproductive justice (Riggs & Bartholomaeus, 2019). Likewise, queer and reproductive justice theories offer distinct yet complementary lenses through which to consider common issues and the dialogue between the approaches is only beginning (Stacey, 2018). Such a conversation has the potential to greatly benefit both theoretical and empirical scholarship in reproductive justice.

Geo-politics and transnational perspectives in knowledge production

The emergence and growth of the reproductive justice paradigm has also brought about an expansion in thinking about the interconnections between domestic and global reproductive politics. Such interconnections have, for instance, been highlighted in the policy domain where policies in the wealthier countries can have a tremendous impact on the countries dependant on them for aid (Joffe & Reich, 2015). A good example of this is the US "Mexico City Policy", commonly known as the "global gag rule" for its silencing effect on abortion advocacy. This policy has been retracted and reinstated several times, depending on the political leanings of the current administration. Most recently, in 2021, the policy was rescinded by Democrat President Biden. The policy forbids organisations receiving financial assistance from the US from counselling on abortion, providing abortion, or making referrals to abortion services (except in cases of incest, rape, or endangered life) (Mavodza et al., 2019). It has had significant negative effects on the services offered in low-resource countries and has been described as an assault on sexual and reproductive health and rights (Hawkes & Buse, 2017).

Research also demonstrates the complexity of global power relations and the contradictory effects that these may have. This is illustrated in the work on assisted reproduction and transnational gestational surrogacy, discussed above. Considering potential resolutions to this issue, Fixmer-Oraiz (2013, p. 152) concludes:

For all of their complexities and problematics contemporary practices of assisted reproduction and commercial surrogacy link us to one another in concrete, visible, and profound ways. Perhaps, in leveraging some of these connections both materially and rhetorically, we might move closer to a vision of justice that includes us all.

Her conclusion points to the possibility of areas of common ground around sexual and reproductive injustices. It is upon this common ground that solutions can be generated through alliances built across seemingly disparate positions (Collins, 2017).

To this end, scholars have more recently begun to call for transnational work in reproductive justice that investigates how:

we are linked by common themes of the struggle for bodily autonomy, the residual impacts of colonization and intergenerational trauma, family violence, and a desire for reproductive freedom. Recognizing these connections, across time and space, national boundaries, and various identity categories are vital to building the solidarities necessary to create a more equitable world.

(Bakhru, 2019, p. 4)

The ways that transnational scholarship may contribute to the creation of solidarities is demonstrated by Chiweshe and colleagues' work on abortion decision-making in Zimbabwe and South Africa. Comparing and contrasting the discursive resources drawn on in women's narratives of their abortion decision, the researchers' objective was to highlight cross-cutting commonalities and differences in the data in terms of power relations across the two countries. This, they maintain, situates reproductive issues within the social power relations of particular contexts, identifying cross-cutting, transnational power relations that can be challenged on a broad front, as well as context-specific power relations that require localised strategies. Their analysis works toward producing a contextually-attuned reproductive justice approach to decision-making on pregnancy termination (Chiweshe et al., 2017).

The relatively limited engagement with reproductive justice beyond Euro-America, and questions posed by some writers and activists regarding its utility, prompts reflection on the uses – and perhaps limitations – of reproductive justice as an approach in marginalised regions and contexts. Considering this question, Chiweshe and colleagues have argued that, for the reproductive justice framework to have power and utility in diverse contexts, including geopolitically marginalised locations, researchers need to understand localised power structures and participants' experiences of these, as well as local ways of articulating in/justice. Use of the reproductive justice framework should be grounded in and responsive to such an understanding (Chiweshe et al., 2017; Chiweshe & Macleod, 2018).

The development of reproductive justice as a theoretical framework and analytic lens for application in varied contexts is an avenue for future work. The development and conceptual refinement of reproductive justice theory also requires attention to relatively privileged contexts beyond the USA and Europe and to a wider range of reproductive issues (Macleod et al., 2017). Generating theory from local perspectives for local purposes is important to the broader project of decolonisation.

Conclusion

In this chapter, I have focused on how critical scholarship has addressed questions of power surrounding reproduction as a deeply social, contested, and highly regulated area of health.

Tracing the emergence of the reproductive justice framework from among global perspectives on reproductive health, I have argued that this framework is of particular value to critical scholarship on reproductive health across disciplines and topic areas. The examples in this chapter illustrate why this may be, showing how as an analytic lens reproductive justice is able to highlight the complexity and illuminate nuanced, multi-dimensional power dynamics embedded within reproductive health issues. In consequence, using a reproductive justice framework with its intersectional focus makes it possible to show how the very same practices, interventions, or technologies may be simultaneously liberatory and oppressive, as well as how they may uncover potential common ground upon which to fashion solutions to reproductive injustice.

Thus, as a significant paradigm shift in thinking and scholarship on reproductive health, reproductive justice can provide a much-needed catalyst for reproductive research as well as a rich perspective for advocacy, policy reform, and intervention. Nevertheless, as I have discussed in this chapter, there is still work to be done, not only in terms of applying the framework to diverse topics, populations, and contexts, but also in relation to the conceptual refinement of reproductive justice as an analytical lens that may be suited to a range of settings. At the height of neoliberal capitalism, in the face of growing backlash and reproductive oppression, the need for such work is more pressing than ever.

References

Alan Guttmacher Institute. (2003). *In their own right: Addressing the sexual and reproductive health needs of American men.* https://www.guttmacher.org/pubs/us_men.pd

Asian Communities for Reproductive Justice (ACRJ). (2005). *A new vision for advancing our movement for reproductive health, reproductive rights and reproductive justice.* ACRJ & SisterSong. https://forwardtogether.org/wp-content/uploads/2017/12/ACRJ-A-New-Vision.pdf

Bakhru, T. S. (2019). Thinking transnationally: Reproductive justice in a globalized era. In T. S. Bakhru (Ed.), *Reproductive justice and sexual rights: Transnational perspectives* (pp. 3–12). Taylor and Francis Group.

Chiweshe, M., & Macleod, C. (2018). Cultural de-colonization versus liberal approaches to abortion in Africa : The politics of representation and voice. *African Journal of Reproductive Health, 22,* 49–59. doi:10.29063/ajrh2018/v22i2.5

Chiweshe, M., Mavuso, J., & Macleod, C. I. (2017). Reproductive justice in context: South African and Zimbabwean women's narratives of their abortion decision. *Feminism & Psychology, 27*(2), 2013–2224. doi:10.1177/0959353517699234

Collins, P. H. (1991). *Black feminist thought: Knowledge, consciousness, and the politics of empowerment* (2nd ed.). Routledge.

Collins, P. H. (2017). On violence, intersectionality and transversal politics. *Ethnic and Racial Studies, 40*(9), 1460–1473. doi:10.1080/01419870.2017.1317827

Cornwall, A., & Esplen, E. (2010). Women's empowerment: What do men have to do with it? *Contestations: Dialogues on Women's Empowerment, 3.* https://www.contestations.net/issues/issue-3/womens-empowerment-what-do-men-have-to-do-with-it/

Crenshaw, K. (1989). Demarginalizing the intersection of race and sex: A Black Feminist critique of antidiscrimination doctrine, feminist theory and antiracist politics. *University of Chicago Legal Forum, 1989,* 139–167.

Eager, P. W. (2017). *Global population policy: From population control to reproductive rights.* Routledge.

Figueroa-Pera, J. G. (2003). A gendered perspective on men's reproductive health. *International Journal of Men's Health, 2*(2), 111–130.

Fixmer-Oraiz, N. (2013). Speaking of solidarity: Transnational gestational surrogacy and the rhetorics of reproductive (in)justice. *Frontiers, 34*(3), 126–163. doi:10.5250/fronjwomestud.34.3.0126

Flores, B. F., González-Rojas, J., & Henriquez, S. (2011). *LGBTQ Latin@s and reproductive justice.* http://www.latinainstitute.org

Ghebreyesus, T. A., & Kanem, N. (2018). Defining sexual and reproductive health and rights for all. *The Lancet, 391*(10140), 2583–2585. doi:10.1016/S0140-6736(18)30901-2

Gilliam, M. L., Neustadt, A., & Gordon, R. (2009). A call to incorporate a reproductive justice agenda into reproductive health clinical practice and policy. *Contraception, 79*(4), 243–246. doi:10.1016/j.contraception.2008.12.004

Hawkes, S., & Buse, K. (2017). Trumped again: Reinstating the global gag rule. *BMJ (Online), 356*, j654. doi:10.1136/bmj.j654

Honkasalo, J. (2018). Unfit for parenthood? Compulsory sterilization and transgender reproductive justice in Finland. *Journal of International Women's Studies, 20*(1), 40–52.

Joffe, C., & Reich, J. (2015). Introduction: Reproduction and the public interest in private acts. In C. Joffe & J. Reich (Eds.), *Reproduction and society: Interdisciplinary readings* (pp. 1–12). Routledge. doi:10.4324/9781315754222

Luna, Z., & Luker, K. (2013). Reproductive justice. *Annual Review of Law and Social Science, 9*, 327–352. doi:10.1146/annurev-lawsocsci-102612-134037

Macleod, C. I. (2012). Feminist health psychology and abortion: Towards a politics of transversal relations of commonality. In C. Horrocks & S. Johnson (Eds.), *Advances in health psychology* (pp. 153–168). Palgrave Macmillan.

Macleod, C. I., Beynon-Jones, S., & Toerien, M. (2017). Articulating reproductive justice through reparative justice: Case studies of abortion in Great Britain and South Africa. *Culture, Health & Sexuality, 19*(5), 601–615. doi:10.1080/13691058.2016.1257738

Macleod, C. I., & Morison, T. (2020). Fertility, childbirth and parenting: Defining sexual and gender relations. In F. Cheung & D. Halpern (Eds.), *Cambridge international handbook on psychology of women*. Cambridge University Press.

Mamo, L., & Alston-Stepnitz, E. (2015). Queer intimacies and structural inequalities: New directions in stratified reproduction. *Journal of Family Issues, 36*(4), 519–540. doi:10.1177/0192513X14563796

Mavodza, C., Goldman, R., & Cooper, B. (2019). The impacts of the global gag rule on global health: A scoping review. *Global Health Research and Policy, 4*(1), 1–21. doi:10.1186/s41256-019-0113-3

Mohapatra, S. (2012). Achieving reproductive justice in the international surrogacy market. *Annals of Health Law, 21*(1), 191–200.

Mohapatra, S. (2019). Law in the time of Zika: Disability rights and reproductive justice collide. *Brooklyn Law Review, 84*(2), 325–364.

Morison, T., & Lynch, I. (2019). "Living two lives" and "blending in": Reproductive citizenship and belonging in the parenthood narratives of gay men. In *Queer kinship: South African perspectives on the sexual politics of family-making and belonging* (pp. 167–189). Routledge; Unisa Press.

Morison, T., Lynch, I., & Reddy, V. (2019). *Queer kinship: South African perspectives on the sexual politics of family-making and belonging*. Routledge; Unisa Press.

Morison, T., & Macleod, C. I. (2015). *Men's pathways to parenthood: Silence and heterosexual gendered norms*. HSRC Press.

Nixon, L. (2013). The right to (trans) parent: A reproductive justice approach to reproductive rights, fertility, and family-building issues facing transgender people. *William & Mary Journal of Women and the Law, 20*(1), 73–103.

Perez, M. Z. (2007, 31 May). Queering reproductive justice. *Rewire News*, 1–3. doi:10.2307/j.ctt1pwt8jh.9

Price, K. (2010). What is reproductive justice? How women of color activists are redefining the pro-choice paradigm. *Meridians, 10*(2), 42–65.

Price, K. (2019). Queering reproductive justice in the Trump era: A note on political intersectionality. *Politics & Gender, 14*(2018), 581–601. doi:10.1017/S1743923X18000776

Rabionet, S. E., Zorilla, C. D., Rivera-Vinas, J. I., & Guerra-Sanchez, Y. (2018). Pregnancy and Zika: The quest for quality care and reproductive justice. *Puerto Rico Health Sciences Journal, 37*(S1), S45–S50.

Rebouché, R. (2017). Reproducing rights: The intersection of reproductive justice and human rights. *U.C. Irvine Law Review, 7*, 579–609.

Richardson, D. (2000). Constructing sexual citizenship: Theorizing sexual rights. *Critical Social Policy, 20*(1), 105–135. doi:10.1177/026101830002000105

Riggs, D. W., & Bartholomaeus, C. (2019). Toward trans reproductive justice: A qualitative analysis of views on fertility preservation for Australian transgender and non-binary people. *Journal of Social Issues*, 1–24. doi:10.1111/josi.12364

Ross, L. J. (2017a). Conceptualising reproductive justice theory: A manifesto for activism. In L. Ross, E. Derkas, W. Peoples, L. Roberts, P. Bridgewater, & D. Roberts (Eds.), *Radical reproductive justice: Foundation, theory, practice, critique*. Feminist Press at CUNY.

Ross, L. J. (2017b). Reproductive justice as intersectional feminist activism. *Souls, 19*(3), 286–314. doi:10.1 080/10999949.2017.1389634

Ross, L. J., Roberts, L., Derkas, E., Peoples, W., & Bridgewater, P. D. (Eds.). (2017). *Radical reproductive justice: Foundations, theory, practice, critique.* Feminist Press at CUNY.

Ross, L. J., & Solinger, R. (2017). *Reproductive justice: An introduction.* University of California Press.

Saravanan, S. (2016). "Humanitarian" thresholds of the fundamental feminist ideologies: Evidence from surrogacy arrangements in India. *Analize: Journal of Gender and Feminist Studies, 6,* 66–88.

SisterSong. (2007). *Reproductive justice briefing book: A primer on reproductive justice and social change.* SisterSong. https://www.law.berkeley.edu/php-programs/courses/fileDL.php?fID=4051

Stacey, J. (2018). Queer reproductive justice? *Reproductive Biomedicine and Society Online, 7,* 4–7. doi:10.1016/j. rbms.2018.06.004

Stern, O., Peacock, D., & Alexander, H. (2009). *Working with men and boys: Emerging strategies from across Africa to address gender-based violence and HIV/AIDS.* Sonke Gender Justice Network and MenEngage Network. https://genderjustice.org.za/publication/working-with-men-and-boys/

The LGBT Community Center. (n.d.). *Causes in common: Reproductive Justice and LGBT liberation.* Lesbian, Gay, Bisexual & Transgender Community Centre. http://www.causesincommon.org

Thompson, B. Y. (2017). Centering reproductive justice: Transitioning from abortion rights to social justice. In L. J. Ross, L. Roberts, E. Derkas, W. Peoples, & P. B. Toure (Eds.), *Radical reproductive justice: Foundation, theory, practice, critique.* Feminist Press.

United Nations Population Fund (UNPF). (1994a). *Cairo declaration on population & development* (pp. 1–7). United Nations Population Fund. https://www.unfpa.org/resources/cairo-declaration-population -development

United Nations Population Fund (UNPF). (1994b). *Programme of action* (pp. 1–296). United Nations Population Fund. https://www.unfpa.org/sites/default/files/pub-pdf/programme_of_action_Web ENGLISH.pdf

Ussher, J. M., Chrisler, J. C., & Perz, J. (2020). *Routledge international handbook of women's sexual and reproductive health.* Routledge.

Wanhalla, A. (2007). To "better the breed of men": Women and eugenics in New Zealand, 1900–1935. *Women's History Review, 16*(2), 163–182. doi:10.1080/09612020601048779

15

ETHNICITY AND HEALTH

Dharmi Kapadia and Hannah Bradby

Introduction

The field of ethnicity and health research has grown dramatically over the last few decades, both theoretically and empirically. Theoretically, there is a critical awareness of the use of ethnic categories in research, and more explicitly developed understandings of what it means to belong, or be seen to belong, to a particular ethnic group, both in terms of personal identity and how such socially constructed groupings reflect the social circumstances influencing the incidence, progression, and treatment of illnesses. In some contexts, these theoretical understandings of ethnicity have translated well into empirical work, with responsible and reflective operationalisations of ethnicity, and with the betterment of ethnic minority people's health as part of progressive public health research agendas. Ethnicity is a complex concept that is meaningful in terms of both identity and structure: it can be a component of identity at the individual and at the group level, as well as a structural dimension of society that determines access to resources and influence. The significance of the identity and structural dimensions of ethnicity are historically and politically contingent, so they cannot be read from appearance in any simple fashion. Ethnicity may be strongly and positively identified with by individuals; it may be the basis of group solidarity, and, through a process of racialisation, may also be the basis of discrimination. Furthermore, since ethnic group classifications are used in some settings as a variable in state-level administrative datasets, then ethnicity can work as a structural feature of society, which influences access to resources.

Ethnicity: an ever-changing, approximate concept

Unsurprisingly, the definitions and usage of ethnicity terminology and classifications vary by place, time, and political regime. Ethnic group classifications are used in routine administrative data collection in the UK and the Netherlands, although race has never been classified in legal or administrative terms. By contrast, in other countries, such as the United States and South Africa, race categories are used in official data, sometimes in combination with ethnic groupings. In Sweden and France, data on the religious, cultural, or ethnic background of the population are not collected as part of statutory data, because principled decisions have been taken to avoid such classifications on the grounds that they are inherently racist and therefore divisive. However, in countries where data on ethnic groupings are not officially gathered, other proxies have developed which are similar to ethnicity variables elsewhere. For instance, in Sweden and Germany "migrant background" is used as a classification, variously defined, but based on the individual's country of birth and/or their parents' and grandparents' countries of birth.

Classifications of ethnic and racial groups and their proxies, as used in service provision, research, and routine data, vary in how they are defined and operationalised, not to mention how they are used in the analysis. In Anglophone quantitative health research, the ethnic categories that are deemed suitable for analysis vary from study to study, making comparisons problematic, particularly since the construction and use of categories are rarely explicitly justified. While the lack of stable and widely shared definitions of ethnicity for health research is problematic, it is also a reflection of the contingent, complex nature of ethnicity as a quality that operates on different levels and in particular historical and political conditions. A single operationalisable definition of what ethnicity means in critical health research across the world is perhaps unrealistic, given that the meaning of ethnic classifications is so context-dependent.

Ethnic minority health disadvantage

Despite the epistemological uncertainties of conceptualising and operationalising ethnicity, empirical research to date has nonetheless provided compelling evidence that in many countries, ethnic minority groups are at a health disadvantage compared with White majority groups. The ethnic minority health burden, compared with local White majority populations is seen for both physical and mental health problems, and also manifests itself in access to, and experience of, good quality healthcare. Documented ethnic health inequalities have been attributed to racist experiences over the lifecourse at both interpersonal and institutional levels and to socioeconomic disadvantage. Explaining how these inequalities are produced and maintained in the context of other forms of health inequality is a neglected research agenda, despite the widening of some of these inequalities in recent decades. This calls into question the willingness of public institutions such as health services, the criminal justice system and education to listen to the research evidence and create, adopt and implement policies to tackle racism in combination with other forms of structural and individual discrimination, to reduce ethnic inequalities in health.

This chapter has five aims. First, we critically discuss how ethnicity is conceptualised by researchers and practitioners in the field of ethnicity and health, including how definitions of ethnicity are related to the concepts of race and racialisation, and the implications of using ethnic categories in health research. Second, we describe some of the ways that ethnic inequalities in health at various points in the lifecourse for different health conditions are evident in research findings, and synthesise the main causes of ethnic inequalities that have been proffered by experts in the field, under the headings of racism and socioeconomic explanations. Third, we turn our attention to ethnic inequalities in mental illness, since this is where harm from racialisation, stigma, and discrimination have been shown to be clearly damaging. Fourth, we consider how ethnic minority people's experience of healthcare provided primarily by state institutions has highlighted the ways in which racialisation of ethnic minority groups has adversely affected their quality of care, and ultimately their health. Fifth, we conclude the chapter with reflections on how researchers can responsibly theorise ethnicity in research studies without compounding racialisation and essentialisation, and highlight the current challenges to ensuring research knowledge informs policy and practice in the area.

What do we mean when we talk about ethnicity?

Much research into ethnicity and health has been driven by a progressive intention to uncover unjust health inequalities, to benefit marginalised groups, and to promote social justice. However, not all researchers are working from the same foundation, as the specific details of what ethnicity means as a social category has divided opinion in the field (Bhopal, 2007; Nazroo, 2003). When we (academics, health practitioners, lay people) use the term "ethnicity", there are a number of aspects of a person's identity that are alluded to including, but not limited to, country of birth, parents' country of birth, languages spoken, cultural and family practices, skin colour, dress, religion, and diet. Additionally, there is an assumption of common origins (Bradby, 1995) for people belonging to the same ethnic group, but in reality people belonging to the same socially constructed ethnic group can have very different migration and family histories; for example, people classified as "South Asian" in the UK may have migrated from East Africa. Ethnicity is a quality that is inherited vertically down generations, unlike, for instance sexual identity, and this expectation defines some of the limits of ethnicity. While ethnic identities may be claimed, amplified, and refuted such that their prominence can vary dramatically, there are limits to this, as illustrated by the notorious case of Rachel Dolezal, an American civil rights activist and teacher who identified as Black despite being born to White American parents of German heritage (Brubaker, 2016).

So far throughout this chapter we have predominantly used the term ethnicity or ethnic group, but these terms are not used in some countries, with the term "race" being co-opted instead. Generally, when used in official or administrative data, "race" is used as a synonym for ethnic group and does not refer to the historical notion of biological race, which has been widely discredited. In addition to the differences in overarching terms used to describe ethnic groupings, there are variations in the state-level descriptors of ethnic/racial groups. For example, there is a contrast between the US where there are 15 possible self-assigned race options on the most recent census (2020) form (White; Black, African American or Negro; American Indian or Alaska Native; Asian Indian; Chinese; Filipino; Other Asian; Japanese; Korean; Vietnamese; Native Hawaiian; Guamanian or Chamorro; Samoan; Other Pacific Islander; some other race) and Brazil, where there are only five options on the 2010 census form (White; Black, Yellow, Brown; Indigenous). Of course, these differences reflect colonial and migration histories specific to each country, but these examples also serve to highlight that ideas of skin colour, country of origin, and Indigenous status are used unsystematically in these top-down formulations of ethnicity and race. The UK 2011 census ethnic group categories suffer from the same conflation, whereby some of the 18 ethnic groups available for self-identification, are bound to skin colour and whereas others represent nationality or country of origin (Jivraj & Simpson, 2015).

Reification and racialisation

The differences in ethnic categories across countries and time serve to highlight that ethnic groups are not fixed entities; these groups are created for specific purposes, at particular times, in different contexts, and moreover these brief descriptors do not capture the heterogeneity of people within any one single ethnic group, e.g. the experiences of a particular ethnic minority group living in a sparsely populated rural area differs greatly from people from that same ethnic group living in a densely populated urban setting. Further, ethnic categorisations change over time to reflect the changing demographics within a country. For example, in the UK, we have seen the number of ethnic groups on the national census form increase from 7 in 1991, to 16 in 2001, to 18 in the most recent census in 2011 and additional ethnic groups (e.g. Roma,

Somali) proposed for the 2021 census (at the time of writing). This increase may be interpreted as evidence of the dynamic nature of ethnicity and also indicates its uncertain ontological status. Researchers that favour well-developed and theoretically explicit notions of ethnicity do not necessarily evoke ethnicity as a real entity that exists "out there" and it is acknowledged that the exercise of defining and using ethnic categories in analysis amplifies their reification (Nazroo, 2001). The argument that making ethnic classifications has, not only a reifying effect on ethnicity as a category, but also a racialising effect underpins the reluctance of, for instance, Swedish healthcare systems, to use any such categorisations: to enact ethnic differentiation in any form is seen as racist in and of itself. The counter-argument is that creating ethnic categories and monitoring health outcomes by those categories has allowed the identification of ethnic health inequalities that may otherwise have remained hidden. While there are no ethnicity data in Swedish official statistics, there is evidence of inequalities in access to treatment and health outcomes. For instance, in one of the largest Swedish cities, women of African origin had perinatal mortality outcomes markedly poorer than native Swedes and these differences could not be explained by known risk factors (Essén, Hanson, Ostergren, Lindquist, & Gudmundsson, 2000). In the absence of monitoring by ethnic group, it is impossible to know whether Swedish-born women of African origin also show this type of perinatal mortality burden and to check any changes in the perinatal rates for women of African origin over time. However, by the same token, ethnic categories are sometimes presumed to be pseudonyms for the defunct biological construction of race (Bradby & Chandola, 2007), and their use in official data can unintentionally reinforce the idea of innate or inherent ethnic divisions that can form the basis for racial discrimination and stigma.

The "racialisation" of certain ethnic groups in terms of their (ill) health involves the problematic assumption that negative health outcomes and health behaviours are inherent to a particular ethnic group (Bradby & Nazroo, 2021), failing to take account of the effects of socioeconomic conditions for that group. To illustrate, over the past 30 years, a particular narrative about the health behaviours of South Asian women in the UK has emerged. This narrative racialises South Asian women in two ways. First, it blames South Asian culture (e.g. lifestyle, beliefs, supposed cultural practices associated with being South Asian), for the incidence and progression of physical and mental health problems; the way South Asian women live their lives *makes* them more likely to become ill in the first instance. For example, one UK qualitative study of 29 mental health professionals' views of South Asian women (Burr, 2002) showed that some professionals thought that one of the reasons South Asian women became depressed was due to living isolated, subordinate lives in a patriarchal South Asian cultural system. Mental health professionals homogenised and pathologised South Asian cultures in their explanations and painted them in juxtaposition to the presumed sociable, liberal cultural system in which White women live. Such stereotypical and racist explanations ignore the substantial proportions of South Asian women (particularly Pakistani and Bangladeshi women) who live in poverty, a known correlate of poor health, as well as downplaying or simply disregarding these women's experiences of racism and discrimination, which also explains their high levels of poor health (Karlsen & Nazroo, 2002). Second, when South Asian women do become ill, this narrative negatively portrays this group as less likely to access appropriate health services due to their "cultural" beliefs, ultimately contributing to higher rates of morbidity and mortality for this group. This is illustrated in Bowler's (1993) ethnographic study of interactions between midwives and South Asian women on a maternity ward, where staff often referred to women as non-compliant because of their low attendance at antenatal classes, which they thought led to less maternal understanding in the delivery room. Again, a reluctance to attend appointments is posited as characteristic of South Asian culture, based on beliefs surrounding mistrust of health professionals, or preferences to use familial sources of support for prenatal healthcare. In both of these examples, the assumptions made about South Asian women were used by health professionals to make decisions about their healthcare, leading to racialised and inequitable treatment.

There are undoubtedly dilemmas in the deployment of ethnicity as a category in research and in health service provision, in terms of the reification of fixed ethnic categories that can become the basis for racialised thinking and discrimination. In research, ethnic groupings can become reductionist in quantitative studies, and there is the danger of "ethnicity" per se having explanatory power, when in fact it is the experiences of racism and other disadvantages that ethnic minority groups face that provide the real explanation. Qualitative studies can be better designed to both give prominence to lived experience and to pay attention to a range of co-constitutive characteristics (e.g. gender, sexuality, disability) and structural features of society that create ethnic inequalities in health. However, in the absence of a measurement of ethnicity, health disadvantages accruing to specific groups defined by a common culture, place of origin, and structural position, remain invisible. The increased speed and scope of globalised migration-driven diversity, as well as the labile nature of the meaning of ethnicity results in official categories that measure ethnic group becoming rapidly out-dated. However, if there is no attempt to capture the effects of ethnicity on health outcomes, we risk failing to address the damage that social, economic and political processes inflict on ethnic minority groups.

Ethnic health inequalities over the lifecourse

In efforts to minimise further compounding the racialisation of ethnic minority people, many researchers have sought to take a holistic and intersectional approach to ethnicity and health research, to provide contextual explanations of why so many ethnic minority people suffer from poor health. Two major explanations for why ethnic inequalities in health arise are (1) the disadvantaged socioeconomic position of ethnic minority people, and (2) experiences of interpersonal and institutional racism, which lead to poor health outcomes. We refer to both of these in the following paragraphs, in our explanation of ethnic health inequalities that manifest across the lifecourse.

Early life ethnic health inequalities

Ethnic inequalities in health outcomes are evident at every stage throughout the lifecourse, from birth to death. In the UK, low birth weight, a known risk factor for chronic disease later in life, occurs more frequently in ethnic minority groups (Kelly et al., 2009), with Pakistani, Bangladeshi, Indian, Black Caribbean, and Black African mothers 2.5 times as likely to birth babies that are deemed to be low birth weight, constituting a difference of up to 300g, compared with White mothers (Harding, Rosato, & Cruickshank, 2004). This trend for lower birth weight in ethnic minority groups is also evident in the US (Almeida, Bécares, Erbetta, Bettegowda, & Ahluwalia, 2018) and in both countries there has been very little, if any, change in these inequalities over time. In terms of how ethnic inequalities play out among young children, one recent important development in the field is the study of how family members' experience of racism (vicarious racism) has a detrimental effect on children's psychosocial development and wellbeing. A systematic review of 30 studies (Heard-Garris, Cale, Camaj, Hamati, & Dominguez, 2018) showed how vicarious racism operates through two major pathways: by increasing stress during pregnancy and worsening maternal health and increasing risks in childbirth, and by children witnessing experiences of racism and internalising these experiences, to the detriment of their own health (Bécares, Nazroo, & Kelly, 2015); an effect that may be exacerbated by the negative effect of racist experiences on parental health. This "linked lives" approach (Gee, Walsemann, & Brondolo, 2012) to studying how racism affects the health of close family members, as well as those experiencing discrimination, is a noteworthy development, giving due consideration to how experiences of discrimination must be viewed within the whole context of a person's life (over time and across social connections). In adolescence, there are some physical health conditions (high blood pressure, obesity, and asthma) for which there is a clear health disadvantage for some ethnic minority groups (Harding et al., 2015), whilst other UK evidence shows that some ethnic minority adolescents have better mental health than their White counterparts (Astell-Burt, Maynard, Lenguerrand, & Harding, 2012). This health advantage may be due to the protective effect of high levels of ethnic density – the proportion of people of the same ethnic group living in your area. This same protective effect has been found for ethnic minority adults' mental health, particularly of Bangladeshi background, in the UK (Das-Munshi et al., 2012), highlighting the need to consider important geographical and spatial influences in the relationship between ethnicity and health.

The persistence of health inequalities into adulthood

Adulthood is the lifecourse phase where the greatest amount of research evidence has been generated. The health disadvantage for ethnic minority people in the US has been shown for cardiovascular disease (CVD), mental illness, and overall mortality rates (Williams, Lawrence, & Davis, 2019). For example, Black Americans were found to have higher systolic blood pressure (a known risk factor for the development of CVD) than White Americans (Krieger & Sidney, 1996). Research has linked such ethnic health disparities to experiences of racism (Bailey et al., 2017), and the effect of racism on health persists over and above socioeconomic effects on health. Most of the research that examines links between racism and health has been carried out in the US (see Paradies et al., 2015 for a systematic review), but there is also a smaller body of evidence from other countries. Studies from New Zealand have shown Māori are more likely to have poorer physical and mental health, higher rates of CVD and higher rates of smoking than the general population (Harris et al., 2006), and in the UK, national community studies, and census data have been analysed to show worse mental and physical health outcomes for ethnic minority groups (Bécares, 2015; Weich et al., 2004).

The onset of the COVID-19 pandemic in early 2020 has further highlighted the effects of contemporary and historical racism on health. In the UK, ethnic minority people were one of the worst affected groups at the start of the pandemic, with higher mortality and infection rates (ONS, 2020), and many ethnic groups have been disproportionately affected by the lockdowns (local and national) and associated restrictions which have further hampered their health (Nazroo et al., 2020; Platt & Warwick, 2020). The evidence to date shows that the ethnic minority groups (Pakistani, Bangladeshi, Black African, and Black Caribbean groups) that are most likely to suffer poor health outcomes in the pandemic, are also those that have been persistently shown over the last few decades to be suffering from the worst health and are most disadvantaged socially and economically (Byrne, Alexander, Khan, Nazroo, & Shankley, 2020). This evidence suggests that poor COVID-19 outcomes are not only a result of contemporary conditions, such as elevated exposure to the virus through disproportionately high employment rates in occupations working with the public, but also historical deprivation and marginalisation. In Sweden, where ethnicity is not measured, a 220% excess in mortality was recorded in the spring of 2020 among adults born in countries from which many refugees have recently arrived (Hansson, Albin, Rasmussen, & Jakobsson, 2020).

Cumulative disadvantage

There is evidence that disadvantageous experiences throughout the lifecourse in the form of racism and other forms of discrimination have a cumulative effect on health, with a dose-response relationship. A UK longitudinal study by Wallace and colleagues (2016) found that for each incident of racist discrimination there was an incremental negative effect on mental health. This emerging work on cumulative disadvantage in the ethnicity and health field provides two areas for further exploration. First, it throws a spotlight on ethnicity and health research at older ages, as this is where we should see the greatest effects of disadvantage accumulated over the lifecourse. Research in the UK and US suggests that ethnic health inequalities at older ages are much worse than for younger ages – as ethnic minority adults age, they can expect to have even worse health than their White counterparts (Nazroo, 2006). However, such work is sparse and the health of older ethnic minority people has been largely neglected both in ethnicity and race research and in the social gerontology field (Phillipson, 2016), and quantitative studies in the UK are particularly sparse, due to the lack of substantially large samples for data analysis (Bécares, Kapadia, & Nazroo, 2020). Given that globally, populations are living longer, this presents an area of research that requires development. Second, the cumulative disadvantage model requires us to think through how time is theorised in studies of ethnic health inequalities. Recent theoretical advancements in the field call for us to think about time in a multidimensional way and not constrain ourselves to biological and (Western) chronological notions of time (Gee, Hing, Mohammed, Tabor, & Williams, 2019). For example, there may be critical time periods in the lifecourse when economic disadvantage or racist experiences are particularly detrimental for the subsequent development of health.

Mental illness

Mental illness is, arguably, the health problem for which there are the most unjust and stark inequities for ethnic minority populations. In this illness context, racism (both interpersonal and institutional), socioeconomic inequalities and disadvantage over the lifecourse, and at key junctures in life, can be observed in interplay, resulting in dire health outcomes for ethnic minority people. In the UK context, the over-use of coercive mental health treatment under mental health law for Black Caribbean and Black African groups (Halvorsrud, Nazroo, Otis, Brown Hajdukova, & Bhui, 2018) and the under-use of specialist mental health services by South Asian (Indian, Pakistani, and Bangladeshi) groups (Kapadia, Nazroo, & Tranmer, 2018) have been two of the main concerns articulated by health policy commentators, clinicians, and health researchers. In recent years, we have also seen new forms of racial discrimination emerging in the treatment of mental illness with the implementation of the UK government's Prevent agenda, in the wake of a series of terrorist attacks in the 2000s, leading to the securitisation of mental illness (Younis & Jadhav, 2020). The mental health consultation room has become a site for detecting people at risk of radicalisation, alongside treatment for mental illness. And it is Muslims that are disproportionately subjected to these insidious and covert assessments (Younis & Jadhav, 2019). In this section, we focus on the over-use of coercive mental health treatment for Black Caribbean and Black African groups and the under-use of specialist mental health services by South Asians.

The first of these concerns is perhaps the more serious, with findings from numerous studies showing both increased rates of mental illness for Black Caribbean and Black African men (Bhui, Halvorsrud, & Nazroo, 2018), and systematic persecution from psychiatric services and criminal justice systems, with these groups much more likely to be subjected to coercive treatments such as involuntary admission to mental health wards, Community Treatment Orders, and violence from state systems (Barnett et al., 2019). Black patients in the UK are also subject to more intrusive treatments, such as injectable anti-psychotics, and are less likely to be offered talking treatment for severe mental illness (Das-Munshi, Bhugra, & Crawford, 2018). Thus, it is not surprising that the psychiatric system has been accused on numerous occasions, by academics and activists, of institutional racism (Fernando, 2017), a term that was brought into mainstream use in the UK after the McPherson inquiry into the racially motivated murder of Stephen Lawrence, a young Black man who was killed in London (Bradby, 2010). Despite the overwhelming research evidence of racist treatment of Black populations by the UK mental healthcare system, a recent review of the Mental Health Act (Department of Health and Social Care, 2018) gave only cursory attention to race inequalities, thereby neglecting a real opportunity to address the institutional racism evident in the psychiatric care system.

Stigma as deflection

In the second of these concerns, we see under-use of mental health services by South Asian (mainly comprised of Indian, Pakistani, and Bangladeshi people) groups in the UK, despite very high rates of engagement and consultation with primary care services (Nazroo, Falaschetti, Pierce, & Primatesta, 2009), suggesting a lack of referral to appropriate secondary services, perhaps due to racial stereotyping of people in this group (Burr, 2002). However, it is also likely that some ethnic minority groups are reluctant to seek help from mental health services due to a fear of discriminatory treatment, based on their previous interactions with health professionals (Bowl, 2007). In the context of this under-utilisation of mental health services, there is also a widespread assumption of greater mental illness stigma in ethnic minority groups, as compared to the general population. There is said to be higher levels of stigma against mentally ill persons among minority ethnic groups due to certain religious, spiritual, or traditional beliefs about mental illness and the stigma that seeking help for these problems entails. These explanations are widely shared, not only amongst psychiatrists and other mental health professionals, but also amongst people who are suffering, or who have suffered, with mental illness, their family members, charities and advocacy groups working with marginalised ethnic minority groups (Anglin, Link, & Phelan, 2006; Conner et al., 2010; Corrigan & Watson, 2007; Nadeem et al., 2007).

There is some evidence in the US that ethnic minority people with mental illness may feel more stigma from their family members than White people do (Anglin et al., 2006), and there is some emerging evidence from the UK and other countries (Bhavsar, Schofield, Das-Munshi, & Henderson, 2019; Eylem et al., 2020). But most of the qualitative studies (Knifton, 2012; Shefer et al., 2013) that purport to show greater levels of stigma in ethnic minority populations focus their analysis on minority samples, without a comparative White British sample, but nonetheless make baseless comparative statements (Kapadia, Brooks, Nazroo, & Tranmer, 2017). What has been skewed in the academic debate, and in the public consciousness, is the idea that mental illness stigma is so great in ethnic minority populations that it can account for a lot of the disparities we see, including those in access to talking treatments (comparative to White groups), recovery rates and satisfaction with mental health services, use of crisis mental health services, and detainment under the Mental Health Act (McManus, Bebbington, Jenkins, & Brugha, 2016). The intense focus on stigma in ethnic minority groups (but not in White majority groups) as a reason for lack of help-seeking and poorer mental health outcomes is a deflection away from other problems that affect ethnic minority groups in the pursuit of improving their mental health. Using mental illness stigma as a deflection, in this way, is damaging to ethnic minority people's health, as it focuses undue attention on reducing mental illness stigma within ethnic minority groups at the expense of ignoring other, greater structural problems that affect the poorer quality of mental health treatment that ethnic minority groups receive. In particular racial discrimination from health professionals has been downplayed as a major reason for under-use of mental health services.

Addressing ethnic health inequalities through healthcare practices

Having laid out the reasons for ethnic inequalities in health, we now turn our attention to efforts to translate research findings into practice, to address these inequalities within healthcare settings. Initiatives that have sought to tackle ethnic disparities in health suffer from the same dilemmas we have raised regarding the construction of ethnic group categories: reification, calcification, and, potentially, racialisation. As a socially, politically, historically, and culturally contingent category, ethnicity is highly labile, whereas categories of official data collection tend to calcify, allowing ethnicity to be seen as a fixed, essentialist quality. This can mean that some interventions to un-do ethnic health inequalities can have a negative effect, by further racialising, and "othering" ethnic minority populations, with detrimental consequences for health and wellbeing.

Race-specific prescribing

Take, for example, BiDiL, the first drug in the history of prescribing in the US to be recommended by the Food and Drug Administration (FDA) in 2005 for the treatment of hypertension in African Americans only. This drug caused substantial controversy, when, in an attempt to reduce racial inequalities, the FDA "unscientifically endorsed a biological model of race" (Bibbins-Domingo & Fernandez, 2005, p. 54). But the drug trial, on which the recommendation was based, consisted of only self-identified Black or African American patients. Hence, differential responses to the drug by racial group were not tested, and the resultant conclusion of greater efficacy in Black patients was scientifically incorrect (Kahn, 2005). The correct conclusion would have been to assert the efficacy of BiDiL for the whole US population, as has been done for previous US drug trials performed with exclusively majority White, male samples. In departing from a whole population approach, and endorsing race-specific prescribing, the FDA had unequivocally alluded to racial variations in the underlying biological mechanisms in how patients' bodies respond to BiDiL, without an evidence base. This has added to the racialisation of Black people as it assumes that BiDiL works for Black patients simply *because they are Black*, or more precisely, because they self-identify as Black. With this kind of reasoning, the battle to combat health disparities becomes reduced to simply treating patients on an individual, biological level with minimal attention paid to structural and economic factors that contribute to the higher incidence of hypertension in Black adults.

Despite refutations of the research evidence for the use of BiDiL for only Black patients, the recommendation was also adopted by the National Institute for Health and Care Excellence (NICE), the UK body responsible for clinical guidelines. Recent analysis of the thought processes underpinning both the production of these guidelines and how practitioners understand them, highlights the contentious nature of both what it means to belong to a specific ethnic group, and the criteria that are used to determine this (Smart & Weiner, 2018). In clinical settings, there is real uncertainty, ambiguity, and inconsistency in the way clinicians implement these guidelines, with varying ways that patients' Blackness is ascertained, by asking patients to self-identify (recommended by NICE) using pre-defined categories, or by "eyeballing" patients (clinicians' best guess). Clinicians often defined "mixed-race" (White and Black) patients as

"Black" contrary to NICE guidelines. One notable omission from Smart and Weiner's study is the lack of reflection from clinicians on how racial prescribing perpetuates essentialist notions of ethnicity and race.

Racialisation of female genital cutting (FGC)

Another example where attention to ethnic minority health concerns has had equivocal effects concerns a focus on female genital cutting/circumcision (FGC) or mutilation (FGM) and its link with poor perinatal outcomes of migrants from Somalia to Sweden. There is no evidence to link the perinatal outcomes of women of Somali birth in Sweden to the effects of FGC, although this link is regularly presumed in research (Humphris & Bradby, 2017). However, there is evidence that a number of aspects of poor access to healthcare and poor quality healthcare have negative effects on the perinatal outcomes of Somali-born women in Sweden, including delay in seeking healthcare, refusal of caesarean sections, insufficient surveillance of intrauterine growth restriction, inadequate medication, misinterpretation of cardiography, poor interpersonal communication (Essén et al., 2002), and the under-reporting of sexual violence (Byrskog, Olsson, Essén, & Allvin, 2015). Despite the lack of evidence that scar tissue from circumcision obstructs or otherwise impedes labour, healthcare professionals nonetheless attribute poor outcomes to the aftereffects of FGC, rather than to the quality of healthcare and the ease of accessing that care. The presumption that FGC determines poor birth outcomes for women of Somali origin in Sweden effectively releases the healthcare system from the need to reconfigure how obstetric care is organised for immigrants. An interview study with obstetricians found very little consensus about what constitutes good obstetric care for women with FGC or how care should be provided, as demonstrated by inconsistent policy and praxis, difficulties in monitoring labour and foetal status as well as inhibited communication (Widmark, Levál, Tishelman, & Ahlberg, 2010). The historical establishment of FGC among people of East Africa was tightly bound up with the colonial administrations of the early 20th century (Boddy, 2007), yet today, in a European context, cutting is presumed to be an expression of culture. In contemporary Sweden, FGC has become a sign of the cultural and possibly inherent inferiority of women of Somali origin, thereby contributing to the racialisation of African women, and providing a rationale for discrimination. While in no way supporting it as a practice, we point here to the indirect, as well as direct damage that genital cutting does to ethnic minority women in healthcare settings. In providing an example of the presumed inferiority of particular minority cultures, the high profile of research around FGM cements a pathologisation of minority cultures more generally, facilitating an erosion of minority women's dignity and a lack of trust in healthcare (Hamed, Thapar-Bjorkert, Bradby, & Ahlberg, 2020)

Conclusions

Our understanding of the ever-changing and approximate nature of ethnicity as both structural and individual characteristics informs how it can be used progressively to critically inform research and healthcare provision. The persistent and global nature of ethnic minority group health disadvantage speaks to the need to develop ways of conceptualising the role of ethnicity in both health status and healthcare access to combat the social injustice of cumulative health damage through socioeconomic disadvantage and the effects of racism. However, the racialisation of classifications of an ethnic group or migrant background carries the risk of essentialising measurable difference and thereafter attributing cause for any health deficits to features of ethnic minorities. In research settings, there is a need to be explicit about how ethnicity variables are constructed and how they are related to the research question under consideration. Where health burdens by ethnic group (or some other proxy of ethnicity) are revealed by research, there is a public health need to address those inequalities. Where ethnic group inequalities are demonstrated, for instance, in terms of mental health or obstetric outcomes, the routine collection of data around ethnicity is warranted for monitoring whether the inequalities are reduced. The collection of ethnicity data for monitoring purposes can only hope to have a progressive effect if undertaken in the context of a commitment to anti-racism, which in turn suggests a willingness and a vocabulary to identify discriminatory effects of healthcare provision and an agreed framework in which to tackle those effects at local and national levels. The commitment to tackle ethnic inequalities in health of course varies globally, and is driven by presiding governments. For example, in the UK, there has been a government commitment to document and highlight race disparities in health and other areas of social and economic life, yet there is very little evidence that this translates into practice and policies to transform healthcare, as increasingly it seems that race is dropped from the healthcare agenda. Where countries have a measurement of ethnicity or race, stark inequalities have been apparent in COVID-19 infection and mortality rates. Early attempts to account for disparities in the UK suggest that a range of different factors need to be taken into account, including how ethnicity and gender interact with occupational structures, migration status, wealth, family obligations, housing, and existing chronic illness. What is clear is that the challenges facing ethnic minority people, including marginalisation and discrimination, have to be included in an equitable and responsive public health agenda. Black Lives Matter demonstrations and discussions have drawn attention to iniquitous racialised inequalities at the hands of statutory authorities world-wide, the momentum of which, it must be hoped, will bring about action to redress long-standing injustices. What constitutes appropriate redress will vary across countries and cultures, given the contextual and historical dimension of how such inequalities have developed and become embedded in healthcare settings.

The ideal of careful and reflective construction of ethnicity variables for use in an anti-racist context is difficult to realise at a time when anti-immigrant, xenophobic, and nationalist politics are thriving. The welfarist attitudes which question the entitlement of ethnic minority and migrant people's access to good healthcare have negative effects on ethnic minority individuals' wellbeing (Bradby, Liabo, Ingold, & Roberts, 2017) and ability to access healthcare (Bradby, Humphris, & Padilla, 2018). A society's collective ability to provide equitable healthcare to the population, in a way that undoes existing health inequalities, is part of a wider politics of health, which sees ethnicity as one of a number of intersecting dimensions influencing health. Attending to ethnicity as a variable in health inequalities does not imply assuming it to be an immutably dominant factor across all cultures, and this perhaps represents the most challenging feature of thinking through the relationship between ethnicity, racism and health. To develop models that allow for the contingencies of how socially constructed categories play out over time and across cultures, means maintaining a contextual and flexible perspective that is not easy within the context of day-to-day healthcare provision.

References

Almeida, J., Bécares, L., Erbetta, K., Bettegowda, V. R., & Ahluwalia, I. B. (2018). Racial ethnic inequities in low birth weight and preterm birth: the role of multiple forms of stress. *Maternal and Child Health Journal*, *22*, 1154–1163.

Anglin, D. M., Link, B. G., & Phelan, J. (2006). Racial differences in stigmatizing attitudes toward people with mental illness. *Psychiatric Services*, *57*(6), 857–862.

Astell-Burt, T., Maynard, M. J., Lenguerrand, E., & Harding, S. (2012). Racism, ethnic density and psychological wellbeing through adolescence: Evidence from the determinants of adolescent social wellbeing and health longitudinal study. *Ethnicity & Health, 17*(1–2), 71–87.

Bailey, Z. D., Krieger, N., Agénor, M., Graves, J., Linos, N., & Bassett, M. T. (2017). Structural racism and health inequities in the USA: Evidence and interventions. *The Lancet, 389*, 1453–1463.

Barnett, P., Mackay, E., Matthews, H., Gate, R., Greenwood, H., Ariyo, K., … Smith, S. (2019). Ethnic variations in compulsory detention under the Mental Health Act: A systematic review and meta-analysis of international data. *The Lancet Psychiatry, 6*(4), 305–317.

Bécares, L. (2015). Which ethnic groups have the poorest health? In S. Jivraj & L. Simpson (Eds.), *Ethnic identity and inequalities in Britain* (pp. 123–140). Bristol: Policy Press.

Bécares, L., Kapadia, D., & Nazroo, J. (2020). Neglect of older ethnic minority people in UK research and policy. *British Medical Journal, 368* (February), 11–12. doi:10.1136/bmj.m212

Bécares, L., Nazroo, J., & Kelly, Y. (2015). A longitudinal examination of maternal, family, and area-level experiences of racism on children's socioemotional development: Patterns and possible explanations. *Social Science & Medicine, 142*, 128–135.

Bhavsar, V., Schofield, P., Das-Munshi, J., & Henderson, C. (2019). Regional differences in mental health stigma – Analysis of nationally representative data from the Health Survey for England, 2014. *PLoS ONE, 14*(1), 1–16.

Bhopal, R. (2007). *Ethnicity, race, and health in multicultural societies: Foundations for better epidemiology, public health, and health care*. Oxford: Oxford University Press.

Bhui, K. S., Halvorsrud, K., & Nazroo, J. (2018). Making a difference: Ethnic inequality and severe mental illness. *British Journal of Psychiatry, 213*, 574–578.

Bibbins-Domingo, K., & Fernandez, A. (2005). In the balance BiDiL for heart failure in black patients: Implications of the U. S. Food and Drug Administration approval. *Annals of Internal Medicine, 146*, 52–56.

Boddy, J. P. (2007). *Civilizing women: British crusades in colonial Sudan*. Princeton, NJ: Princeton University Press.

Bowl, R. (2007). Responding to ethnic diversity: Black service users' views of mental health services in the UK. *Diversity in Health and Social Care, 4*, 201–210.

Bowler, I. (1993). "They're not the same as us": Midwives' stereotypes of South Asian descent maternity patients. *Sociology of Health and Illness, 15*(2), 157–178.

Bradby, H. (1995). Ethnicity: Not a black and white issue. A research note. *Sociology of Health and Illness, 17*(3), 405–417.

Bradby, H. (2010). Institutional racism in mental health services: The consequences of compromised conceptualisation. *Sociological Research Online, 15*(3), 8.

Bradby, H., & Chandola, T. (2007). Ethnicity and racism in the politics of health. In A. Scriven & S. Garman (Eds.), *Public health: Social context and action*. Maidenhead: Open University Press.

Bradby, H., Humphris, R., & Padilla, B. (2018). Universalism, diversity and norms: Gratitude, healthcare and welfare chauvinism. *Critical Public Health*, 1–13. doi:10.1080/09581596.2018.1522420

Bradby, H., Liabo, K., Ingold, A., & Roberts, H. (2017). Visibility, resilience, vulnerability in young migrants. *Health*, 1–18. doi:10.1177/1363459317739441

Bradby, H., & Nazroo, J. (2021). Health, ethnicity and race. In W. C. Cockerham (Ed.), *The new companion to medical sociology* (pp. 113–129). Malden, MA: Blackwell.

Brubaker, R. (2016). The Dolezal affair: Race, gender, and the micropolitics of identity. *Ethnic and Racial Studies, 39*(3), 414–448.

Burr, J. (2002). Cultural stereotypes of women from South Asian communities: Mental health care professionals' explanations for patterns of suicide and depression. *Social Science & Medicine, 55*(5), 835–845.

Byrne, B., Alexander, C., Khan, O., Nazroo, J., & Shankley, W. (2020). *Ethnicity, race and inequality in the UK: State of the nation*. Bristol: Policy Press.

Byrskog, U., Olsson, P., Essén, B., & Allvin, M. K. (2015). Being a bridge: Swedish antenatal care midwives' encounters with Somali-born women and questions of violence; a qualitative study. *BMC Pregnancy and Childbirth, 15*(1), 1–11.

Conner, K. O., Copeland, V. C., Grote, N. K., Koeske, G., Rosen, D., Reynolds, C. F., & Brown, C. (2010). Mental health treatment seeking among older adults with depression: The impact of stigma and race. *American Journal of Geriatric Psychiatry, 18*(6), 531–543.

Corrigan, P. W., & Watson, A. C. (2007). The stigma of psychiatric disorders and the gender, ethnicity, and education of the perceiver. *Community Mental Health Journal, 43*(5), 439–458.

Das-Munshi, J., Bécares, L., Boydell, J. E., Dewey, M. E., Morgan, C., Stansfeld, S. A., & Prince, M. J. (2012). Ethnic density as a buffer for psychotic experiences: Findings from a national survey (EMPIRIC). *British Journal of Psychiatry*, *201*(4), 282–290.

Das-Munshi, J., Bhugra, D., & Crawford, M. J. (2018). Ethnic minority inequalities in access to treatments for schizophrenia and schizoaffective disorders: Findings from a nationally representative cross-sectional study. *BMC Medical Research Methodology*, *16*(55), 1–10.

Department of Health and Social Care. (2018). *Modernising the Mental Health Act: Increasing choice, reducing compulsion*. Department of Health and Social Care. Retrieved from https://www.gov.uk/government/publications/modernising-the-mental-health-act-final-report-from-the-independent-review

Essén, B., Bödker, B., Sjöberg, N. O., Gudmundsson, S., Östergren, P. O., & Langhoff-Roos, J. (2002). Is there an association between female circumcision and perinatal death? *Bulletin of the World Health Organization*, *80*(8), 629–632.

Essén, B., Hanson, B. S., Ostergren, P. O., Lindquist, P. G., & Gudmundsson, S. (2000). Increased perinatal mortality among sub-Saharan immigrants in a city-population in Sweden. *Acta Obstetricia et Gynecologica Scandinavica*, *79*(9), 737–743.

Eylem, O., De Wit, L., Van Straten, A., Steubl, L., Melissourgaki, Z., Danlşman, G. T., … Cuijpers, P. (2020). Stigma for common mental disorders in racial minorities and majorities a systematic review and meta-analysis. *BMC Public Health*, *20*(1), 1–20. doi:10.1186/s12889-020-08964-3

Fernando, S. (2017). *Institutional racism in psychiatry and clinical psychology: Race matters in mental health*. Palgrave Macmillan.

Gee, G. C., Hing, A., Mohammed, S., Tabor, D. C., & Williams, D. R. (2019). Racism and the life course: Taking time seriously. *American Journal of Public Health*, *109*(S1), S43–S47.

Gee, G. C., Walsemann, K. M., & Brondolo, E. (2012). A life course perspective on how racism may be related to health inequities. *American Journal of Public Health*, *102*(5), 967–974.

Halvorsrud, K., Nazroo, J., Otis, M., Brown Hajdukova, E., & Bhui, K. S. (2018). Ethnic inequalities and pathways to care in psychosis in England: A systematic review and meta-analysis. *BMC Medicine*, *16*(1), 1–17.

Hamed, S., Thapar-Bjorkert, S., Bradby, H., & Ahlberg, B. M. (2020). Racism in European health care: Structural violence and beyond. *Qualitative Health Research*, *30*(11), 1662–1673.

Hansson, E., Albin, M., Rasmussen, M., & Jakobsson, K. (2020). Stora skillnader i överdödlighet våren 2020 utifrån födelseland. *Läkartidningen*, *117*(20113).

Harding, S., Read, U. M., Molaodi, O. R., Cassidy, A., Maynard, M. J., Lenguerrand, E., … Enayat, Z. E. (2015). The determinants of young adult social wellbeing and health (DASH) study: Diversity, psycho-social determinants and health. *Social Psychiatry and Psychiatric Epidemiology*, *50*, 1173–1188.

Harding, S., Rosato, M. G., & Cruickshank, J. K. (2004). Lack of change in birthweights of infants by generational status among Indian, Pakistani, Bangladeshi, Black Caribbean, and Black African mothers in a British cohort study. *International Journal of Epidemiology*, *33*, 1279–1285.

Harris, R., Tobias, M., Jeffreys, M., Waldegrave, K., Karlsen, S., & Nazroo, J. (2006). Effects of self-reported racial discrimination and deprivation on Māori health and inequalities in New Zealand: Cross-sectional study. *Lancet*, *367*, 2005–2009.

Heard-Garris, N. J., Cale, M., Camaj, L., Hamati, M. C., & Dominguez, T. P. (2018). Transmitting trauma: A systematic review of vicarious racism and child health. *Social Science & Medicine*, *199*, 230–240.

Humphris, R., & Bradby, H. (2017). Health status of refugees and asylum seekers in Europe. In *Oxford Research Encyclopedia of Global Public Health*. Oxford University Press. Retrieved from doi:10.1093/acrefore/9780190632366.013.8

Jivraj, S., & Simpson, L. (2015). *Ethnic identity and inequalities in Britain. The dynamics of diversity*. Bristol: Policy Press.

Kahn, J. (2005). Misreading race and genomics after BiDil. *Nature*, *37*(7), 655–656.

Kapadia, D., Brooks, H. L., Nazroo, J., & Tranmer, M. (2017). Pakistani women's use of mental health services and the role of social networks: A systematic review of quantitative and qualitative research. *Health and Social Care in the Community*, *25*(4), 1304–1317.

Kapadia, D., Nazroo, J., & Tranmer, M. (2018). Ethnic differences in women's use of mental health services: Do social networks play a role? Findings from a national survey. *Ethnicity and Health*, *23*(3), 293–306.

Karlsen, S., & Nazroo, J. (2002). Agency and structure: The impact of ethnic identity and racism on the health of ethnic minority people. *Sociology of Health & Illness*, *24*(1), 1–20.

Kelly, Y., Panico, L., Bartley, M., Marmot, M., Nazroo, J., & Sacker, A. (2009). Why does birthweight vary among ethnic groups in the UK? Findings from the Millennium Cohort Study. *Journal of Public Health*, *31*(1), 131–137.

Knifton, L. (2012). Understanding and addressing the stigma of mental illness with ethnic minority communities. *Health Sociology Review*, *21*(3), 287–298.

Krieger, N., & Sidney, S. (1996). Racial discrimination and blood pressure: The CARDIA study of young black and white adults. *American Journal of Public Health*, *86*(10), 1370–1378.

McManus, S., Bebbington, P., Jenkins, R., & Brugha, T. (2016). *Mental health and wellbeing in England: Adult psychiatric morbidity survey 2014*. Leeds: NHS Digital.

Nadeem, E., Lange, J. M., Edge, D., Fongwa, M., Belin, T., & Miranda, J. (2007). Does stigma keep poor young immigrant and U.S.-born black and Latina women from seeking mental health care? *Psychiatric Services*, *58*(12), 1547–1554.

Nazroo, J. (2001). *Ethnicity, class and health*. London: Policy Studies Institute.

Nazroo, J. (2003). The structuring of ethnic inequalities in health: Economic position, racial discrimination, and racism. *American Journal of Public Health*, *93*(2), 277–284.

Nazroo, J. (2006). Ethnicity and old age. In J. A. Vincent, C. Phillipson, & M. Downs (Eds.), *The futures of old age* (pp. 65–76). London: SAGE.

Nazroo, J., Falaschetti, E., Pierce, M., & Primatesta, P. (2009). Ethnic inequalities in access to and outcomes of healthcare: Analysis of the health survey for England. *Journal of Epidemiology & Community Health*, *63*(12), 1022–1027.

Nazroo, J., Murray, K., Taylor, H., Becares, L., Field, Y., Kapadia, D., & Rolston, Y. (2020). Rapid evidence review: Inequalities in relation to COVID-19 and their effects on London. London: Greater London Authority. Retrieved from https://data.london.gov.uk/dataset/rapid-evidence-review-inequalities-in-relation-to-covid-19-and-their-effects-on-london

ONS. (2020). Coronavirus (COVID-19) related deaths by ethnic group, England and Wales – Office for National Statistics. *Office for National Statistics*, (April), 1–10. Retrieved from https://www.ons.gov.uk/peoplepopulationandcommunity/birthsdeathsandmarriages/deaths/articles/coronavirusrelateddeathsbyethnicgroupenglandandwales/2march2020to10april2020%0Ahttps://www.http://ons.gov.uk/peoplepopulationandcommunity/birthsdeathsandmarriages/deaths

Paradies, Y., Ben, J., Denson, N., Elias, A., Priest, N., Pieterse, A., … Gee, G. (2015). Racism as a determinant of health: A systematic review and meta-analysis. *PLoS ONE*, *10*(9), 1–48.

Phillipson, C. (2016). Placing ethnicity at the centre of studies of later life: Theoretical perspectives and empirical challenges. *Ageing & Society*, *35*(2015), 917–934.

Platt, L., & Warwick, R. (2020). Are some ethnic groups more vulnerable to COVID-19 than others? *Institute for Fiscal Studies*. Retrieved from https://www.ifs.org.uk/inequality/chapter/are-some-ethnic-groups-more-vulnerable-to-covid-19-than-others/

Shefer, G., Rose, D., Nellums, L., Thornicroft, G., Henderson, C., & Evans-Lacko, S. (2013). "Our community is the worst": The influence of cultural beliefs on stigma, relationships with family and help-seeking in three ethnic communities in London. *International Journal of Social Psychiatry*, *59*(6), 535–544.

Smart, A., & Weiner, K. (2018). Racialised prescribing: Enacting race/ethnicity in clinical practice guidelines and in accounts of clinical practice. *Sociology of Health & Illness*, *40*(5), 843–858.

Wallace, S., Nazroo, J., & Bécares, L. (2016). Cumulative effect of racial discrimination on the mental health of ethnic minorities in the United Kingdom. *American Journal of Public Health*, *106*(7), 1294–1300.

Weich, S., Nazroo, J., Sproston, K., McManus, S., Blanchard, M., Erens, B., … Tyrer, P. (2004). Common mental disorders and ethnicity in England: The EMPIRIC study. *Psychological Medicine*, *34*(8), 1543–1551.

Widmark, C., Levál, A., Tishelman, C., & Ahlberg, B. M. (2010). Obstetric care at the intersection of science and culture: Swedish doctors' perspectives on obstetric care of women who have undergone female genital cutting. *Journal of Obstetrics and Gynaecology*, *30*(6), 553–558.

Williams, D. R., Lawrence, J. A., & Davis, B. A. (2019). Racism and health: Evidence and needed research. *Annual Review of Public Health*, *40*, 105–125.

Younis, T., & Jadhav, S. (2019). Keeping our mouths shut: The fear and racialized self-censorship of British healthcare professionals. *Culture, Medicine and Psychiatry*, *43*, 404–424.

Younis, T., & Jadhav, S. (2020). Islamophobia in the National Health Service: An ethnography of institutional racism in PREVENT's counter-radicalisation policy. *Sociology of Health & Illness*, *42*(3), 610–626.

16

INDIGENEITY AND WELLNESS

Critically understanding the health of Indigenous peoples and communities

Sarah de Leeuw, Margo Greenwood, and May Farrales

Introduction, overview, and key terms

Writing, thinking about, and practicing Indigenous health and wellness are not straightforward tasks. What does "Indigenous" mean? For whom does it have that meaning? What do "health" and "illness" really mean and, again, for whom? How did contemporary understandings about the meaning of these words, and all that they signify, come into being? Who writes about these words and concepts? Why? How are the concepts studied? Taught about? Put into professional or clinical practice? In this chapter, we answer some of these questions. If we do not *fully* answer all of these questions (and others), it is in part because we believe that to suggest totality in critical investigations of contested concepts is, unto itself, an erroneous colonial conceit. Our efforts are thus to delve critically into terrains of Indigenous peoples' health with a partialness that invites further and future efforts of innovative analytical – and hopefully anti-colonial – investigation.

Before we begin our exploration of Indigenous health, however, we briefly place ourselves: The act of *placing* authors within knowledge production and publication is itself a process we urge more health and medical researchers and clinicians to undertake, as this chapter intermittently suggests. So, to begin: We three authors are a unique combination of Indigenous and non-Indigenous identities. Margo is a Cree woman hailing from Treaty 8 in Alberta, Canada, who has spent much of her life on Dekelh territory in north-central British Columbia and on Sylx territory in the central Okanagan region of the province. She is a mother of three sons and an internationally established scholar whose work on Indigenous health and children has always been anchored in community wellbeing. Sarah was born to a Dutch father and a Canadian mother of Scottish and Irish heritage and grew up in remote northern geographies on Haida Gwaii and Tsimshian territories of British Columbia. She is a feminist activist, poet, and humanities scholar, employed in a faculty of medicine, whose work focuses on colonial violence and health inequities. May's parents migrated to unceded Musqueam territory from the Philippines during the early stages of President Ferdinand Marcos's Martial Law period. Since beginning to organise among racialised immigrants and migrants on Coast Salish territories, May has been learning about the importance of place, politics, and overlapping responsibilities from immigrants as well as from Indigenous peoples and communities. We hope that by writing this chapter *together*, we are taking an anti-colonial stance against colonial modalities that insist on dualities and opposition and do not recognise the complexity and slippery intersectionality (Tuck & Yang, 2012). In our effort of working together as diverse Indigenous peoples and diverse settlers, we are taking seriously the concepts of relationality, of being in relationship with "all our relations" – a teaching that insists not only upon the interconnectedness and responsibility of all humans to both each other and to nonhuman beings, but also upon forging new ways of being together (Beniuk, 2016).

As we have written about elsewhere (de Leeuw & Hunt, 2018), if one is to critically understand complicated concepts (such as Indigenous health), one must begin by understanding that the epistemologies, lexicons, and discursive terrains that comprise complicated concepts are, themselves, socially and culturally constituted. People make up knowledge. People have assumptions, positionalities, values, biases, understandings, fluencies, and logics that (perhaps even unconsciously) can be maintained when we author and produce knowledge. This conceptualisation of knowledge production (as inherently biased and never objective, neutral, or impartial) is an orientation that has been increasingly acknowledged by Indigenous scholars, including Indigenous health scholars and scholars of critical Indigeneity (Hunt, 2014). Many critical Indigenous scholars and anti-colonial scholars also insist that coloniality and colonial power are upheld, in great part, by discursive knowledge terrains produced almost exclusively by settler scholars and theorists, most of whom are White (de Leeuw & Hunt, 2018; Simpson, 2017). It should be noted that we purposefully use the concept of anti-colonial here, as opposed to "post" colonial. As we have written elsewhere, and other scholars also argue, settler-colonial geographies like Australia, Canada, the United States or Aotearoa/New Zealand are not "post" colonial places since colonial powers and a state of coloniality still dominates (de Leeuw and Hunt, 2018).

Having now ushered in terms such as "settler" and "Indigenous", let us turn to definitions and meanings of key words deployed throughout this chapter. While it sometimes feels like the word "Indigenous" is in use all around us, the word is actually a relatively recent one – especially to those of us in progressive healthcare or post-secondary educational environments. Moreover, the word Indigenous is neither uncontested nor circulated unproblematically. Indeed, in Australia there have been fierce debates about settler rights to claim "indigenousness" in efforts to assert rights of belonging, especially in land-based ways (Anderson & Taylor, 2005). In Global South countries and other national spaces where neoliberal policies – including those, for instance, of the International Monetary Fund (IMF) – are shifting in response to pressures of the United Nations Declaration on the Rights of Indigenous Peoples (UNDRIP), individuals' claims to Indigenous identity are incrementally shifting over time. These shifts respond in part to growing international recognition that Indigenous peoples have unique and protected claims to land and resources. Consequently, some marginalised peoples have come to realise the economic potential in an Indigenous lineage, particularly if they can claim the genealogy as a "pure subject" (Li, 2007, p. 185).

Claims about the "pureness" and "authenticity" of Indigenous identity are divisive and hurtful; they are often the outcome of violent colonial taxonomies and hierarchies that systematically privilege whiteness. In Canada and the United States, peoples once incongruously categorised as "Indian" – because of the colonial conceit and error that Columbus had discovered India upon arrival in the America – have rightfully argued for the more accurate moniker of "Indigenous" or sometimes "First Peoples" while simultaneously demanding, again rightfully, a return to non-colonial nomenclatures of local geographies. Thus, while there are *Indigenous* peoples around the world, from the Circumpolar North to Japan, from Central and South America to New Zealand/Aotearoa, from Canada to Australia and back again, it is always best, when referring to Indigenous peoples, to be as geographically and linguistically specific as possible. For instance, three groups of Indigenous peoples (First Nations, Inuit, and Métis) are constitutionally recognised in Canada. While all three Indigenous groups of Indigenous peoples are dispersed across Canada, Inuit people hail principally from the Circumpolar North regions of the country. Métis are people of mixed European and Indigenous ancestry with distinct and unique socio-cultural customs and traditions alongside a common language. First Nations are neither Métis nor Inuit, although multiple identities are possible so that a person can easily be of First Nations and Métis heritage. First Nations people are original inhabitants of the geographies that are now Canada and, originally categorised as "Indians", were the first to encounter sustained European contact, settlement, and trade. In north-western Canada alone, however, the populations are remarkably diverse, including Nisga'a, Haida, Dene, Gitxsan, Dakalth, and Wet'suwet'en First Nations who, in turn, live alongside Métis people and, further north (or even in some urban geographies), Inuit people. These diverse people also live in distinct and varied geographies, from no-road-access communities to cities with more than a million people.

When thinking, writing, or practicing in areas of Indigenous peoples' health and illness, it is important to understand and capture these complexities: To do otherwise is to risk pan-Indigenising or falling into problematic colonial lexicons. Following eminent Indigenous Māori scholar and activist Linda Tuhiwai Smith (2013), and recognising Indigenous peoples are contemporary global subjects who move and migrate and live across diverse spaces, we understand and use the word and concept "Indigenous" to denote people who *self-identify as having no homeland other than the homeland to which they claim an Indigenous ancestral tie*. This is not a singular definition, and it remains fluid, but it is a definition we have found helpful.

Similar to the complexities associated with the word Indigenous, tensions also exist with reference to the increasingly popular word "settler". Like the word Indigenous, the term and concept of "settler" is not a singular or homogeneous catchall term. For example, in settler-colonial contexts like that of Turtle Island (also known as "North America"), settler colonialism is theorised as a project inherently and fundamentally tied to settler (often White) acquisition of Indigenous lands. Kahnawake Mohawk scholar, Audra Simpson (2014), explains: "Although the settler variety is acquisitive, unlike other colonialisms, it is not labour but territory it seeks. Because 'Indigenous' peoples are tied to the desired territories, they must be 'eliminated'" (p. 19). Therefore, the concept "settler" can be understood less as an "identity" and more as a means of describing one's relationship to the ongoing project of settler colonialism.

Most problematically, and often with reference to Indigenous peoples and places, "settler" is too often used as a shorthand reference for *White* people of often Euro-global-north ancestry. Such homogenisations erase gradations of racialisation and power that structure settler people and settler geographies. While people who are *not* Indigenous to an area can, correctly, be referred to as settlers, not all settlers are equally implicated in coloniality. In Canada and the United States, for instance, Black-Afro-Caribbean-American peoples, and many people from mainland China, were forcibly traded as slaves, imported as bonded workers, and relocated from their native homes in order to fulfil needs for cheap exploitable labour (see also Kobayashi & de Leeuw, 2010). Increasingly, alliances and allyships between Indigenous peoples and Black and People of Colour (BIPOC) are seen to be some of the most fertile grounds for fighting coloniality, racism, and White supremacy (see, for instance, Farrales, 2019; Simpson, 2017; Walia, 2013). Finally, undergirding the broad concepts of both Indigenous and settler are complexities of sexuality, gender, age, dis/ability, economic status, and even geographic location. It cannot be emphasised strongly enough that understanding Indigenous health and wellness from a critical anti-colonial perspective must take intersectionality into account: In terms of the ways that health, wellness, or illness are navigated and lived by Indigenous peoples, great differences exist between, for example, an Indigenous trans-woman in a remote northern community and an economically prosperous, cisgendered, heterosexual Indigenous man in a large global city.

If the words and concepts of "Indigenous" and "settler" are slippery, so too are ideas such as health and illness. Indeed, as has been eloquently evidenced elsewhere (Fadiman, 1999), what one person or community might see as a strength and a blessing, a different person or community might understand (and even diagnose) as a tragic illness. Such tensions in concepts of illness and wellness are especially urgent for Indigenous peoples because, often as an outcome of homogenised pan-Indigenising by often White settlers, many Indigenous peoples and communities have been pathologised or conceptualised through deficit-lenses of illness and disorder that result in muddled understandings about how to address urgent needs (Greenwood et al., 2015). For instance, much media and academic scholarship – including health and medical scholarship – circulates the idea that there is a "suicide epidemic" among Indigenous peoples, especially Indigenous youth, in Canada. While from a population-based perspective (e.g. based on census data that conflates all First Nations, Inuit, and Métis people) rates of suicide among Indigenous youth are higher than among non-Indigenous settler youth, mass characterisations such as this mask important and informative differences between Indigenous peoples and communities, including important evidence about what factors lead to *lower* rates of suicide (as compared with the broader settler populations) in some First Nations (Chandler & Lalonde, 1998).

Indeed, it may be impossible to accurately assess the health of Indigenous individuals, or even individual communities, based on aggregated, collective, population, or census-based data. This is because population or census-based data speak to systemic realities, but those realities may not accurately portray any individual Indigenous person, family, or community. Such challenges in understanding health profiles of Indigenous peoples – from an individual, to a community, to a population – pose additional challenges when critically thinking about or practicing healthcare with Indigenous peoples and communities. Additionally, and as some Indigenous scholars and activists (e.g. Cree Elder Willie Ermine) have pointed out, there is an inherent bias in much of the literature written about Indigenous peoples' health and wellness. After all, much of the literature about Indigenous people's health is written by non-Indigenous (often White) "experts", many of whom are deeply vested in pathologising Indigenous peoples and communities in order to continue a colonialist paradigm of settlers paternalistically saving Indigenous peoples, especially from their deviant selves (Ermine et al., 2004; see also de Leeuw, Greenwood, & Cameron, 2010).

Critically thinking about and practicing in areas of Indigenous health, wellness, and illness is, as outlined, complicated business. The very words that are used, the positionalities of the people implicated, the spaces and times of ideas and practices involved: All these are slippery and changing, and all are germane to the conversation. Keeping all this in hand might feel a little daunting, especially for non-Indigenous settler readers. Consequently, and in an effort to encourage fewer frustrations or feelings of helplessness, we turn now to some more known, knowable, and concrete parameters of thinking about Indigenous health. We begin by presenting these parameters with a degree of uniformity that stands somewhat in tension with the slippery complexity just outlined. We then move, therefore, onto anti-colonial critiques of these broad parameters, thus opening new ways of thinking about and practicing within Indigenous peoples' health in both specific, local geographies and across broader scales globally.

Local, global, and everything in-between: Indigenous health across different times and spaces

Indigenous peoples' health, wellness, and illness is addressed across multiple scales and jurisdictions. The United Nations' recent Declaration on the Rights of Indigenous Peoples states that Indigenous peoples have the right to health improvements, free from discrimination (United

Nations, 2007, see articles 21, 22, 29). That wording, along with numerous other expressions about the rights to health restoration, the rights to self-determination in health provision, and the rights to improved health status, clearly signals broad global truths about Indigenous peoples' health. Indigenous peoples currently face discrimination in areas of health, many Indigenous peoples do not have self-determination when it comes to health and wellness, and Indigenous peoples on the whole, compared with non-Indigenous peoples, live with diminished health and wellbeing that require attention and restoration (Marmot, 2015). While UNDRIP is responding to global scales and international realities of Indigenous peoples, the United Nations declaration reflects realities at scales of individual nation-states and the smaller geographies (provinces, territories, and municipalities) of which nation-states are composed. Canada, Australia, and New Zealand/Aotearoa have all, over the past several decades, released population-based reports anchored in census data that reveal that Indigenous peoples live with disproportionally high burdens of illness and poor health, including (when compared with non-Indigenous populations) lowered life expectancies, higher rates of chronic disease and infant mortality, and elevated levels of mental illness and addiction (Anderson, 2019; Australian Bureau of Statistics, 2016; Stas NZ, 2019). Studies of Indigenous peoples of the Circumpolar North (Russia, Scandinavia, and Canada's far north) reveal that while infectious diseases have seen decreases since the 19th century, there are significant rates of increase in chronic diseases and in "pathologies" such as violence, substance misuse, and preventable accidents (Bjerregaard, Young, Dewailly, & Ebbesson, 2004). While it is impossible to generalise, many Indigenous peoples around the world – from the Inagno in Colombia to the Igbo in Nigeria, from the Maasai in Kenya to the Awajun in Peru, from the Karen in Thailand to the Dalit in India – face similar health challenges with regards to higher rates of chronic disease and illnesses related to social and environmental influences (Bjerregaard et al., 2004). Again, broadly speaking, these profile similarities in Indigenous peoples' illness and burdens of poor health have some shared underlying factors that, increasingly, are being addressed through common frameworks of understandings.

In 2008, the World Health Organization (WHO) released a seminal report that showed that it was not individual peoples' decisions or actions about their health that resulted in the greatest health disparities; instead, it was "social injustice … killing on a grand scale, with a toxic combination of poor social policies and [programmes], unfair economic arrangements, and bad politics … responsible for producing and reinforcing health inequalities" (Marmot & Bell, 2012, p. 4). These factors – economic status, gender, race, etc. – are called "social determinants of health" (SDoH), and the inequalities within them stem from socio-cultural norms and education, both of which may be grounded in or supported by governmental policies. Thus, the victim of poor health is less to blame than hegemonic socio-cultural forces bearing down unevenly on certain peoples and communities; that is, the "causes of the causes" of poor health must take precedence over the nature of the poor health itself in a consideration of health inequities (Braveman & Gottlieb, 2014). SDoH frameworks, which are being adopted by a growing and influential number of Indigenous peoples around the world, have been transformative for many Indigenous peoples. These frameworks have offered the individuals who fall under this term a new lens by and through which to theorise, understand, and develop solutions to pressing states of health inequalities.

In Canada, for instance, the country's recent Truth and Reconciliation Commission (TRC) Final Report (2015) stated that the country's colonialist residential school system, a system almost identical in nature to "civilising" educational efforts in Australia, New Zealand/Aotearoa, and the United States that were all designed to eradicate Indigenous identity and culture, is unquestionably a contributor to poor health status among present-day Indigenous peoples (TRC, 2015). Such understandings of health inequities quickly opened the door for Indigenous scholars, healthcare practitioners, activists, and community members to argue that colonialism and ongoing states of coloniality are possibly the greatest contributors to rates of poor Indigenous health (Reading & Wien, 2009).

Recognising colonialism as a key determinant of Indigenous peoples' health has resulted in new understandings about how Indigenous health statuses have been arrived at from historical standpoints. It has likewise issued in novel understandings about the current state of Indigenous peoples' health and illness and about how to remedy inequities in the future. Many Indigenous health experts around the world have observed that, prior to colonial interruption in the form of diseases, violence, suppression, and enforced othering of peoples and places (often not White), Indigenous peoples were healthy, self-sustaining, and self-determining (see, for example, National Inquiry into Missing and Murdered Indigenous Women and Girls, 2019; Smith, 2013). Successive waves of diseases, both prior to settler landfall and during settler expansion, decimated Indigenous populations across the Americas and Polynesia, around the Circumpolar North, and deep into most island nations. With much knowledge about wellness (in the form of healers, health and medicine experts, or knowledge keepers) eradicated from waves of disease, Indigenous peoples were often left with only sparse expertise to remain free from (or combat) sicknesses that, until then, they had often never encountered or even heard of. Such failings to stave off these new illnesses only reinforced colonial conceits that Indigenous peoples were dying populations. Assumptions such as this were entrenched in Euro-colonial ideologies that formed the foundation of eradication or assimilation policies premised on beliefs that Indigenous peoples were inherently flawed and inferior, and that they required salvation (Simpson, 2017; Million, 2013; Lawrence, 2000). Indeed, increasing bodies of evidence suggest that early colonial ideologies and conceits about the poor health and savagery of Indigenous peoples formed powerful foundations of settler assumptions about and dealings with Indigenous peoples. These foundations persist, broadly anchored in White supremacy (a sometimes unconscious and sometimes conscious bias about the superiority of whiteness) and continually position Indigenous peoples as needing settler salvation, as problematic populations standing in the way of logic and progress (including in realms of health and medicine); and as ultimately othered subjects in settler-colonial nation-states (Moreton-Robinson, 2015; Smith, 2013).

More recently, and with a particular ascendance in Canada, New Zealand/Aotearoa, and Australia, evidence about colonialism being a key social determinant of Indigenous peoples' health has given way to even more pointed discussions about why Indigenous peoples live contemporaneously with greater burdens of ill health. Anti-Indigenous racism is rooted in and fundamental to colonialism and coloniality. A result is that many Indigenous peoples not only feel unsafe in healthcare settings but also face discrimination by healthcare providers. What is more, anti-Indigenous racism stands as a barrier to Indigenous peoples' entering healthcare professions (Allan & Smylie, 2015). Racism of all incarnations is anchored in taxonomic orderings, associated with the Swedish botanist and physician Carl Lineaus, which imagine differences between subjects as inherently tethered to worthiness and hierarchies of superiority: nonhuman animals, for instance, are less worthy than human animals but worthier than plants; amongst humans, males (usually White) are worthier and more "developed" than females. These are, at a very basic level, the logics of racism: people who are imagined as morally and physically fit are understood to be of a higher, and thus more deserving, order than subjects who are sick, poor, racialised, or "difficult". People who fall into these "lower" categories – those who have been historically constructed by colonialist ideologies as savage, unfit, lazy, undeserving, and sick – are then seen (and "read") in contemporary healthcare settings to be overly demanding and irresponsible drains on the healthcare system. Indigenous peoples are read through racist lenses as peoples who unfairly demand to be served and who are problematic, noncompliant, complaining patients who cannot be assuaged or ever fully treated. Such stereotypes and imaginings are deeply rooted in historical constructions and narratives about Indigenous peoples: the contemporary results, however, are myriad communities of Indigenous peoples feeling alienated from healthcare systems that seem to denigrate their cultures and realities.

As a consequence of feeling unsafe and discriminated against in healthcare settings, many Indigenous peoples simply avoid them entirely. Indeed, avoidance is another well-documented social determinant of health (Dolezal & Lyons, 2017; Monchalin, Smylie, & Nowgesic, 2020). If people are not accessing services that could improve their wellbeing, the likelihood of poor health outcomes for those people increases. For many, that avoidance is the result of racism. Indeed, the reality of anti-Indigenous racism in healthcare systems is well-documented internationally: in New Zealand/Aotearoa, efforts to address anti-Indigenous racism sparked the "cultural competency" revolution (Papps et al., 1996). Cultural competency, which has now expanded around the world and evolved into movements such as cultural humility and cultural safety (Isaacson, 2014), all have one thing in common: an understanding that health and wellness, especially for Indigenous peoples, hinge on a non-judgemental recognition of power dynamics and cultural diversity. This understanding must be grounded in an awareness of the antecedents that may be resulting in their poor health and must be backed by an ability and willingness, especially by health professionals or researchers to work in relationship with and treat peoples of different cultural backgrounds (Campinha-Bacote, 2002). Cultural safety, competency, and humility as responses to Indigenous-led critiques about healthcare practices and research exemplify how Indigenous and non-Indigenous activists, researchers, patients, and clinicians are increasingly and globally working together, often with a focus on the social determinants of health, to address the pressing reality of poor health outcomes in Indigenous peoples around the world. The rise of cultural safety, competency, and humility makes clear that change is possible; however, such change must be deeply and fundamentally anchored in anti-colonial frameworks that are informed by Indigenous peoples. Cultural safety, competency, and humility also confront historical social constructions of Indigenous peoples as inherently flawed, pathologised, sick, and lesser subjects either requiring constant settler salvation or being unworthy of healthcare. They replace such flawed perceptions with anti-colonial visions, and voices.

Nothing about us without us: Transformations in Indigenous wellness

There exists, around the world, what many Indigenous peoples are calling an Indigenous resurgence. While forms and movements of resurgence vary and are highly context- and place-based, resurgence is often tied to questions of land and communities' multiple and multi-layered relationships to ancestral lands, waterways, each other and other-than-human relations (see, for example, Simpson, 2017; Daigle, 2016; Coulthard, 2014). This resurgence is often anchored in an internationalisation of Indigenous resistance and the development of allyships between and within Indigenous peoples and communities and/or between Indigenous peoples, communities, and non-White settler communities (Simpson, 2017; Walia, 2013). Many of these connections and allyships surface and focus on a few – but powerfully incontrovertible – demands: 1) Indigenous peoples are strong; 2) they are knowledgeable about ideas, innovations, solutions, and their own potential; 3) knowledge about Indigenous peoples must be informed, if not led by, Indigenous peoples; 4) coloniality must be confronted by anticolonialism; 5) dispossession of Indigenous lands, bodies, and their self-determining authorities must be understood in relation to questions of Indigenous sovereignty; and 6) the world will be richer with healthier and ever-vibrant Indigenous peoples. These powerful contentions are, increasingly, the foundations on which change in health research and healthcare practice is being constructed. For instance, a resurgence in scholarship on Indigenous peoples' health and wellness is increasingly being driven by Indigenous peoples (Simpson, 2014; Simpson, 2017), a point that aligns these studies with feminist, queer, and anti-racist scholarship that has for many years pointed out that medical and healthcare research should not continue to be penned by White, straight, cisgendered men. Indigenous scholars, activists, and clinicians are observing that research is still too often done about them, usually without them, and often with no applicability to the health priorities of Indigenous peoples and communities (Simpson, 2014; Simpson, 2017). Many Indigenous peoples and communities around the world are evidencing that health research, and by extension healthcare practices, has rendered and constructed Indigenous peoples as perpetually sick, as needing healthcare they (as Indigenous peoples) have not been a part of developing, and as tending to see Indigenous peoples and realities as subjects of, rather than participants in, related research. These observations are linked to other increasingly-argued positions by Indigenous peoples: health and medical research and practices are often extractive as opposed to generative with regard to Indigenous peoples and, relatedly, inquiries and scholarship about Indigenous peoples' health and wellness are often anchored in protocols (e.g. research ethics and standards of scholarship) that reflect (often White) settler norms as opposed to Indigenous ways of knowing and being (Came, Gifford, & Wilson, 2019; Morton Ninomiya, & Pollock, 2017; Ermine, Sinclair, & Jeffery, 2004).

In response to these entrenched hegemonic, colonial ways of producing knowledge that then structure health and medical practices, Indigenous peoples (increasingly in concert with critical radicalised and racialised activists and scholars also pushing against established norms) are proposing new, innovative, and transformative ways of thinking about Indigenous health and wellness. Many of these emerging ideas are tethered to traditional ways of knowing and being. Furthermore, they are anchored in cultural strength, and they demand both conceptual and applied changes in thinking about and practicing healthcare with Indigenous peoples and communities (Simpson, 2014; Simpson, 2017). For instance, through the Institute of Indigenous Peoples Health within the Canadian Institutes for Health Research (CIHR), Indigenous peoples authored one chapter of Canada's largest research and ethics governing body, the *Tri-council policy statement: Ethical conduct for research involving humans* (TCPS-2, 2014). Aimed squarely at the way health research is conducted in Canada, this chapter in the TCPS-2 acknowledges early on that health research about Indigenous peoples:

> has been defined and carried out primarily by non-Aboriginal researchers. The approaches used have not generally reflected Aboriginal world views, and the research has not necessarily benefited Aboriginal peoples or communities. As a result, Aboriginal peoples continue to regard research, particularly research originating outside their communities, with a certain apprehension or mistrust.
>
> *(para. 3)*

This acknowledgement is followed by concrete demands for change. The authors note that research concerning Indigenous peoples must engage Indigenous peoples and acknowledge Indigenous governance structures alongside cultural protocols. Summarised as "OCAP" principles, the chapter provides clear direction about research concerning Indigenous peoples (and especially health research) must observe that Indigenous communities should have Ownership, Control, Access, and Possession of all research and data produced with reference to them. These parameters are ensuring the kinds of health research being produced about Indigenous peoples are shifting, including Indigenous health research having utility for Indigenous communities and Indigenous health research being owned and authored by Indigenous peoples themselves.

At more applied and practical levels, many training and educational spaces for future health-care professionals are proactively recruiting Indigenous trainees and learners. In Canada's second-largest faculty of medicine, for instance, there has been concentrated and targeted efforts to recruit and graduate Indigenous physicians. Having more Indigenous physicians practicing in the healthcare system is evidenced and understood to ensure a healthcare system that will one day be more accessible to and welcoming of Indigenous patients. And, if Indigenous patients feel more recognised and supported by healthcare systems, they will be more likely to use and trust those systems. This will, over time, lead to better outcomes for Indigenous peoples.

At the same time, the growing numbers of Indigenous physicians are transforming the ways that medicine and healthcare are practised. The vision of the Indigenous Physicians Association of Canada (IPAC), stated on their website, is:

> Healthy and vibrant Indigenous nations, communities, families and individuals – *supported by **Indigenous physicians and others who are contributing to** the physical, mental, emotional and spiritual well-being of our people and having a positive impact on the social determinants of Indigenous health.*
>
> *(emphasis added)*

The IPAC's clear commitment to the emotional and spiritual wellbeing of patients demonstrates how Indigenous physicians are slowly but surely transforming the very foundations of how health is addressed through and in clinical practice. IPAC offers a strongly articulated statement that health and wellness are not, for Indigenous peoples, simply about an absence of disease or a diagnosis and treatment of physical ailments. Instead, they relate to a holistic state of being in the world. Indigenous leaders and scholars are also articulating different ways of conceptualising and then practicing Indigenous health and healthcare. The Native Youth Sexual Health Network in Canada, for example, theorises links between resource extractive industries and projects on Indigenous lands on the one hand and the health of Indigenous peoples and communities on the other:

> If discussions are taking place about violations of industry on Indigenous lands, we should also be talking about the violations of people's bodies. We cannot have healthy families, communities, and nations on the land while people's bodies continue to experience violence. It is through listening to survivors of violence, asking them about solutions to land violations, and building in teachings about consent that we will have healthy nations.
>
> *(Women's Earth Alliance & Native Youth Sexual*
> *Health Network, 2016)*

New generations of Indigenous youth leaders, activists, and scholars are rightfully demanding recognition that Indigenous health is inherently and inextricably tied to the land, that Indigenous health and wellness have to be firmly rooted in the knowledge terrains of Elders, and that refusing settler-colonial narratives and norms and declaring health sovereignty and self-determination are important acts of wellness for individuals, communities, nations, and cultures (Simpson, 2014; Simpson, 2017). These kinds of transformative visions about Indigenous health and wellness are changing and altering not only how Indigenous peoples are understood within healthcare research but also, and importantly, the way Indigenous peoples can expect to be treated and engaged when seeking medical or clinical care.

For far too long, the health and wellness of Indigenous peoples around the world have been compromised by negation, most frequently by non-Indigenous people self-defining as experts in Indigenous strength and knowledge systems. This negation has been exacerbated and amplified for Indigenous peoples because (often White) settler-colonial healthcare researchers and clinicians have ignored colonial violence and ongoing states of racism and coloniality as fundamental determinants of Indigenous health. Simultaneously, they have authored the research and practised the clinical work ostensibly designed to heal, cure, fix, and address ongoing issues of health disparities and illness experienced by so many Indigenous peoples and communities.

Yet, a time of transformation in Indigenous health and wellness has arrived. Increasing critical and radical thinking and practice, often led by Indigenous leaders and activists, is making clear that Indigenous health and wellness are pressing issues that must be informed and led by Indigenous experts and Indigenous ways of knowing and being. The very languages used to consider Indigenous health and wellness are changing, as are the authors and theorists using those languages and ideas. Relatedly, the drivers of clinical practices in the realm of Indigenous health and wellness are increasingly Indigenous clinicians and healers. Finally, there is an ever-growing understanding that "health" is not simply an absence of disease at the scale of the cell or the human body. Instead, Indigenous health and wellness are intimately tied to community, land, culture, and family, all of which colonialism and colonial violence have disrupted. Restoring and celebrating Indigenous health and wellness means unsettling ongoing colonial incursions into Indigenous communities, lands, cultures, and families. Understanding Indigenous health and wellness, in other words, is complicated, shifting, changing, and difficult – the very point with which we began this chapter.

Conclusions without endings: Decolonising understandings about Indigenous health and wellness and what we can do

This chapter offered a broad, high-level overview of Indigenous health and wellness from a critical and questioning perceptive. Penned by both Indigenous and non-Indigenous scholars, it aims to invite other scholars, students, researchers, activists, and clinicians from multivariant backgrounds and walks of life to carefully and reflexively consider ways of transforming understandings about Indigenous health and wellness. Such transformations will hopefully lead to changes in professional practice. The two transformations – understanding and practice – in combination could conceivably result in a world in which Indigenous peoples' health and wellness flourish.

In a nutshell, we hope this chapter offers the theoretical, historical, and analytical foundations for people to rethink, and to practice anew in, Indigenous health and wellness. If, however, someone is left wanting concrete "how-tos" and "takeaways", we offer here a short set of suggested actions, in no particular order, that we suspect everyone can undertake in personal, scholarly, and professional contexts. We end on these in the spirit of hopefulness that centuries of colonial hegemony can be unsettled and disrupted if only we all set our minds and hearts to the task.

Our suggested actions are: Do your best to understand the history of colonialism and how it relates to Indigenous health and wellness (or barriers to wellbeing). Get actively involved in Indigenous health and wellness. Ensure your active involvement is welcome. Be humble and generous when considering Indigenous peoples, communities, and nations; extend this spirit of humility and generosity to understanding topics related to Indigenous health and wellness. Write and conduct research about Indigenous health and wellness, in partnership with Indigenous peoples and communities, and practice in these areas as if lives depend on it –

because they do. Always make time and space for Indigenous peoples' abundant expertise; it's everyone's job to seek it out and lift up that experience, and partnership is key. Strive to unsettle yourself every day: coloniality is a human-manufactured state of being that can – and must – be unmade. Speak out whenever you see or perceive anti-Indigenous racism; remember, lives depend on your action. Practice your daily tasks with an open heart and open mind: you have much to learn, especially in consultation and in reference to Indigenous knowledges and ways of being. Be self-reflective. Have empathy but never patronise. Celebrate strengths. Acknowledge diversity. Know everything is changing, all the time. Be committed to always doing your best. Be humbly critical and kindly inquisitive.

References

Allan, B., & Smylie, J. (2015). *First peoples, second class treatment: The role of racism in the health and well-being of Indigenous peoples in Canada.* Discussion Paper, Wellesley Institute. Available: http://www.wellesleyinsti tute.com/wp-content/uploads/2015/02/Summary-First-Peoples-Second-Class-Treatment-Final.pdf

Anderson, K., & Taylor, A. (2005). Exclusionary politics and the question of national belonging: Australian ethnicities in "multiscalar" focus. *Ethnicities, 5*(4), 460–485.

Anderson, T. (2019). Results from the 2016 census: Housing, income and residential dissimilarity among Indigenous people in Canadian cities. *Insights on Canadian Society,* 10 Dec. Ottawa, ON: Statistics Canada.

Australian Bureau of Statistics. (2016). Census of population and housing: Characteristics of Aboriginal and Torres strait islander Australians. https://www.abs.gov.au/statistics/people/aboriginal-and-torres -strait-islander-peoples/census-population-and-housing-characteristics-aboriginal-and-torres-strait-isl ander-australians/latest-release

Beniuk, J. (2016). All my relations: Reclaiming the stories of our Indigenous grandmothers. *Atlantis: Critical Studies in Gender, Culture & Social Justice, 37*(2), 161–172.

Bjerregaard, P., Kue Young, T., Dewailly, E., & Ebbesson, S. O. (2004). Indigenous health in the Arctic: An overview of the circumpolar Inuit population. *Scandinavian Journal of Public Health, 32*(5), 390–395.

Braveman, P., & Gottlieb, L. (2014). The social determinants of health: It's time to consider the causes of the causes. *Public Health Reports, 129*(Suppl. 2), 19–31. doi:10.1177%2F00333549141291S206.

Came, H., Gifford, H., & Wilson, D. (2019). Indigenous public health: Nothing about us without us! *Public Health, 176,* 2–3.

Campinha-Bacote, J. (2002). The process of cultural competence in the delivery of healthcare services: A model of care. *Journal of Transcultural Nursing, 13*(3), 181–184.

Canadian Institutes of Health Research, Natural Sciences and Engineering Research Council of Canada, and Social Sciences and Humanities Research Council. (2018). *Tri-council policy statement: Ethical conduct for research involving humans,* Chapter 9: *Research involving the first nations, Inuit and Métis peoples of Canada. Panel on research ethics.* Retrieved from http://www.pre.ethics.gc.ca/eng/tcps2-eptc2_chapter9-chapitr e9.html

Chandler, M. J., & Lalonde, C. (1998). Cultural continuity as a hedge against suicide in Canada's First Nations. *Transcultural Psychiatry, 35*(2), 191–219.

Coulthard, G. S. (2014). *Red skin, white masks: Rejecting the colonial politics of recognition.* Minneapolis, MN: University of Minnesota Press.

Daigle, M. (2016). Awawanenitakik: The spatial politics of recognition and relational geographies of Indigenous self-determination. *The Canadian Geographer/Le Géographe Canadien, 60*(2), 259–269. doi:10.1111/cag.12260

De Leeuw, S., Greenwood, M., & Cameron, E. (2010). Deviant constructions: How governments preserve colonial narratives of addictions and poor mental health to intervene into the lives of Indigenous children and families in Canada. *International Journal of Mental Health and Addiction, 8*(2), 282–295.

De Leeuw, S., & Hunt, S. (2018). Unsettling decolonizing geographies. *Geography Compass, 12*(7), e12376.

Dolezal, L., & Lyons, B. (2017). Health-related shame: An effective determinant of health? *Medical Humanities, 43,* 257–263. doi:10.1136/medium-2017-011186

Ermine, W., Sinclair, R., & Jeffery, B. (2004). *The ethics of research involving Indigenous peoples: Report of the Indigenous peoples' health research centre to the Interagency Advisory Panel on research ethics.* Saskatoon: Indigenous Peoples' Health Research Centre. http://iphrc.ca/pub/documents/ethics_review:iphrc.pdf.

Fadiman, A. (1999). *The spirit catches you and you fall down.* New York: Noonday.

Farrales, M. (2019). Repurposing beauty pageants: The colonial geographies of Filipina pageants in Canada. *Environment and Planning D: Society and Space, 37*(1), 46–64.

Greenwood, M., De Leeuw, S., Lindsay, N. M., & Reading, C. (Eds.). (2015). *Determinants of indigenous peoples' health in Canada: Beyond the social.* Toronto: Canadian Scholars' Press.

Hunt, S. (2014). Ontologies of indigeneity: The politics of embodying a concept. *Cultural Geographies, 21*(1), 27–32. doi:10.1177/1474474013500226

Isaacson, M. (2014). Clarifying concepts: Cultural humility or competency. *Journal of Professional Nursing, 30*(3), 251–258.

Kobayashi, A., & De Leeuw, S. (2010). Colonialism and the tensioned landscapes of Indigeneity. In S. Smith (Ed.), *The Sage handbook of social geographies* (pp. 118–138). London: SAGE.

Lawrence, J. (2000). The Indian Health Service and the sterilization of Native American women. *American Indian Quarterly, 24*(3), 400–419.

Li, T. M. (2007). *The will to improve: Governmentality, development, and the practice of politics.* Duke University Press.

Marmot, M. (2015). The health gap: The challenge of an unequal world. *The Lancet, 386*(10011), 2442–2444.

Marmot, M., & Bell, R. (2012). Fair society, healthy lives. *Public health, 126*(Supplement 1), S4–S10.

Million, D. (2013). *Therapeutic nations: Healing in an age of Indigenous human rights.* University of Arizona Press.

Monchalin, R., Smylie, J., & Nowgesic, E. (2020). "I guess I shouldn't come back here": Racism and discrimination as a barrier to accessing health and social services for urban Métis women in Toronto, Canada. *Journal of Racial and Ethnic Health Disparities, 7*, 251–261.

Moreton-Robinson, A. (2015). *The White possessive: Property, power, and Indigenous sovereignty.* Minneapolis, MN: University of Minnesota Press.

Morton Ninomiya, M.E., & Pollock, N.J. (2017). Reconciling community-based Indigenous research and academic practices: Knowing principles is not always enough. *Social Science & Medicine, 172*, 28–36.

National Inquiry into Missing and Murdered Indigenous Women and Girls. (2019). *Reclaiming power and place: The final report of the national Inquiry into missing and murdered Indigenous women and girls, Volume 1a.* Retrieved from https://login.proxy.bib.uottawa.ca/login?url=http://www.deslibris.ca/ID/10100806

Papps, E., & Ramsden, I. (1996). Cultural safety in nursing: The New Zealand experience. *International Journal of Quality in Health Care, 8*, 491–497. doi: 10.1093/intqhc/8.5.491

Reading, C. L., & Wien, F. (2009). *Health inequalities and the social determinants of Aboriginal peoples' health.* Prince George, BC: National Collaborating Centre for Aboriginal Health.

Simpson, A. (2014). *Mohawk interruptus: Political life across the borders of settler states.* Duke University Press.

Simpson, L. B. (2017). *As we have always done: Indigenous freedom through radical resistance.* Minneapolis, MN: University of Minnesota Press.

Smith, L. T. (2013). *Decolonizing methodologies: Research and indigenous peoples.* Zed Books.

Stats NZ. (2019). *New Zealand as a village of 100 people: Our population.* Wellington, NZ: Author. https://www.stats.govt.nz/infographics/new-zealand-as-a-village-of-100-people-2018-census-data

Truth and Reconciliation Commission of Canada. (2015). *Honouring the truth, reconciling for the future: Summary of the final report of the Truth and Reconciliation Commission of Canada.* Retrieved from http://epe.lac-bac.gc.ca/100/201/301/weekly_acquisition_lists/2015/w15-24-F-E.html/collections/collection_2015/trc/IR4-7-2015-eng.pdf

Tuck, E., & Yang, K. W. (2012). Decolonization is not a metaphor. *Decolonization: Indigeneity, Education & Society, 1*(1), 1–40.

United Nations. (2007). United Nations declaration on the rights of Indigenous peoples. *GA Res. 61/295,* 13 Sept. Retrieved from https://www.un.org/development/desa/indigenouspeoples/wp-content/uploads/sites/19/2018/11/UNDRIP_E_web.pdf

Walia, H. (2013). *Undoing border imperialism.* AK Press.

Women's Earth Alliance & Native Youth Sexual Health Network. (2016). *Violence on the land, violence on our bodies: Building an Indigenous response to environmental violence.* Retrieved from http://landbodydefense.org/uploads/files/VLVBReportToolkit2016.pdf

17

DISABILITY, TECHNOLOGY, AND HEALTH

Dan Goodley, Rebecca Lawthom, and Katherine Runswick-Cole

Introduction

This chapter situates disability in a complex web of social, technical, and cultural networks. We find this writing slotted into a section of this book entitled *life contexts*. We appreciate the editors' choice of disability being given a *context* (one that should be beyond the body and mind, reaching out to wider social, cultural, and economic factors that influence how disability emerges in the world) and associating disability with life (a welcome antidote to the usual tendency to equate disability with literal and social death). And we want to build on this appreciation by considering some critical issues in health and illness as they relate to disabled people and their wider engagements with a rapidly changing, increasingly chaotic, and toxic world. The starting point in thinking together is clear: the life chances, health, and wellbeing of all human beings are under threat in these uncertain economic times entangled with political moments of post-welfare, post-austerity, and a global pandemic. And these threats are acutely felt by disabled people. We use an expansive definition of disability to represent people with physical, sensory, and cognitive impairments as well as those with mental health issues. And we approach the very concept of health from a salutogenic stance; the conviction being that our affects, feelings, embodiment, ills, wellbeing, state of mind, physiology, psychology, epistemology, ontology, and subjectivity are knotted up with our personal, relational, social, cultural, economic, and political realities. Address these realities and, we would argue, one can address health and wellbeing. We will develop the argument that an analysis of the intersections of disability, health, and illness must adequately contextualise the lives of disabled people and sit with these intersections to offer emancipatory responses. Thus, with these ambitions in mind, the chapter unpacks two critical issues impacting on the health of disabled people; the demands of Industry 4.0 (late capitalism and technologically advanced economies) and the material conditions of disablism (which describes the social, economic, and cultural exclusion of disabled people). We then consider three potentially affirmative responses (assistive technologies, collaborative robotics, and DIY makerspaces). We conclude with an appeal to the development of a critical posthumanites that puts disabled people at its centre.

Contextualising the health and illness of disabled people

The dominant hegemony, at least in the UK context from which this is written, understands disability as an individual pathology, a failing of mind or body, a medical, individual, or psychological problem requiring treatment, rehabilitation, or cure. A counter-hegemonic move is permitted through the interventions of critical disability studies (e.g. Campbell, 2009; Meekosha & Shuttleworth, 2009; Shildrick, 2012; Mallett & Runswick-Cole, 2014; Goodley, 2014, 2016). This trans-disciplinary community of activism, scholarship, and art, demands a de-individualisation of disability. Traditional perspectives on disability tend to focus on individualistic preoccupations, including studies of co-morbidity (connecting the individualised troubles of impairment with other health conditions), probings of the embodied effects of the impairment (based on the assumption that the presence of impairment inevitably creates illness and incapacity) and fixations on the subjective and personal impacts of living a disabled life (automatically assumed to be a limited form of personhood). Critical disability studies does something radically different. It demands us to consider the ways in which social, cultural, and economic conditions have enormous causal impacts on the health and wellbeing of disabled people. Critical disability studies is an approach – or perhaps more fairly a collection of approaches – in touch with the critical impulse of this text. This handbook, and this chapter, have a connected ambition relating to the politicisation of health and illness. So, let us survey the socio-political terrain with a specific focus on the place of disabled people.

The demands of Industry 4.0

The health and illness of disabled people needs to be understood in direct relationship to disablism and the exacting demands of advanced capitalism framed in terms of Industry 4.0 (Schwab, 2016); an historical period of advanced capitalism marked by rolled back government, rampant individualisation, and national isolationism where nation-states and their social policies demand their citizens to be highly skilled and able in body and mind (Goodley, 2014; Mitchell & Snyder, 2015). These times create opportunities to augment human abilities across a range of domains through the use of robotics, artificial intelligence, digitalisation, the Internet of Things, and automation. In times of rapid scientific, cultural, and economic change, enhancing and governing human ability have become key concerns of nation-states as they respond to the volatile demands of the knowledge economy (Vercellone, 2007). One might argue that we have entered an era of cognitive capitalism where "peoples' competences, mediated by technological progress, are a deciding factor in a nation's wealth" (Rindermann & Thompson, 2011, p. 754). The importance of an individual's abilities takes on greater significance as governments reduce welfare spending and nations become more isolated and insular. Technology is often held up as *the* route towards human enhancement. While global citizens are increasingly expected to be self-sufficient and entrepreneurial then technologies are rolled in as the means to boost the productivity of these citizens. Being able is not simply something to desire; it is a necessity if one is to survive and thrive in the world (Goodley, 2020). Industry 4.0 places further demands on citizens. While opportunities are offered for raising human capacities through the input of technological and digital advances (Bostrom & Sandberg, 2009), questions are raised about those who benefit from these developments and those who are side-lined. The "Me Generation" of the 1970s (Wolfe, 1976) and the "Transhuman Generation" of the noughties (Fukuyama, 2004) were distinct historical epochs that affirmed an individualistic trope of the human being thriving or failing in an increasingly competitive capitalist system of labour and consumption (Bradbury & Robert-Holmes, 2017). Such ideas favoured some sections of the population and devalued others.

Indeed, in the contemporary geopolitical moment, Brexit, Trump, and the rise of alt-right nationalism interpolate citizens into cultural imaginaries associated with autonomy and self-governance (Goodley & Lawthom, 2019). This retrenchment back to a celebration of individualism occurs precisely at the same time as powerful new technological interventions in biology, brain, and behaviour reinvent what it means to be human (Hogle, 2005; Clark, 2007). Examples include pharmacologies and physical devices to improve physical and cognitive abilities (Coveney, Willams, & Gabe, 2011; Gimlin, 2013) and an amalgamation of neuroscientific, epigenetic, and biotechnologies focused on enhancing human performance (Latour, 1988; Shonkoff & Phillips, 2000; Carey, 2011; Meloni & Testa, 2014). The centrality of these scientific developments in everyday life have created new ways of understanding what it means to be human, ranging from posthuman (Fukuyama, 2002; Braidotti, 2019) to cyborg identities (Haraway, 1991). Being technologically enhanced might in some ways be deemed the new normal (Verlager, 2004; Bostrom, 2005; Rose, 2007; Wolbring, 2008; Persson & Savulescu, 2012). Nation-states have, understandably, embraced these new technological possibilities, especially around productivity, knowledge exchange, research and innovations. For example, the United Kingdom's Research and Innovation's (2018) mission is "to push the frontiers of human knowledge … to become enriched, healthier, more resilient and sustainable". These ambitions are laudable but also based upon a technologically souped-up version of human knowledge exchange. As the UK government's Industrial Strategy outlines: the aim is to make industry and public services more productive and "go beyond human limits" through the use of such advanced technologies (Innovate UK and BEIS, 2017). The emphasis on the use of technologies and their impact on human development and wellbeing have been rolled out in government research and innovation priorities such as mental health and wellbeing, education, and work (DoH, 2018; DoE, 2018; UKRI, 2018).

We need to recognise that human progression and technological augmentation are far from being benign practices. Global digital divides exist between the rich and the poor, those living in the Global North and Global South and between disabled and non-disabled people (MacDonald & Clayton, 2013; Duplage, 2017). For the critical disability studies scholars, Mitchell and Snyder (2015), the optimism of a new technological age risks collapsing into a melancholy for disabled people, as they find themselves left behind by socio-technical practices that privilege the non-disabled. The evidence is clear: disabled people have been historically excluded from employment opportunities associated with new technologies (Roulstone, 1998; Goggin & Newell, 2003, 2007; Goggin, 2018). Further, new technologies of human augmentation tend to be gendered and racialised in ways that benefit those already successfully engaging in labour and consumption (namely, white, non-disabled, male citizens). Disabled people are often marginalised consumers and conspicuously absent from places of work. The realities of this exclusion is readily associated with ontological experiences of marginalisation, and this can be experienced as lowered mental health and wellbeing. Industry 4.0 is demanding physically and cognitively, especially for those who live on the edges of our societies.

The material conditions of disablism

Just as ability has become a central plank of contemporary notions of human and social worth, so disability has become equally ubiquitous, modified, and recalibrated. The WHO and World Bank (2011) recognised over one billion disabled people in the world, making disabled people the world's biggest minority group. More and more human beings are being diagnosed with disability categories. We live in a contradictory contemporary moment. Human ability is centralised as the attribute through which individual and societal progress occurs. Technologies are drawn in as the means by which human abilities can be enhanced. Yet, at the very same time disability has never been so conspicuous. Disabled people consistently score lower on measures of health and wellbeing, educational achievement, community participation, and economic performance than their non-disabled peers (World Bank/WHO, 2011). The lowering of expenditure in healthcare and social care – often as a consequence of austerity – has created a substantial mortality gap between disabled and non-disabled people (Watkins et al., 2018). The Equality and Human Rights Commission (2018) found that, of the 14 million disabled people in Britain, many live in poverty; endure poor health conditions; lack access to suitable housing and are excluded from education, communities, and work. The critical issues of health and illness for disabled people relate to their systemic exclusion from mainstream society – or what Thomas (2007) defines as disablism, the material oppression of disabled people that potentially leads to a host of negative psycho-emotional impacts. The shift from Disability Living Allowance to the Personal Independence Payment; the reduction of Employment and Support Allowance and the introduction of the "Bedroom tax" are all high profile examples of changes to disability benefits and social policies that have had devastating impacts on the everyday lives of disabled people. Disabled people's lives are routinely devalued across the world (WHO, 2011). The interplay of disability, health, and illness must be considered in association with this awareness of systemic disablism. It is impossible to separate disability or health from socio-political considerations. Many health inequities experienced by disabled people are caused by conditions of exclusion and oppression that are simply not experienced by non-disabled people.

Critical disability studies

Critical disability studies start with a disability but never end with it (Goodley, 2013). By this, we mean that while disability is the driving subject of our analysis we soon find that we connect with a host of other social concerns. As this contributors to this volume consistently demonstrate health, illness, and wellbeing can never be isolated from their wider social, cultural, and economic contexts. Disability too is a deeply social phenomenon: constituted in the relationships between humans and non-humans, defined by formal, national, and supranational discourses and experienced in embodied and psychological ways by those with and without impairments. A critical disability studies approach seeks to explore two key processes: how disability is constituted in the world and the difference that disability makes in the world. We want to explore, then, how disability is manufactured in a highly technologically mediated society such as ours precisely at the same time as we want to understand what disability does to this society. Disability is not a passive object or creation of society. Disability is a dynamic entity that changes society by its very presence.

Technological responses to the health and illness of disabled people

The key question – and perhaps the more complex question – relates to how we should respond to the conditions of inequity experienced by disabled people. In this section, we want to tease out three socio-technical affirmative responses placing technologies in the foreground of consideration. We do so fully cognizant that these responses are not without problems or controversy. We write not as technophiles but as critical disability studies researchers acknowledging the centrality, meaning, and influence of technology in the lives of disabled people. And we seek to consider what these technological responses give and take away. Our ambitions are to explore the technological potential in affirming the health and wellbeing of disabled people in relational ways through these interventions. We explore below three technologies below: assistive technologies, robotics and automation and DIY makerspaces. These are chosen because of their close association with practices that seek to improve the health and wellbeing of disabled people. While some of these technologies are associated with traditional models of rehabilitative science, others have the potential to draw in disabled people as the designers of technology. Through the discussion we are interested in the relative weight that is given to the contributions of disabled people and the possible implications this might have in improving their lives in times of Industry 4.0.

Assistive technologies

Numerous disabled people's health and wellbeing are tied to their daily use of Augmentative and Alternative Communication (AAC), Environmental Controls (EC), and Dignity Assistive Technologies (DAT). There is a huge body of literature that documents the many positive impacts of these technologies on disabled people (O'Keefe et al., 2007; Baxter et al., 2012; Hynan et al., 2015; Goggin, 2018; Ellis, 2018). The influence includes the use of control home devices (including TVs, lights, telephones, doors, curtains, and windows) – which we now understand as smart homes – through to practices that are worked via speech and movement and communication in absolute and digital communities. For many years disabled people have excelled in their use of new technologies. However, because the provision and design of these technologies have occurred in specialist, assistive, and rehabilitative contexts, many of the revolutionary impacts of this tech has remained outside of the mainstream conscience. Indeed, as Cowan et al. (2015) note, while clinical engineers and medical technologists have worked hard to join up technological platforms, there is still often a lack of fit between specialist assistive and mainstream technologies (Judge, 2018). There is also a conceptual gap in the communication chain between those living and using assistive technologies (such as disabled people) and those advocates of technological human enhancement. Hence, while a disabled person might be a proficient users of AAC, their experiences of being augmented by this technology are rarely included in more mainstream (and controversial) debates associated with human enhancement, perfection, and utopian future human-technology imaginaries (Grüber & Rehmann-Sutter, 2014). As many accessibility features become normalised in the design of products by big tech companies such as Google and Apple, disabled consumers, and users are clearly in the minds of many manufacturers. The extent to which disabled users of assistive and inclusive technologies are brought into wider debates about human enhancement remains questionable. Furthermore, the discourse that underpins human augmentation is often framed in deeply exclusionary ways (Goodley, 2014). Transhumanist organisations such as Humanity+ (https://humanityplus.org/) laud the influence of technological interventions as forms of augmentation that move beyond the human, excitedly citing examples that cure disability and impairment. It is absolutely essential, then, in these times of Industry 4.0 that disabled people are brought front and centre into any discussions of technological enablement. This means reminding us all that technologies can offer essential pathways to improving health and wellbeing in mundane, everyday contexts, including bathing, eating, and communicating. And while it is tempting to be seduced by the futuristic possibilities of technological improvement we need to recognise that many disabled people across the globe live in conditions of poverty where they cannot access AAC (Light & McNaughton, 2015), while these very technologies do not even some of the most basic health needs of their users (Light et al., 2019). One key question relating to health, wellbeing, and technology is: to what extent do developments in assistive and mainstream technologies improve the independent living skills of disabled people? And by independence we are not asserting an individualist nor the traditionally psychological concept of autonomy. Instead, we are interested in the potential of new technologies to improve the daily lives of disabled people, enhance their support mechanisms and augment their interdependencies with human and non-human others.

Robotics and automation

The critical disability studies literature has exposed the deeply disablist premise that paid work is *the* signifier of human value (Bates et al., 2017). Too often, the lives and un/paid labours of disabled people have been ignored in mainstream debates (Goodley, 2016). The global COVID-19 pandemic follows close on the heels of the ideologically-driven practices of austerity politics. As a result, we are all experiencing precarity in relation to the labour market (Puar, 2012). And yet, while the white middle classes are experiencing a deepening sense of precarity as a new ontology, disabled people have a long history of living with this precarity. Despite the promise of paid work having been held up as the object of desire by successive governments, paid employment remains stubbornly out of reach for many disabled people. Storied as a "wicked" policy problem, the disability employment gap persists; currently, the UK employment rate for disabled people in the UK is 53.2% compared to 81.8% for non-disabled people (Office for National Statistics, 2019.) This economic backdrop needs to be kept in mind when we consider the positive correlation between positive health and experiences of work. New technologies pose a particular challenge to this health-work relationship. NESTA (2017) has predicted that two-thirds of children of primary school age now will work in jobs that do not currently exist. This prediction reveals the extraordinary impacts of Industry 4.0 on human skills and abilities (Deloitte, 2016; Goldin & Katz, 2009). Across various sectors of industry, robotic, and digital technologies are transforming the practice and meaning of work (Royal Society, 2017; Waterstone, 2018). We know that automation and labour are understood to complement one another. AI, robotics, and automated practices have the potential to increase human productivity, while the emergence of collaborative robotics (or cobots) have been shown to maximise the abilities of both humans and machines (Autor, 2015; Law & Maple, 2016). However, the skill-sets demanded by these rapidly developing industries are often absent in certain sectors of the working-age population (Waterstone, 2018). Class, geographical location, age, and disability are just some of the human factors that interact with automation in the workplace. We know that the participation and exclusion of disabled people in these technological developments remains under-researched and in need of further consideration. Because disabled people already occupy peripheral places on the edges of the workforce there is a real danger that they are not included in deliberations about policies, practices, and provision of automation and robotics. Yet again, there is a real danger that disabled people are left behind in contemporary debates about health, wellbeing, and technology. The technologisation of the workforce creates a double-edged sword. On one side there is potential: the opening up of labour practices to different kinds of bodies and abilities as a consequence of the empowering impacts of automation. On the other side is danger: the increased exclusion of disabled people from a labour force already grappling with the need for increased knowledge and technical skills. A critical disability studies perspective would place disability in the foreground of any debate about work and automation.

DIY makerspaces

There has been a persistent tendency to conceptualise disabled people as the end-users of new technologies (if they are considered at all). In terms of exploring the links between health and technology, it is crucial that we reposition disabled people as co-designers and makers of technology. Barba (2015) argues for the democratisation of technological design, and from a critical disability studies perspective we agree with this requirement to centralise disabled people as active participants in the development of technological design. We are witnessing a global renaissance in democratic making processes in the makerspace movement. Nascimento and Pólvora (2018, p. 930) define makerspaces as the coming together of:

> professional and amateur inventors, crafters, hackers, entrepreneurs, artists, scientists, engineers, designers, teachers, or activists, from nearly all ages and backgrounds, are currently not only thinking about how to transform their material environments, but also taking their own steps in that direction by learning how and choosing to modify, assemble, create, disassemble, recreate, duplicate, and sharing objects and systems through open and collaborative networks from their homes, garages, schools, businesses, museums, libraries, makerspaces, hackerspaces, Fab Labs, and other emerging innovation-oriented spaces.

Dougherty (2012) conceptualises as open and optimistic spaces for democratic design (Blikstein, 2013; Rose, 2014). And yet, as Brady et al. (2014) have found, many makerspaces are inaccessible to disabled people. Nevertheless, the potential of opening up these spaces in accessible ways is huge as is evident in recent work at the University of Sheffield developed in relation to the Hackcessible workshops https://www.hackcessible.org/about/. As the website explains:

> Sheffield is a city of makers, with a tremendous history of technology talent and ingenuity. We are a group of students and staff based at The University of Sheffield with a deep passion for developing technology for good and a firm belief that science, engineering and design should be used to make the world a better place for all. Inspired by the likes of the AT-Hack at MIT, one of the first disability-related hackathons, and the popular BBC programme "The Big Life Fix", we are planning our first disability-focused make-a-thon
>
> **What is Hackcessible?** Hackcessible is a make-a-thon that brings together engineers, designers, computer scientists, students and others to collaborate with individuals with disabilities and create workable products that support their needs.
>
> **What makes us different?** We want to put end-users at the heart of the make-a-thon and invite them to lead the project as "Co-designers" to ensure we design products that are useful and effective in solving everyday challenges.
>
> **Why take part?**
> You are guaranteed to learn and apply new skills.
>
> A golden opportunity to build a great network and make new friends.
> Gain experience in turning concepts into actions.
> You'll have built something by the end of the weekend! It may not be completely finished, but you should have an early prototype solution to present.
> Make a difference and change lives.
> You could get external recognition – be part of something that may be considered for commercialisation.
> Win prizes.
> Have fun!

This attempt to democratise makerspace culture seeks to put disabled people at the centre of product design, research, and innovation. Hackcessible demonstrates that through inclusive social, cultural, technological, and material practices, the capacities of disabled people can be strengthened

(Roulstone, 1998). There has recently been an upsurge of interest in the place of disabled people in the design and development of digital practice (Jaeger, 2010; Lewthwaite, 2014; Goggin & Newell, 2003, 2007) and universal and inclusive design (Pullin, 2011; Boys, 2014; Hamraie, 2017). The potential for engaging with health through technological design is incredibly important not least in further enhancing the interdependent relationships of disabled people (Reindall, 1999). In many ways one might read inclusive makerspaces as an extension of the already extended interrelations that disabled people have with other people, non-humans, and machines. Disability disrupts the very idea of human independence through notions of distributed competence (Booth & Booth, 1998), the idea that our cognitive, emotional, and health competences merge through our relationships with other humans and non-humans. Disability provides an opportunity to collectivise the very notions of health and wellbeing. This move from individualistic understandings of wellbeing to collectivist models of health resonate with recent literatures associated with relational ethics (Shakespeare, 2000), crip communities (Kafer, 2013; Mitchell & Syner, 2018), feminist ethics of care (Kittay, 2002), digital connectivity (Trevisan, 2017), and human–animal-machine assemblages (Shildrick, 2009; Feely, 2016). Each of these approaches, in their own specific way, consider the possibilities for human sustainability and growth that are found in our entanglements with others. And the makerspace is but another place through which to probe the possibilities of interdependence. In considering health, disability, and technology we are permitted to explore the ways in which human capacities are embedded in our technological entanglements, and it is possible to do so without lapsing into technological determinism and normalisation (Morse, 2005, 2006). Disabled people are the inventors, makers, designers, and end-users of new technologies as revealed in emancipatory, participatory, and co-production approaches to disability research (Roulstone, 2016; Goggin, 2018).

Conclusion – Towards a critical posthumanities

In this chapter we have explored health and wellbeing in the lives of disabled people through reference to a number of technological possibilities. One helpful way of theorising the rich interconnections of technology and humanity is found in posthuman philosophy (Renold & Ivinson, 2014; Braidotti, 2019, 2018; Braidotti & Regan, 2017; Bozalek, 2018; Braidotti & Hlavajova, 2018). Posthuman approaches emphasise the ways in which personhood, psychology, health, and wellbeing are mediated through the blurring of the wetware of bodies with the hardware of machines. The posthuman citizen is an amalgamation of biology, technology, and culture where some people are given a central place and others a more peripheral position. A posthuman condition demands, understandably, a posthuman theoretical arena. As we have traced through our discussion of disability, health, work, industry, technology then this leaves us with a number of questions – three of which we present here:

1. How might we conceive of health, illness and disability in a manner that keeps us firmly attached to political, economic and cultural registers?
2. To what extent can we converse about health, illness and disability in ways that do not individualise, pathologise, nor disconnect these phenomena?
3. In what ways might we foreground disability as a central affirmative phenomenon through which to think through health, illness and society?

These questions merge neatly into a form of study that Braidotti (2018) defines as the critical posthumanities: an interdisciplinary space that identifies and addresses disparities by being open to minoritarian knowledge. This space, following Muñoz (2005), brings together analyses at the intersections of black, feminist, indigenous, queer, trans, disabled, and displaced studies (see also Baynton, 2001; Wynter, 2003). This is a rich community of politicised scholars that are committed to responding to the dizzying implications of the political turbulence in which we live. Tapping into inequities of the posthuman epoch is urgently required. And disability offers one productive and reproductive response.

References

Autor, D. (2015). Why are there still so many jobs? The history and future of workplace automation. *Journal of Economic Perspectives, 29*(3), 3–30.

Barba, E. (2015). Cultural change in the twenty-first century shop class. *Design Issues, 31*(4), 79–90.

Bates, K., Goodley, D., & Runswick-Cole, K. (2017). Precarious lives and resistant possibilities: The labour of people with learning disabilities in times of austerity. *Disability & Society, 32*(2), 160–175.

Baxter, S., Enderby, P., Evans, P., & Judge, S. (2012). Interventions using high-technology communication devices: A state of the art review. *Folia Phoniatr Logop, 64*, 137–144. doi: 10.1159/000338250.

Baynton, D. (2001). Disability and the justification of inequality in American history. In P. Longmore & L. Umansky (Eds.), *The new disability history: American perspectives* (pp. 33–57). New York: New York University Press.

Blikstein, P. (2013). Digital fabrication and "making" in education: The democratization of invention. In J. Walter-Herrmann & C. Büching (Eds.), *FabLab: Of machines, makers and inventors* (pp. 203–222). Bielefeld: Transcript Publishers.

Booth, T., & Booth, W. (1998). *Parenting under pressure.* Buckingham: Open University Press.

Bostrom, N. (2005). A history of transhumanist thought. *Journal of Evolution and Technology, 14*(1), 1–30.

Bostrom, N., & Sandberg, A. (2009). Cognitive enhancement: Methods, ethics, regulatory challenges. *Science and Engineering Ethics, 15*(3), 311–341.

Bradbury, A., & Roberts-Holmes, G. (2017). *Grouping in the early years and key stage: A necessary evil?* Final report. London: National Education Union.

Brady, T. Salas, C. Nuriddin, A. Rodgers, W & Subramaniam, M. (2014). MakeAbility: Creating Accessible Makerspace Events in a Public Library. *Public Library Quarterly, 33*(4), 330–347.

Braidotti, R. (2013). *The posthuman.* London: Polity.

Braidotti, R. (2019). A theoretical framework for the critical posthumanities. *Theory, Culture & Society, 36*(6), 31–61.

Braidotti, E., & Hlavajova, M. (Eds). (2018). *Posthuman glossary.* London: Bloomsbury.

Braidotti, R., & Regan, L. (2017). Our times are always out of joint: Feminist relational ethics in and of the world today: an interview with Rosi Braidotti. *Women: A Cultural Review, 28*(3), 171–192.

Bozalek, V., Braidotti, R., Zembylas, M., & Shefer, T. (Eds). (2018). *Socially just pedagogies posthumanist, feminist and materialist perspectives in higher education.* London: Bloomsbury.

Campbell, F. K. (2009). *Contours of ableism: The production of disability and abledness.* Basingstoke: Palgrave Macmillan.

Carey, N. (2011). *The epigenetics revolution: How modern biology is rewriting our understanding of genetics, disease and inheritance.* London: Icon Books.

Clark, A. (2007). Reinventing ourselves: The plasticity of embodiment, sensing, and mind. *Journal of Medicine and Philosophy, 32*(3), 263–282.

Coveney, C. M., Williams, S. J., & Gabe. J. (2011). The sociology of cognitive enhancement: Medicalisation and beyond. *Health Sociology Review, 20*(4), 378–390.

Cowan, D., Cudd, P., & Judge, S. (2015). Over a decade of developing the assistive technology field in the UK. *Technology and Disability, 27*, 1–3.

Deloitte. (2016). Talent for survival | Essential skills for humans working in the machine – advances in technology age. Accessed on 14 November 2018: https://www2.deloitte.com/content/dam/Deloitte/uk/Documents/Growth/deloitte-uk-talent-for-survival-report.pdf

Department for Education. (2018). *Areas of research interest: May 2018.* London: Crown Copyright.

Department for Health. (2018). *Areas of research interest: May 2018.* London: Crown Copyright.

Dougherty, D. (2012). The maker movement. *Innovations, 7*(3), 11–14.

Duplaga, M. (2017). Digital divide among people with disabilities: Analysis of data from a nationwide study for determinants of Internet use and activities performed online. *PLoS ONE, 12*(6). doi: 10.1371/journal.pone.0179825

Ellis, K. (2018). A media manifesto. In K. Ellis, R. Garland-Thomson, M. Kent, & R. Robertson (Eds.), *Manifestos for the future of critical disability studies* (pp. 92–107). London: Routledge.

Equality and Human Rights Commission. (2018). Is Britain fairer? The state of equality and human rights in 2018. Accessed on 1 December 2018: https://www.equalityhumanrights.com/en/britain-fairer/b ritain-fairer-2018-supporting-data

Feely, M. (2016). Disability studies after the ontological turn: A return to the material world and material bodies without a return to essentialism. *Disability & Society, 31*(7), 863–883.

Fukuyama, F. (2002). *Our posthuman future: Consequences of the biotechnology revolution.* London: Profile.

Fukuyama, F. (2004). Transhumanism. *Foreign Policy, 144*(Sep–Oct), 42–43.

Gimlin, D. L. (2013). Too good to be real: The obviously augmented breast in women's narratives of cosmetic surgery. *Gender and Society, 27*, 913–934.

Googin, G. (2018). Technology and social futures. In K. Ellis, R. Garland-Thomson, M. Kent, & R. Robertson (Eds.), *Manifestos for the future of critical disability studies* (pp. 79–90). London: Routledge.

Goggin, G., & Newell, C. (2003). *Digital disability: The social construction of disability in new media.* Lanham, MD: Rowman & Littlefield.

Goggin, G., & Newell, C. (2007). The business of digital disability. *The Information Society, 24*(2), 159–168.

Goldin, C., & Katz, L. F. (2009). *The race between education and technology.* Cambridge, MA: Harvard University Press.

Goodley, D. (2013). Dis/entangling critical disability studies. *Disability & Society, 28*(5), 631–644.

Goodley, D. (2014). *Dis/ability studies.* London: Routledge.

Goodley, D. (2016). *Disability studies: An interdisciplinary introduction* (2nd ed.). London: SAGE.

Goodley, D. (2020). *Disability and other human questions.* London: Emerald Publishing Limited.

Goodley, D., & Lawthom, R. (2019). Critical disability studies, Brexit and Trump: A time of neoliberal–ableism. *Rethinking History, 23*(2), 233–251.

Grüber and Rehmann-Sutter (Eds.). (2014). The human enhancement debate and disability: New bodies for a better life. Basingstoke: Palgrave Macmillan.

Hamraie, A. (2017). *Building access: Universal design and the politics of disability.* Minneapolis, MN: University of Minnesota Press.

Haraway, D. J. (1991). *Simians, cyborgs and women: The reinvention of nature.* London: FA Books.

Hogle, L. (2005). Enhancement technologies and the body. *Annual Review of Anthropology, 34*, 695–716

Hynan, A., Goldbart, A., & Murray, J. (2015). A grounded theory of Internet and social media use by young people who use augmentative and alternative communication (AAC). *Disability and Rehabilitation, 37*(17), 1559–1575.

Innovate UK and Department for Business, Energy & Industrial Strategy. (2017). Robotics and AI: Apply in the industrial strategy challenge fund. London: Crown Copyright. 13 June 2017.

Jaeger (2010). Disability and the internet. Boulder, CO: Lynne Rienner.

Judge, S. (2018). Assistive technology integration and accessibility. In L. Najafi & D. Cowan (Eds.), Handbook of electronic assistive technology. 1st Edition. Cambridge, MA: Academic Press.

Judge, S., Hawley, M., Cunningham, S., & Kirton, A. (2015). What is the potential for context aware communication aids? *Journal of Medical Engineering & Technology, 39*(7), 448–453.

Kafer, A. (2013). Feminist queer crip. Bloomington, IN: Indiana University Press.

Kittay, E. F. (2002). When caring is just and justice is caring: Justice and mental retardation. In Kittay, E. F., & Feder, E. K. (Eds.), The subject of care: Feminist perspectives on dependency. Oxford: Rowan and Littlefield Publishers.

Latour, B. (1988). Mixing humans and non-humans together: The sociology of a door-closer. *Social Problems, 35*, 298–310.

Law, J., & Maple, C. (2016). *Manufacturing robotics – The next robotic industrial Revolution.* UK-RAS Network: UK-RAS White Paper.

Lewthwaite, S. (2014). Web accessibility standards and disability: Developing critical perspectives on accessibility. *Disability and Rehabilitation, 36*(16), 1375–1383.

Light, J., & McNaughton, D. (2015). Designing AAC research and intervention to improve outcomes for individuals with complex communication needs. *Augmentative and Alternative Communication, 31*(2), 85–96.

Light, J., McNaughton, D., Beukelman, D., Koch Fager, S., Fried-Oken, M., Jakobs, T., & Jakobs, E. (2019). Challenges and opportunities in augmentative and alternative communication: Research and technology development to enhance communication and participation for individuals with complex communication needs. *Augmentative and Alternative Communication, 35*(1), 1–12.

Macdonald, S. J., & Clayton, J. (2013). Back to the future, disability and the digital divide. *Disability & Society*, *28*(5), 702–718.

Mallett, R., & Runswick-Cole, K. (2014). *Approaching disability: Critical issues and perspectives*. Abingdon: Routledge.

Meekosha, H., & Shuttleworth. R. (2009). "What's so 'critical' about critical disability studies?" *Australian Journal of Human Rights*, *15*(1), 47–75.

Meloni, M., & Testa, G. (2014). Scrutinizing the epigenetics revolution. *BioSocieties*, *9*, 431–456.

Mitchell, D. T., & Snyder, S. L. (2015). *Biopolitics of disability: Neoliberalism, able-nationalism, and peripheral embodiment*. Ann Arbor, MI: University of Michigan Press.

Moser, I. (2005). On becoming disabled and articulating differences. *Cultural Studies*, *19*(6), 667–700.

Moser, I. (2006). Disability and the promises of technology: Technology, subjectivity and embodiment within an order of the normal. *Information, Communication & Society*, *9*(3), 373–395.

Muñoz, J. E. (2005). Teaching, minoritarian knowledge, and love. *Women & Performance: A Journal of Feminist Theory*, *14*(2), 117–121.

Nascimento, S., & Pólvora, A. (2018). Maker cultures and the prospects for technological action. *Science and Engineering Ethics*, *24*, 927–946.

NESTA. (2017). *Employment in 2030: Skills, competencies and the implications for learning*. Accessed on 3 January 2020: https://www.nesta.org.uk/report/the-future-of-skills-employment-in-2030/

Office for National Statistics. (2019). *Disability and employment, UK – 2019*. Accessed on 6 May 2020: https://www.ons.gov.uk/peoplepopulationandcommunity/healthandsocialcare/disability/bulletins/disabilityandemploymentuk/2019#employment-by-disability.

O'Keefe, B. M., Kozak, N. B., & Schuller, R. (2007). Research priorities in augmentative and alternative communication as identified by people who use AAC and their facilitators. *Augmentative and Alternative Communication*, *23*, 89–96.

Persson, I., & Savulescu, J. (2012). *Unfit for the future? The need for moral enhancement*. Oxford: Oxford University Press.

Puar. (2012). Precarity talk: A virtual roundtable with Lauren Berlant. Judith Butler, Bojana Cvejic, Isabell Lorey, Jasbir Puar, and Ana Vujanovic, TDR: The Drama Review, *56*(4), 163–177.

Pullin, G. (2011). *Design meets disability*. Cambridge, MA: MIT Press.

Reindall, S. M. (1999). Independence, dependence, interdependence: Some reflections on the subject and personal autonomy. *Disability & Society*, *14*(3), 353–367.

Renold, E., & Ivinson, G. (2014). Horse-girl assemblages: Towards a posthuman cartography of girls' desire in an ex-mining valleys community, *Discourse: Studies in the Cultural Politics of Education*, *35*(3), 361–376.

Rindermann, H., & Thompson, J. (2011). Cognitive capitalism: The effect of cognitive ability on wealth, as mediated through. *Psychology Science*, *22*(6), 754–763.

Rose, M. (2014). Not your father's shop class: Bridging the academic-vocational divide. *American Educator*, *38*(3), 12–17.

Rose, N. (2007). *The politics of life itself: Biomedicine, power and subjectivity in the twenty-first century*. Oxford: Princeton University Press.

Roulstone, A. (1998). *Enabling technology: Disabled people, work, and new technology*. Buckingham: Open University Press.

Roulstone, A. (2016). *Disability and technology: International and interdisciplinary perspectives*. Basingstoke: Palgrave.

Royal Society. (2017). *After the reboot – Computing education in UK schools*. London: Royal Society. Accessed on 4 January 2018: https://royalsociety.org/~/media/policy/projects/computing-education/computing-education-report.pdf

Schwab. (2016). The Fourth Industrial Revolution. Geneva, Switzerland: World Economic Forum.

Shakespeare, T. (2000). *Help*. Birmingham: Venture Press.

Shildrick, M. (2009). *Dangerous discourses of disability, subjectivity and sexuality*. London: Palgrave Macmillan.

Shildrick, M. (2012). Critical disability studies: Rethinking the conventions for the age of postmodernity. In N. Watson, A. Roulstone, & C. Thomas (Eds.), *Routledge handbook of disability studies* (pp. 30–41). London: Routledge.

Shonkoff, J. P., & Phillips, D. (2000). *From neurons to neighborhoods: The science of early childhood development*. Washington, DC: National Academy Press.

Thomas, C. (2007). *Sociologies of disability and illness: Contested ideas in disability studies and medical sociology*. Basingstoke: Palgrave Macmillan.

Trevisan, F. (2017). *Disability rights advocacy online. Voice, empowerment and global connectivity*. London: Routledge.

UK Research and Innovation. (2018). *Strategic prospectus: Building the UKRI strategy. Insight, inspiration, impact*. Polaris House Swindon: UKRI.

Vercellone, C. (2007). From formal subsumption to general intellect: Elements for a Marxist reading of the theory of cognitive capitalism. *Historical Materialism, 15*(1), 13–36.

Verlager, A. K. (2004). *Decloaking disability: Images of disability and technology in science fiction media*. University of Massachusetts, Boston. Unpublished B.A. English Masters dissertation.

Waterstone, R. (2018). *Skills and education for robotics and AI (SERAI): A report for Sheffield robotics*. Sheffield: University of Sheffield.

Watkins, J., Wulaningsih, W., Zhou, D., Marshall, C., Sylianteng, D., Rosa, C. D., Miguel, P., Raine, V., King, R., & Maruthappu, M. (2018). Effects of health and social care spending constraints on mortality in England: A time trend analysis. *BMJ Open*, 7, e017722. doi:10.1136/ bmjopen-2017-017722

Wolbring, G. (2008). The politics of ableism. *Development, 5*(1), 252–258.

Wolfe, T. (1976). The "me" decade and the third great awakening. *New York Magazine* (August 23).

World Health Organization and The World Bank. (2011). *World report on disability*. Geneva, Switzerland: World Health Organization.

Wynter, S. (2003). Unsettling the coloniality of being/power/truth/freedom. Towards the human, after man, its overrepresentation – An argument. *The New Centennial Review, 3*(3), 257–337.

18

HEALTH AND ILLNESS AMONG OLDER PEOPLE

What has age got to do with it?

Christine Stephens

Introduction

This chapter broadly addresses the apparent conundrum involved in recognising the diverse experiences of health and ageing, while maintaining an interest in the health of all older people as an important focus for research and practice. At a population level, older people are more likely than younger adults to become ill; however, there is a great diversity of health experiences within ageing populations, and age itself is not an indication of health status. At the same time, there has been insufficient research attention paid to healthcare needs and health-related policy for older people. The chapter briefly covers illness among older people and ageism in healthcare to introduce the negative impacts of treating older people as "other", rather than as members of society with diverse healthcare needs. The recognition that our populations are ageing has further intensified the homogenising and "othering" of older people. To counteract these ageist assumptions, I include sections focusing on diversity among older people, particularly regarding health inequalities. To address the issues raised by the critiques of ageism and homogenising of older people, I introduce new frameworks for health promotion and care among older people. In conclusion, the contribution of a critical approach to recognising diversity while focusing on the needs of older people, as a group, is discussed.

Illness and ageism in healthcare

As people age, they are more likely, as a population group, to suffer more illnesses. Prince and colleagues (2015) noted that 23% of the total global experience of disease is borne by people aged 60 years and older and an increased proportion of morbidity and mortality due to chronic diseases occurs in this age group. The diseases most likely to be experienced are cardiovascular diseases, malignant neoplasms, chronic respiratory diseases, musculoskeletal diseases, and neurological and mental disorders. The most common disorders of older age (dementia, stroke, chronic obstructive pulmonary disease, and vision impairment) result in ongoing disability rather than mortality, and older people are also more likely to suffer from multiple illnesses (Prince et al., 2015).

According to Beard and Bloom (2015), improved healthcare systems are required to manage chronic illness and its consequences. Older people who become ill are more likely to have multiple, coexistent, issues (multi-morbidity), which is more likely to lead to frailty, mobility problems, and impaired cognition (Prince et al., 2015). Comprehensive and coordinated care will provide the best support for healthy functioning; however, these more holistic perspectives are not common in the treatment of older people. One of the major causes of failures to provide appropriate medical care is pervasive ageist attitudes which have been identified across many fields of treatment and care, and infiltrate all aspects of the health of older people. Broad assumptions about the relationships between age and health, and concerns about the economic effects of an ageing population, have contributed to ageist constructions of older people as globally unhealthy and a burden to society. Ageist stereotypes have also been shown to influence the treatment of older people in research, diagnosis, and clinical care. Commonly held beliefs that ill health is inevitable for all older people, that interventions are ineffective, and older people are not worth the use of healthcare resources, are widespread among health professionals and among older people themselves.

Older people have long been rendered invisible in medical and social research. They have been systematically excluded from clinical research on diseases that specifically affect older people, such as diabetes mellitus, cancer, or heart failure (Witham & McMurdo, 2007). Although cardiovascular disease is the major cause of death and disability in aged patients, older people have been generally excluded from clinical trials. This has in turn resulted in an inadequate evidence base to support the care of older patients with heart disease (Gurwitz & Goldberg, 2011). There is also evidence that older patients are poorly represented in the randomised controlled trials of medications that are frequently prescribed for older patients with chronic illnesses (Konrat et al., 2012) or insomnia (Roehrs, Verster, Koshorek, Withrow, & Roth, 2018).

Older people are also often ignored regarding health-related behaviours. Although alcohol is commonly used by older adults, the New Zealand Alcohol and Drug use Survey included only adults up to the age of 64 (Ministry of Health, 2010). This has not only excluded valuable information from the findings (such as high levels of alcohol use by some older people) (Stevenson, Stephens, Dulin, Kostick, & Alpass, 2015), but perpetuates assumptions around older people as a homogenous group with low alcohol use. Because ageing brings changes in physiological functioning, such as the ability to metabolise alcohol (Dufour & Fuller, 1995) or decreased immune functioning (Yung, 2000), the evidence from younger samples may not be appropriate for the treatment of complex interactions in older age groups, and these gaps between research and treatment needs have been generally ignored.

Treating older people as a category or group with particular characteristics, impacts directly on the treatment of their physical or mental health problems by health professionals in many hospital settings (Latimer, 1997). Safiliou-Rothschild (2009) reviewed healthcare for elders in several European countries to show that older patients are less likely to be provided with appropriate treatment. In addition to non-representation in clinical trials, older patients were discriminated against because physicians were less prepared to risk treatment, and insurers were unwilling to risk expenses. More recently, Prince et al. (2015) have cited evidence of age discrimination in the treatment of cardiovascular disease, stroke, and access to surgical procedures; fewer diagnostic procedures and evidence-based treatments are given to older people in cancer care. Illnesses that affect any age group, such as deafness, poor sight, depression, anxiety, insomnia, and various chronic illnesses among the frail and old, may not be taken seriously by health professionals, or their treatment among older people may be considered from a different perspective. Many common problems, such as alcohol abuse by older patients are overlooked by physicians because of assumptions about age-related behaviours (Berks & McCormick, 2008). Similarly, older people are often regarded as sexually inactive (Beard & Bloom, 2015) and hence excluded from screening programmes or advice around sexually transmitted diseases.

Nurse researchers have shown considerable concern about ageist attitudes among those caring for older people; ageism among health professionals in caring roles has been discussed and described in many different ways, including loss of dignity by and respect for older patients and resulting dismissal of patient concerns and symptoms by carers (Chrisler, Barney, & Palatino, 2016; Kagan & Melendez-Torres, 2015). Lothian and Philp (2001) reviewed a range of qualitative data and surveys to find many examples of older people or their carers reporting insensitive and disrespectful treatment by nursing staff and stereotypical views held by nurses. Although there has been a high level of concern over the years, a critical review of reviews of nursing and healthcare ageism (Wilson et al., 2017) concluded that the reviews provided neither sufficient information to determine the impact of ageism, nor how to address it. The diversity in the literature is a problem in itself, and the authors were only able to suggest that nurses need to be aware of ageism and its potential problematic impacts. These findings do not deny the widespread existence of and impact of ageism which leads to systematically poor care for older people, but they point to the need for more considered research efforts if changes are to be made.

Ageist stereotypes are also taken up by older people themselves and have been shown to have a negative influence on their mental and physical health. Internalised negative stereotypes lead to poor health, impaired memory, and dependency, impaired recovery from illness and decreased longevity (Chrisler et al., 2016; Nelson, 2016). At the institutional level, practices of ageism provide particular identities for older people, which have very practical consequences for physical functioning. Latimer (1999) described how health professionals in an acute hospital ward worked to assign identities and categorise older people in terms of their problems as medical or otherwise to determine their access to treatment. This identity assignment in turn affected the conduct of patients.

Latimer described the ways in which this realisation led to people "lying low" or effacing their own social identity in order to assume a valued clinical identity and access to medical care. Reed and Clarke (1999) have provided an analysis of the ways in which the construction of older people as a problem, because of physical impairment and costs to the public healthcare system, shaped the provision of nursing care through social policy and professional practice. These authors described a system that provided home support according to bureaucratic requirements, rather than older people's everyday needs such as, to stay in their life-long home or for a couple to spend the evening together. They show how these attitudes create a pathway to unnecessary and disabling institutionalisation of frail older people. Angus and Reeve (2006) describe the marginalising effects of such ageism on those who would benefit from physical assistance in very old age. They describe older people who were isolating themselves from any social or physical support owing to fear of the total loss of independence and self-hood signified by hospitalisation. Angus and Reeve note that an ageist society has produced a problem for older people who fail to age successfully and must "access punitive and fragmented service systems" (p. 143). These ageist stereotypes function to disempower older people and deprive them of basic rights in social and institutional settings such as healthcare.

Accordingly, ageism affects how individual old people are viewed by society and how they are treated in social spaces, including healthcare and support service settings, and how they see themselves. The stereotypes of ageism are part of the social world and drawn on by older people themselves to construct their identity. Ageist assumptions work to exclude older people from participation as active and respected social participants and are the reason that older people may be discriminated against, excluded, and subordinated, to the detriment of their health.

The ageing population and health

Recognition that older people are now a much greater proportion of the whole population has resulted in a greater focus on the health of older people. The third United Nations Sustainable Development Goal is good health and wellbeing for all and the achievement of this important goal must include attention to the needs of older adults (Suzman, Beard, Boerma, & Chatterji, 2015). People aged over 60 years comprise 13% of the global population and this age group is growing at about 3% per year. By 2050 the UN estimates that all regions of the world except Africa will have nearly a quarter or more of their populations aged 60 and above (United Nations, 2017). This rapidly changing demographic profile, more older people and fewer children, is due to both global improvements in health resulting in increasing longevity, and reduced fertility in many countries. However, as the world population ages, a new focus on the health needs of older people has led to public and government concern about the burden on healthcare systems and future societal healthcare costs. The recognition of these needs has resulted in alarm and a great deal of discussion about the ageing population as a burden on society.

The shifts in the shape of the population are often described in terms of the proportion of older versus younger people and increased "dependency ratios", which are calculated in terms of the proportion of older and younger people in the population. As such, understandings of these changes are described as an intergenerational burden in terms of an unsupportable explosion of medical care costs for society (Binstock, 2010; Prince et al., 2015; Yang, Norton, & Stearns, 2003). In response, older people are often portrayed as some sort of universal "other" in the media or in policy statements where images such as a "silver tsunami" or "tidal wave" of ageing people about to descend upon "us" are used (e.g. Martin, Williams, & O'Neill, 2009). Ann Robertson (1997) has critically named this the "apocalyptic demography" scenario in which the growing older population, with its ailing, retired bodies and high healthcare costs, drains the larger society and brings economic and social catastrophe.

Such apocalyptic constructions are based in medical and epidemiological literature, which is subject to growing critique. For example, in an article entitled, "Population Ageing: the time bomb that isn't?" Spijker and MacInnes (2013) highlighted the problem of focusing on chronological age to characterise a very large group of people. They suggest that an age dependency ratio merely takes a single cut point and assigns all adults to one or other side of the ratio, which is a very poor measure of the potential burden of an ageing population. They also point to alternative ways of understanding ageing and illness in general. In the public health literature, researchers discuss these alternative futures for the health of the current ageing cohort in terms of three main hypotheses: "compression of morbidity", which suggests that the onset of morbidity is delayed as life expectancy rises, so that older people become ill only at the very end of longer lives; "expansion of morbidity" maintaining that increases in life expectancy mean longer periods of late-life morbidity; and an "equilibrium" hypothesis suggesting that as health improves severe morbidity is replaced by a rise in moderate morbidity (Chatterji, Byles, Cutler, Seeman, & Verdes, 2015). Chatterji and colleagues reviewed recent studies to find no consistent support for any of these theories and concluded that the issue of whether rising life expectancies across the world will be accompanied by lesser or greater morbidity is still open. Apart from methodological issues, there was conflicting evidence across countries with different levels of wealth and development. Such findings point to ongoing problems with the use of broad-based measurement. This approach is based on underlying assumptions about the homogeneity of older people, under which average scores can provide us with prediction and understanding of future needs. These assumptions are located within a biomedical model of ageing.

Estes and Binney (1989) described the ways in which ageing, and health have been captured by a biomedical model in which ageing itself becomes a medical problem and influences the treatment of ageing people. In research, the focus of medicalised interest is on outcomes measured in terms of morbidity, life expectancy, falls, and disability. Franco et al. (2009) described a common definition of ageing as "the progressive loss of function accompanied by increasing morbidity and decreasing fertility", and healthy ageing defined as "the condition of being alive, while having highly preserved functioning metabolic, hormonal and neuroendocrine control systems at the organ, tissue and molecular levels" (p. 15). In this way, a biomedical model frames "normal ageing" in terms of biological processes with a focus on the diseases of ageing, and old age as a process of biological and psychological decline and disability. This approach reduces people to their deficiencies and individualises their treatment by divorcing health from social and material life. Antonovsky (1993) described this process this way: "When we focus on risk factors, on a disease, and on its pathologic development, we are pressured to identify the person with the disease". Johnson (1995) described how this approach to "healthy ageing" has more generally promoted ageist attitudes in Western society through which older people are seen as "other" to be segregated, cared for and controlled. More recently, in light of concerns about medical costs, we can add, "feared". While focusing on achievements in conquering diseases and extending individual lives, the dominance of a biomedical model has prevented attention to the wider lifetime and social aspects of ageing and wellbeing.

The claims that a population top-heavy with sicker older people will necessarily result in shortfalls in medical care and a failure to provide good health to all, has depended on assumptions about the nature of illness and the nature of healthcare. A medicalised focus on life expectancy and illness as characteristics of ageing has resulted in predictions of failures to provide adequate healthcare and resulting in serious economic implications. There are a growing number of voices to counter this view. For example, Bloom and colleagues (2015) suggested other ways to construct the health needs of older people from a public health perspective. These include population-level responses to prevent chronic disease and modification of the physical and social environment to support older people to remain engaged in society as their bodies change. These changes must include shifts in the ways in which we construct older people as individuals and as a group. Treating chronological age as a cut-off point at which a whole population becomes assigned to a problematic category; using population averages across countries without accounting for economic and cultural differences, and generally disregarding the social and cultural location of illness and healthcare, has led to the construction of older people as one large homogenous group.

Diverse experiences of health

In talking about "older people" as a population group to be studied, we tend to forget that "age" is only about the number of years lived. Based on a lifetime of transitions and experiences, people who have lived more years become increasingly diverse (Minkler, 1996). Different identities, health-related behaviours, and varying social situations are related to very broad differences in health in older age. For example, analysis of the psychological wellbeing of people aged 70 to 100 years, in just one city, in the Berlin Aging Study identified nine very different sub-groups ranging from those who were "cognitively very fit and vitally involved" to those who showed "cognitive impairment, withdrawn, in despair" (Smith & Gerstorf, 2006). Different identities, health-related behaviours, and social situations are related to very broad differences in health in older age (Victor, 2010). Conversely, treating all old people as one group has led to equating old age with disability when the general population of older people is generally far less disabled than stereotypes suggest (Reed & Clarke, 1999). For all people, ageing is a developmental process that goes on across a lifetime, so that "ageing" is not the equivalent of being an aged person. All people aged 65 to 95 years of age represent a 30+ year age span (comparable to the developmental differences between 10 and 40 years of age). Debates about the age at which people may be labelled "old" will never be resolved, as the characteristics of certain age groups keep changing, as universal health improves, the age of eligibility for pensions shifts, and social constructions of "elderly" or "old" change.

To acknowledge diversity among population samples, a report from the Health Work and Retirement (HWR) longitudinal study in New Zealand (Stephens et al., 2018) identified groups of older people with similar health trajectories across ten years (2006–2016). This analytic strategy acknowledged the diversity of health experiences by identifying clusters of people (aged from 65–80 years in 2016) with similar health trajectories across time. This allowed the researchers to include and highlight the experiences of small groups of people, which would be lost by averaging the data for overall trends. This strategy also ensured that those who face barriers to participating in such surveys, such as poor health, were represented.

The analytic approach additionally acknowledged that "healthy ageing" is not well represented by physical wellbeing alone. The Constitution of the World Health Organisation (WHO) defines health as "a state of complete physical, mental and social wellbeing and not merely the absence of disease or infirmity", highlighting health as a physical, mental and social experience. This multi-dimensional view, emphasising broader definitions of health is particularly pertinent for studies of ageing, in which physical health changes may be considered a normal part of ageing and are not the sole focus of assessments of health (Marengoni et al., 2011). The HWR longitudinal study identified five distinct profiles of older New Zealanders based on changes in their physical health, mental health, and social provisions over ten years. These were labelled as:

- *Vulnerable health*: the smallest group (8.7%) who reported very poor physical and mental health, and low social provisions.
- *Mental and social health limitations*: 11.8% of participants reported good physical health but poor mental health along with low social provisions.
- *Declining physical health*: 17.5% of participants had good mental health and social provisions, but their physical health declined over time.
- *Average good health*: approximately one-third of participants (31.4%) had average physical and mental health, which remained stable over time. Their social provisions were slightly lower than the average.
- *Robust health*: another third of the participants (30.6%) reported good physical and mental health and high levels of social wellbeing across ten years.

An important observation is that over 60% of these older New Zealanders (from a population sample) reported good health. Furthermore, a substantial proportion with physical health problems, disabilities or other physical limitations reported healthy social provisions and good mental health; approximately 85% of older adults in the study maintained good mental health and social provisions over the ten-year period. Having physical health problems did not mean poor overall health.

Identifying different profiles showed that the tendency for physical health to decline with age, was reflected most strongly in one smaller group whose physical health declined across the ten years. Otherwise, the physical, mental and social health status of people within each of these groups showed very little change. People who entered the study in 2006 with poor physical, social and mental health remained in *vulnerable health*. Those who reported *robust health* by the time they were 80 years old had begun the study in good shape. These aspects point to the importance of earlier lifetime influences on health and illness in old age.

The study findings indicated some of the lifecourse factors that shape wellbeing. Membership in the five health profiles was related to possession of economic resources, employment, caregiving, housing ownership, and housing quality, revealing inequalities across different aspects of life that are related to health in older age. For example, participants in *robust health* were generally the best off economically. They reported the most formal education, followed by those with *average good health*, *declining health*, and *social and mental health limitations*. Participants characterised by a *vulnerable health* profile had the least formal education, and few reported good economic living standards. Homeownership is high and stable in the whole HWR sample, reflecting the circumstances for this cohort in New Zealand. However, those whose physical, mental and social wellbeing was consistently poor across time (*vulnerable health*) were more likely to be renting and most likely to report problems with safety, keeping warm, and house maintenance.

The different profiles were also related to other health issues, including early mortality, cognitive functioning, and health-related behaviours. Analyses indicated that those with a *vulnerable health* profile were at a disproportionately higher risk of mortality than older adults in any other group. Those with a *robust health* profile were more likely to survive, followed, in order, by those in groups reporting *average good health*, *limitations in mental and social health*, and *declining physical health*. This suggests that limitations in physical health, mental health, and social provisions represent risk factors with multiplicative effects. Those categorised as being in *robust* and *average good health* showed advantages in cognitive performance compared to other groups, with evidence of lower memory and verbal fluency performance for *vulnerable* older adults.

This approach to analysing population-level data makes three important points. First, the experiences of health among older people are diverse. A large proportion of older people may maintain good health for many years as they age. Many people over the age of 65 are well and maintain their activities as contributing citizens, and this must be acknowledged when considering the role of these members of an ageing population. Many people also report good quality of life and high levels of wellbeing, while coping with physical disabilities. Second, the different health trajectories shown by these groups are not due to having suddenly become old. Those who were more socially, mentally, and physically vulnerable and more likely to die across ten years entered old age with these disabilities. Third, consideration of social and demographic factors showed that factors developed over a lifetime such as education, and standard of living are related to health in older age. This supports the recognition that people arrive at an older age with different levels of health and functioning that are the result of a lifetime of structural and physical effects. A consideration of diversity among older people shows the need to consider inequalities in ageing experiences as important factors across the lifecourse that predict health and illness in older age.

Lifecourse inequalities

The older we are in years, the closer to death and the more at risk of illness and infirmity we become. However, there are such broad variations in who gets ill, which illnesses we might contract, and at what age biological ageing occurs, that age in years is not a good indicator of health. There is a rapidly growing recognition of the important contribution of the whole lifecourse in shaping the health and wellbeing of people as they age, and that inequalities in life chances that contribute to good or poor health continue to widen as people grow older.

Beard and Bloom (2015) drew on evidence to suggest that, allowing for a genetic determination of 25% of heterogeneity in health in older age, the remainder is the cumulative effect of health inequities across the lifecourse. "Thus, someone born into a poor family with limited access to education, or in a marginalised cultural group, is likely to have poor health in older age and earlier mortality" (p. 658). Homogenising practices take little account of such life-long inequalities and different opportunities for different groups of people to age in good health.

Several authors (e.g. Estes, Biggs, & Phillipson, 2003; Minkler & Estes, 1999; Portacol, 2011; Walker, 2009) have pointed to the influence of economic, political, and social processes on the health of older people. Age intersects with other inequalities such as socioeconomic status (Victor, 2010), gender (Calasanti, 2007) and minority group status (Bin-Sallik & Ranzijn, 2001), to shape the health chances of people throughout life, and these inequalities are exacerbated in old age (Dannefer, 2003; Ferraro & Shippee, 2009). Critical gerontologists such as Stoller and Gibson (2000) focus on structural influences to explain these life-long effects. Discernible groups in any population (e.g. those characterised by gender, socioeconomic status, ethnicity, sexuality, or intersections of these characteristics) have shared experiences of advantage or disadvantage across the lifecourse and these experiences are seen as properties of the social system within which certain groups age, rather than qualities of individuals. Accordingly, particular demographic groups are understood to share the effects of inequalities on their health and wellbeing. Those older people who have experienced a lifetime of poor health and low wage insecure employment, are most likely to reach later life least physically and financially able to maintain their own wellbeing. Ignoring these differences reinforces the poor health of marginalised older people.

To address the social, rather than individual behavioural, determinants of health in older age, broader societal action, rather than individually focussed education and intervention, is needed to create a social environment that supports and maintains good health for all. It is particularly important to understand the breadth and impact of inequalities on the health of current cohorts of elders, so that their damaging effects are not reinforced by present policies and practices. For example, active ageing policies (WHO, 2002) that include broad-based interventions to encourage participation, such as raising the retirement age, or encouraging volunteering to improve health, place many older people in demanding situations that exacerbate their health issues (Beard & Bloom, 2015; Stephens, Breheny, & Mansvelt, 2015; Walker, 2013). Public health responses to issues around the health of older people must include recognition of the broad diversity of health, circumstances, and life-long inequalities.

Health promotion

Disorders that become more frequent for many in older age include chronic conditions, non-communicable diseases, hearing loss, and musculoskeletal disorders (Beard, Officer, & Cassels, 2016). These conditions are preventable or amenable to amelioration from a public health perspective, and from the late 20th century, health promotion practice in many countries shifted towards encouraging participation, independence, and good health with the aim of reducing the potential burden of older people on health and welfare systems (Stenner, McFarquhar, & Bowling, 2011). The "successful" ageing model (Rowe & Khan, 1997), which focuses on avoiding disease and disability, maintaining high mental and physical functioning, and remaining socially engaged, has been an important influence on research, intervention, and public policy around ageing. The World Health Organisation's Active Ageing policy framework (WHO, 2002) further influenced the shift to public policies described as "successful", "active", "healthy", or "positive" ageing strategies.

Such positive changes from a previous focus on decline and dependence, with recognition of the need to foster participation and active contribution, are beneficial for many older people. However, several critiques (e.g. Estes, Biggs, & Phillipson, 2003; Martinson & Berridge, 2015; Minkler & Estes, 1999; Portacolone, 2011; Rubinstein & de Medeiros, 2015; Stephens, 2017) have shown that the successful ageing model is problematic owing to a focus on individual responsibility, support for oppressive ideals, and denial of death. "Successful ageing" discourse positions older people as personally responsible for engaging in exercise, diet, and social engagement prescriptions to produce good health. These ideals are oppressive when they take little account of opportunities for different groups of people to achieve them. "Successful ageing" works very well for those who are already advantaged, while those who are already disabled or already suffering poor health are seen as ageing unsuccessfully. This approach encourages surveillance and blaming (Breheny & Stephens, 2010). Furthermore, the biomedical focus on prolonging healthy life is unable to encompass embodied ageing; "successful ageing" ignores the fact that we will physically decline and die. The effect of this sort of denial is to pathologise ageing bodies. Suggestions that relentless activity and virtuous diets might allow us to live forever create difficulties for older people who are experiencing changes in energy and strength levels (Pond et al., 2010).

These critiques are now well known; however, many researchers have responded within the terms of the successful ageing model. Investigations attempting to adapt the conceptualisation of "success" to multiple lives, cultures and ages, confuse our understandings of "successful" ageing, rather than clarifying it. To work toward useful policy and practice to support the wellbeing of all older people in our societies we need a completely different framework that conceptually includes diversity, values, and the importance of social location in our understanding of healthy ageing.

A capability approach

To respond to the need for a new framework, the World Health Organization (WHO) released the first "World report on ageing and health" (World Health Organisation, 2015). The report outlines a public health framework for *healthy ageing* that is built around the concept of functional ability. Drawing on Sen's (1987) Capability Approach, the functional ability is defined as "the health-related attributes that enable people to be and to do what they have reason to value" (p. 227). A capability approach provides a broader basis for understanding health and focusses on the environmental and structural basis of wellbeing (Stephens, 2017; Stephens & Breheny, 2018). By focusing on valued functions (what people wish to be and do), the Capability Approach provides a theoretical framework that takes into account the different material and social situations of people's lives, and accounts for different culturally-based ideals. Rather than focus on individual responsibility for health with its moral implications, it focuses on the importance of the social and environmental context of ageing and health, the environmental context that can support or obstruct valued functions. Accordingly, from a capabilities perspective, rather than individual responsibility for maintaining health, the structural and environmental obstacles to healthy ageing become the focus of policy and practice. Inequalities in access to transport and warm housing may be understood in relation to the policies, practices and structures of public and private sector organisations. Within this framework, inequalities in health are not explained by individual abilities or choices, but by inequalities in capability and the impact of social arrangements on the freedom of people to live a life they value (Alkire, 2005). A capability approach provides a radical shift in thinking about healthy ageing to focus on the social and material environments that support valued capabilities.

Within this framework, health may be viewed in a way that is relevant to all older people. Rather than prescriptions for certain levels of physical, cognitive, and social wellbeing, health promotion would be focussed on supporting everybody's ability to achieve their valued levels of functioning, regardless of economic resources or physical impairment. Environments that do not support the desired functioning are seen as disabling (Beard et al., 2016) and interventions focus on creating environments (housing, employment, transport, and social protection) that support all older people to function well. For example, the WHO Global Network of Age-Friendly Cities and Communities (World Health Organisation, 2016) focuses on changing many aspects of built environments which can include quite simple changes such as access to buildings and public toilets and seating in public spaces or access to affordable transport as important aspects of wellbeing. A capabilities framework shifts research attention toward the impact of housing and neighbourhoods as important determinants of the health of older people (Stephens & Breheny, 2018; Stephens, Szabó, Allen, & Alpass, 2019a, 2019b). In general, it shifts conceptualisations of health in older age from a focus on the presence or absence of disease, to a focus on functioning, including recognition that both the individual's capacity and their environment have a role in determining healthy functioning in older age.

Conclusion

Current dominant discourses of ageing within which older people are positioned as a homogenous group based on age, as a burden on society (from which they are excluded) and as non-important subjects of research and healthcare are damaging and exclusionary. Recognition of diversity raises the anomaly involved in discussing the needs of older people in general. If we recognise that older people are very diverse, that chronological age does not describe health status at all (a closer look into the physiological change literature reveals even greater diversity), and that this sort of characterisation leads to damaging constructions, then why should we discuss older people and their needs as a group at all? What is the purpose of this chapter focusing on health and illness among older people as a group, if it only serves to contribute to ageist practices?

A critical perspective provides us with two interrelated views of ageing and health. First, a separate chapter in a book on illness and health does recognise that growing older as a human being brings us closer to death and that this inevitably brings embodied change. At some point, as we age, the physical changes, which are the precursor of death, mean that most of us will need some care at some time. Although the experiences and final causes of death are hugely diverse, an ageing body is a common experience and ageing as a stage in life cannot be ignored. Attention to ageing and the needs of older people recognises this common need. Second, a critical look at practices of homogenising, attributing, and assigning prescriptions and treatment shows that research attention to ageing and health as a category must consider the social and material situation, the capabilities, and the views and needs of older people themselves. Critical research has shown that in addition to care for physical health, those needs include full acceptance of all older people as participating members of their society and recognition of people's social, cultural and spiritual values as important aspects of their health and healthcare.

References

Alkire, S. (2005). Why the capability approach? *Journal of Human Development, 6*(1), 115–135.

Angus, J., & Reeve, P. (2006). Ageism: A threat to "aging well" in the 21st century. *Journal of Applied Gerontology, 25*(2), 137–152.

Antonovsky, A. (1993). *The Salutogenic Approach to Ageing.* Address to University of California, Berkeley, 21 January 1993. Retrieved from http://www.angelfire.com/ok/soc/a-berkeley.html

Beard, J. R., & Bloom, D. E. (2015). Towards a comprehensive public health response to population ageing. *The Lancet, 385*(9968), 658–661. doi:10.1016/S0140-6736(14)61461-6

Beard, J. R., Officer, A. M., & Cassels, A. K. (2016). The world report on ageing and health. *The Gerontologist, 56* Supplement 2(Suppl_2), S163–S166. doi:10.1093/geront/gnw037

Berks, J., & McCormick, R. (2008). Screening for alcohol misuse in elderly primary care patients: A systematic literature review. *International Psychogeriatrics, 20*(6), 1090–1103.

Bin-Sallik, M. A., & Ranzijn, R. (2001). *Report on a scoping study into the needs of Indigenous aged care in South Australia.* University of South Australia, Adelaide: College of Indigenous Education. Retrieved from http://www.sapo.org.au

Binstock, R. H. (2010). From compassionate ageism to intergenerational conflict? *Gerontologist, 50*(5), 574–585. doi:10.1093/geront/gnq056

Bloom, D. E., Chatterji, S., Kowal, P., Lloyd-Sherlock, P., McKee, M., Rechel, B., … Smith, J. P. (2015). Macroeconomic implications of population ageing and selected policy responses. *The Lancet, 385*(9968), 649–657. doi:10.1016/S0140-6736(14)61464-1

Breheny, M., & Stephens, C. (2010). Ageing in a material world. *New Zealand Journal of Psychology, 39*(2), 41–48.

Calasanti, T. (2007). Bodacious berry, potency wood and the aging monster: Gender and age relations in anti-aging ads. *Social Forces, 86*(1), 335–355. doi:10.1353/sof.2007.0091

Chatterji, S., Byles, J., Cutler, D., Seeman, T., & Verdes, E. (2015). Health, functioning, and disability in older adults – present status and future implications. *The Lancet, 385*(9967), 563–575. doi:10.1016/S0140-6736(14)61462-8

Chrisler, J. C., Barney, A., & Palatino, B. (2016). Ageism can be hazardous to women's health: Ageism, sexism, and stereotypes of older women in the healthcare system. *Journal of Social Issues, 72*(1), 86–104.

Dannefer, D. (2003). Cumulative advantage/disadvantage and the life course: Cross-fertilizing age and social science theory. *Journals of Gerontology. Series B – Psychological Sciences and Social Sciences, 58*(6), S327–S337. doi:10.1093/geronb/58.6.S327

Dufour, M., Mary, M. P. H., Fuller, M., & Richard, K. (1995). Alcohol in the elderly. *Annual Review of Medicine, 46*(1), 123–132.

Estes, C. L., Biggs, S., & Phillipson, C. (2003). *Social theory, social policy and ageing. A critical introduction.* Maidenhead: Open University Press.

Estes, C. L., & Binney, E. A. (1989). The biomedicalization of aging: Dangers and dilemmas. *The Gerontologist, 29*(5), 587–596.

Ferraro, K. F., & Shippee, T. P. (2009). Aging and cumulative inequality: How does inequality get under the skin? *The Gerontologist, 49*(3), 333–343.

Franco, O. H., Karnik, K., Osborne, G., Ordovas, J. M., Catt, M., & van der Ouderaa, F. (2009). Changing course in ageing research: The healthy ageing phenotype. *Maturitas, 63*(1), 13–19.

Gurwitz, J. H., & Goldberg, R. J. (2011). Age-based exclusions from cardiovascular clinical trials: Implications for elderly individuals (and for all of us): Comment on "the persistent exclusion of older patients from ongoing clinical trials regarding heart failure". *Archives of Internal Medicine, 171*(6), 557–558.

Johnson, T. F. (1995). Aging well in contemporary society: Introduction. *American Behavioral Scientist, 39*(2), 120–130. doi:10.1177/0002764295039002003

Kagan, S. H., & Melendez-Torres, G. J. (2015). Ageism in nursing. *Journal of Nursing Management, 23*(5), 644–650. doi:10.1111/jonm.12191

Konrat, C., Boutron, I., Trinquart, L., Auleley, G.-R., Ricordeau, P., & Ravaud, P. (2012). Underrepresentation of elderly people in randomised controlled trials. The example of trials of 4 widely prescribed drugs. *PloS one, 7*(3), e33559.

Latimer, J. (1997). Figuring identities: Older people, medicine and time. In A. Jamieson, S. Harper, & C. Victor (Eds.), *Critical approaches to ageing and later life* (pp. 143–159). Buckingham: Open University Press.

Latimer, J. (1999). The dark at the bottom of the stair: Participation and performance of older people in hospital. *Medical Anthropology Quarterly, 13*(2), 186–213.

Lothian, K., & Philp, I. (2001). Care of older people: Maintaining the dignity and autonomy of older people in the healthcare setting. *BMJ, 322*(7287), 668–670. doi:10.1136/bmj.322.7287.668

Marengoni, A., Angleman, S., Melis, R., Mangialasche, F., Karp, A., Garmen, A., … Fratiglioni, L. (2011). Aging with multi-morbidity: A systematic review of the literature. *Ageing Research Reviews, 10*(4), 430–439.

Martin, R., Williams, C., & O'Neill, D. (2009). Retrospective analysis of attitudes to ageing in the Economist: Apocalyptic demography for opinion formers? *BMJ, 339*, b4914. doi: 10.1136/bmj.b4914

Martinson, M., & Berridge, C. (2015). Successful aging and its discontents: A systematic review of the social gerontology literature. *The Gerontologist, 55*(1), 58–69.

Ministry of Health, N. Z. (2010). *Drug use in New Zealand: Key results of the 2007/08 New Zealand alcohol and drug use survey.* Wellington: Ministry of Health.

Minkler, M. (1996). Critical perspectives on ageing: New challenges for gerontology. *Ageing & Society, 16*(04), 467–487. doi:10.1017/S0144686X00003639

Minkler, M., & Estes, C. L. (1999). *Critical gerontology: Perspectives from political and moral economy.* Amityville, NY: Baywood.

Nelson, T. D. (2016). Promoting healthy aging by confronting ageism. *American Psychologist, 71*(4), 276.

Pond, R., Stephens, C., & Alpass, F. (2010). Virtuously watching one's health older adults' regulation of self in the pursuit of health. *Journal of Health Psychology, 15*(5), 734–743.

Portacolone, E. (2011). The myth of independence for older Americans living alone in the Bay Area of San Francisco: A critical reflection. *Ageing & Society, 31*(05), 803–828. doi:10.1017/S0144686X10001169

Prince, M. J., Wu, F., Guo, Y., Robledo, L. M. G., O'Donnell, M., Sullivan, R., & Yusuf, S. (2015). The burden of disease in older people and implications for health policy and practice. *The Lancet, 385*(9967), 549–562.

Reed, J., & Clarke, C. L. (1999). Nursing older people: Constructing need and care. *Nursing Inquiry, 6*(3), 208–215. doi:10.1046/j.1440-1800.1999.00033.x

Robertson, A. N. N. (1997). Beyond apocalyptic demography: Towards a moral economy of interdependence. *Ageing & Society, 17*(04), 425–446.

Roehrs, T., Verster, J., Koshorek, G., Withrow, D., & Roth, T. (2018). How representative are insomnia clinical trials? *Sleep Medicine, 51*, 118–123.

Rowe, J. W., & Kahn, R. L. (1997). Successful aging. *Gerontologist, 37*(4), 433–440.

Rubinstein, R. L., & de Medeiros, K. (2015). "Successful aging", gerontological theory and neoliberalism: A qualitative critique. *The Gerontologist, 55*(1), 34–42. doi:10.1093/geront/gnu080

Safiliou-Rothschild, C. (2009). Are older people responsible for high healthcare costs? *CESifo Forum, 10*(1), 57–64.

Sen, A. (1987). *The standard of living (the tanner lectures)* (G. Hawthorne Ed.). Cambridge: Cambridge University Press.

Smith, J., & Gerstorf, D. (2006). Ageing differently: Potential and limits. In S. O. Daatland & S. Biggs (Eds.), *Ageing and diversity: Multiple pathways and cultural migrations* (pp. 13–28). Bristol: Policy Press.

Spijker, J., & MacInnes, J. (2013). Population ageing: The timebomb that isn't? *BMJ, 347*, f6598. doi:10.1136/bmj.f6598

Stenner, P., McFarquhar, T., & Bowling, A. (2011). Older people and "active ageing": Subjective aspects of ageing actively. *Journal of Health Psychology, 16*(3), 467–477. doi:10.1177/1359105310384298

Stephens, C. (2017). From success to capability for healthy ageing: Shifting the lens to include all older people. *Critical Public Health, 27*(4), 490–498. doi:10.1080/09581596.2016.1192583

Stephens, C., Alpass, F., Allen, J., Szabo, A., Stevenson, B., & Towers, A. (2018). *The New Zealand Health, Work & Retirement Longitudinal Study 2006–2016.* Palmerston North: Health and Ageing Research Team, Massey University. Retrieved from http://www.massey.ac.nz/hart/

Stephens, C., & Breheny, M. (2018). *Healthy ageing: A capability approach to inclusive policy and practice.* London: Routledge.

Stephens, C., Breheny, M., & Mansvelt, J. (2015). Volunteering as reciprocity: Beneficial and harmful effects of social policies to encourage contribution in older age. *Journal of Aging Studies, 33*, 22–27. doi:10.1016/j.jaging.2015.02.003

Stephens, C., Szabó, Á., Allen, J., & Alpass, F. (2019a). A capabilities approach to unequal trajectories of healthy ageing: The importance of the environment. *Journal of Aging and Health, 31*(9), 1527–1548.

Stephens, C., Szabó, Á., Allen, J., & Alpass, F. (2019b). Livable environments and the quality of life of older people: An ecological perspective. *The Gerontologist. 39*(4), 675–685. 10.1093/geront/gny043

Stevenson, B. S., Stephens, C., Dulin, P., Kostick, M., & Alpass, F. (2015). Alcohol consumption among older adults in Aotearoa/New Zealand: A comparison of "baby boomers" and "over-65s". *Health Psychology and Behavioral Medicine, 3*(1), 366–378.

Stoller, E. P., & Gibson, R. (2000). Advantages of using the life course framework in studying aging. In E. Stoller & R. Gibson (Eds.), *Worlds of difference: Inequality in the aging experience* (pp. 19–33). Thousand Oaks, CA: Pine Forge Press.

Suzman, R., Beard, J. R., Boerma, T., & Chatterji, S. (2015). Health in an ageing world – what do we know? *The Lancet, 385*(9967), 484–486. doi:10.1016/S0140-6736(14)61597-X

United Nations, D. o. E. a. S. A., Population Division. (2017). *World population prospects: The 2017 revision, volume II: Demographic profiles (ST/ESA/SER.A/400)*. Retrieved from https://population.un.org/wpp/Publications/Files/WPP2017_Volume-II-Demographic-Profiles.pdf

Victor, C. (2010). *Ageing, health and care*. Bristol: Policy Press.

Walker, A. (2009). Why is ageing so unequal? In P. Cann & M. Dean (Eds.), *Unequal ageing*. Bristol: Policy Press.

Walker, A. (2013). *Active ageing: A policy for all ages?* Paper presented at the 20th IAGG World Congress of Gerontology and Geriatrics (IAGG June 2013), Seoul, South Korea.

Wilson, D. M., Nam, M. A., Murphy, J., Victorino, J. P., Gondim, E. C., & Low, G. (2017). A critical review of published research literature reviews on nursing and healthcare ageism. *Journal of Clinical Nursing, 26*(23–24), 3881–3892. doi:10.1111/jocn.13803

Witham, M. D., & McMurdo, M. E. (2007). How to get older people included in clinical studies. *Drugs & Aging, 24*(3), 187–196.

World Health Organisation. (2002). *Active ageing: A policy framework*. Retrieved from http://whqlibdoc.who.int/hq/2002/who_nmh_nph_02.8.pdf

World Health Organisation. (2015). *World report on ageing and health*. Retrieved from http://www.who.int/ageing/events/world-report-2015-launch/en/.

World Health Organisation. (2016). *Age-friendly cities and communities*. Retrieved from http://www.who.int/ageing/projects/age-friendly-cities-communities/en/

Yang, Z., Norton, E. C., & Stearns, S. C. (2003). Longevity and health care expenditures: The real reasons older people spend more. *Journals of Gerontology. Series B – Psychological Sciences and Social Sciences, 58*(1), S2–S10.

Yung, R. L. (2000). Changes in immune function with age. *Rheumatic Disease Clinics of North America, 26*(3), 455–473.

19

DEATH, DYING, AND END-OF-LIFE CARE

Erica Borgstrom

Introduction

Common sayings in English about death imply that it is one of life's only certainties and that it is an equaliser amongst people; these sayings imply that death is a universal experience. However, how death comes about, and is experienced, is neither certain nor equal. Examining the variability in death and dying through a critical lens enables an understanding about how even in death there is inequality, and how managing dying and death is a political act. Thinking about death is not new to politicians; Foucault pointed out how death and dying are influential to political power and the shaping of our social world, especially through medicine (Foucault, 1973, 1977). Much of medical care – from international aid to improve infant mortality rates to advances in life-support technologies – is designed to prevent death. This implies that some forms of death are deemed to be "better" or "worse" than others, even if we all eventually have to die. Consequently, these interventions have led to increasing life expectancy on a global scale and an increased global population, which is now also causing a rise in the total number of deaths each year (Ritchie & Roser, 2019). This rise has led to questions about what can be done about and with all the people who are dying. For some, the care of the dying is viewed as an indicator of how a society cares for sick and vulnerable people and a litmus test for health and social care services (England Department of Health, 2008). So if death is both common and variable, how might one critically understand current contexts of dying?

Such questions and assertions lead to considerations about the contexts in which death and dying are considered to be "good" and "done well". The purpose of this chapter is to illustrate some of the diversity surrounding death and dying in different contexts, and explore some of the trends that affect how deaths come to be evaluated as "good". In this chapter I use the concept of "good death" to highlight the importance of thinking about the structural and political elements that affect death and dying. The first section of the chapter provides a brief overview of the literature on good death, emphasising its usefulness as an analytical tool rather than empirical reality. Using this concept in this way invites an examination of how death and dying are positioned within "Western" society, rather than evaluating individual circumstances of death.

There are entire tomes related to the study of death, dying, and bereavement, so a single chapter cannot possibly cover all the topics related to this field, nor can it be an in-depth critical analysis of each of these subjects. The chapter therefore focuses on three aspects of death and dying: end-of-life care, assisting both life-extensions and dying, and changing mortality trends. By discussing these contemporary, global issues this chapter reveals how thinking about these issues critically illuminates that the social context of death is not as universal or equalising as it is sometimes presumed to be.

Good death

What is a good death? Set out like this, the concept of death appears as if it can be defined, providing a category to evaluate an individual's dying experience or moment of death. The concept of "good death" has been used to distinguish between types of death (Jacobsen, 2017) and to reflect on the organisation of end-of-life care (McNamara, Waddell, & Colvin, 1994). It has also been used to discuss meaning making through organ donation (Simpson, 2001), responses to grief (Seal, Murray, & Seddon, 2014), and funerary practices (van der Geest, 2004). In an analysis of policy documents about end-of-life care, it was noted that whilst a "good death" was explicitly framed as an event, the focus was often on the dying process (Borgstrom, 2020). During the COVID-19 pandemic, the research highlighted that what a "good death" looks like varies across community groups even when people are dying from the same disease and are affected by identical social restrictions within one country (Bear et al., 2020). So whilst at first the concept of a "good death" appears self-explanatory, it also contains considerable diversity and versatility (Green, 2008) and is sometimes used interchangeably to refer to the dying process or the event of death even though these may be evaluated differently. Attending to the concept of "good death" in this chapter allows a critical understanding of how individual experiences of death and dying are shaped by societal forces as well as how societal changes are responding to a search for particular versions of "good death".

There have been several attempts to define "good death", including reviews of existing literature and research (Cottrell et al., 2016; Meier et al., 2016a). Often these attempts collate a list of features, including themes like notions of control, comfort, closure, dignity, awareness of impending death, and the presence of family. For example, people may describe a "good death" as one where the person died at home as they wished, with no distressing symptoms or pain, surrounded by their family, and after having sorted their will. Others may describe a "good death" as one after every medical intervention has been attempted, which therefore may occur in the hospital. In my own research experience in England, asking people what they think would be a good death for them often brought up the notion of dying in one's sleep or dying suddenly; however, deaths by accident (which could also be sudden) were less desirable. When discussing their deaths in the context of end-of-life care – where they were more likely to think of good death as the process of dying rather than just the event of death – their responses indicated wanting to be comfortable and have some sense of control.

Within the sociological and anthropological literature it has been acknowledged that what constitutes a good death has changed over time (Walter, 2003). Today, within Western societies, it is accepted that deaths may be highly individualised to reflect personal perspectives and experiences (Kehl, 2006). Nonetheless, most people attempt to achieve a death reflecting wider social values and scripts (Seale, 1998). Medical staff strive to provide deaths that conform with these notions, or at least a "good enough death", in that they attempt to meet as many of the patient's preferences as possible (McNamara, 2004). A normative concept of "good death" is used to justify policy interventions in end-of-life care (Borgstrom, 2016). So whilst there may be variability in how people define a death as "good", there are also social norms and practices that contribute to how different deaths are evaluated or experienced as "good".

Despite understandings of a "good death" being variable and pluralistic, it is used in health policy, practice, or research as if it were unproblematic (e.g. Ellershaw, Dewar, & Murphy, 2010). The concept of a good death has been identified as an ideology that underpins the modern hospice movement and end-of-life care (Hart, Sainsbury, & Short, 1998). Because of this, for some authors, it is considered a vital concept for discussing dying, at least from a European perspective (Howarth, 2011). Yet, activities that rank countries internationally, like the Quality of Death Index (Economist Intelligence Unit, 2015) suggest that the salience of the concept extends more globally.

Whilst the concept of a good death is prevalent, it is not without critique. First, the terminology of a "good death" implies that there is a singular understanding of "good", and therefore the concept does not adequately reflect the multiple ways of dying (Green, 2008). Moreover, there are several studies that illustrate how different groups evaluate the concept differently (e.g. Long, 2004; Semino, Demjen, & Koller, 2014), even if from the same "cultural background" (Meier et al., 2016). Research into "good death" in medical contexts illuminate many of the challenges of current medical practice and the complexity of the process of dying (Masson, 2002); and that a "good death" does not necessarily mean "good dying" (Sandman, 2005). Lastly, when the concept of "good death" is used uncritically, there is failure to question for whom must a death be good and from what perspective is this evaluation being made (Hart et al., 1998).

It is important to keep these critiques in mind because they help illustrate a critical way of thinking about death and dying. In this chapter, I am not using the concept of a good death to say that there is one way to die that is best, or that there is an ultimate kind of good death, or that all deaths should feature certain criteria. Instead, I have included the concept here to raise attention to the fact that death is often evaluated – both individually and societally – and that this process of judgement affects how dying is done, reacted to, and ultimately managed. Using the concept invites you, the reader, to think about what criteria may be utilised in different contexts, who are making these judgements, and how explicit this is. In turn, it challenges you to think about what kinds of deaths and experiences of dying are being privileged or disadvantaged, and if this disparity matters. The next section discusses changes in mortality over time and across places to illustrate the variability in contemporary contexts of death and dying and how these implicitly affect the potential to experience "good" deaths.

End-of-life care

With an increase in deaths from non-communicable diseases, there has been increased attention on how people die, instead of focusing primarily on what people die from. This has led to the rise in the recognition of end-of-life care as a legitimate element of healthcare (Seymour, 2012). End-of-life care is broadly understood as the support, treatment, and care provided to people in the last months of their lives, often upon recognising that they are dying or that the condition they have is terminal. It can be provided to anyone from any age; however, policy guidelines in many countries, including the UK, distinguish between paediatric and adult end-of-life care.

The principles behind current end-of-life care are attributed to the development of the modern hospice movement and palliative care in the 1960s. The founding of the modern hospice movement is credited to Dame Cicely Saunders, who set up a dedicated space for the care of the dying at St Christopher's Hospice in London in 1967 (Clark, 2010). At the time, she felt that the care given to dying people marginalised and stigmatised them, particularly within hospitals. Instead, she was committed to an entirely open approach in which death and dying were discussed with terminally-ill people and the significant others in their lives. She devised care that was focused on the whole person, which is understood to be holistic by encompassing physical, social, psychological, and spiritual elements (Clark, 2000). This is an example of how a particular vision about what a "good death" should be has changed the way dying people are cared for.

Since the 1960s, an acknowledged set of palliative care standards, along with a hospice-building programme that includes an underlying philosophy of whole-person care, has been developed and disseminated to many areas around the globe (Clark, 2007). As such, the modern hospice movement has grown into a global social movement that has supported policymakers to view end-of-life care as a human right (Seymour, 2012). Interestingly, whilst the modern hospice movement was originally designed to de-medicalise death, in countries such as the UK, USA, and Australia, palliative and end-of-life care have since become embedded within medical care. This is partially due to how policy and funding has categorised palliative care as healthcare (James & Field, 1992). End-of-life care in these countries is therefore considered to be medical-ised (Zimmermann & Wennberg, 2006), even when death occurs within a hospice or a person's home, and that medical involvement is part of a "good death". This idea that end-of-life care is supported by and within a medical system is part of the expansion of palliative and end-of-life care both nationally and internationally (Economist Intelligence Unit, 2015).

Yet, embedding end-of-life care within healthcare systems means that access to end-of-life care can be inequitable and variable. For example, the UK is currently ranked as a world leader in end-of-life care provision, due to the history of the modern hospice movement in the UK and recent policy developments promoting end-of-life care (Economist Intelligence Unit, 2015). Nevertheless, various reports indicate that within the UK, as in other countries, access to good multi-professional end-of-life care is not guaranteed for every person dying (Burles, Peternelj-Taylor, & Holtslander, 2016; Walshe, Todd, Caress, & Chew-Graham, 2009). Research indicates that many people throughout the UK who would benefit from palliative-focused end-of-life care are not receiving it (Dixon et al., 2015). On a global scale, inequalities in the receipt of end-of-life care are also noted (Connor, 2020; Singer & Bowman, 2002). This can be caused by policy differences (e.g. restricted access to certain medications in some countries), differences in healthcare financing and infrastructure, and cultural differences in discussing and planning for death (Economist Intelligence Unit, 2015).

In a wide range of countries, there are certain groups of people who tend to be dispropor-tionally disadvantaged in receiving end-of-life care, particularly in receiving specialist end-of-life care. These include older people (particularly those living in nursing and residential homes), people from ethnic minority groups, homeless people, or those living in prisons, and people from socioeconomically deprived geographical areas (e.g. Haines et al., 2018; Rosenwax & McNamara, 2006; Stajduhar et al., 2019). People may experience a double-disadvantage in accessing end-of-life care if they belong to more than one of these groups, such as having dementia and being from an ethnic minority background (Connolly, Sampson, & Purandare, 2012). People from different religious backgrounds, the LGBT+ community, and people who have mental health issues may also anticipate discrimination, which can affect if and how they access end-of-life care services. Overall, people who may be generally marginalised in healthcare systems are also disadvantaged in terms of accessing and receiving end-of-life care.

Because of the variability in access to end-of-life care, there have been attempts to widen access to it, both within countries and internationally (e.g. Gott & Ingleton, 2011). For example, organisations like International Association for Hospice and Palliative Care support the develop-ment of hospices in countries where they may not otherwise exist. However, as with the global variations in epidemiological transitions discussed in the previous section, there are some con-cerns about the assumption that all countries should have a particular form of end-of-life care that is based on the modern hospice movement (Zaman, Inbadas, Whitelaw, & Clark, 2017). In contrast to attempts to rank countries based on their end-of-life provision, such as the Quality of Death Index, this approach argues that we must accept the plurality of context-specific challenges to end-of-life care provision and how these may be overcome. This also means accepting that there is variability in how a "good death" is understood and how it may not be a goal for every country, society, person, or family. This variation is exemplified in how end-of-life care is defined differently in different contexts and places, including variations in what length of time is included and what kinds of care are covered.

The issue of variability has also resulted in several attempts to re-design end-of-life care. One example is the shift in viewing end-of-life care as something not exclusively provided by specialist palliative care to care that can, and should be, provided by a wider range of people and services (Nevin, Smith, & Hynes, 2019). For example, within UK healthcare policy, there is a saying that end-of-life care is "everybody's business". Another initiative is viewing end-of-life care from a public health perspective. To date, the most cited example of a public health approach has been the development of compassionate communities or cities. Compassionate cities provide a community-based approach to support people who are dying or are bereaved, involving families, neighbours, local organisations, and businesses, as well as more formal care providers. The philosophy behind compassionate communities is that dying is a social issue and something that can involve everyone (Kellehear, 2005). Compassionate communities actively involve local citizens to build partnerships between organisations and services. Compassionate communities can be found around the world and each area has developed their own network to support their local population. The most famous is in Kerala, India, where an extensive network of volunteers provides care in people's homes (Sallnow, Kumar, & Numpeli, 2010). It is likely that palliative and end-of-life care will continue to change as new innovations are designed to address the needs of individuals and populations.

In the last century, changes to the way dying people were cared for created the field of palliative care and hospice. It was driven by healthcare professionals seeking to improve the quality of people's care and experiences of dying, primarily through reducing suffering and pain. This approach has been largely drawn on to inform what is now known as end-of-life care, situating care of the dying people within healthcare systems. Because of the challenges faced in provided end-of-life care in such systems, and acknowledging the diversity in how care can be provided and deaths can be considered "good", communities, charities, and a wide range of designers and academics are involved in re-envisioning what care and dying can be like. In doing so, they maintain that dying is about more than just the physical decline of an individual's body, and affects not just the dying person but those around them as well. At the core of thinking about how end-of-life care can be done differently is a concern with what a good death – both as a process and event – looks like and how it can be best supported.

Medical technology: Dual processes of extending life and assisting dying

In an earlier section, I outlined how, generally, people's lives are getting longer and that the kinds of deaths people are dying from are changing over time. One explanation for this is the use of medical interventions and clinical care to sustain life. On the one hand, it can be a positive thing that people are able to live longer and are less likely to die suddenly. On the other hand, people are also experiencing living longer with disabilities and reporting a lower quality of life, particularly in the last few years of life (Kaufman, 2000). This has opened up a space to think about how societies care for people towards the end of their lives. The previous section outlined how this is done largely under the rubric of end-of-life care, drawing on palliative and hospice care. This section looks more closely at two processes that can affect what is considered a "good death" in this context of extended lives: the use of medical treatment to further extend life and the use of medicines for assisted dying to purposefully shorten a life. Both of these bring to fore the question: what is the role of medicine in death?

The role of medical treatment, and the conundrum of the possibility of too much treatment in the context of living longer with disabilities, is summed up by medical anthropologist Sharon Kaufman:

> When faced with a life-threatening disease, most of us want the miracles of medicine to extend our lives into a vaguely perceived open-ended future. Yet we don't want to live too long, that is, into a medically prolonged period of suffering or suspension in some limbo, no longer who we were but not yet dead. The big problem, the intractable, increasingly apparent problem is that few know when that line between life-giving therapies and too much treatment is about to be crossed.
>
> *(Kaufman, 2015, p. 2)*

Kaufman argues that through advancements in medicine, the standards of care are constantly changing, and therefore the level of treatment is increasing. In her book *Ordinary Medicine*, she uses the example of technological advancements in devices that treat abnormal heart rhythms – the ICD (implantable cardioverter defibrillator, or "pacemaker") – to describe how what was once new medical technology to save lives has become routine in the USA. Towards the end of life it can become problematic because it typically has to be turned off to enable a person "to die" or it will otherwise keep shocking their heart. Implementing technology as standard to save or extend life, which is often viewed as unproblematically positive, therefore also creates the need to think about when such technologies can be turned off, withdrawn, or withheld.

From a philosophical standpoint, withholding life-extending treatment is often viewed as less morally problematic than withdrawing treatment once started, which is the problem Kaufman is highlighting. The main reason seems to be that withholding treatment does not involve taking any action, whereas withdrawing treatment does (British Medical Association, 2007). For example, if tubes are removed, a ventilator is turned off or antibiotics are withdrawn, that involves doing something that can result in death. On the other hand, if the decision is made not to insert the tubes in the first place, not to put someone on a ventilator, or begin a course of antibiotics, this is understood as omitting to do something, thereby allowing death. This line of thought derives from the acts/omissions doctrine, which holds that acts are morally more important than omissions. Furthermore, this doctrine allows that withdrawing treatment (that is, acting) is morally worse than withholding it (that is, omitting to act). In these circumstances, health professionals might be seen as less morally responsible for the outcome if they withhold treatment than if they withdraw it.

Yet sometimes the acts/omissions doctrine can be difficult to justify. Indeed, basing decisions on this moral distinction between withdrawing and withholding treatment can lead to consequences that might not be in the best interests of the dying person. For example, as implied by Kaufman's phrase "where to draw the line", it can lead to the under-treatment or, somewhat paradoxically, the over-treatment of dying people. If treatment is started, and then found to be ineffective or to have intolerable side effects, doctors might be reluctant to withdraw it on the grounds that, although it would have been morally acceptable not to start it, it is morally wrong to withdraw it once started. In this case, they risk over-treating, and thereby creating needless stress for the dying person. Furthermore, using limited resources to treat someone who is not benefiting from treatment deprives someone who might benefit. Maintaining a moral distinction between withholding and withdrawing treatment means that doctors will be reluctant to start a treatment unless it clearly benefits the dying person. With some medical procedures, however, health professionals cannot know in advance the right course of action for a particular dying person without first seeing how they respond to treatment. Thus, if doctors are reluctant to start treatment because they consider it wrong to withdraw treatment once started, they run the risk of undertreating the dying person because they are not sure in advance how beneficial it will be. Some professionals find these permissible ethical boundaries difficult to navigate, and this can lead to them feeling distressed (Dzeng et al., 2016).

Discussions about the use of medical technology to extend or end life can also highlight global differences and inequalities in the access to such technologies. In some countries, such as Japan, it is considered culturally appropriate to use life-extending technology up until death as a way of respecting a person and "doing all that is possible" (Lock, 2002; Long, 2004). However, other countries have restrictions on the use of different technologies and medications. For example, opioid-based medication – often used in end-of-life care to treat pain – is tightly regulated in many countries, such as in Egypt, China, and Ecuador, making it difficult to pre-scribe and access (Cherny et al., 2013). Reasons for this include that there is a concern about the potential addictive nature of the drug and that it may be used to shorten life without the person's permission via terminal sedation (Lamas & Rosenbaum, 2012). This means that the standard treatment or care varies cross-culturally, and leads to different interpretations in the role of such technologies as part of a good death.

The role of medicine and technology to extend life is further highlighted in societal debates around assisted dying. Arguments for assisted dying can include appealing to notions that lives primarily supported through medical technology may not be valued by all individuals (Cox et al., 2013), and therefore death is preferable to "too much treatment" to borrow Kaufman's phras-ing. Although not always acknowledged within palliative care, contemporary interpretations of a good death are historically linked to euthanasia – a form of assisted dying – and ideas of dying with one's personal affairs in order (Kellehear, 2007). In this sense, a good death is a managed death where the person has some level of control.

Assisted dying is not legal in most countries, although this is changing with local and national referendums and law changes in different states and countries throughout the globe. Where it is, it is offered alongside palliative and end-of-life care (e.g. in the Netherlands and Switzerland, as two long-standing jurisdictions permitting assisted death). Some people argue that if end-of-life care were better, people would then not want assisted dying because their pain and other symptoms, including psychological and social, would be managed. Others argue that even with such holistic care, some individuals may wish to choose when and how they die (Bernheim & Raus, 2017). However, research suggests that requests for assisted dying (or euthanasia, depend-ing on how it is classified and if the person is considered to have the ability to consent) actually increase among people receiving hospice (i.e. end-of-life) care (Chapple, Ziebland, McPherson, & Herxheimer, 2006). A number of reasons for this have been suggested, including the greater openness of expression encouraged in hospices, the distress of witnessing other people's deaths and wanting to avoid a similar experience, and the wish to remain physically independent and "in control" (Chapple et al., 2006). In countries where assisted dying is legal, there is some evidence to suggest that not everyone who requests assisted dying follows through with the act (Warnes, 2014). A core theme in this research suggests that the individual's perception that they can control when to "draw the line" is important, rather than if they act on it or not.

From both of these approaches, there is the concern that withdrawing/withholding treat-ment or assisted dying may negatively impact the lives of certain groups, such as people with pre-existing disabilities or dementia (Jackson & Keown, 2012). This is because there is a concern that biases, implicit or explicit, about the quality of a person's life may cause medical profession-als to shorten their life without their explicit informed consent.

The issues raised by advances in medical technology and questions around where to draw the line on assisted dying and the use of medicine and technology to extend life are likely to continue, both within individual countries and internationally. This is because of increasing life expectancies, including living longer with co-morbidities, increasing technological advancements and research into medication use at the end of life, societal discussions around the value of life and quality of living, and increasing uptake of advance care planning in some countries. These issues directly relate to how death can be judged as good, or made good, through different practices, and because of this, why such issues can be intensely debated and vary cross-culturally.

The demographics of death

How people die has changed over time, and the demographics of who is dying are shifting. In his discussion of the history of death, Kellehear notes that how, on the whole for humanity, there has been a shift from sudden deaths in the Stone Age to an increase in a dying phase characterised by poor health and the involvement of institutions (Kellehear, 2009). His analysis echoes the arguments made by both Illich (1976) and Aries (1981) that death in European societies has gone through "historical stages"; ultimately arguing that death was once more public – and people knew how to die through this regular exposure – and is now medicalised and hidden, resulting in a crisis for society in knowing how to die well. These analyses map onto an understanding of the epidemiological transitions in "Western" countries, where these demographic shifts are considered to impact where people die (Kalseth & Theisen, 2017). There is some debate about whether all countries globally experience – or will experience – the same changes in death rates, causes of death, and location of death. Due to this, some argue that the theory of epidemiological transitions does not adequately account for inequality (McKeown, 2009; Santosa, Wall, Fottrell, Högberg, & Byass, 2014). Whilst these analyses are Eurocentric, a core argument from all of these authors is that how death is commonly experienced at any one historical moment influences how individuals and society generally think about death and dying. What we "know" about death – and how it affects us – is not a universal given, but informed by our socio-cultural and historical context. Mortality statistics[1] provide one way of describing this context whilst also illustrating the variability in the reported cause of death that occurs.

One of the ways of understanding changing societal experiences of death is by examining the demographic shifts that societies have experienced in terms of who is dying at what age and from what. Internationally, most countries have experienced a rise in life expectancy over the last 100 years: this means that, on average, people are dying later in life. At the time of writing, the latest statistics indicate that the average life expectancy globally has risen by 5.5 years between 2009 and 2016. This has been the fastest increase since the 1960s. This rise in life expectancy is attributed to reduced child mortality and greater access to medication (WHO, 2018).

Such global rates hide the variety between and within countries. It is not uncommon for people in the USA, UK, or Australia to expect to live into their late 70s and early 80s. However, there is a great diversity of life expectancy between countries. For example, the highest life expectancy is estimated to be in Monaco (89.4 years) and the lowest in Chad (50.6 years) (CIA, 2016). Moreover, within countries, there can be considerable variation, both between the sexes (e.g. women often have a higher life expectancy than men) and between places and socioeconomic classes. Within the UK, this variation is most marked by observing the difference in life expectancy of males: data from 2014–2016 indicate that males living in the most affluent 10% of areas in England and Wales could expect to live almost a decade longer than males living in the 10% of most deprived areas (ONS, 2018). Recognising that there is inequality in life expectancy is a useful reminder that despite great advances in improving the lives of people, such as through medical intervention and public health, these "advances" do not necessarily reduce inequality across the lifetime (Abramson, 2015). This inequality is often intersectional, related to issues like, but not limited to, relative poverty and socioeconomic status, structural racism and sexism, and healthcare literacy and access to healthcare.

A rise in life expectancy is considered to be linked to a change in what people are dying from: largely a shift from "treatable" infections to conditions that people may live with for years. More than 70% of deaths globally are now being caused by non-communicable diseases, such as cardiovascular disease and cancer (Ritchie & Roser, 2019).[2] This change is generally welcomed as a positive one, with death later in life considered to be "good". Whilst non-communicable diseases are the primary cause of death globally, and especially in high-income countries, infectious disease, maternal and neonatal deaths, and malnutrition are still prevalent in many countries, particularly in Africa.[3] For example, in Kenya, the leading cause of death remains diarrheal diseases, and for South Africa and Botswana the leading cause of death remains HIV/AIDS (Ritchie & Roser, 2019). Moreover, the rise of antimicrobial resistance means that infections that have become treatable in the last century may again become deadly (O'Neill, 2014). Similarly, the COVID-19 pandemic has illustrated how infectious diseases can still have a global impact and that different political decisions can influence infection and death rates (Balmford, Annan, Hargreaves, Altoè, & Bateman, 2020). This means that the kinds of death that have become to be understood as good – death happening later in life and not from an infection, accident or natural disaster – are not necessarily the kinds of death everyone will experience.[4]

Another challenge to the simplistic view that death later in life is inherently a better death is that, although life expectancy has been rising, healthy life expectancy, especially in countries like the UK, is not keeping pace (Raleigh, 2018). This means that more people are living longer in poor health, often living with illness and disability rather than dying from them at a younger age. For some countries, this trend is expected to continue with more people living longer in ill-health (Matthijs, Neels, Timmerman, Haers, & Mels, 2016). This has important implications for how care is delivered to people by thinking about the longer-term process of dying, and with the potential to identify dying trajectories (Lunney, Lynn, Foley, Lipson, & Guralnik, 2003). Not only does this pose practical implications but also raises societal and moral discussions about what kinds of dying society supports.

At the beginning of this section, I outlined how generally the experience of death is considered to be changing. There is the expectation that more people will die later in life in a medicalised setting following a period of ill-health in older age. Whilst on the one hand, dying later in life might be considered "good", this section has briefly illustrated how such broad trends do not reflect the variability between and within countries. For many people in the world, there is the high likelihood that they may have a death that does not neatly fit within individual and societal understandings of a "good death": whether it be from an infectious disease or dying due to a complication of birth. Nevertheless, the general shift to more people dying later in life from accumulative ill-health has led to considerations about how the dying process can be managed.

Concluding statements

This chapter has considered several themes about death and dying in the contemporary era, using the concept of "good death" to critically examine how death and dying are done and made sense of. In doing so, it is evident that not all deaths are "equal" or that each society manages dying in the same way – death and dying are therefore shaped by political and societal factors. With an increase in the numbers of people dying globally, and medical advancements allowing for both the extending and shortening of lives, it is becoming increasingly imperative for policymakers, healthcare professionals, and societies to consider to what extent there is a desire and need to manage dying. Some countries have started this through an increased provision of end-of-life care, which is likely to continue and evolve in different cultural contexts. However, there are several potential challenges on the horizon that may destabilise a palliative care approach to end-of-life care, such as the increasing need for care later in life, changing disease patterns, including antimicrobial resistance and viral outbreaks, which may shorten lives earlier on, or even the threat of more natural disasters with climate collapse and increase in deaths related to this. These potential challenges serve as a useful reminder that how death is experienced is neither certain nor equal.

Notes

1 Statistics about death are collected for different purposes and there is variability in how they are collected in different countries. Mortality statistics – who is dying from what – are often gleaned from death certificates and may not be accurate, entirely comparable, or up-to-date. Nevertheless, they can be useful in seeing trends over time.
2 This website it contains information about causes of death in a wide range of countries.
3 It is beyond the scope of this chapter to discuss on different causes of death can impact grief. See Wijngaards-De Meij et al., 2008 for an example of such a discussion in the context of the death of children.
4 Deaths through terrorism and natural disasters can be significant in some countries even if globally they only account for 0.1% of deaths in 2016. For instance, deaths from terrorism were the 6th most common reason of death in Iraq in 2016, and ranked within the top ten causes of death in Syria and Libya (Ritchie, Hasell, Apple, & Roser, 2019).

References

Abramson, C. M. (2015). *The end game*. Cambridge, MA: Harvard University Press.

Aries, P. (1981). *The hour of our death*. New York: Alfred A Knopf.

Balmford, B., Annan, J. D., Hargreaves, J. C., Altoè, M., & Bateman, I. J. (2020). Cross-country comparisons of Covid-19: Policy, politics and the price of life. *Environmental and Resource Economics*, *76*(4), 525–551. doi:10.1007/s10640-020-00466-5

Bear, L., Simpson, N., Angland, M., Bhogal, J. K., Bowers, R., Cannell, F., ... Zidaru-Barbulescu, T. (2020). *"A good death" during the Covid-19 pandemic in the UK: A report on key findings and recommendations*. Retrieved from London School of Economics and Political Science website: http://eprints.lse.ac.uk/104143/4/GoodDeath_Report_FINAL.pdf

Bernheim, J. L., & Raus, K. (2017). Euthanasia embedded in palliative care. Responses to essentialistic criticisms of the Belgian model of integral end-of-life care. *Journal of Medical Ethics*. doi:10.1136/medethics-2016-103511

Borgstrom, E. (2016). End of life care strategy and the Coalition Government. In L. Foster & K. Woodthrope (Eds.), *Death and social policy in challenging times* (2016). Basingstoke: Palgrave Macmillan.

Borgstrom, E. (2020). What is a good death? A critical discourse policy analysis. *BMJ Supportive & Palliative Care, Online First*, bmjspcare-2019-002173. doi:10.1136/bmjspcare-2019-002173

British Medical Association. (2007). *Withholding and withdrawing life-prolonging medical treatment: Guidance for decision making*. Oxford.

Burles, M. C., Peternelj-Taylor, C. A., & Holtslander, L. (2016). A "good death" for all?: Examining issues for palliative care in correctional settings. *Mortality*, *21*(2), 93–111. doi:10.1080/13576275.2015.1098602

Chapple, A., Ziebland, S., McPherson, A., & Herxheimer, A. (2006). What people close to death say about euthanasia and assisted suicide: A qualitative study. *Journal of Medical Ethics*, *32*(12), 706–710. doi:10.1136/jme.2006.015883

Cherny, N. I., Cleary, J., Andre, F., Hatake, F. K., C Pestalozzi, J. B., Antman, S. K., ... Ohtsu, I. A. (2013). Opioid availability and accessibility for the relief of cancer pain in Africa, Asia, India, the Middle East,

Latin America and the Caribbean: Final report of the international collaborative project. *Annals of Oncology, 24*(Supplement 11), xi7–xi64.

CIA. (2016). *World factbook 2016–2017*. Retrieved from https://www.cia.gov/library/publications/the-world-factbook/rankorder/2102rank.html

Clark, D. (2000). *Total pain: The work of Cicely Saunders and the hospice movement*. Retrieved from http://eprints.gla.ac.uk/56632/

Clark, D. (2007). From margins to centre: A review of the history of palliative care in cancer. *Lancet Oncology, 8*, 430–438.

Clark, D. (2010). Originating a movement: Cicely Saunders and the development of St Christopher's Hospice, 1957–1967. *Mortality, 3*(1), 43–63. doi:10.1080/713685885

Connolly, A., Sampson, E. L., & Purandare, N. (2012). End-of-life care for people with dementia from ethnic minority groups: A systematic review. *Journal of the American Geriatrics Society, 60*(2), 351–360. doi:10.1111/j.1532-5415.2011.03754.x

Connor, S. R. (2020). *Global atlas of palliative care* (2nd ed.). Retrieved from http://www.thewhpca.org/resources/global-atlas-on-end-of-life-care

Cottrell, L., Duggleby, W., Balducci, L., Bendle, M. F., Borbasi, S., Wotton, K., … Zimmermann, C. (2016). The "good death": An integrative literature review. *Palliative and Supportive Care, 14*(06), 686–712. doi:10.1017/S1478951515001285

Cox, K., Bird, L., Arthur, A., Kennedy, S., Pollock, K., Kumar, A., … Seymour, J. (2013). Public attitudes to death and dying in the UK: A review of published literature. *BMJ Supportive & Palliative Care, 3*(1), 37–45. doi:10.1136/bmjspcare-2012-000203

Dixon, J., King, D., Matosevic, T., Clark, M., & Knapp, M. (2015). *Equity in the provision of palliative care in the UK: Review of evidence*. Retrieved from http://www.pssru.ac.uk/archive/pdf/4962.pdf

Dzeng, E., Colaianni, A., Roland, M., Levine, D., Kelly, M. P., Barclay, S., & Smith, T. J. (2016). Moral distress amongst American Physician Trainees regarding futile treatments at the end of life: A qualitative study. *Journal of General Internal Medicine, 31*(1), 93–99. doi:10.1007/s11606-015-3505-1

Economist Intelligence Unit. (2015). *The 2015 quality of death index*. London.

Ellershaw, J., Dewar, S., & Murphy, D. (2010). Achieving a good death for all. *BMJ (Clinical Research Ed.), 341*(sep16_2), c4861. doi:10.1136/bmj.c4861

England Department of Health. (2008). *End of life care strategy: Executive summary*. Retrieved from https://www.gov.uk/government/uploads/system/uploads/attachment_data/file/136443/EOLC_exec_summ.pdf

Foucault, M. (1973). *The birth of the clinic*. London: Routledge.

Foucault, M. (1977). *Discipline and punish: The birth of the prison*. London: Penguin.

Gott, M., & Ingleton, C. (2011). How can we improve palliative care provision for older people? Global perspectives. *BMJ Supportive & Palliative Care, 1*(2), 115–116. doi:10.1136/bmjspcare-2011-000088

Green, J. W. (2008). *Beyond the good death: The anthropology of modern dying*. Philadelphia, PA: University of Pennsylvania Press.

Haines, K. L., Jung, H. S., Zens, T., Turner, S., Warner-Hillard, C., & Agarwal, S. (2018). Barriers to hospice care in trauma patients: The disparities in end-of-life care. *American Journal of Hospice and Palliative Medicine, 35*(8), 1081–1084. doi:10.1177/1049909117753377

Hart, B., Sainsbury, P., & Short, S. (1998). Whose dying? A sociological critique of the "good death". *Mortality, 3*(1), 65–77.

Howarth, G. (2011). The emergence of new forms of dying in contemporary societies. In D. Oliviere, B. Monroe, & S. Payne (Eds.), *Death, dying and social differences*. Oxford: Oxford University Press.

Illich, I. (1976). *Limits to medicine; medical nemesis: The expropriation of health*. Harmondsworth: Penguin.

Jackson, E., & Keown, J. (2012). *Debating euthanasia*. Oxford: Hart.

Jacobsen, M. H. (2017). *"The bad death": Deciphering and developing the dominant discourse on "The Good Death"*. doi:10.1007/978-3-319-55759-5_18

James, N., & Field, D. (1992). The routinization of hospice: Charisma and bureaucratization. *Social Science & Medicine, 34*(12), 1363–1375.

Kalseth, J., & Theisen, O. M. (2017). Trends in place of death: The role of demographic and epidemiological shifts in end-of-life care policy. *Palliative Medicine, 31*(10), 964–974. doi:10.1177/0269216317691259

Kaufman, S. R. (2000). Senescence, decline, and the quest for a good death: Contemporary dilemmas and historical antecedents. *Journal of Aging Studies, 14*(1), 1–23. doi:10.1016/S0890-4065(00)80013-4

Kaufman, S. R. (2015). *Ordinary medicine: Extraordinary treatments, longer lives and where to draw the line*. Duke University Press.

Kehl, K. A. (2006). Moving toward peace: An analysis of the concept of good death. *American Journal of Hospice and Palliative Medicine, 23*(4), 277–286.

Kellehear, A. (2005). *Compassionate cities*. London: Routledge.

Kellehear, A. (2007). *A social history of dying*. Cambridge: Cambridge University Press.

Kellehear, A. (2009). *The study of dying*. Cambridge: Cambridge University Press.

Lamas, D., & Rosenbaum, L. (2012). Painful inequities – Palliative care in developing countries. *New England Journal of Medicine, 366*(3), 199–201. doi:10.1056/NEJMp1113622

Lock, M. (2002). *Twice dead: Organ transplants and the reinvention of death*. Berkeley, CA: University of California Press.

Long, S. O. (2004). Cultural scripts for a good death in Japan and the United States: Similarities and differences. *Social Science & Medicine, 58*(5), 913–928.

Lunney, J. R., Lynn, J., Foley, D. J., Lipson, S., & Guralnik, J. M. (2003). Patterns of functional decline at the end of life. *Journal of the American Medical Association, 289*(18), 2387–2392.

Masson, John D. (2002). Non-professional perceptions of 'good death': A study of the views of hospice care patients and relatives of deceased hospice care patients. *Mortality*, 7(2), 191–209, DOI: 10.1080/13576270220136294

Matthijs, K., Neels, K., Timmerman, C., Haers, J., & Mels, S. (2016). *Population change in Europe, the Middle-East and North Africa : Beyond the demographic divide*. London: Routledge.

McKeown, R. E. (2009). The epidemiologic transition: Changing patterns of mortality and population dynamics. *American Journal of Lifestyle Medicine, 3* Supplement(1_suppl), 19S–26S. doi:10.1177/1559827609335350

McNamara, B. (2004). Good enough death: Autonomy and choice in Australian palliative care. *Social Science & Medicine, 58*(5), 929–938. doi:10.1016/j.socscimed.2003.10.042

McNamara, B., Waddell, C., & Colvin, M. (1994). The institutionalization of the good death. *Social Science & Medicine, 39*(11), 1501–1508. Retrieved from http://www.sciencedirect.com/science/article/B6VBF-4656DBR-6T/2/77136570f9f36e6ad666f80242262c98

Meier, E. A., Gallegos, J. V., Thomas, L. P. M., Depp, C. A., Irwin, S. A., Jeste, D. V., et al. (2016). Defining a good death (successful dying): Literature review and a call for research and public dialogue. *American Journal of Geriatric Psychiatry, 24*(4), 261–271. doi:10.1016/j.jagp.2016.01.135

Nevin, M., Smith, V., & Hynes, G. (2019). Non-specialist palliative care: A principle-based concept analysis. *Palliative Medicine*, 026921631984096. doi:10.1177/0269216319840963

O'Neill, J. (2014). *Antimicrobial resistance: Tackling a crisis for the health and wealth of nations*. Retrieved from https://amr-review.org/sites/default/files/AMR Review Paper – Tackling a crisis for the health and wealth of nations_1.pdf

ONS. (2018). Health state life expectancies by national deprivation deciles, England and Wales – Office for National Statistics. Retrieved 24 June 2019, from https://www.ons.gov.uk/peoplepopulationandcommunity/healthandsocialcare/healthinequalities/bulletins/healthstatelifeexpectanciesbyindexofmultipledeprivationimd/englandandwales2014to2016

Raleigh, V. (2018). *What is happening to life expectancy in the UK?* London: The King's Fund.

Ritchie, H., Hasell, J., Apple, C., & Roser, M. (2019). Terrorism. Retrieved 2 November 2020, from Our World in Data website: https://ourworldindata.org/terrorism

Ritchie, H., & Roser, M. (2019). Causes of death. Retrieved 2 May 2019, from Our World in Data website: https://ourworldindata.org/causes-of-death

Rosenwax, L., & McNamara, B. (2006). Who receives specialist palliative care in Western Australia – and who misses out. *Palliative Medicine, 20*(4), 439–445. doi:10.1191/0269216306pm1146oa

Sallnow, L., Kumar, S., & Numpeli, M. (2010). Home-based palliative care in Kerala, India: The neighbourhood network in palliative care. *Progress in Palliative Care, 18*(1), 14–17. doi:10.1179/096992610X12624290276142

Sandman, L. (2005). *A good death: On the value of death and dying*. Milton Keynes: Open University Press.

Santosa, A., Wall, S., Fottrell, E., Högberg, U., & Byass, P. (2014). The development and experience of epidemiological transition theory over four decades: A systematic review. *Global Health Action*, 7(1), 23574. doi:10.3402/gha.v7.23574

Seal, K., Murray, C. D., & Seddon, L. (2014). Family stories of end-of-life cancer care when unable to fulfill a loved one's wish to die at home. *Palliative & Supportive Care*, 1–11. doi:10.1017/S1478951514000017

Seale, C. (1998). *Constructing death: The sociology of dying and bereavement*. Cambridge: Cambridge University Press.

Semino, E., Demjen, Z., & Koller, V. (2014). "Good" and "bad" deaths: Narratives and professional identities in interviews with hospice managers. *Discourse Studies, 16*(5), 667–685. doi:10.1177/1461445614538566

Seymour, J. (2012). Looking back, looking forward: The evolution of palliative and end-of-life care in England. *Mortality, 17*(1), 1–17.

Simpson, B. (2001). Making "bad" deaths "good": The kinship consequences of posthumous conception. *Journal of the Royal Anthropological Institute, 7*(1), 1–18. doi:10.1111/1467-9655.00047

Singer, P. A., & Bowman, K. W. (2002). Quality care at the end of life. *BMJ (Clinical Research Ed.), 324*(7349), 1291–1292. doi:10.1136/bmj.324.7349.1291

Stajduhar, K. I., Mollison, A., Giesbrecht, M., McNeil, R., Pauly, B., Reimer-Kirkham, S., … Rounds, K. (2019). "Just too busy living in the moment and surviving": Barriers to accessing health care for structurally vulnerable populations at end-of-life. *BMC Palliative Care, 18*(1), 11. doi:10.1186/s12904-019-0396-7

van der Geest, S. (2004). Dying peacefully: Considering good death and bad death in Kwahu-Tafo, Ghana. *Social Science & Medicine, 58*(5), 899–911.

Walshe, C., Todd, C., Caress, A., & Chew-Graham, C. (2009). Patterns of access to community palliative care services: A literature review. *Journal of Pain and Symptom Management, 37*(5), 884–912. doi:10.1016/j.jpainsymman.2008.05.004

Walter, T. (2003). Historical and cultural variants on the good death. *BMJ, 327*(7408).

Warnes, S. (2014). How many people choose assisted suicide where it is legal? | News | *The Guardian*. Retrieved 20 October 2017, from The Guardian website: https://www.theguardian.com/news/datablog/2014/jul/18/how-many-people-choose-assisted-suicide-where-it-is-legal

WHO. (2018). WHO | Life expectancy. Retrieved from https://www.who.int/gho/mortality_burden_disease/life_tables/situation_trends_text/en/

Wijngaards-De Meij, L., Stroebe, M., Stroebe, W., Schut, H., Van Den Bout, J., Van Der Heijden, P. G. M., & Dijkstra, I. (2008). The impact of circumstances surrounding the death of a child on parents' grief. *Death Studies, 32*(3), 237–252. doi:10.1080/07481180701881263

Zaman, S., Inbadas, H., Whitelaw, A., & Clark, D. (2017). Common or multiple futures for end of life care around the world? Ideas from the "waiting room of history". *Social Science & Medicine, 172*, 72–79. doi:10.1016/j.socscimed.2016.11.012

Zimmermann, C., & Wennberg, R. (2006). Integrating palliative care: A postmodern perspective. *American Journal of Hospice and Palliative Medicine, 23*(4), 255–258. doi:10.1177/1049909106290242

PART III

Shifting contextual domains

20

BIOETHICS

Critical reflections and future directions

Kathryn MacKay and Angus Dawson

Introduction

Ethics is the study of what we ought to do and how we ought to live our lives as individuals and as communities. It seeks to answer questions about what is valuable (what is good) and what is permissible, acceptable, or obligatory (what is right). Ethics can thus be described as a *normative* discipline, focused on studying prescriptive claims about what we should or should not do. Such claims of ethics, about what is good or right, of course, often involve an appeal to empirical evidence. This provides three grounds for potential dispute when an ethical argument is advanced. First, is a focus on the ethical claim and the normative reasons that seek to provide justification for the view presented. Second, is a potential dispute about the empirical evidence (its nature, relevance, and quality). Third, is the exact relationship between the first two. Since David Hume (1978 [1739]) distinguished between *is* and *ought* claims it has been widely accepted that we need to take care in our arguments to ensure that we do not, problematically, derive a normative conclusion (an *ought*) from purely empirical premises (from *is*, claims about how things are). On this view, we cannot (and, therefore, should not) explore ethical issues using purely empirical methods. An ethical argument, about what we ought to do, must be grounded in moral reasons. Such reasons can be justificatory (tell us why we ought to do something), deliberative (tell us how we ought to go about making a decision), or explanatory (setting out why someone was acting in the way that they did). All three sets of reasons are important, but it is justificatory reasons that are at the heart of arguments in bioethics because bioethics, as a part of ethics, is a normative discipline.

To see how bioethics fits into the broader discipline of ethics, the study of ethics can be divided into three overlapping categories of study. The first is metaethics, which focuses on the nature and meaning of ethical judgements. The second is normative theory because it studies the theories that attempt to set out in a systematic way what is morally justified and why it is so (e.g. consequentialism, deontology and virtue ethics, etc.). The third category is practical ethics, which applies the theories and understandings of the other two categories to particular contexts. Bioethics is one branch among many of this applied field. Other branches of practical ethics include animal ethics, legal ethics, military ethics, environmental ethics, business ethics, and professional ethics. The nature, extent and remit of bioethics is contested. Some see bioethics as, largely, interchangeable with medical ethics (Beauchamp & Childress, 2019; Veatch

& Guidry-Grimes, 2019). We prefer a broader view, one that seeks to discuss all ethical issues within the health and life sciences. This view, which goes back to the origins of bioethics as an area of explicit academic discussion, takes seriously the idea of *bio* meaning life (Potter, 1971). Bioethics, on this view, involves not just the traditional dilemmas of medical ethics (e.g. euthanasia, abortion, etc.) or issues about the relationship between healthcare workers and patients (e.g. informed consent, confidentiality, etc.), but will include a much broader set of ethical issues relating to health systems, public health, and global health, as well as at least some environmental and ecological matters.

Building upon this broader account of bioethics, we aim, in this chapter, to provide a critical review of the current state of the field of bioethics (at least within a Western, English-language context). We will outline the main current areas of activity within the field, setting out what we see as their limitations, before discussing some areas of recent theoretical and methodological innovation that provide the basis for some optimism for the future.

The current state of bioethics

There is certainly some outstanding bioethics scholarship currently being produced (Voigt, 2010; Smith, 2015; Eckenwiler, 2018). This work makes a difference to academic debate, but also to how people live their lives. However, much of bioethics is stale, disengaged and formulaic. In this section we map out what we see as a series of problems visible in much recent work. In the following section, we are more positive and outline some ethical traditions and philosophical theories that can be seen as providing the basis for a broader understanding of the human experience of health and illness and, thereby, potential sources for reinvigorating bioethics as a discipline and area of practice. But first: what is wrong with much current bioethics? In this section we cover three key issues: a tendency to focus on a limited range of topics, a narrowness in values, and some problems with method.

As suggested above, we favour a broader account of bioethics. It is true that over the last ten years the range of topics covered within mainstream bioethics has expanded, but much of it is still dominated by a fairly narrow focus on questions that dominate the issues discussed in textbooks and journals. These include, for example, issues relating to patient confidentiality and privacy in clinical settings; opposition to paternalism; issues of access to healthcare; issues related to consent for treatment and research; questions around assisted reproduction and genetic enhancement; questions about data collection and use; and questions about end of life care and physician-assisted death. The work that bioethicists have done on these topics has been extremely important. It is no overstatement to claim that bioethicists have played an important role in changing harmful practices within clinical and research settings, as well as oppressive laws, over the past 50 years. However, the range of topics considered remains slight because the narrow account of bioethics remains dominant. Areas of bioethics that have emerged more recently, such as the issues covered by neuro-ethics and mental health ethics, public health ethics, climate change and environmental aspects of healthcare, health issues that emerge in the context of migration, emergencies, disasters and war, organisational ethics and healthcare systems, globalisation and inequalities, and so on, all tend to continue to be seen as marginal.

The first problem of a narrow range of topics can be explained, at least partly, by appeal to the second problem of a narrow range of values. Western approaches to ethics dominate global discussion in bioethics, and we can see this reflected in the individualistic orientation to values that govern current discussions. The language used may appear to be diverse, appealing to different concepts such as individual rights, preferences and choices, ideas of dignity or, most often, ideas of autonomy and liberty, but the focus is centred upon individuals. The dominant list of topics in bioethics and the key individualistic values used in their discussion reinforce one another. The dominant value in much of this work is autonomy, where the standard view (called hereafter *liberal autonomy*) draws from the political and moral traditions of both liberalism and social contract models of the state, and imagines each person to be an independent actor, sovereign over their bodies, choices, preferences, and beliefs. Immanuel Kant (1996 [1797]) linked his account of autonomy to the idea of responsibility and legislating the rational *moral law* (Ross, 1954; see also Christman, 2018). By contrast, John Stuart Mill's (2015 [1859]) influential idea of liberty suggests the justification of only a minimal set of restrictions on freedom of thought and action (e.g. where actions may harm others). This is usually interpreted as promoting minimal state or collective action. Although these approaches are very different, and are justified in distinct ways, this is elided in the role that autonomy tends to play in bioethical discussions. As mentioned above, bioethics has made enormous progress in improving the ways in which patients and research participants are treated over the past decades. However, the narrow scope of attention of much bioethics in terms of topics is framed by its continuing reliance on individual liberty and liberal autonomy as central values.

The particular interpretations of liberty and autonomy that are at the centre of bioethical reasoning, and the sort of solutions that are offered, tend to be restricted to forms of non-interference, such as providing information, often with the aim of educating or empowering people (in a neutral way). Of course, this rational choice model is common because the assumption is that those provided with this information will then go on to make the correct decision to guide their actions: their actual choices will align with the ideally rational agent. In cases where this does not happen, we are encouraged to accept the individual's choice, *because* it is their choice (even if it contrary to their interests) or to see what they choose (whatever it may be) as being, by definition, what *is* in their interests. Otherwise, we may consider the individual to be incompetent to choose, or to be lacking proper information, or suffering some other defect of reasoning that could warrant intervention (Benson, 2000; Kukla, 2006). This approach reveals that much of bioethics is undertaken with the core assumption that we can understand an agent's health-related actions and decisions as functions of individuals as a locus for consumer-oriented rational choice processes, isolated from relationships with other people, their particular social contexts, and their experiences of the burden and pain of illness (Brownell, 2010; MacKay, 2019).

The third problem in current bioethics is that of method. As we stated above, there are different ways to contest bioethical issues, and this is an important reason why there is no agreed methodology. Some work in bioethics uses philosophical methods of analysis and argumentation, with little or no discussion of relevant empirical considerations. Some of the material that uses such an approach is oriented to producing subtle and relevant ethical discussions that can help us to make better decisions and live good lives. However, such work can also, too often, be abstract and disengaged from the complexity of the relevant domain of practice. Part of the problem here is the assumption that bioethics is literally a type of *applied* ethics, where we straightforwardly apply our favourite normative moral theory in a top-down manner. Such an approach has the advantage that it can help us with deliberative reasons (it tells us, allegedly, what we should do), but it has the disadvantage that it may have nothing to say to anyone who favours an alternative normative theory. This encourages the idea of perpetual conflict between theories, locking in fragmentation and incommensurability, rather than focusing on the provision of justificatory reasons that may provide common ground. One trend in recent bioethics, within this more philosophical tradition, that provides considerable promise is an alternative idea of working bottom-up. This approach suggests that we need to understand the complexity of the particular set of issues we are seeking to explore. This pushes us to understand and engage more with the relevant empirical issues, but still allows us to use the resources of normative analysis and argumentation. On this view, we cannot just read-off the answer from our theory. We need to do the work at the level of the example, both understanding the context and providing justificatory solutions (Kihlbom, 2004).

An alternative method that has become influential over the last 20 years or so is the use of empirical methods, particularly from the social sciences, to explore bioethical questions (Ives et al., 2017). The best of this work results in bioethical discussions that are both sensitive to context but also informed by philosophically sophisticated ideas. At its worst, such work can be just a mundane and superficial description of a problem with little exploration of relevant assumptions and no normative bite. Empirical bioethics needs to articulate and justify the use of relevant empirical methods and explain how it will answer the kinds of normative research questions that drive discussions in bioethics. In addition, empirical bioethics needs to take care around the is/ought issue mentioned in the introduction to this chapter. Too often, it is left unclear how the empirical part of a project relates to the normative. It is not enough to just skip over this with a vague wave in the direction of so-called reflective equilibrium, the idea that the empirical and normative are somehow mutually supporting within a coherentist approach to epistemology (Daniels, 1996). Central issues remain around what role, if any, public attitudes may play in the formation of normative positions. It is certainly the case that public attitudes are relevant to policy formation, at least in the sense that we should not propose positions that are broadly unacceptable. However, it is quite another thing to suggest that what the majority of people think should be the case determines what we should do. Such a view requires articulation of quite a contested set of meta-ethical views. Public opinion on a topic can be used to explain policy, but it is quite another to use it to justify particular answers.

Other methodological issues include a strong current of work that focuses on solutions, pragmatics, or the practical. At its best, such work encourages us to think about the process of deliberation, which values are relevant to consider, and how we ought to make decisions in response to our bioethical issues. However, too often such approaches just ignore, consciously or not, complex but relevant philosophical issues. A good example of the problems of such solution-focused work in bioethics is the appeal of principlism, most famously presented in Beauchamp and Childress's *Principles of Biomedical Ethics* (originally published in 1979, now in its eighth edition (2019)). The attraction of such an approach, often taught in courses in health, nursing, and medicine, is that the so-called four *principles* – respect for autonomy (defined as liberal autonomy), beneficence (doing good), non-maleficence (do no harm), and justice – can be presented in a single digestible slide during a lecture about ethics. Some have also seen the four *principles* as an essential distillation of other moral theories, or indeed universal moral concepts, into a simple and intuitive framework (Gillon, 2003).

However, critics can argue that the focus on such a practical heuristic is not the answer to our bioethical issues if it just chooses to skip over relevant normative and meta-ethical disagreements. For example, are the four *principles* supposed to be seen as being of equal value (as Beauchamp and Childress claim), with decisions about priority to be assigned in response to an individual situation, or is autonomy to be given a prior and primary importance as claimed by Gillon (2003)? Or, to focus on a different issue, the four *principles* do not seem to capture all relevant values, nor do they seem well-suited to the discussion of bioethical questions outside of the limits of clinical encounters. They do not seem well-suited to helping us to deliberate about issues in public health, nor to respond to structural injustice at the level of health systems, or issues such as climate change.

In conclusion to this section, as we have seen, there are a number of problems with bioethics as it is currently conducted. In the sections that follow, we argue that other theoretical approaches such as feminist moral theory, public health ethics, and non-Western philosophical traditions all offer alternatives to the individualistic preoccupations of much current bioethics. We argue that the liberal interpretations of autonomy and liberty, so central to much bioethical reasoning, are problematic, and this troubles the arguments that bioethics offers, insofar as they rely on incomplete (or incorrect) interpretations of such values. In order to remain relevant and useful, bioethics must adapt and take seriously other, perhaps more important, values to reflect alternative perspectives on human interaction, and to capture the depth and richness of human agency and our relations with each other and the world.

Reinvigorating bioethics through reaching out to diverse alternatives

In this section, we consider some ways in which bioethics can be rejuvenated by incorporating the theory, knowledge, and perspectives of other fields of inquiry, and thereby demonstrate the richness of understanding and problem-solving that can come from using these different theoretical and conceptual tools. In this section, we will present bioethical perspectives from feminist philosophy, public health ethics, global health and ecological perspectives, and philosophical traditions from selected non-Western sources. There are many beyond these, but for reasons of space we limit our discussion to these few.

Feminist ethics

Developments within social philosophy and feminist theory have begun to guide a refocusing of bioethics, and to contribute toward developing a broader base from which to explore ethical issues. Much work within feminist philosophy begins with explaining and highlighting the situatedness or relational nature of human beings as social creatures. As humans are necessarily connected to each other and other species, for bodily and psychological wellbeing, feminist thought has focused on understanding people within their family, peer, and social networks and environments. In recognising the fundamental interconnectedness of persons, feminist moral theory has established a more complete interpretation of autonomy, widely known as relational autonomy, which highlights two important ideas (Mackenzie & Stoljar, 2000).

The first idea is that the term autonomy is a kind of master concept, which includes within it a wide array of values, skills, and capacities. Some of the procedural components have been mentioned above, such as rationality and judgement, but other substantive components include self-regarding attitudes, evaluation of one's own abilities, and confidence in making certain kinds of choices (Mackenzie, 2014; McLeod, 2002; Stoljar, 2000). As such, autonomy is something that a person develops as they grow to adulthood, learning the skills and abilities to make choices and coming to hold the sorts of attitudes that give a person confidence to make them. This takes practice in reasoning and weighing options, and it also takes coming to see oneself as the sort of person who is capable of making good choices in various circumstances.

Feminist theorists have argued that autonomy is a matter of degree and related to the particular realm of activity. One can be autonomous in some areas of one's life and not in others, and at certain times of one's life and not at others (Meyers, 1989). So, we are all less autonomous as children, and we may be less autonomous through periods of our lives that involve unemployment, illness, or injury, and we may further become less autonomous as we grow old. It is also the case that while a person could be very autonomous when it comes to making financial decisions, because they have an excellent understanding of the market and of financial risk, they may be far less autonomous when it comes to making decisions about having their car fixed, because they have very little understanding of how an engine works or how the computer in their car is programmed. As such, even as the most skilled, capable, and rational adults, there may be a variety of realms in which we are confident to different degrees in our individual ability to make good autonomous decisions.

The second idea to come from feminist bioethics is connected to the idea of autonomy as a set of skills, abilities, and attitudes; it is that one is not born an independent, rational actor, but one becomes autonomous over time. In order to accrue the capacities and skills to become autonomous, one must learn these in connection with other people. These other people will impact the degree to which one's autonomy develops, and the ways in which one feels confident employing the skills involved (Benson, 1994; Khader, 2011; Meyers, 1987). Relationships with others thus form the foundations upon which we become relatively (but never entirely) independent, autonomous agents in the world.

Relational theories of autonomy have implications for bioethical questions regarding matters like informed consent or patient decision-making. It highlights, especially, that people are not isolated decision-makers, but parts of networks that may involve multiple people in health decisions (McLeod & Sherwin, 2000). In fact, in making the most important decisions in healthcare contexts, it may be most rational to have the help of our closest friends and family, as in models of shared-decision-making. In standard discussions of autonomy in bioethics, there can be a tendency to separate the individual from important familial or friend relations in the interest of protecting the patient's autonomous decision-making. Liberal autonomy considers important interpersonal relations as possible sources of interference with the patient's supposedly real decisions or interests. Relational autonomy, on the other hand, sees these relations as a possible source of value, identity, and resilience. However, they can also be oppressive, and this approach seeks to take seriously the individual injustice within relationships (e.g. domestic violence) and the broader societal structures that deny or limit autonomy (e.g. racism, sexism, ageism, or ableism within the health system). Rather than seek to separate the individual from their network of relations, which feminist ethicists argue is impossible, we should seek to understand more about the positive and negative features of such relations and act to ensure that they are just.

Public health ethics

Within the broad sphere of bioethics, the sub-field of public health ethics can also be informative in broadening and refocusing our attention on ethical issues. Similar to those theorists working on relational autonomy, public health ethics places values like solidarity, community, sustainability, trust, and social justice, which until recently had little role in bioethics, to the fore. Such values are more social in orientation and offer a critique of the individual values of traditional bioethics, as we saw above (Baylis et al., 2008; Dawson, 2010). Solidarity and justice, for example, are concepts that inherently involve exploring ethical issues within a context of groups, communities, and societies. Bioethics, on such a view, must include more political issues about how we live with other people to further collective ends. This approach also has the advantage that we can begin to think about how ecological contexts ought to be valued and thereby involve other people, beings, and elements, and their interaction in our bioethics (Rock & Degeling, 2015) as well as values such as sustainability and consideration of our collective obligations to future generations in relation to climate change.

There are many kinds of health concerns that can only be addressed collectively, and it is specifically in the face of these kinds of issues that public health ethics can contribute important values and approaches to guide policies and collective action. An individual's health status is not merely an issue within the control of that individual. Factors such as when and where you are born, your social and economic circumstances, the opportunities and obstacles that emerge in your life, all shape your health status (Chaufan et al., 2015; Warin, 2014). If you live in a place where water and air are contaminated by pollutants, there is little you can do as an individual. Your whole life can be impacted by childhood experiences such as particulates in the air damaging your developing lungs. You may not have access to fresh fruit and vegetables due to poverty and may instead live in a country with aggressive advertising from global corporations selling you food that will impact negatively upon your health. You may live in a country with a history of racism and colonisation, and this may impact your health, as you do not have the same access to healthcare, or your community may be plagued by the trauma of children having been taken from families so that they could be "educated" and "socialised" into the dominant culture (Australian Institute of Health & Welfare, 2018). Such injustices have lasting impacts in terms of drug and alcohol misuse and mental issues, including high rates of suicide (Dawson & Silva, 2009). Mainstream bioethics is largely uninterested in such issues, and approaches such as the *principles* do not provide the resources to discuss them adequately. Such wrongs and the necessary solutions are often collective in nature and require societal mobilisation in response, not just respect for an individual's informed consent (Goldberg, 2009).

Public health uses epidemiology to attempt to explore the reasons for population-level health issues by investigating differences in groups within society (Broadbent, 2013). The focus of such work is not merely to describe the differences but then to propose ways to bring about equality for disadvantaged groups. Public health activity is motivated by trying to bring about change at the level of society, with an appeal to ideas of social justice. For example, it is important to know that tuberculosis is largely a disease of poverty, exacerbated by poor nutrition, housing, and work conditions (Selgelid, 2008). In higher-income countries those with TB are overwhelmingly migrants (through exposure prior to movement), marginalised groups such as First Nations communities, and those who are homeless. Public health ethics, as part of bioethics, focuses on such examples as a way to seek to not just discuss concepts such as solidarity and justice but also to motivate action and change. Preventing and tackling such health issues requires the active intervention of governments, pushing back against the non-interventionist paradigms that have dominated political debate for the last 40 years. Public health, and therefore public health ethics, also has an interest in exploring the idea of health promotion. This involves having a robust idea of what constitutes the nature of, and conditions for, health and seeking to provide opportunities for all to achieve this goal (Carter, 2017; Baum, 2017). On this view, health is, again, a public and collective endeavour. We flourish as individuals and communities where we work together to provide the grounds for every individual to live the life they wish to pursue.

Once inherently interpersonal or social values, such as relational autonomy or solidarity, are given greater attention in moral deliberations, it is less likely that we will fall into patterns of reasoning in which we place ourselves or our social group in isolation from others, or in positions of hierarchy with the natural world or with each other. This also encourages moral reasoning to begin from the collective or group level, to see individuals as part of a network of relations between kin, friendship, and place, rather than to begin with the individual as if they were an isolated being. Insights from feminist philosophy and public health ethics allow a shift towards a more critical bioethical investigation, and a refocusing on the kinds of questions that we ask in moral deliberation and how we should approach their solution.

Global and First Nation ethics

Just as individuals do not stand alone and unconnected, neither do nations. A globalised world raises many bioethical issues: an infectious disease can spread around the world in a matter of weeks, no country can stand against climate change alone, global capital uses supply chains shaped by bonded and slave labour, Western tobacco companies shift their marketing to low-income countries as high-income countries offer greater public health protections, etc. Action and inaction in one country has implications for others. We must respond to such issues urgently, but they have been neglected within bioethics. These are global health issues, but we can also think about how bioethics may seek a greater understanding of, and uses for, the vast range of ethical, religious, and cultural traditions from across the world. A global world need not just appeal to values derived from a limited range dominated by Western individualism and professional medical traditions. A global bioethics need not consist of an aggressively marketed US manufactured product arriving on the shelves of even the remotest parts of every other nation. Most people in the world live within more community oriented sets of values, and Western bioethics has, potentially, much to learn from such approaches. Sources of inspiration are too numerous to cover here, but we illustrate our point by saying a few brief words about two of them: some African ideas about the importance of character and Aboriginal ideas of connection.

Africa has a rich ethical tradition that is largely ignored in the West (Gyekye, 2010). Mainstream bioethics still tends to discuss issues in an African context using the usual set of individualistic values. We should take care to see African ethics as a family of theories, open to the same diversity of interpretations and variants as those of Western ethical traditions. Gyeke's summary, focused mainly on Akran thought, articulates a set of obligations related to connections with others captured by a broad idea of humanity. The focus is on developing one's character and habits in the right kinds of ways, with some striking parallels to those articulated in Aristotelian virtue ethics. The way that this is filled out means that the atomistic individualism of so much Western ethics and bioethics is challenged. Gyeke refers to an Akran art motif that represents a crocodile with two heads and one stomach. He uses this to explore the idea and importance of the common good. The two heads represent two individuals, but the single stomach emphasises the common. It is perhaps significant that this links to the idea of food and nutrition and how the securing of food and other essential goods in life often involve joint activity. The benefits to one are not divisible from benefits to others. This whole approach to ethics is one of focusing on ideas of working together, of the social and the *we*, not the *I*.

Connection is also at the heart of much Aboriginal thought (Graham, 2008). However, here the connection is not just to other humans, although that is crucial, but to all aspects of the environment. Connections exist with others through family, kinship, community, but also to ancestors, and to those to come in the future, to animals, plants, and to country. These ways of thinking have a profound metaphysical impact on connection to place and others through space and time. These links provide grounds for deep ideas of responsibility to care for the land as a shared inheritance and common resource that must be preserved for those who come afterwards (Dodson & Williamson, 1999; Behrendt, 2015). Such ideas of sustainability and the obligation to respect and live with the environment rather than treat it as a private resource to be exploited, provide inspiration for thinking about more ecological approaches to health and illness.

The point, here, is not to argue that Western bioethics should simply adopt an alternative approach to ethical thought. It is rather to see that many cultures have ways to explore and provide rich input into our common questions. There seems no good reason to ignore such alternative ways of thinking and remain locked into the dominant Western individualistic approach as if it had some higher-level value. A recent example of how non-Western ways of thinking about ethics can be a source of knowledge and a resource for everyone is provided by the reform to the Aotearoa/New Zealand research ethics framework, where Māori concepts are integrated into the national guidance for all (National Ethics Advisory Committee, 2019). Non-Western traditions can be linked to some of the more marginal concepts in current bioethics, such as the values of community, sustainability, solidarity, trust, reciprocity, and social justice. The common theme of all the critical perspectives we have reviewed in this section is connection, not difference and isolation.

Critical questioning

In this section, we present an example of how discussion of issues in bioethics can be transformed by stepping outside existing dominant bioethical approaches. New advances in health technology or research are sometimes treated as simply new opportunities for applying the same old theory or framework. However, there are many cases in which this leads to unsatisfying approaches that lack nuance and relevance and leave important power structures and relations unexamined. An approach that leaves these untouched is not fit for purpose. Bioethics must be able to, and must commit to, examining these structures and relations, and explore them using the broader resources that we outline above.

Patient data research

Some of the limitations of standard bioethics approaches (especially when applying an approach such as the *principles*) are revealed by examining developing areas of health research at the population level, such as patient data research. In the burgeoning field of data research, which makes use of patient information mined from places like clinical records, personal fitness tracking devices, internet histories, or biobanks, the values and priorities of traditional bioethics are not well-suited to provide adequate moral guidance (Ballantyne, 2019). However, bioethics is slow to adjust to new problems, and so we often see the appeal to the same values (autonomy, privacy, etc.), see the same method of crudely applying ethical principles to a new context with unsatisfying results, and tend not to get a fair appreciation for the possible benefits (e.g. pharmacovigilance, etc.) that may emerge from pooling data if relevant protections are in place.

Some of these issues are manifest in two recent guidelines for research ethics: the World Medical Association's *Declaration of Taipei on ethical considerations regarding health databases and biobanks* (WMA, 2016) and the Council for International Organizations of Medical Sciences' *International ethical guidelines for health-related research involving humans* (CIOMS, 2016). Both of these documents focused their ethical guidance for using patient data or human research participants on consent and individual control of data use. While this approach may have been satisfactory in the past, in the current context the nature of some kinds of health data, as well as some current and future uses of it, make individual consent impractical, and in some cases impossible. It is, therefore, a poor basis for policy formation (Ballantyne, 2019). For example, it may in the past have been quite straightforward in the medical research context to control a patient's health information in their medical record, to destroy certain information upon their request, or withdraw their information from the study if they withdrew consent to participate. To the degree that this was ever possible, it is no longer. A person's health data may be held in a country different from their own nation; it may be used for purposes of which they are unaware (which may still be covered by an initial consent process), and it may be impossible to destroy an individual's data if it has been aggregated into particular data sets. Further, given the complexity of this new area of research, it is unclear what an individual could reasonably be considered to consent to when it comes to the uses of their data. While an individual may consent to participate in a study based on risks or benefits to themselves, "many of the risks of secondary data use apply to communities and stakeholders rather than individual data subjects" (Ballantyne, 2019). So, consent from one person may be insufficient, even inappropriate, as it can put an entire group at risk

(Dodson & Williamson, 1999). We are then pushed to engage with more social values again and think about new structures to address these potential ethical problems.

Critiquing power structures

Shifting from traditional bioethics to a focus informed by public health ethics highlights the issues that a model based on patient autonomy in clinical encounters simply misses. For example, public health ethics has the resources to consider how the benefits and burdens of data use is distributed, how data research can (dis)empower communities, and ask questions about who holds legitimate decision-making capacity over research proposals (Esteal et al., 2020). Such questions emphasise the limited ability of traditional bioethical approaches to answer important issues related to shared interests. Ballantyne (2019) argues that a public health ethics perspective, with a focus on the values of proportionality, equity, trust, and accountability is better suited to providing answers about the ethical uses of health data. One advantage of taking a public health ethics view of questions related to data research is that we are better equipped to interrogate issues of power, justice, and equity from this perspective. Data has greater meaning and power when it is considered not just at the individual level but within the context of groups. This requires us to think about potential group benefits and harms and how new forms of protection may have to be put in place (Easteal et al., 2020; Neuhaus, 2020). Here is a place where bioethics may have to look more towards non-Western approaches to ethics, more community than individualistic approaches, for inspiration. What can bioethics learn from the ideas of collective knowledge and values present within African and First Nations perspectives? Is this a way for contemporary bioethics to step away from the tired and legalistic obsession with individualistic property rights and consent?

Conclusion

So, what sorts of questions should bioethics attend to? Bioethics should (and does) have something to say about all of the topics covered within this handbook. Bioethics has positive resources to bring to these and other questions, but it must develop beyond the traditional liberal bioethics, as it has been shaped by medical – and especially clinical – encounters. In this chapter, we argue for an understanding of bioethics as much broader than the standard set of topics (such as autonomy, consent, or privacy), as interested in more than clinical ethics or research ethics, and as more varied than an application of the *principles*.

Bioethics, when re-investigated by ideas of social connection and justice derived from feminist, public health, global, and First Nations health ethics perspectives, it can recapture its analytical bite. With a broader focus, bioethics can contribute to bigger-picture questions, rather than remaining trapped in micro-debates within the discipline. On the model of bioethical inquiry we are proposing, which is already happening in many corners of the field, bioethics becomes a practical but critical discipline. Rather than a monolith with a few set ideas about health or wellbeing, bioethics can – and should – become nimble, lively and varied, and thereby contribute to the major issues of collective action and public interest facing us all today.

References

Australian Institute of Health & Welfare. (2018). Aboriginal and Torres Strait islander stolen generations and descendants: Numbers, demographic characteristics and selected outcomes. Cat. no. IHW 195.

Canberra, ACT: AIHW. Available: https://www.aihw.gov.au/getmedia/a6c077c3-e1af-40de-847f-e8a3e3456c44/aihw-ihw-195.pdf.aspx?inline=true

Ballantyne, A. (2019). Adjusting the focus: A public health ethics approach to data research. *Bioethics, 33*(3), 357–366.

Baum, F. (2017). *The new public health* (4th ed.). Melbourne, AU: Oxford University Press.

Baylis, F., Kenny, N. P., & Sherwin, S. (2008). A relational account of public health ethics. *Public Health Ethics, 1*(3), 196–209.

Beauchamp, T., & Childress, J. (2019). *Principles of biomedical ethics* (8th ed.). New York: Oxford University Press.

Behrendt, L. (2015). Happiness born of connectedness lifts up Aboriginal Australians. *The Conversation Australia*. 24 June. https://theconversation.com/happiness-born-of-connectedness-lifts-up-aboriginal-australians-42896

Benson, P. (1994). Free agency and self-worth. *Journal of Philosophy, 91*(12), 650–668.

Benson, P. (2000). Feeling crazy: Self-worth and the social character of responsibility. In Mackenzie, C., & Stoljar, N. (Eds.), *Relational autonomy: Feminist perspectives on autonomy, agency, and the social self* (pp. 72–93). Oxford: Oxford University Press.

Broadbent, A. (2013). *Philosophy of epidemiology*. Basingstoke: Palgrave Macmillan.

Brownell, K. D., Kersh, R., Ludwig, D. S., Post, R. C., Puhl, R. M., Schwartz, M. B., & Willett, W. C. (2010). Personal responsibility and obesity: A constructive approach to a controversial issue. *Health Affairs, 29*(3), 379–387.

Carter, S. M. (2017). Ethics and health promotion. In S. R. Quah (Ed.), *International encyclopedia of public health* (2nd ed.) (pp. 1–6). Oxford: Academic Press.

Chaufan C., Yeh, J., Ross, L., & Fox, P. (2015). You can't walk or bike yourself out of the health effects of poverty: Active school transport, child obesity, and blind spots in the public health literature. *Critical Public Health, 25*(1), 32–47.

Christman, J. (2018). Autonomy in moral and political philosophy. *The Stanford encyclopedia of philosophy (Spring 2018 Ed.)*, Edward N. Zalta (Ed.). https://plato.stanford.edu/archives/spr2018/entries/autonomy-moral

Council for International Organizations of Medical Sciences. (2016). *International ethical guidelines for health-related research involving humans*. Geneva: World Health Organisation.

Daniels, N. (1996). *Justice and justification: Reflective equilibrium in theory and practice*. New York: Cambridge University Press.

Dawson, A. (2010). The future of bioethics: Three dogmas and a cup of hemlock. *Bioethics, 24*(5), 218–225.

Dawson, A., & Silva, D. (2009). Suicide prevention: A task for public health? *Journal of Public Mental Health, 8*(3), 4–6.

Dodson, W., & Williamson, R. (1999). Indigenous peoples and the morality of the human genome diversity project. *Journal of Medical Ethics, 25*(2), 204–208.

Eckenwiler, L. (2018). Displacement and solidarity: An ethics of place-making. *Bioethics, 32*(9), 562–568.

Easteal, A., et al. (2020). Equitable expanded carrier screening needs Indigenous clinical and population genomic data. *American Journal of Human Genetics, 107*(2), 175–182.

Gillon, R. (2003). Ethics needs principles – four can encompass the rest – and respect for autonomy should be "first among equals". *Journal of Medical Ethics, 29*, 307–312.

Goldberg, D. S. (2009). In support of a broad model of public health: Disparities, social epidemiology and public health causation. *Public Health Ethics, 2*(1), 70–83.

Graham, M. (2008). Some thoughts about the philosophical underpinnings of Aboriginal worldviews. *Australian Humanities Review, 45*, 181–194.

Gyekye, K. (2010). African ethics. *The Stanford encyclopedia of philosophy (Fall 2011 Ed.)*. Edward N. Zalta (Ed.). https://plato.stanford.edu/archives/fall2011/entries/african-ethics/ (Accessed: 13/12/20).

Hume, D. (1978 [1739]). *A treatise on human nature* (2nd ed.). Edited by Selby-Bigge, L. A., & Nidditch, P. H. Oxford: Oxford University Press.

Ives, J., Dunn, M., & Cribb, A. (2017) *Empirical bioethics: Theoretical and practical perspectives*. Cambridge: Cambridge University Press.

Kant, I. (1996 [1797]). *The metaphysics of morals*. Trans. M. Gregor. Cambridge: Cambridge University Press.

Khader, Serene. (2011). *Adaptive preferences and women's empowerment*. New York: Oxford University Press.

Kihlbom, U. (2004). Guidance and justification in particularistic ethics. *Bioethics, 14*(4), 287–309.

Kukla, R. (2006). Ethics and ideology in breastfeeding advocacy campaigns. *Hypatia, 21*(1), 157–180.

MacKay, K. (2019). Reflections on responsibility and the prospect of a long life. *Public Health Ethics*, *12*(2), 130–132.

Mackenzie, C. (2014). Three dimensions of autonomy: A relational analysis. In A. Veltman & M. Piper (Eds.), *Autonomy, oppression, and gender* (pp. 15–41). New York: Oxford University Press.

Mackenzie, C., & Stoljar, N. (2000). *Relational autonomy: Feminist perspectives on autonomy, agency, and the social self*. Oxford: Oxford University Press.

McLeod, C. (2002). *Self-trust and reproductive autonomy*. Cambridge, MA: MIT Press.

McLeod, C., & Sherwin, S. (2000). Relational autonomy, self-trust, and health care for patients who are oppressed. In C. Mackenzie & N. Stoljar (Eds.), *Relational autonomy: Feminist perspectives on autonomy, agency, and the social self* (pp. 259–279). Oxford: Oxford University Press.

Meyers, D. T. (1987). Personal autonomy and the paradox of feminine socialization. *Journal of Philosophy*, *84*(11), 619–628.

Meyers, D. T. (1989). *Self, society, and personal choice*. New York: Columbia University Press.

Mill, J. S. (2015 [1859]). *On liberty* (2nd ed.). Edited by Philp, M., & Rosen, F. Oxford: Oxford University Press.

National Ethics Advisory Committee. (2019). National ethical standards for health and disability research and quality improvement. Wellington: New Zealand Ministry of Health. Available: https://neac.health.govt.nz/national-ethical-standards-health-and-disability-research-and-quality-improvement (Accessed: 13 December 2020).

Neuhaus, C. (2020). Does solidarity require "all of us" to participate in genomics research? *Hastings Center Report*, *50*(S1), S62–S69.

Potter, V. R. (1971). *Bioethics: Bridge to the future*. Englewood Cliffs, NJ: Prentice-Hall.

Rock, M., & Degeling, C. (2015). Public health ethics and more-than-human solidarity. *Social Science & Medicine*, *129*, 61–67.

Ross, W. D. (1954). *Kant's ethical theory*. Oxford: Clarendon Press.

Selgelid, M. J. (2008). Ethics, tuberculosis and globalization. *Public Health Ethics*, *1*(1), 10–20.

Smith, M. J. (2015). Health equity in public health: Clarifying our commitment. *Public Health Ethics*, *8*(2), 173–184.

Stoljar, N. (2000). Autonomy and the feminist intuition. In C. Mackenzie & N. Stoljar, (Eds.), *Relational autonomy: Feminist perspectives on autonomy, agency, and the social self* (pp. 94–111). Oxford: Oxford University Press.

Veatch, R., & Guidry-Grimes, L. (2019). *The basics of bioethics* (4th ed.). New York: Routledge Press.

Voigt, K. (2010). Smoking and social justice. *Public Health Ethics*, *3*(2), 91–106.

Warin, M. (2014). Material feminism, obesity science and the limits of discursive critique. *Body & Society*, *21*(4), 48–76.

World Medical Association. (2016). *Declaration of Taipei on ethical considerations regarding health databases and biobanks*. Revision October 2016. Taipei, Taiwan. https://www.wma.net/policies-post/wma-declaration-of-taipei-on-ethical-considerations-regarding-health-databases-and-biobanks/

21

DIGITAL HEALTH

Benjamin Marent and Flis Henwood

Overview

This chapter provides an up-to-date overview of the current state of knowledge about how digital technologies are embedded within practices of health and illness. This is a vast field that has grown exponentially over the last 40 years and is located within and across a range of disciplines (health informatics, sociology, science and technology studies (STS), and media studies) that are more or less critical in focus. Any overview must therefore be very selective and clear in its goals. Our own work sits at the boundary of medical sociology and STS (Henwood & Marent, 2019) and explores digital technologies as embedded in practices of healthcare. This provides the framework for our overview and critique here.

We start by presenting an overview of four broad areas of digital health practice that have emerged since the 1980s – telemedicine, eHealth, mHealth, and algorithmic medicine – to give a sense of the heterogeneity now associated with the term "digital health". Second, we reflect on the normative arguments and imaginaries through which digital health has gained momentum as a new phenomenon. In the third section, we offer a brief overview of some key overarching social theories that have sought to explain the growth of the "information", "network", or "digital" society and explore two examples of what are often considered to be important societal level implications of the emergence of digital health – the growth of a "health data economy" and threats to "health data privacy". In the final section, we introduce the more empirically-driven socio-technical approaches to studying digital health, especially those which emphasise the importance of avoiding generalised accounts of the implications of digital health technologies and instead focus on understanding the situated character of digital health, including the specificities of technologies, relationships, and embedding environments. We illustrate the value of these approaches through our analysis of three central aspects of digitalisation: quantification, connectivity, and instantaneity. Using a socio-technical lens, we illustrate how these are associated with the (re)configuration of knowledge about health and illness, relationships between patients and healthcare professionals, and practices of providing or engaging in care and we highlight the continued ambivalences associated with digital health, across a range of situated practices.

The selection of issues and approaches covered in this chapter is necessarily limited and partial, but our aim is to capture a sense of the current state of the "field" of digital health research that is produced and read by critical social scientists, in particular.

Digital health practices – From telemedicine to algorithmic medicine

In this section, we identify and introduce four broad areas of digital health practice that have emerged since the 1980s – telemedicine, eHealth, mHealth, and algorithmic medicine. Although presented as analytically separate and somewhat temporal, they overlap both empirically and temporally and, together, may be understood as constituting the current field of digital health. Here, we aim, simply, to give a sense of the heterogeneity that characterises the field of digital health and of the broad questions and concerns being raised by critical social scientists examining the field. Later sections explore more specific configurations of digital health and the conceptual and social issues they raise.

Telemedicine

In the 1980s, the implementation of personal computers and early videoconferencing technologies converged to enable the emergence of telemedicine, which supported healthcare at a distance. Early telemedicine applications were designed to enable communication between health professionals to facilitate clinical care in remote communities and/or in the context of rare conditions where specialist input was needed but not locally available (Finch, Mort, Mair, & May, 2008; May, Finch, Mair, & Mort, 2005). Later applications supported remote doctor–patient consultations and even remote monitoring practices – usually of chronically ill people living at home – that have come to be referred to as "telecare". For example, Oudshoorn's study of telecare in the context of people with heart disease showed how electrocardiogram (ECG) recorders are worn at home by patients to diagnose heart-rhythm irregularities with results being monitored remotely by telecare workers (Oudshoorn, 2012). Telemedicine and telecare might therefore be seen as increasing access to health services for patients living in remote areas and as supporting those living with chronic diseases to have greater autonomy and independence. However, these new practices of remote care also fundamentally reconfigure not only the spaces of care but the nature of care work and the responsibilities for care, having implications for professionals, patients and carers. In teleconsultations, the doctor and patient are no longer in physical proximity and the sensory richness of mutual perception, often experienced in face-to-face consultations, may be significantly reduced. Therefore, telecare involves multifaceted invisible work by professionals and patients with both being required to establish new practices to articulate and identify symptoms and concerns and to create intimacy and good relationships at a distance (Håland & Melby, 2015; Oudshoorn, 2008). Furthermore, these new forms of digitally mediated care do not simply liberate the patient from the clinic but may actually be experienced as bringing the clinic into the home in ways that may be disrupting or invading patients' everyday lives (Oudshoorn, 2011; Pols, 2012).

eHealth

The introduction of the World Wide Web in the 1990s made health information potentially more accessible for patients and citizens and offered new forums and platforms for sharing health and illness experiences. Health information websites like healthline.com attract many millions of visitors per month, and social media sites like Facebook, YouTube, or Twitter have become important platforms for people to exchange health experiences. eHealth researchers have investigated how the internet is used to access and share health information and services online. Early research in this area explored the challenges faced by different social groups accessing health information and highlighted the resources and competences that are needed in order to navigate, evaluate and negotiate different sources and types of knowledge and avoid the reproduction of health inequalities via digital inequalities (Wathen, Wyatt, & Harris, 2008). Another related strand of eHealth research examined how the new information landscape, whereby medical knowledge had "e-scaped" from its traditional boundaries (Nettleton, 2004), provided a challenge to medical authority that could lead to the recalibration of traditional doctor–patient relationships and its inherent asymmetries (Hardey, 1999; Kivits, 2009; Ziebland & Wyke, 2012). While health information may well provide a rich source for patients to actively negotiate their treatment, empirical research over many years suggests a wide range of potential possibilities here. Trust has been shown to remain an important factor in determining if, where, and how patients access and use health information sourced online and health professionals have also been shown to act, and react, differently to the challenges of the new health information landscape (Renahy, Parizot, & Chauvin, 2008; Stevenson et al., 2019). For example, Stevenson et al. (2019) highlighted how some general practitioners used the internet to check information during consultations while others translated online health information to offer more detailed explanations to patients or signposted them towards resources or self-help outside the consultation. Another strand of eHealth research has drawn attention to the ways in which dominant interests come to shape how health information is portrayed and disseminated by the internet. For example, Lupton (2018a) outlines how search engines like Google can manipulate their software and algorithms to privilege some type of health information over others, especially where companies pay to have their website up-front in search returns. Critical research like this has led scholars to argue that the new information environment raises questions not only about the skills and competencies needed by individuals to become "informed patients" and good neo-liberal citizens, but also about the more critical engagement with the politics of health information needed for the emergence of more active "health e-citizens" (Henwood, Carlin, Guy, Marshall, & Smith, 2010).

mHealth

The notion of mHealth is quite recent and signifies health practices that rely on mobile technologies such as sensors and geolocation devices (e.g. Fitbit or Apple Watch), smart textiles, and smartphone applications. These technologies are often worn on the body (mobile), connected to other digital devices and media (interactive), and allow instant access from any location (ubiquitous). By such characteristics, these technologies have the potential to monitor bodies, analyse the development of health conditions and promote healthy behaviour, on the move. Personal activity trackers and smartphone apps allow individuals to keep a record of everyday activities (e.g. sleep, physical activities, nutrition intake) and are therefore often seen as facilitating self-care for specific chronic conditions, such as diabetes (e.g. record glucose levels in the blood) or HIV care (e.g. record treatment adherence). mHealth technologies have made biomedical data collection easier, leading to arguments that self-tracking is increasingly becoming ordinary and mundane (Pink, Sumartojo, Lupton, & Heyes La Bond, 2017). The often-claimed "power" of mHealth relies in the logic of quantification by which fitness targets or health behaviours can be visualised by simple graphs or colours and cross-referenced and benchmarked with peers or population groups. Furthermore, people engaging in self-tracking often aim to discover correlations, for example, by comparing their sleep with their running performance. Lupton (2016) has elaborated different modes by which people engage in self-tracking – it can be done as a private activity to enhance self-awareness and improve one's life, or, communally, with people sharing their data with others on social media in order to experience themselves as part of a community. In many cases, there is a push for self-tracking from external agencies such as governments, employers, or insurance companies (see also: Pols, Willems, & Aanestadt, 2019; Till, 2018) that have an interest in healthier citizens or employees and/or in viewing and using participants' personal data. Lupton's (2016) "exploited self-tracking" indicates a mode where personal health data is overtly or covertly collected and commercialised by external agencies such as marketing companies that have an interest in harvesting or selling consumer data.

Algorithmic medicine

Recent advances in computing have seen an increasing capacity for the production, storing, and sharing of data – often referred to as the era of "big data", which, in a health context, has led to the claims that we are seeing a "datafication of health" (Ruckenstein & Schüll, 2017). In this environment, algorithms, which have the capacity to filter, sort, and process data and automate reasoning, have been regarded as the main drivers that will revolutionise medicine (Obermeyer & Emanuel, 2016). The production and use of big health data sets in the fields such as genomic biobanks (Petersen, 2019, Chapter 3) or reproductive medicine (van de Wiel, 2019) require novel technologies such as predictive analytics and machine learning. In the context of reproductive health and embryo selection, van de Wiel (2019) outlined how embryologists' manual appraisals of embryos *in vitro* are being displaced by a new "*in silico* vision". This builds on visual information produced through time-lapse embryo imaging and uses algorithmic analysis to correlate data with temporally and spatially disperse embryo cohorts in order to predict embryo viability. What van de Wiel refers to as an "algorithmic way of seeing" has penetrated many areas of healthcare, where algorithms are used to predict and diagnose risks of diseases within individuals or population groups and to select or implement treatment regimens. Other examples are the World Health Organisation's mhGAP-IG algorithm that has been implemented on a global scale to enable non-specialists to diagnose mental health disorders (Mills & Hilberg, 2019) and an algorithmic-based "virtual trainer", implemented in a physiotherapy context in Denmark (Schwennesen, 2019). These forms of algorithmic medicine may reconfigure the ways in which medical knowledge is produced and social relations are shaped.

The four broad areas of digital health practice we have proffered above are intended to be neither chronological nor necessarily empirically separate from one another – telemedicine and telecare applications are increasingly mobile, with ambulatory monitors, internet connections, and GPS technologies enabling telecare beyond the confines of the home; health information searching and health community building can just as easily be undertaken on a smartphone while on the move as while sitting at a laptop or desktop in the home or office. Later, we explore some of the more specific configurations of digital health, but first we want to draw attention to another context within which such developments need to be understood – the normative claims and promissory discourses that tend not only to generalise about the likely impact of digital health developments but also help constitute the field of digital health itself.

The promissory discourse of digital health

Great claims have been made about medicine facing its "Gutenberg moment" (Topol, 2015), a revolution driven by the novel digital health practices outlined above. Digital health technologies are widely advocated by policymakers (European Commission, 2014; Topol, 2019; WHO, 2016) as a solution to the complex challenges facing healthcare systems across the developed countries in the aftermath of the economic crisis (De Vogli, 2011), the ageing population (Rechel et al., 2013), and the rise of chronic diseases (Holman, 2005). The "sociology of expectations" literature (Brown & Michael, 2003) provides a useful lens through which to reconstruct the ways in which digital health and new ventures in technology development gain momentum through promissory discourses. In government health and digital policies as well as in associated research and innovation policies, the notions of telemedicine, eHealth, mHealth, and algorithmic medicine are often used as part of what Pickersgill (2019) calls "performative nominalism". Pickersgill outlines how the articulation of neologisms, along with the explicit or implicit extolment of specific virtues and expectations, contributes significantly towards the constitution of purportedly novel fields of medical practice that are often vested with interests in expanding professional projects or commercial markets. We argue that "digital health" is a case in point (Henwood & Marent, 2019). Below, we outline two key arguments that are mobilised in support of digital health to encourage and support the utilisation of digital technologies in healthcare. The *utilitarian argument* underlines the potential of digital technologies to increase the efficiency, effectiveness, and quality of health services, while the *empowerment argument* highlights the opportunities that digital technologies create for citizens and patients to participate in their own care.

The utilitarian argument

From a utilitarian perspective, digital technologies are seen as a way to increase the efficiency, effectiveness, and quality of health services. We can illustrate this through discussion of our EU-funded "Research and Innovation" project, EmERGE (emergeproject.eu), where an mHealth platform for HIV care has been developed, implemented, and evaluated across five clinical sites in the EU (Marent, Henwood, Darking, & EmERGE Consortium, 2018a, 2018b; Marent, Henwood, & EmERGE Consortium, 2021). The platform is being implemented as part of a "reduced visit pathway" that, it is expected, will increase efficiency for clinics while facilitating greater self-management for patients. The platform offers patients a smartphone application where they can access test results along with messages from clinicians, as well as information about medications and appointments. This digital care pathway is seen as a more convenient and efficient way for stable HIV patients to receive routine care as it reduces the number of visits to the clinic. Furthermore, by receiving reminders for medication intake and notification for health-related appointments, patients are expected to improve their treatment adherence, thereby increasing the effectiveness of care. For doctors, who analyse and push blood test results, messages, and prescriptions (encrypted and without identifiable information) through a clinical web application to patients' smartphones, this new pathway is expected to increase efficiency via leaner and more flexible workload allocation, including fewer appointments for stable patients and more time with patients with complex needs.

Many critical digital health scholars have outlined how digital technologies cannot be understood as simple solutions to current health challenges. Socio-technical approaches, which we will introduce in more detail below, have been adopted to better reveal the heterogeneity and complexity of "technologies-in-practice" (Henwood & Marent, 2019; Lupton, 2018b; Petersen, 2019). In the case of the EmERGE platform, introduced above, the reduction of face-to-face visits embedded within the new care pathway was not experienced by all as quality improvement. Patients, particularly those who were socially isolated, often experienced their face-to-face visits as a meaningful opportunity not just to collect blood test results but to discuss these alongside broader issues such as engaging in intimate relationships or managing emotions (Marent et al., 2018a; Marent et al., 2021). Both clinicians and patients may resist the adoption of mHealth applications that, despite being seen as efficient in the use of resources, may nevertheless be perceived as a threat towards their understanding of what counts as "good care".

The empowerment argument

The empowerment argument claims that digital technologies provide patients and citizens with personal health data and timely feedback by which they can gain a better understanding of their medical condition and are better placed to manage and participate in their health (Flores, Glusman, Brogaard, Price, & Hood, 2013; Swan, 2012; Topol, 2015). Thus, according to Swan (2012, p. 108), novel digital technologies will lead to a paradigm shift and towards an emancipated patient who is thinking: "My health is my responsibility, and I have the tools to manage it". Such promissory expectations that emphasise the emergence of informed, activated, and connected patients have been deconstructed by critical digital health studies as part of "techno-utopian" discourses that ignore social and political dimensions that are part of how people engage with digital technologies (Lupton, 2013; Petrakaki, Hilberg, & Waring, 2018). For example, such promissory expectations ignore how digital health technologies may act as "inscription devices" (Latour & Woolgar, 1979) that reify medical conditions in a particular way. In the case of the EmERGE mHealth platform, introduced above, specific biomedical measures like viral load and CD4 come to define what constitutes HIV health, while less attention is given to the importance of experiential knowledge and peer-support. While such technologies may increase a particular form of knowledge and place some patients in a better position to negotiate their treatment with healthcare professionals, it also has to be recognised that some population groups, often those with poorer health as well as poorer health and information literacy, will be excluded. In particular, the empowerment argument often ignores the importance of the material resources (e.g. owning a smartphone or other digital device), competencies (e.g. digital literacy) and knowledge (e.g. understanding of medical measures) that are needed to better self-manage one's health. Therefore, digital health developments may contribute to further entrenching disadvantages amongst vulnerable groups who are less likely to access and benefit from advances in digital technologies.

In the next section, we introduce key theoretical approaches that challenge promissory discourse, both at the societal level and at the level of practice.

Challenging promissory discourse – "Societal implications" and "socio-technical practices"

The promissory discourse of digital health has been challenged at two levels. At the societal level, social theory has focused on the disruptions caused by the increasing use of digital technologies sometimes mirroring promissory discourse, at least in their generalisations and implicit technological determinism. In more empirically-driven theories at the practice level, challenges seek to move away from overarching claims, including the language of promises and threats, to examine situated digital health practices in ways that can offer more nuance regarding the intersection of digital technologies and healthcare in specific environments.

The societal implications of digital health

In societal level theories, the introduction of new digital technologies has been conceptualised not as a solution to facilitate information exchange or a way to empower individuals but as an evolutionary stage with disruptive societal consequences. Technological innovations in data processing, digital networks, and opportunities for instantaneous information exchange have been understood as creating an epochal shift, leaving the modern industrial era behind (Luhmann, 2012), and giving rise to a new "network" society (Castells, 2011) or an "information" age (McLuhan, 1994). These theories have made important contributions to our understanding of how digital data and digital connections, which are increasingly present, come to influence cultural forms and ways of reasoning (Luhmann, 2012), societal power structures (Castells, 2011) and media ecologies (McLuhan, 1994). The increasing ubiquity of digital technologies is considered to have broad societal implications in terms of distributions of power and inequalities, capitalisation of economic interests, and the penetration of personal privacy. Such societal level implications can be illustrated by reference to two interrelated aspects of the emergence of digital health – the growth of a "health data economy" and threats to "health data privacy".

Health data economy

The heterogeneous practices of tracking physical activities (e.g. via Fitbit), submitting saliva samples for analysis to a personal genome database (e.g. via 23andMe), or sharing patient experiences online (e.g. via PatientsLikeMe.com) provide digital platforms with potentially huge amounts of data that may be transformed into new kinds of value as platforms sell this data to technology, pharmaceutical, advertising, and insurance companies who then use the data to create consumer profiles, calculate cost-benefit analyses, or generate predictive health scores, generating further market value. For this reason, van Dijck and Poell (2016) have argued that understanding the operation of digital health platforms involves understanding processes of both "datafication" and "commodification". Furthermore, while digital platforms are based on business models that aim to transform personal data into financial commodities, critical scholars have argued that such business models are often hidden on platform websites by being overlaid by a normative discourse that seeks to persuade people to donate and upload their personal data either for personal gain (for example, via personalised and fine-grained overviews of their state of health), or for the good of society at large (by outlining how the resulting "big data" can transform and improve health research, education and care provision for society as a whole) (Lupton, 2014; Sharon, 2018; Van Dijck & Poell, 2016). The "public service" benefit promises are powerfully illustrated by text on the website of the genetic testing platform 23andMe:

> We are building a powerful, diverse, and ever-growing *resource for research* that combines advances in genetic analysis with the power of the Internet … So when you send in that DNA sample, you're not only learning about yourself, you're *joining a community of motivated individuals* who can *collectively impact research* and basic human understanding.
> *(23andMe Core Values, quoted and emphases added*
> *in van Dijck & Poell, 2016)*

In their detailed analysis of three different health platforms, van Dijck and Poell have outlined how terms like "sharing", "communities", and "partners" are used to attract and convince people to provide their data. Others have pointed to how, by collecting and uploading their data onto such platforms, individuals engage in "digital labour" that is largely unpaid and invisible in this new health data economy (Lupton, 2018b) and how restrictions on the use of such data and products are creating a new "big data divide" (Andrejevic, 2014) between large commercial interests who have access to and control over data flows and individual citizens who provide the data in the first place but do not have access. Moreover, platforms such as 23andMe do not provide enough transparency about how data is sold or reused by contracting partners.

Health data privacy

The increased collection and sharing of health data within and across digital platforms has also given rise to discussions about the implications for privacy and security. Recent incidents of data breaches and scandals gave rise to strong public concerns regarding the utilisation of cloud computing and big data in health. In England, for example, the care.data programme was launched by the NHS to collect and store patient data from GPs around the country in a central database with the aim of improving health services and outcomes (Carter, Graeme, & Dixon-Woods, 2015). The initiative triggered strong public debate regarding data privacy and the involvement of commercial interests. Patients were particularly concerned about the NHS' ambition to sell its big data sets to commercial entities. These entities were expected to apply data mining methods and data profiling that could create potential for the re-identification of anonymised data. Due to these strong public reactions, the programme had to be abandoned in 2016. Such examples highlight the importance of implementing basic principles of informed consent, data governance, and quality and data security to build public trust and transparency regarding the use of health data (Blasimme, Fadda, Schneider, & Vayena, 2018; Jacobs & Popma, 2019). However, these mechanisms become extremely stretched in a digital environment. Informed consent requires informing people about the consequences of providing their data, about data uses and protection measures, and about options to erase data. The big data environment challenges informed consent practices as it is difficult to make up-front decisions on possible future uses of data. This requires new procedures that enable case-by-case deliberations alongside the various potential uses of data (Blasimme et al., 2018). By data mining and profiling through the combination of diverse data sets, very detailed and sensitive information about individuals can be revealed (Lupton, 2018b). This requires increased investments in data protection where innovations in advanced cryptography and blockchain technology could be used to streamline data sharing and traceability and reduce risks of data breaches and misuse (Blasimme et al., 2018).

While these broad and often very general accounts of the societal transformation brought about by digitalisation are important for stimulating thinking and identifying areas for further research, they have been criticised for implying a more or less subtle form of technological determinism – reading off from the functionalities of technologies to the likely social implications.

Socio-technical approaches to digital health practices

A second and different approach to challenging promissory discourse has been offered by more empirically-driven theories at the practice level. These seek to move beyond universalising claims – whether promises or threats – and examine, instead, situated cases of digital health practices that can offer more nuance regarding the intersection of digital technologies and healthcare in specific environments.

Scholars working within science and technology studies have, for many years, pointed out that the "social" cannot be separated or read off from the "technical" and instead have pointed to the mutually constitutive relationship between technology and the social (Bijker, Hughes, Pinch, & Douglas, 1987). From this perspective, technologies have "interpretive flexibility" as they develop and become embedded in different contexts of use with different social groups using technologies in different ways, leading to multiple variations and ongoing reconfigurations of "technologies-in-practice". In more recent, posthumanist, accounts of the socio-technical, the unit of analysis is the relational and heterogeneous practices that are formed of assemblages of human and non-human actors (see, for example, actor-network-theory (Latour, 2005) and new materialism (Barad, 2007; Fox & Alldred, 2016)). The emphasis of these theories is on the "performativity" of the socio-technical assemblages. Below, we illustrate the value of socio-technical approaches through our analysis of three central aspects of digitalisation: quantification, connectivity, and instantaneity. Using a socio-technical lens, we illustrate how these are associated with the (re)configuration of healthcare practices in three dimensions – knowledge about health and illness, healthcare interactions, and new forms of control enabled through instant feedback and alerts. We highlight how such approaches can help avoid universalising claims about digital health developments and highlight the continued ambivalences associated with digital health, across a range of situated practices.

Quantification and the reconfiguration of knowledge

The long-standing debate about digital health and the emergence of a new information and knowledge environment, discussed under "eHealth" above has, in recent years, become much more focused on quantification and the implications of this for how knowledge is configured in specific health practices. An obvious example here is the body of research generated in response to the growth of the quantified self movement (Schüll, 2016; Sharon, 2017). Smartphone apps, smartwatches, personal activity trackers (e.g. Fitbit), or smart textiles that have inbuilt sensors and geolocation functions that can produce a detailed and, as many argue, "objective" portrait of the user. These are powerful technologies because they make data collection as simple and mundane as never before and they use specific visualisation tools to indicate whether intended targets in terms of hours of sleep or walked steps have been reached (Pink et al., 2017). They also enable users to cross-reference and to benchmark their performance with peers and friends and allow for the discovery of correlations, for example, between sleep patterns and running performance. However, while the functionalities of these "self-tracking" devices are crucial to understanding the new practices that may emerge around them, they do not determine such outcomes in any straightforward way. Socio-technical accounts, often focusing on user engagement with such devices, have shown that data will often be incomplete – either "broken" and requiring "repair work" (Pink, Ruckenstein, Willim, & Duque, 2018) or simply "partial" as users are often inconsistent in their collection and recording of self-monitoring data (Weiner, Will, Henwood, & Williams, 2020). Quantified data have also been conceptualised as "lively" because they are continuously shifting and recombining their meanings across different assemblages and life situations. Thus, from a socio-technical lens, we can question the circumstances and relationships in and through which data become insightful or not and what forms of knowledge about ourselves and our bodies are eclipsed by digital data.

In the EmERGE project (introduced earlier) that focused on using digital technologies to self-manage HIV (Marent et al., 2018a), we found that the years since diagnosis with HIV and the relative stability of the HIV condition was central to understanding how users felt about having access to quantified data. In the case of newly diagnosed and unstable HIV conditions, direct access to numbers (before consulting a clinician) was associated with bringing anxiety and uncertainty into care practices because patients were unable to make sense of strong fluctuations of numbers due to their unstable medical conditions. Experienced and stable HIV patients, on the other hand, were confident in reading blood test results and having access to historic overviews of the development of medical parameters was seen as a way to increase knowledge about one's condition, leaving them feeling more in control of their own condition and care.

Critical scholars have also highlighted how quantified health data are, by necessity, produced through reductive and normative means and may render the understanding of health and the body in specific ways (Lupton, 2018b; Sharon, 2017). In particular, the new obsession with "objective" data has been criticised for undermining people's awareness of the haptic sensations of their bodies which may lead to a reductionist understanding of the self and its complex health conditions (Maturo & Setiffi, 2016; Rich & Miah, 2016).

Digital connections and shifting relationships

Close face-to-face interactions, where professionals become acquainted with patients and apply their abstract knowledge in concrete ways, have traditionally been considered central to medical practice (Abbott, 1988). Being in each other's physical proximity, doctors and patients find themselves accessible to their naked senses (Goffman, 1983). The intimacy of the consultation room creates an empirically rich space for experiencing visual body language, human voice, touch, and smell, which is of central importance to conduct examination and consultation. This interaction order is also constituted through a concurrent time frame, where doctors and patients are simultaneous present and can coordinate their activities through immediate reciprocity. This spatiotemporal ordering of doctor–patient interactions is significantly reconfigured through digital technologies and new forms of mediated interactions involved, but the specificities of the technologies, relations and embedding environments are central to understanding these reconfigurations. This can be illustrated by comparing two different cases- the EmERGE case of HIV care, already introduced, and the case of digitally mediated diabetes care (Piras & Miele, 2019).

Through the EmERGE platform (Marent et al., 2021), digital connectivity was designed as facilitating only asynchronous communication where blood test results are analysed by clinicians and sent directly to patients, together with a reassuring message or, where there were concerns, a request to call the clinic. Clinicians were ambivalent about the loss of synchronicity here. On the one hand, it allowed them for more flexibility and better coordination of their work practices – for example, fewer interruptions as the need for routine phone calls to deliver results was eliminated. On the other hand, the asynchronous mode of communication embedded in the new platform and care pathway was experienced as restricting opportunities for reciprocity, something patients also mentioned. Clinicians were uncertain whether a message has been received and appropriately understood by patients and patients were frustrated that the app did not allow them to send questions back to clinicians. Both patients and clinicians argued that "real" conversations and immediate reciprocal communicative accounts enabled them much better to gain a feeling of how utterances have been understood. Particularly urgent and complex health issues required immediate reciprocity and patients and clinicians both outlined how they moved from the asynchronous platform to synchronous modes of interactions (like phone calls or face-to-face visits to the clinic) to negotiate and deliberate such issues.

In a contrasting case, a digital health platform created more opportunities to facilitate reciprocity and connections. In their study of digitally mediated diabetes care, Piras and Miele (2019) found that digital connections can generate new forms of digital intimacy through the continuity of care (in-between clinic visits) and by complementing abstract medical knowledge with an exchange of personal messages that allowed clinicians to better understand the life situations and condition of their diabetes patients. This was facilitated by the design of the platform that, unlike the EmERGE case, allowed two-way communication in a rather unstructured form. The remote monitoring in this case was experienced as fostering greater intimacy between patients and care providers and as increasing both the quantity and quality of communication.

Instantaneity and the reconfiguration of control

Digital technologies often confront us with instantaneity and the potential for new real-time relations. Self-tracking devices, for example, can provide immediate feedback during and between exercises and activities, confronting users with their current running pace, and sending alerts about dietary targets or medication reminders. Through notifications on the screen or via sounds and/or vibrations, digital devices can be set to attract the user's immediate attention that may then lead them to outsource control over the accomplishment of health tasks, such as taking or ordering medications and booking appointments. In the case of the EmERGE app, we found that certain health practices were reconfigured as attentive responses to prompts from the digital device (Marent et al., 2018a). Self-care and health no longer occupied a clearly demarcated space in the temporal structuring of everyday life (e.g. person takes medications as part of a morning routine) but, rather, were accomplished as "layered simultaneity" alongside other social activities. For example, a person is at work while the smartphone app buzzes with a medication reminder; the reminder gains immediate attention and is followed by action, whereby the tablet is taken, and, subsequently, the work is continued. The socio-technical assemblages formed in such human–technology interactions create ambivalence regarding the question of whether they bring forth active patients/citizens that take control over their health, or, conversely, create passive patients/citizens that are being controlled by the technical device (Marent et al., 2018a).

In a different case, Lomborg and colleagues (2018), conducting qualitative research with self-trackers in the context of exercise and mood tracking, demonstrated how the instantaneous feedback offered via tracking devices was akin to having a personal coach that takes over the responsibility for monitoring and supports users in accomplishing health tasks and targets. However, as they also observed, users' attachment to such temporal tracking regimes, especially when combined with overly frequent and negative feedback, could be experienced as a distraction and a source of frustration.

Exploring the temporal flows within socio-technical assemblages offers a fruitful lens for observing the control and regulating mechanisms that individuals operate on and to which they are subjected. The control projects facilitated through socio-technical assemblages may come with benefits and risks. They may liberate the individual from the burden of information storage and produce a cognitive agility to exploit opportunities within specific situations (Serres, 2014), but they can also create dependencies, negative experiences, and unhealthy practices. In this way, Schwennesen (2019) outlined how algorithmic systems, assisting in conducting physiotherapy, needed to be creatively adjusted and repaired by its users in order to enable a productive relationship between the system and the body exercising and performing therapeutic sessions. In cases where users followed the system too rigidly, they overstrained some muscles and were training too much. Critical to engaging in distributed forms of control in socio-technical assemblages might be a continuous switch between engagement and disengagement, or, in the words of Michel Foucault (2007, p. 45), a mode of reflexivity that can be simply called "the art of not being governed quite so much".

Conclusion

Digital health is a fast-moving field of research. The current COVID-19 pandemic, in particular, has contributed to a rapid increase in the utilisation of digital health technologies for accessing health information and care providers (Hollander & Carr, 2020). It will be crucial to understand how these new interactional forms between doctors and patients, which are now becoming so widely adopted, may reconfigure roles and relationships and understandings of what constitutes "good care". The socio-technical approach, outlined in this chapter, offers promising avenues to investigate how new ways of knowing (saturated by quantified data), reciprocity (afforded by digital connections) and temporality (shaped by instantaneous algorithmic calculations) are enacted in digital health practice.

It is also important, however, to recognise that practices are shaping and being shaped by wider material and social structures. This has been illustrated in this chapter by the discussion of the health platform economy, which exploits new business models and market principles for growth and expansion. Platform organisations have developed comprehensive strategies to capture consumer data and commodification mechanisms that help transform almost any "behavioural surplus" (from tracking a run through Fitbit to liking a post on Instagram) into economic value (Zuboff, 2019). The underlying business models and flows of data remain largely opaque and raise significant concerns regarding the public values at stake. How do health platforms and apps protect privacy? How do they contribute to equality in health and treatment? How do they enable informed consent regarding the reuse of citizens' data? These questions necessitate the development of new governance frameworks that guide the value-centric design of the emerging platform society (Van Dijck, Poell, & de Waal, 2018). Such governance frameworks need to go beyond the focus on specific digital health devices and address the wider platform ecosystem, because the infrastructure upon which digital health operates is largely owned by a few big technology companies who run search engines (Google), cloud spaces (Amazon), app stores (Apple) and operating systems (Microsoft).

The term "digital health" captures a range of diverse and complex socio-technical practices and therefore needs to be understood as far more than a set of technological solutions to particular health problems or tools to bring about efficient healthcare provision. Digital health raises critical issues concerning how knowledge, relationships and control are reconfigured in specific use contexts and can inspire social scientists to engage with public stakeholders in both better understanding of these contexts and in co-designing appropriate models and pathways for future care delivery.

References

Abbott, A. (1988). *The system of professions: An essay on the division of expert labor.* Chicago, IL: University of Chicago Press.

Andrejevic, M. (2014). The big data divide. *International Journal of Communications, 8*, 1673–1689.

Barad, K. (2007). *Meeting the universe halfway: Quantum physics and the entanglement of matter and meaning.* Durham, NC: Duke University Press.

Bijker, W. E., Hughes, T. P., Pinch, T., & Douglas, D. G. (1987). *The social construction of technological systems: New directions in the sociology and history of technology.* MIT Press.

Blasimme, A., Fadda, M., Schneider, M., & Vayena, E. (2018). Data sharing for precision medicine: Policy lessons and future directions. *Health Affairs, 37*(5), 702–709.

Brown, N., & Michael, M. (2003). A sociology of expectations: Retrospecting prospects and prospecting retrospects. *Technology Analysis & Strategic Management, 15*, 3–18.

Carter, P., Graeme, L. T., & Dixon-Woods, M. (2015). The social licence for research: Why care. Data ran into trouble. *Journal of Medical Ethics, 41*(5), 404–409.

Castells, M. (2011). *The rise of the network society. The information age: Economy, society, and culture* (2 ed. Vol. 1). Oxford: John Wiley & Sons.

De Vogli, R. (2011). Neoliberal globalisation and health in a time of economic crisis. *Social Theory & Health, 9*(4), 311–325.

European Commission. (2014). *Green paper on mobile health (mHealth).* Retrieved from http://ec.europa.eu/digital-agenda/en/news/green-paper-mobile-health-mhealth

Finch, T. L., Mort, M., Mair, F. S., & May, C. R. (2008). Future patients? Telehealthcare, roles and responsibilities. *Health & Social Care in the Community, 16*(1), 86–95.

Flores, M., Glusman, G., Brogaard, K., Price, N. D., & Hood, L. (2013). P4 medicine: How systems medicine will transform the healthcare sector and society. *Personalized Medicine, 10*(6), 565–576.

Foucault, M. (2007). What is critique? In S. Lotringer (Ed.), *The politics of truth* (pp. 42–82). Los Angeles, CA: Semiotext(e).

Fox, N. J., & Alldred, P. (2016). *Sociology and the new materialism: Theory, research, action.* SAGE.

Goffman, E. (1983). The interaction order. *American Sociological Review, 48*(1), 1–17.

Håland, E., & Melby, L. (2015). Negotiating technology-mediated interaction in health care. *Social Theory & Health, 13*(1), 78–98.

Hardey, M. (1999). Doctor in the house: The Internet as a source of lay health knowledge and the challenge to expertise. *Sociology of Health & Illness, 21*(6), 15.

Henwood, F., Carlin, L., Guy, E. S., Marshall, A. M., & Smith, H. (2010). Working (IT) out together: Engaging the community in e-health developments for obesity management. In R. Harris, C. N. Wathen, & S. Wyatt (Eds.), *Reconfiguring health consumers: Health work and the imperative of personal responsibility.* Basingstoke: Palgrave Macmillan.

Henwood, F., & Marent, B. (2019). Understanding digital health: Productive tensions at the intersection of sociology of health and science and technology studies. *Sociology of Health and Illness, 41*(S1), 1–15. doi:10.1111/1467-9566.12898

Hollander, J. E., & Carr, B. G. (2020). Virtually perfect? Telemedicine for COVID-19. *New England Journal of Medicine, 382*(18), 1679–1681.

Holman, H. R. (2005). Chronic disease and the healthcare crisis. *Chronic Illness, 1*(4), 265–274.

Jacobs, B., & Popma, J. (2019). Medical research, Big Data and the need for privacy by design. *Big Data & Society.* doi:10.1177/2053951718824352

Kivits, J. (2009). Everyday health and the internet: A mediated health perspective on health information seeking. *Sociology of Health & Illness, 31*(5), 673–687. doi:10.1111/j.1467-9566.2008.01153.x

Latour, B. (2005). *Reassembling the social: An introduction to actor-network-theory.* Oxford: Oxford University Press.

Latour, B., & Woolgar, S. (1979). *Laboratory life: The construction of scientific facts.* Princeton, NJ: Princeton University Press.

Lomborg, S., Thylstrup, N. B., & Schwartz, J. (2018). The temporal flows of self-tracking: Checking in, moving on, staying hooked. *New Media & Society, 20*(12), 4590–4607.

Luhmann, N. (2012). *Theory of society* (R. Barrett, Trans. Vol. 1). Stanford, CA: Stanford University Press.

Lupton, D. (2013). The digitally engaged patient: Self-monitoring and self-care in the digital health era. *Social Theory & Health, 11*(3), 256–270.

Lupton, D. (2014). The commodification of patient opinion: The digital patient experience economy in the age of big data. *Sociology of Health & Illness, 36*(6), 856–869. doi:10.1111/1467-9566.12109

Lupton, D. (2016). The diverse domains of quantified selves: Self-tracking modes and dataveillance. *Economy and Society, 45*(1), 101–122.

Lupton, D. (2018a). Digital health and health care. In G. Scambler (Ed.), *Sociology as applied to health and medicine.* London: Palgrave.

Lupton, D. (2018b). *Digital health: Critical and cross-disciplinary perspectives.* New York: Routledge.

Marent, B., Henwood, F., & EmERGE Consortium. (2021). Platform encounters: A study of digitised patient follow-up in HIV care. *Sociology of Health & Illness.* Doi 10.1111/1467-9566.13274

Marent, B., Henwood, F., Darking, M., & EmERGE Consortium. (2018a). Ambivalence in digital health. Co-designing an mHealth platform for HIV care. *Social Science & Medicine, 215*, 133–141.

Marent, B., Henwood, F., Darking, M., & EmERGE Consortium. (2018b). Development of an mHealth platform for HIV care: Gathering user perspectives through co-design workshops and interviews. *JMIR mHealth and uHealth, 6*(10), e184.

Maturo, A., & Setiffi, F. (2016). The gamification of risk: How health apps foster self-confidence and why this is not enough. *Health, Risk & Society, 17*(7–8), 477–494.

May, C., Finch, T., Mair, F., & Mort, M. (2005). Towards a wireless patient: Chronic illness, scarce care and technological innovation in the United Kingdom. *Social Science & Medicine, 61*(7), 1485–1494. doi:10.1016/j.socscimed.2005.03.008

McLuhan, M. (1994). *Understanding media: The extensions of man.* Cambridge, MA: MIT Press.

Mills, C., & Hilberg, E. (2019). "Built for expansion": The "social life" of the WHO's mental health GAP Intervention Guide. *Sociology of Health and Illness, 41*(S1), 162–175.

Nettleton, S. (2004). The emergence of E-scaped medicine? *Sociology, 38*(4), 661–679.

Obermeyer, Z., & Emanuel, E. J. (2016). Predicting the future – big data, machine learning, and clinical medicine. *New England Journal of Medicine, 375*(13), 1216–1219.

Oudshoorn, N. (2008). Diagnosis at a distance: The invisible work of patients and healthcare professionals in cardiac telemonitoring technology. *Sociology of Health & Illness, 30*(2), 272–288.

Oudshoorn, N. (2011). *Telecare technologies and the transformation of healthcare*: Palgrave Macmillan.

Oudshoorn, N. (2012). How places matter: Telecare technologies and the changing spatial dimensions of healthcare. *Social Studies of Science, 42*(1), 121–142.

Petersen, A. (2019). *Digital health and technological promise: A sociological inquiry*. Abingdon: Routledge.

Petrakaki, D., Hilberg, E., & Waring, J. (2018). Between empowerment and self-discipline: Governing patients' conduct through technological self-care. *Social Science & Medicine, 213*, 146–153.

Pickersgill, M. (2019). Digitising psychiatry? Sociotechnical expectations, performative nominalism and biomedical virtue in (digital) psychiatric praxis. *Sociology of Health and Illness, 41*(S1), 16–30. doi: 10.1111/1467-9566.12811

Pink, S., Ruckenstein, M., Willim, R., & Duque, M. (2018). Broken data: Conceptualising data in an emerging world. *Big Data & Society, 5*(1), 2053951717753228.

Pink, S., Sumartojo, S., Lupton, D., & Heyes La Bond, C. (2017). Mundane data: The routines, contingencies and accomplishments of digital living. *Big Data & Society, 4*(1), 2053951717700924.

Piras, E. M., & Miele, F. (2019). On digital intimacy: Redefining provider-patient relationships in remote monitoring. *Sociology of Health and Illness, 41*(S1), 116–131.

Pols, J. (2012). *Care at a distance: On the closeness of technology*. Amsterdam: Amsterdam University Press.

Pols, J., Willems, D., & Aanestadt, M. (2019). Making sense with numbers. Unraveling ethico-psychological subjects in practices of self-quantification. *Sociology of Health and Illness, 41*(S1), 98–115.

Rechel, B., Grundy, E., Robine, J.-M., Cylus, J., Mackenbach, J. P., Knai, C., & McKee, M. (2013). Ageing in the European union. *The Lancet, 381*(9874), 1312–1322.

Renahy, E., Parizot, I., & Chauvin, P. (2008). Health information seeking on the Internet: A double divide? Results from a representative survey in the Paris metropolitan area, France, 2005–2006. *BMC Public Health, 8*(69). doi:10.1186/1471-2458-8-69

Rich, E., & Miah, A. (2016). Mobile, wearable and ingestible health technologies: Towards a critical research agenda. *Health Sociology Review, 26*(1), 84–97.

Ruckenstein, M., & Schüll, N. D. (2017). The datafication of health. *Annual Review of Anthropology, 46*, 261–278.

Schüll, N. D. (2016). Data for life: Wearable technology and the design of self-care. *Biosocieties, 11*(3), 317–333.

Schwennesen, N. (2019). Algorithmic assemblages of care: Imaginaries, epistemologies and repair work. *Sociology of Health and Illness, 41*(S1), 176–192.

Serres, M. (2014). *Thumbelina: The culture and technology of millennials*. Lanham, MD: Rowman & Littlefield.

Sharon, T. (2017). Self-tracking for health and the quantified self: Re-articulating autonomy, solidarity, and authenticity in an age of personalized healthcare. *Philosophy & Technology, 30*(1), 93–121.

Sharon, T. (2018). When digital health meets digital capitalism, how many common goods are at stake? *Big Data & Society*. doi:10.1177/2053951718819032

Stevenson, F., Hall, L., Sequin, M., Atherton, H., Barnes, R., Leydon, G., … Ziebland, S. (2019). General practitioner's use of online resources during medical visits: Managing the boundary between inside and outside the clinic. *Sociology of Health and Illness, 41*(S1), 65–81. doi:10.1111/1467-9566.12833

Swan, M. (2012). Health 2050: The realization of personalized medicine through crowdsourcing, the quantified self, and the participatory biocitizen. *Journal of Personalized Medicine, 2*(3), 93–118.

Till, C. (2018). Self-tracking as the mobilisation of the social for capital accumulation. In B. Ajana (Ed.), *Self-tracking. Empirical and philosophical investigations*. Basingstoke: Palgrave Macmillan.

Topol, E. (2015). *The patient will see you now: The future of medicine is in your hands*. New York: Basic Books.

Topol, E. (2019). *The Topol Review: Preparing the healthcare workforce to deliver the digital future*. Leeds, UK: Health Education England. Retrieved from https://topol.hee.nhs.uk/.

van de Wiel, L. (2019). The datafication of reproduction: Time-lapse embryo imaging and the commercialisation of IVF. *Sociology of Health and Illness, 41*(S1), 193–209.

Van Dijck, J., & Poell, T. (2016). Understanding the promises and premises of online health platforms. *Big Data & Society, 3*(1), 2053951716654173.

Van Dijck, J., Poell, T., & de Waal, M. (2018). *The platform society. Public values in a connective world*. Oxford: Oxford University Press.

Wathen, C. N., Wyatt, S., & Harris, R. (Eds.). (2008). *Mediating health information: The go-betweens in a changing sociotechnical landscape*. Basingstoke: Palgrave Macmillan.

Weiner, K., Will, C., Henwood, F., & Williams, R. (2020). Everyday curation? Attending to data, records and record keeping in the practices of self-monitoring. *Big Data & Society*, 71(1), 1–15.

WHO. (2016). *FROM INNOVATION TO IMPLEMENTATION eHealth in the WHO European region*. Copenhagen: WHO Europe.

Ziebland, S., & Wyke, S. (2012). Health and illness in a connected world: How might sharing experiences on the internet affect people's health? *Milbank Quarterly*, *90*(2), 219–249.

Zuboff, S. (2019). *The age of surveillance capitalism: The fight for a human future at the new frontier of power*. London: Profile Books.

22

MIGRATION AND HEALTH

Heide Castañeda

Far back enough in time, we are all migrants. Migration is part of what it is to be human, with population movements shaping the globe throughout the history of our species; it is a fundamental impulse to seek out better living conditions, whether that means safety and security, adequate resources, or a healthier environment. Yet migration has become a defining global issue of the 21st century, despite the fact that the proportion of the world's migrants has remained relatively consistent over the past three decades at around 3%. The scale and pace have been accelerated by globalisation and technology, while economic inequalities, political conflicts, natural disasters, and environmental change have caused more people to leave their homelands. As a result, migrations are now much more frequent, more rapid, and to more distant places. We are currently witnessing the highest ever-recorded number of international migrants at 258 million, a rapid 49% increase from 173 million at the turn of the century (UN, 2017). If we include internal migration, the number rises to more than 1 billion migrants worldwide, or one in seven people. And of course, the impacts of migration reach beyond this figure to include millions more, as families and wider transnational social networks are separated by borders, and labour markets become increasingly entangled within the wider global political economy (Thomas, 2016).

Thus, while migration is a usual, frequent, and patterned part of the human experience, it is far from "natural". To gloss over the root causes of population movements is an injustice to the people affected by them. Some of the highest levels of forced displacement on record are occurring, with 65.3 million people leaving their homes worldwide. Approximately 21.3 million are refugees, and 10 million are stateless (UNHCR, 2017). Globally, people continue to be displaced by various combinations of violence, choice, and circumstance, challenging the conventional relationship between "voluntary" migrants, who choose to cross borders in search of opportunity, and "involuntary" migrants, who are forced to flee in search of physical security. Even those who move voluntarily generally do so because economically violent circumstances have obstructed life chances for them and their families. Thus, rather than easily characterised as either voluntary or involuntary, the causes of migration are complex and fall along a spectrum (Yarris & Castañeda, 2015).

Global patterns of inequality produce migration and also impact the experiences of migrants in host countries. Social and institutional contexts shape individuals' lives in relation to employment, housing and living conditions, access to food, social isolation, and legal status, with consequences for overall wellbeing. Indeed, patterns of morbidity and mortality follow inequities rooted in conditions produced and reproduced by political economy, such as social structures, policies, and institutions. How we frame the origins and reasons for migration has enormous social and policy implications. When migration is viewed as unusual or even pathological, assumptions are carried over into policy and research practice. If migration is viewed as an expected and necessary response to various forms of violence, it can result in the development of equitable policies to address disparities. This response requires a recognition that the global patterns of inequality fostering migration are not based on cultural difference, but are instead rooted in social, political, and economic conditions produced and reproduced by laws and institutions.

The impact of migration on health is a growing concern worldwide and is increasingly recognised as a global public health priority (Wickramage et al., 2018). However, the relationship between migration and health remains poorly understood. Migration does not always introduce a threat to health; there are opportunities and risks to wellbeing present at the same time. What appears at the outset to be a bidirectional relationship quickly becomes entangled with other aspects of social and political conditions. In order to understand health, we must understand the large-scale social and political forces that impact migrants, including global inequality, political instability, economic insecurity, and climate change (Holmes and Castañeda, 2016).

A critical approach to migrant health focuses on social determinants and particularly how inequality, poverty, institutional constraints, and violence contribute to health disparities. This focus requires us to, first, understand the structural reasons behind people's displacement, and second, recognise the processes of institutional, economic, and political marginalisation that continue after they arrive in a new country. Inequities in the wellbeing of migrants are heavily determined by factors such as exclusionary policies, discrimination and racism, employment in marginal and dangerous jobs, the high cost of healthcare, inadequate housing, and poor access to transportation and other resources. These conditions often emerge from assumptions regarding the root causes of migration, which shape ideas about how deserving of incorporation into the host society a particular immigrant group should be.

The pandemic of SARS-CoV2 (the novel coronavirus that causes COVID-19) has shown us the degree to which health across the world is interconnected. As it unfolded, it highlighted how existing social and economic conditions as well as political decision-making based on nationalist, xenophobic principles rather than public health data can produce unprecedented death and destruction. COVID-19 abruptly halted the movement of people and goods via border shutdowns and travel restrictions implemented by hundreds of countries, some of which barred entry to anyone who is not a citizen or permanent resident, while others suspended the entry of people from certain regions of the world. Thus, in the future the various scales of human, economic, and disease mobility will remain an important area of focus, along with the borders that selectively open and close to them.

Who is a migrant? The importance of terminology

One of the most pressing issues in the world today, migration is frequently referred to as a "crisis". This alarmist framing often provokes extreme political responses and sensationalist media attention. Over the last decade, for instance, the European Union has received unparalleled numbers of migrants, refugees, and asylum seekers, leading some to describe it as a "global migration magnet" (Czaika & Haas, 2014). In other host countries, especially the United States, people speak of a "surge" or "flood" of migrants entering the country, especially via the southern border with Mexico. In the media and in politics, we hear of migration from Africa, the

Middle East, and Latin America described as "swarms," "hordes", and "marauders", and this is not coincidentally occurring at the same time as the rise of isolationist nationalism in many places such as including the United States, Britain, Netherlands, Austria, Italy, and Germany (Lee et al., 2018). These framings serve to produce public and political anxiety and as well as regular "border spectacles" (De Genova, 2017).

Thus, we must begin with the understanding that terminology matters a great deal in discussions on migrant health, and the framing of causes of mobility impacts how a host country views and receives immigrants. While definitions of migrant status vary substantially, the International Organization for Migration defines a migrant as,

> An umbrella term, not defined under international law, reflecting the common lay understanding of a person who moves away from his or her place of usual residence, whether within a country or across an international border, temporarily or permanently, and for a variety of reasons.
>
> *(International Organization for Migration, 2019, p. 132)*

The term, in other words, encompasses a variety of legal categories, including migrant workers, particular types of movements, such as smuggled persons, as well as persons whose movement is not specifically defined under international law, such as students.

Yet migration is not a singular activity but involves a complex set of variables, including different forms of entry and legal status (permanent legal resident, temporary work visa, undocumented), different intentions of settlement (permanent vs. temporary), temporal mobility patterns (seasonal movement of farmworkers vs. continued residence in a single location). As a result, there is a variety of definitions across scholarship. Terms like "migrant" and "im/migrant" (in contrast to "immigrant") explicitly acknowledge this diversity and complexity, and allow us to "problematize the implicitly unilinear teleology of these categories" (De Genova, 2002, p. 420–421), particularly from the perspective of the migrant-receiving societies

The position is similar for those with uncertain legal status. Here I utilise the term "undocumented" when referring to migrants living in a country without legal authorisation, as opposed to irregular, extralegal, unauthorised, or clandestine, all of which are precise in their own ways and in particular contexts. Our attentiveness – and especially to the condition of "illegality" – should not result in constructing people as "passive and agency-less subjects overdetermined by structural conditions, or undocumentedness as a homogeneous and undifferentiated experience" (Sigona, 2012, p. 51). It would be an injustice if we did not also show the ways that people adapt routines and mundane social interactions to the circumstances of their precarious lives.

Another important consideration is: Who, exactly, is considered a refugee? According to the 1951 Convention relating to the Status of Refugees, a refugee is someone who,

> owing to a well-founded fear of persecution for reasons of race, religion, nationality, membership of a particular social group or political opinion, is outside the country of his nationality and is unable or, owing to such fear, is unwilling to avail himself of the protection of that country; or who, not having a nationality and being outside the country of his former habitual residence as a result of such events, is unable or, owing to such fear, is unwilling to return to it.
>
> *(International Organization for Migration, 2019, p. 132)*

But is only someone facing political persecution a "true" refugee, in contrast to those seeking economic opportunity? Some advocate eliminating the distinction between "economic" and "political" refugees in order to highlight the causes of displacement globally, especially national and supranational economic policies, through an explicitly anticolonial perspective (Wright, 2003). At the same time, it is important to consider the impacts of conflating refugees and asylum seekers with other kinds of migrants. While conflating refugees and unauthorised migrants indeed highlights the role of structural economic violence, it can obscure the fact that refugees and asylum seekers generally have some (limited but guaranteed) access to healthcare, in contrast to unauthorised persons. This distinction is crucial in understanding the distribution of rights and resources. Health outcomes across immigrant groups vary by route of entry, impacting experiences during the immigration process and degrees of access to health services in the host country after arrival (Giuntella et al., 2018). In addition, the indiscriminate use of the term "refugee" can further delegitimise the unique forms of suffering for those who had experienced forced migration due to political violence.

It is also important to recognise the intersectional nature of the migrant experience with regards to socio-demographic factors (e.g. gender, race, sexual orientation, etc.) in addition to varied experiences across the lifecourse. This allows for critical insight into "the processes that create and reinforce indicators of social stratification, and the ways that health-related opportunities as well as injustices and inequalities are enacted on a multidimensional basis" (Thomas, 2016, p. 5). In some cases, migration status is conflated with other forms of difference, especially when referencing communities of colour (e.g. those inhabited by racial or ethnic minorities). Despite living there for generations, in some countries, certain ethnic, religious, or tribal groups are still perceived to be "foreign" migrant communities (Lee et al., 2018). The children of immigrants, in particular, have long held a tenuous place in various countries, and are often racialised in a way that they are characterised as perpetual foreigners, even if they are citizens, since whiteness is often the unspoken master narrative about citizenship and belonging. In the United States, for instance, citizen children of immigrants have been derided as "anchor babies" or treated as "suspect citizens" (Chavez, 2017) constructed as a racial threat to the nation. Young Latinos may experience belonging as "citizens, but not Americans" (Flores-González, 2017). Their everyday experiences (including spatial segregation, microaggressions, and anti-Latino rhetoric) belie their status as citizens, underscoring the persistent role of race in notions of belonging to this imagined community. Mae Ngai describes this experience as that of "alien citizens" – that is, citizens by birth but whose immigrant ancestry renders their status as citizens dubious – as they are cast as perpetual foreigners (Ngai, 2014). In Germany, second-, third-, and even fourth-generation individuals born in Germany but with Turkish heritage experience similar exclusions. It is important to recognise that categories used to differentiate between groups of people for a thorough analysis of health inequalities or access barriers are socially constructed and often reproduce "othering" discourses (Wenner et al., 2019). Legitimacy depends on changing and historically produced notions of relative deservingness and emulates distinctions made between citizens and various kinds of "others" in different national settings (Willen, 2010).

Thus, it is important to ask the question: when does a migrant cease to be a migrant and become a "native", or a "citizen"? At the same time, we must recognise that these may be artificial boundaries, since even "natives" or "citizens" may be socially cast as foreigners, particularly if they or their family have any migrant background at all. In addition, in many places we are seeing the rise of mixed-status families, which contain varied constellations of citizens, permanent legal residents, undocumented immigrants, and individuals in legal limbo. All this is to say that it is not facile to draw such lines between migrant and non-migrant, and the disparities they may experience in the forms of inequality, poverty, and institutional constraints still impact health.

Understandably, most scholarly approaches to migration (and especially migrant health) presumes they are disadvantaged in comparison to citizens of the host country. However, we must also acknowledge that not all migrants are poor, disadvantaged, or the targets of discriminated. In many cases – and for a variety of reasons, including dissonance of health understandings or distrust in a different healthcare system – migrants keep ties and engage with health systems and care practices in their country of origin. For instance, Korean migrants to New Zealand may travel to their homeland to obtain medical procedures, based on preferences for decisive and comprehensive treatment in culturally comfortable settings (Lee et al., 2010). Similarly, Mexican migrants in the United States are often able to cross the border and use their earnings to visit private doctors and clinics in Mexico. These medical returns not only provide them access to care that is familiar and viewed as more effective, but also allowed enabled class transformation, as migrants transitioned from poor rural peasants to cash-paying "returning royalty" in their home country (Horton, 2014).

Finally, it is imperative to remember that the term "migrant" usually represents an identity imposed from the outside – by the researcher, the media, or by society at large. Many people identify first and foremost with other characteristics of their lives as lived on a daily basis: mother, daughter, student, artist, engineer, Muslim, neighbour, and so forth. By considering their primary point of reference to be migration status, we create and endorse superficial and reductive identities and perpetuate narratives that reinforce social barriers. Instead, it is important to recognise and reinsert their agency in discussions of their lives, including those that focus on health.

A critical approach to migrant health

Critical perspectives on migrant health have their roots in the tradition of social medicine. Developed in the wake of the industrial revolution in response to increased levels of disease and poverty among its workers, this approach focuses on the socioeconomic conditions affecting health, illness, and the practice of medicine. This critical approach emerges from larger theoretical traditions in the social sciences and is located within a set of broader frameworks and concepts for understanding the effects of social inequality. This perspective challenges us to interrogate assumptions, understand what is socially constructed, and be more precise about how we define the impact of immigration on health or when we are using migration status as a proxy for other social dynamics, such as inequality, marginalisation, or racism.

Being a migrant is not in itself a risk to health; certain vulnerabilities have first to exist. A critical framing of the issue of migrant health focuses on the social origins of illness and the context that precedes them, and particularly how inequality, poverty, institutional constraints, and violence contribute to health disparities. Framing migration as a public health issue may be a bold claim for those who espouse a narrow view of the prevention of disease (Wild & Dawson, 2018). However, a broader, critical approach focuses on the structural factors determined by social and economic policies and institutional contexts that foster unequal effects on health.

Several fields have related theories, models, frameworks, and vocabulary that highlight these issues. Critical public health approaches include a range of overlapping concepts for understanding and responding to the effects of social inequality, including social epidemiology, the eco-social or socio-environmental perspective, eco-epidemiology, and the risk environment framework. A focus on social inequalities can be explored through fundamental social causes, social determinants of health, webs of causation, higher-order causal-level structural factors, upstream factors, and racial disparities in health outcomes. The social sciences have contributed frameworks using political economy, structural violence, symbolic violence, structural vulnerability, syndemic vulnerability, conjugated oppression, hierarchies of embodied suffering, zones of abandonment, intersectionality, and discourses of deservingness.

These concepts have both influenced and emerged from models that focus on the social determinants of health with a focus on upstream fundamental causes, many of which are useful for examining health issues in immigrant populations and for guiding related population-level interventions. These approaches all emphasise the construction and impact of social structures and the relative positions of individuals and communities in stratified hierarchies and power relationships. In addition, these concepts share a concern with the interconnectedness of social, structural, and/or ecological factors that affect health status. The analysis of disease causation, as well as intervention strategies and policy changes to address it, requires an understanding of how social, physical, and biological phenomena interrelate and overlap. As a result, pathways and interactions are understood as multicausal and complex, requiring attention to institutional practices and to the relationships between macrostructural processes and microlevel behaviours. The concept of *syndemics* highlights mutually reinforcing sets of health, environmental, and social problems encountered by specific populations (Alexander and Fernandez, 2014). For example, diabetes has been examined as a syndemic because of its comorbidity with HIV in Kenya, tuberculosis in India, and depression in South Africa. The concept of syndemics highlights interactions between pathophysiology, the structure of healthcare systems, socioeconomic conditions, and cultural context (Mendenhall et al., 2017). These are conceptualised as processes of power that exhibit strong influence over the life chances of migrants and their families, creating obstacles to wellbeing and healthcare access.

Although immigration is a consequence of social determinants, such as poverty, occupational, and educational opportunities, and political persecution, immigration must also be positioned as a social determinant in its own right (Castañeda et al., 2015). Without this perspective, the immigration experience is cast as secondary to more proximal factors such as behaviour, language, norms, income, or education, thus limiting explanatory power and the capacity to create effective interventions that respond to some of the root causes of ill-health in these communities. The enormous consequences of immigration on daily life, and thus on broader health and wellbeing, cannot be reduced simply to a "protective factor" or an acculturative "stressor" that affects health. Rather, immigration must be understood as a broad social determinant of health and wellbeing. Examining immigration through this lens provides a more holistic approach to allow a greater understanding of these complex, interrelated, and far-reaching impacts. A narrow focus on "risk factors" and behavioural or cultural modifications uncritically assumes the unfettered agency of vulnerable populations (Castañeda et al., 2015; Quesada et al., 2011). Responding to individualistic, non-contextualised approaches requires examining the role of social inequality. Social inequality imposes specific risks and constraints on choice. This perspective offers an important corrective for superficial notions of behavioural and cultural difference that rest on static assumptions about migration choice, intergroup relations, and unidirectional advantages of assimilation.

In other words, a critical approach interprets health outcomes by understanding and accounting for the large-scale structures that impact them. More generally, we are talking about living and working conditions, income inequalities and poverty, access to care, immigration policies and enforcement practices, as well as gender, race, and ethnic hierarchies.

Methodological approaches and empirical challenges across disciplines

The study of migrant health presents challenges because migration is a non-linear and dynamic process. It can start and stop or take on circular patterns. As a result, it is not possible to rely on single measures of movement, as these metrics result in contradictory and non-comparable research findings (Vearey, 2016). Another major issue is the causal identification of interconnections with specific health issues, complicated by mechanisms such selection effects of who migrates in the first place, the role of socioeconomic and psychosocial factors, and how health impacts the experience of return. Complicating matters, surveillance systems rarely collect or disaggregate data according to migrant status. The definition of who is considered a migrant varies greatly and is often determined by national legislative, administrative, and policy factors. In addition, there is a lack of data on specific migrant groups, such as those who are undocumented.

A major challenge associated with summarising insights from multiple disciplines comes, of course, from their varied methodologies. Some studies of migrant health are analyses of national-representative surveys, utilise a cross-sectional analytic design, are randomised controlled trials, or incidence/prevalence studies. Others are primarily qualitative, including descriptive, ethnographic, and phenomenological approaches. Some use mixed methods, using embedded or triangulation designs. Furthermore, given the diversity of study types, it is not surprising that sample sizes vary considerably across the existing literature. There are some examples of research that have taken a bi- or multinational approach to understanding migrant health, though these are in the minority. There are many studies that collect primary data in border regions, but fewer conducted outside of these areas, which would add to understanding a broader range of migration experiences. As noted earlier, there is also a bias toward international rather than internal migration.

In order to account for immediate, long-term, and inter-generational impacts on health, research would ideally collect data during the different phases of migration (in the homeland, during transit, after migrating), but this is rarely possible. Instead, there is a heavy reliance on retrospective measures and self-reporting. Methodological innovation is always required.

Concepts used in migrant health

Structural violence and structural vulnerability: *Structural violence* was a concept first introduced by Johan Galtung (1969) and has been built upon by a number of scholars in fields such as medical anthropology, medical sociology, and social epidemiology to explain the processes by which the arrangement of social institutions causes harm by depriving people of resources or preventing them from reaching their potential. It is particularly useful for explaining differential health outcomes among populations as they relate to broader, macro-level social forces. Paul Farmer has argued that:

> (t)he arrangements are structural because they are embedded in the political and economic organization of our social world; they are violent because they cause injury to people ... neither culture nor pure individual will is at fault; rather, historically given (and often economically driven) processes and forces conspire to constrain individual agency. Structural violence is visited upon all those whose social status denies them access to the fruits of scientific and social progress.
>
> *(Farmer, 2001, p. 79)*

Structural vulnerability is an extension of this concept that focuses on one's location in a hierarchical social order defined by the intersection of these larger structural forces. This produces increased suffering and risk for certain diseases, reduced access to care, and poor health outcomes, as such positioning is derived from "forces that constrain decision making, frame choices, and limit life options" (Quesada et al., 2011, p. 3412). Additionally, the experiences of immigrants must also be understood as *intersectional*, since health-related opportunities as well as injustices and inequalities are enacted on a multidimensional basis dependent on factors such as gender, age, country of origin, sexual orientation, and social class (Thomas, 2016, p. 5).

"Illegality" and health: Uncertain legal status, or living as a migrant "without papers" or without a valid residency permit, represents an important factor impacting health, illness, and convalescence. The condition of "illegality", which refers to a socio-political condition, juridical status, and relationship to the state (De Genova, 2002; Ngai, 2004), has a great impact on wellbeing. The choice of terminology for this population is highly varied, including illegal, undocumented, irregular, extralegal, unauthorised, or clandestine, as well as terms such as *sans papiers* in French, *sin papeles* in Spanish, and *ohne Papiere* in German. Additionally, this concept may refer to a variety of circumstances, such as illegal entry to a host country, illegal residency following legal entry, or illegal employment. In other cases, newly rearranged national boundaries may exclude already resident groups as legitimately belonging, essentially "erasing" former identities. While some have stressed that the use of the term "illegal" implies collusion with particular hegemonic constructions, other scholars have advocated retaining the term precisely to indicate this socio-juridical status. They argue that employing the term allows us to (1) deconstruct it as the object of study itself, (2) emphasise the legal context that provides form and content to the everyday lives of migrants, and (3) investigate how this construction implicitly places migrants outside the scope and protection of the rule of law. However, our attentiveness to the condition of "illegality" must not result in constructing people as passive subjects with a homogeneous set of experiences, since people always also adapt their daily lives to the circumstances of precarity and develop a set of strategies.

Migrants without papers face health disadvantages in many nations. The condition of "illegality" influences illness experiences, medical treatment, and convalescence; this ranges from the very types of illnesses they are most likely to encounter because of living and working conditions to a lack of regular access to health services and an inability to afford necessary medications or carry out therapies. While epidemiological data on unauthorised populations in any host nation are scarce, attempts to infer morbidity patterns by examining legal migrants' health patterns result in complex and contradictory data, depending on indices, location, and population (Oropesa et al., 2015; Wenner et al., 2019). Simply put, if a person is undocumented, the social and environmental factors that increase susceptibility to illness, as well as poor access to health services, is considerably greater. Inferences from legally residing migrant populations are insufficient, because migrant illegality represents a factor with separate but largely unexplored effects (Castañeda et al., 2015).

Structural factors impacting access to healthcare

An examination of health disparities requires a careful consideration of legal status as a specific structural constraint, and often the result of the pathogenic role of social inequality. Inequality, poverty, and violence lead to disparities in income, living and working conditions, working alongside other gender, race, and ethnic hierarchies. Barriers to healthcare access for this population have been well-documented and include restrictions based on immigration/citizenship status, lack of insurance, linguistic barriers, lack of transportation, lack of affordable health services, and lack of familiarity with the health system (Castañeda et al., 2015; Quesda et al., 2011; Thomas, 2016; Wickramage et al., 2018). Eligibility for healthcare coverage, or access to state-run health services, is also significantly determined by legal status, as immigration policies and healthcare intersect at numerous junctures. However, these should not be viewed as discrete barriers but as "webs" that create more complex challenges than individual obstacles alone (Heyman et al., 2009).

In many host country settings, care for unauthorised populations is relegated to indigent and charity services, such as community clinics run by various forms of NGO. When they become ill, most unauthorised migrants end up visiting a charity clinic that offers limited services for free or on a sliding scale. The heavy reliance on NGOs and charity care in host countries demands additional attention, because they have resulted in two-tiered health systems and foster only short-term, improvisational remedies. Embedded within these structural concerns are cultural mismatches that further impede access, as in the dissonance of understandings of what constitutes health and illness between migrants and clinicians in the host society (Lawrence & Kearns, 2005). Health practitioners may be unable to sufficiently to meet the needs of migrant patients in an effective and culturally appropriate manner, and often within a limited funding environment.

In response to these limitations to healthcare, other strategies emerge. Sharing medication within the family and larger community is common. Medication practices are socially embedded phenomena, and saving, sharing, and reusing medicines is broadly practised. Sharing medications not only serves the immediate need of treating illness but also creates the obligation of reciprocity between individuals (within a family) and households (within a community), serving as an asset in conditions of scarce resources (Castañeda, 2019). However, it is problematic when, for example, a course of antibiotics is cut in half, rendering it less effective for both persons. Thus, a socially valued and pragmatic act of sharing may in fact lead to twice the negative outcomes; half of an antibiotic regimen may be worse than none at all. Other tactics include those with access to care feigning symptoms to get medicine for siblings or parents or relying on the goodwill of doctors to prescribe "a little extra". Some rely on unlicensed providers operating in the community and willing to treat people at a lower cost (Castañeda, 2019). Finally, some deal with a lack of access to adequate care by using home remedies, alternative approaches, or simply fixing medical problems on their own (Villadrich, 2018).

Precarity and insecurity

In addition to structural constraints creating differential access to resources, the stress of living in fear and insecurity because of one's liminal status is a factor contributing to illness, operating alongside broad-spectrum discrimination and the synergistic effects of class and racism. Studies on the effects of stigma and discrimination on health have focused primarily on minority groups within a single society (e.g. Stuber, Meyer, & Link, 2008), but many of these insights can be applied to the uncertain status of unauthorised migrants. Immigration status affects health though mechanisms including fear, stress, experiences of prejudice and violence, and family separation.

There is little doubt that the rise in anti-immigrant policymaking has fostered an unhealthy environment for this population. Restrictive immigration policies contribute to experiences of racism and discrimination, which are then linked to risk factors that pattern health outcomes. Undocumented immigrants and their family members experience a pervasive fear of deportation that negatively impacts their psychological, emotional, and physical health (Kline & Castañeda, 2019; Martinez et al., 2015; Rhodes et al., 2015). Prolonged and accumulated biological stress associated with persistent hyperarousal may be particularly applicable to the lives of migrants without papers, exacerbating health risks in tandem with other variables such as accessibility, affordability, and willingness to seek care (Stuber et al., 2008; Torres et al., 2018). The effects of migrant "illegality" interact syndemically (Singer, 2009) with other risk factors to increase vulnerability.

Hostile policy environments result in intense feelings of anxiety, fear, and depression, which exacerbate pre-existing health conditions such as high blood pressure and diabetes. The association between worry about the deportation of others (i.e. family members) and cardiovascular risk factors has been quantitatively measured using reference points such as BMI, waist circumference, and continuous measures of systolic and pulse pressure (Torres et al., 2018). Avoidance of health services because of fear of deportation and liminal legal status is a major result.

The physical and mental health consequences associated with heightened anti-immigrant policy environments reach beyond undocumented persons themselves, impacting others in their family and community. Members of mixed-status families – that is, where some family members, often parents, are without papers – report worse physical health compared to their citizen counterparts. Children in these families are more likely to have poor health, lack health insurance, and lack a usual source of care compared to children from non-immigrant households (Vargas & Ybarra, 2016; Yun et al., 2013). Parental immigration status is associated with lower healthcare utilisation in children, especially the legal status of the mother due to women's role as a primary care provider (Oropesa et al., 2015). Using the lens of health, it becomes clear that the "illegality" of just one person in a family can influence resources and practices for all, including legal residents and even citizens (Castañeda, 2019; Dreeby, 2015; Gomberg-Muñoz, 2016).

In recent years, the concept of *precarity* has emerged to describe the multiple forms of dispossession that some populations face as part of lived conditions under regimes of neoliberalism, including increased economic uncertainty, reduced welfare states, violence, political marginalisation, disposability, and injustice. Precarity is not simply a condition but a process built into institutions to create a heightened sense of expendability or disposability for some groups in society (Standing, 2011; Tsing, 2015). In the case of vulnerable legal status, this state of permanent vulnerability and precaritisation translates into deportability (De Genova, 2002). Precarity in relation to health is understood as increased physical and emotional vulnerability, exposure to risk, and instability.

Scholars have only recently begun to systematically measure the health impacts of deportation, including the psychosocial and health consequences for the children of immigrants (Brubeck and Xu, 2010; Chaudry et al., 2010; Gonzales, 2011; Delva et al., 2013). Children in mixed-status families frequently worry about family separation and can exhibit high levels of stress, which may lead to poor mental health (Horner et al., 2014). Scholars studying the health implications of immigration raids have found that the presence of such activities in a community led to higher levels of stress and lower self-related health scores (Lopez et al., 2017). Children whose parents have been deported or detained are more likely to experience a host of social concerns and mental health problems, including decreased school performance, depression and other internalising problems such as anxiety, and externalising problems such as aggression and conduct issues (Allen, Cisneros, & Tellez, 2015; Suárez-Orozco, Todorova, & Louie, 2002; Brabeck, Lykes, & Hunter, 2014). The impact of family separation on children's wellbeing is difficult to overstate. Watching relatives be detained or deported disrupts children's sense of ontological security, or the confidence in the constancy of one's surrounding social and material environments of action (Vaquera, Aranda, & Sousa-Rodriguez, 2017). Especially for adolescents, a parent's deportation takes an enormous emotional toll, and even the threat of deportation has been shown to affect mental health, school performance, and likelihood of experiencing poverty.

Conclusion

Migrants experience unique impacts on health due to restricted access to care, structural constraints related to inequality, poverty, and living and working conditions, as well as the stress associated with precarious legal status. While other specific axes of inequality, such as gender, are well-studied, the absence of migrants without papers in the health disparities literature is noteworthy. This is a hard-to-reach groups for researchers to study, and there is very little reliable epidemiological data for this population, with a reliance on small, local surveys that tend to record access to care rather than long-term health outcomes. These migrants are also frequently excluded precisely because they are located outside the formal system of rights accorded by citizenship and other notions of belonging. However, while some migrants share similar experiences due to their "illegality", local context impacts the everyday experience of how this shared condition is negotiated. Although epidemiological studies indicate that migrants are often among the most disadvantaged populations when it comes to health, empirical evidence also shows lower rates of service utilisation. Even in nations with universal healthcare systems, migrants generally have lower rates of utilisation and unauthorised migrants have little to no access to care.

Researchers and practitioners must be acutely attentive to issues of terminology, because they entail situating oneself in debates on migration and, often, problematising notions of "deservingness". Other specific topical areas remain understudied, such as undocumented migrants' access to expensive but lifesaving care (such as major surgeries or transplants), clinical ethics and practical decision-making by healthcare workers and administrators, unauthorised im/migration and reproductive politics, dental/oral health, and public health threats generated by the denial of healthcare to unauthorised im/migrants. As increased border control and law enforcement activities continue to increase in most host countries, health researchers must examine how migrants' "policeability" impacts health outcomes.

A critical perspective suggests fruitful areas of intervention and explicates future research needs and strategies to tackle the health inequities that affect migrants. This includes the development of "migration-aware" health systems that recognise human mobility as a central concern for care, research, and policy.

References

Alexander, W. L., & Fernandez, M. (2014). Immigration policing and medical care for farmworkers: Uncertainties and anxieties in the East Coast migrant stream. *North American Dialogue, 17*(1), 13–30.

Allen, B., Cisneros, E. M., & Tellez, A. (2015). The children left behind: The impact of parental deportation on mental health. *Journal of Child and Family Studies, 24*(2), 386–392.

Brabeck, K. M., Lykes, M. B., & Hunter, C. (2014). The psychosocial impact of detention and deportation on US migrant children and families. *American Journal of Orthopsychiatry, 84*(5), 496–505.

Brubeck, K., & Xu, Q. (2010). The impact of detention and deportation on Latino immigrant children and families: A quantitative exploration. *Hispanic Journal of Behavioral Sciences, 32*(3), 341–361.

Castañeda, H. (2019). *Borders of belonging: Struggles and solidarity in mixed-status immigrant families*. Stanford, CA: Stanford University Press.

Castañeda, H., Holmes, S. M., Madrigal, D. S., DeTrinidad Young, M.-E., Beyerle, N., & James Quesada, J. (2015). Immigration as a social determinant of health. *Annual Review of Public Health, 36*, 75–392.

Chaudry, A., Capps, R., Pedroza, J., Castañeda, R. M., Santos, R., & Scott, M. M. (2010). *Facing our future: Children in the aftermath of immigration enforcement*. Washington, DC: Urban Institute.

Chavez, L. (2017). *Anchor babies and the challenge of birthright citizenship*. Stanford, CA: Stanford University Press.

Czaika, M., & Haas, H. (2014). The globalization of migration: Has the world become more migratory? *International Migration Review, 48*(2), 283e323.

De Genova, N. (2002). Migrant "illegality" and deportability in everyday life. *Annual Review of Anthropology, 31*, 419–447.

De Genova, N. (Ed.). (2017). *The borders of "Europe": Autonomy of migration, tactics of bordering*. Duke University Press.

Delva, J., Horner, P., Martinez, R., Sanders, L., Lopez, W. D., & Doering-White, J. (2013). Mental health problems of children of undocumented parents in the United States: A hidden crisis. *Journal of Community Positive Practices*, *13*(3), 25–35.

Dreby, J. (2015). *Everyday illegal: When policies undermine immigrant families*. Berkeley, CA: University of California Press.

Farmer, P. (2001). *Infections and inequalities: The modern plagues*. Berkeley, CA: University of California Press.

Flores-González, N. (2017). *Citizens but not Americans: Race and belonging among Latino millennials*. New York: New York University Press.

Galtung, J. (1969). Violence, peace, and peace research. *Journal of Peace Research*, *6*(3), 167–191.

Giuntella, O, Kone, Z. L., Ruiz, I., & Vargas-Silva, C. (2018). Reason for immigration and immigrants' health. *Public Health*, *158*, 102–109.

Gomberg-Muñoz, R. G. (2016). *Becoming legal: Immigration law and mixed-status families*. Oxford: Oxford University Press.

Gonzales, R. G. (2011). Learning to be illegal: Undocumented youth and shifting legal contexts in the transition to adulthood. *American Sociological Review*, *76*(4), 602–619.

Heyman, J. McC., Núñez, G. G., & Talavera, V. (2009). Health care access and barriers for unauthorized immigrants in El Paso County, Texas. *Family and Community Health*, *32*(1), 4–21.

Holmes, S., & Castañeda, H. (2016). Representing the European refugee crisis in Germany and beyond: Deservingness and difference, life and death. *American Ethnologist*, *43*(1), 12–24.

Horner, P., Sanders, L., Martinez, R., Doering-White, J., Lopez, W., & Delva, J. (2014). "I put a mask on": The human side of deportation effects on Latino youth. *Journal of Social Welfare and Human Rights*, *2*(2), 33–47.

Horton, S. (2014). Medical returns as class transformation: Situating Mexican migrants' medical returns within a framework of transnationalism. *Medical Anthropology*, *32*(5), 417–432.

International Organization for Migration. (2019). *Glossary on migration*. https://publications.iom.int/system/files/pdf/iml_34_glossary.pdf

Kline, N., & Castañeda, H. (2019). Immigration enforcement policies and Latino health. In *New and emerging issues in Latina/o health*. Springer.

Lawrence, J., & Kearns, R. A. (2005). Exploring the "fit" between people and providers: Refugee health needs and health care services in Mt Roskill, New Zealand. *Health & Social Care in the Community 13*, 451–461.

Lee, A., Sim, F., & Mackie, P. (2018). Migration and health – Seeing past the hype, hysteria and labels. *Public Health*, *158*, A1–A2.

Lee, J. Y., Kearns, R. A., & Friesen, W. (2010). Seeking affective health care: Korean immigrants' use of homeland medical services. *Health & Place*, *16*, 108–115.

Lopez, W. D., Kruger, D. J., Delva, J., Llanes, M., Ledón, C., Waller, A., Harner, M., Martinez, R., Sanders, L., & Harner, M. (2017). Health implications of an immigration raid: Findings from a Latino community in the midwestern United States. *Journal of Immigrant and Minority Health*, *19*(3), 702–708.

Martinez, O., Wu, E., Sandfort, T., Dodge, B., Carballo-Dieguez, A., & Chavez-Baray, S. (2015). Evaluating the impact of immigration policies on health status among undocumented immigrants: A systematic review. *Journal of Immigrant & Minority Health*, *17*(3), 947–970.

Mendenhall, E., Kohrt, B. A., Norris, S. A., Ndetei, D., & Prabhakaran, D. (2017). Non-communicable disease syndemics: Poverty, depression, and diabetes among low-income populations. *Lancet*, *389*(10072), 951–963.

Ngai, M. (2014). *Impossible subjects: Illegal aliens and the making of modern America*. Princeton, NJ: Princeton University Press.

Oropesa, R. S., Landale, N. S., & Hillemeier, M. M. (2015). Family legal status and health: Measurement dilemmas in studies of Mexican-origin children. *Social Science & Medicine*, *138*, 57–67.

Quesada, J., Hart, L. K., & Philippe B. (2011). Structural vulnerability and health: Latino migrant laborers in the United States. *Medical Anthropology*, *30*(4), 339–362.

Rhodes, S. D., Mann, L., Simán, F. M., Song, E., Alonzo, J., & Hall, M. A. (2015). The impact of local immigration enforcement policies on the health of immigrant hispanics/Latinos in the United States. *American Journal of Public Health*, *105*(2), 329–337.

Sigona, N. (2012). I've too much baggage: The impact of legal status on the social worlds of irregular migrants. *Social Anthropology/Anthropologie Sociale*, *20*(1), 50–65.

Singer, M. (2009). *Introduction to syndemics: A systems approach to public and community health*. San Francisco, CA: Jossey-Bass.

Standing, G. (2011). *The precariat: The new dangerous class*. London: Bloomsbury.

Stuber, J., Meyer, I., & Link, B. (2008). Stigma, prejudice, discrimination, and health. *Social Science and Medicine, 67*(3), 351–357.

Thomas, F. (2016). Migration and health: An introduction. In Felicity Thomas (Ed.), *Handbook of migration and health* (pp. 3–18). Cheltenham: Edward Elgar Publishing.

Torres, J. M., Deardorff, J., Gunier, R. B., Harley, K. G., Alkon, A., Kogut, K., & Eskenazi, B. (2018). Worry about deportation and cardiovascular disease risk factors among adult women: The Center for the Health Assessment of Mothers and Children of Salinas Study. *Annals of Behavioral Medicine, 52*(2), 186–193.

Tsing, A. (2015). *The mushroom at the end of the world: On the possibility of life in capitalist ruins*. Princeton, NJ: Princeton University Press.

United Nations, Department of Economic and Social Affairs, Population Division. (2017). *International migration report 2017*.

United Nations High Commission on Refugees. (2017). http://www.unhcr.org/en-us/figures-at-a-glance.html

Vaquera, E., Aranda E., & Sousa-Rodriguez, I. (2017). Emotional challenges of undocumented young adults: Ontological security, emotional capital, and wellbeing. *Social Problems, 64*(2), 298–314.

Vargas, E. D., & Ybarra, V. D. (2016). U.S. citizen children of undocumented parents: The link between state immigration policy and the health of Latino children. *Journal of Immigrant and Minority Health, 19*(4), 913–920.

Vearey, J. (2016). Mobility, migration and generalised HIV epidemics: A focus on sub-Saharan Africa. In Felicity Thomas (Ed.), *Handbook of migration and health* (pp. 340–356). Cheltenham: Edward Elgar Publishing.

Villadrich, A. (2018). Botanicas unplugged: Latinos' religious healing and the impact of the immigrant continuum. *African Journal of Traditional, Complementary and Alternative Medicines, 15*(1), 188–198.

Wenner, J., Namer, Y., & Razum, O. (2019). Migrants, refugees, asylum seekers: Use and misuse of labels in public health research. In Krämer, A., & Fischer, F. (Eds.), *Refugee migration and health. Migration, minorities and modernity*. Springer.

Wickramage, K., Vearey, J., Zwi, A. B., Robinson, C., & Knipper, M. (2018). Migration and health: A global public health research priority. *BMC Public Health, 18*, 987.

Wild, V., & Dawson, A. (2018). Migration: A core public health ethics issue. *Public Health, 158*, 66–70.

Willen, S. S. (2010). Citizens, real others, and other others: The biopolitics of otherness and the deportation of unauthorised migrant workers from Tel Aviv, Israel. In Nicholas De Genova and Nathalie Peutz (Eds.), *The deportation regime: Sovereignty, space, and the freedom of movement*. Duke: Duke University Press.

Wright, C. (2003). Moments of emergence: Organizing by and with undocumented and non-citizen people in Canada after September 11. *Refuge, 3*(21), 5–15.

Yarris, K., & Castañeda, H. (2015). Discourses of displacement and deservingness: Interrogating distinctions between economic and forced migration. *International Migration, 53*(3), 64–69.

Yun, K., Fuentes-Afflick, E., Curry, L. A., Krumholz, H. M., & Desai, M. M. (2013). Parental immigration status is associated with children's health care utilization: Findings from the 2003 new immigrant survey of US legal permanent residents. *Maternal and Child Health Journal, 17*(10), 1913–1921.

23

MEDICAL TRAVEL

Critical perspectives

Cecilia Vindrola-Padros

Millions of people travel each year to obtain medical care abroad. People decide to engage in travel to obtain cheaper or quicker services, access treatments not available (or legal) near their home, receive a higher quality of care, more culturally appropriate care, or because they do not trust local services. Patients will travel to faraway countries, cross nearby borders, travel within their country, or region or return to their home country for care. Travel for medical services has become a global industry worth billions of dollars and currently affects most healthcare systems across the world. This chapter includes an overview of research on medical travel, outlining its main debates, contributions, and gaps. It explores medical travel from a critical perspective, unpacking power relations, global and local structures, and the (re)production of inequalities in access to care. The chapter outlines the main critical theoretical perspectives used in research to explore the processes of medical travel and identifies future areas of exploration.

Trends in contemporary medical travel

A considerable amount of research has studied medical travel under the concept of "medical tourism", yet many authors have argued that this term alludes to the temporal, elective, one-time and potentially "worry-free" nature of medical travel (Kangas, 2011; Sobo et al., 2011). It also positions patients as consumers and tends to focus primarily on the need to cross national borders to obtain care (Lunt et al., 2014). An in-depth exploration of medical travel experiences across the globe, however, points to the complex and difficult realities faced by many patients who need to seek care away from home, the loss of employment, financial difficulties, feelings of homesickness, and family separation that the need to travel for treatment demands (Kangas, 2007; Vindrola-Padros & Brage, 2017). Medical travel has been proposed as a more "value free" way of thinking about and studying this type of travel (Sobo, 2011). This is the term that will be used throughout the chapter to refer to medical tourism, cross-border care, return tourism, and internal medical travel.

It was estimated that in 2012, almost 1.6 million US patients sought medical services in another country (Keckley & Underwood, 2009), and Thailand reported delivering care to over 1 million patients from the US and Europe per year (Department of Export Promotion, Ministry of Commerce, in Pachanee, 2009). The flows of patients have diversified to include travel from the Global South to the Global North, and vice-versa, as well as North to North and South to

South travel. An increase in intra-regional medical travel (travel within defined regions such as US patients crossing the border to Mexico, Western Europeans travelling to Eastern European countries, and hospitals in Thailand delivering care to patients from neighbouring countries such as Vietnam, Burma, and Cambodia (Cohen, 2010; Lunt et al., 2014)), and even intra-national medical travel (travel within countries) has been documented.

Although economic factors exert some level of influence over patients' decision to travel and their travel destination, empirical research on patients' decision-making processes has indicated that there are a wide range of reasons why patients decide to engage in medical travel (Johnston et al., 2012). Many patients seek treatment abroad to reduce waiting times for procedures (Connell, 2006). This is particularly the case in countries with public healthcare systems (e.g. Canada, UK), which might be overwhelmed by patient demand and suffering from constraints such as staff shortages and other types of limited capacity (Johnston et al., 2012).

Availability of treatment or procedures also plays a role in decisions to engage in medical travel. Availability can mean that the procedure/treatment is not available at all in the home country/region, the procedure/treatment is not legal in the home country/region (Connell, 2006), or the patient has not been able to get a referral or is not able to access the procedure/treatment in the home country/region (for instance, is ineligible due to age or other reasons) (Johnston et al., 2012).

Patients might also be travelling to access more culturally appropriate care or might choose to combine biomedical treatment with other forms of care. In India, for instance, medical travellers are able to access a wide range of allopathic and alternative systems of medicine (Hazarika, 2010). Patients might also travel back to their countries of origin, a process referred to as return medical travel or tourism, to seek care in an environment they are more comfortable with. Inhorn (2011) has written about "diasporic dreaming" in the case of Middle Eastern couples who imagine and plan accessing assisted reproductive technologies back home.

Many patients travel for elective, one-off procedures (such as surgeries), but cases of long-term relocation and multiple trips to the same medical facilities have also been documented (Inhorn, 2015; Speier, 2016; Vindrola-Padros & Whiteford, 2012). In the case of couples seeking assisted reproductive technologies abroad, medical travel experiences are represented as a series of procedures within a given cycle (Speier, 2016). Families from Bolivia and Paraguay seeking oncology treatment for their children in Buenos Aires, Argentina, know they will have to relocate to their destination country at least for a few months, until the child has finished the early stages of treatment (Vindrola-Padros & Whiteford, 2012).

Travel not only affects travelling patients, but also accompanying family members or carers and families left back home. In Kangas's (2007) ethnographic account of Yemeni patients' experiences of international medical travel, she highlights situations where financially abled households who did not send ill family members for medical treatment abroad were criticised. She finds that most families tried to do everything they could to send their ill family members abroad for treatment: "should a patient die abroad, the family could reassure themselves, and others, that they had held nothing back" (Kangas, 2007, p. 299). These families are also responsible for patients and accompanying family members while they are away, extending family loyalty and duties beyond national borders (Kangas, 2007). Family members who remain in the place of origin are also responsible for maintaining employment, caring for children, houses, farms or animals until the ill person and companion return (Vindrola-Padros, 2011).

In sum, medical travel has diversified to include a wide range of travel flows, reasons for travel, types of journeys, and types of treatment sought away from home. The following sections of the chapter include some of the critical perspectives that have been used to examine these trends in contemporary medical travel as well as their implications for medical travel (as an industry) and research on medical travel.

Theoretical frameworks

Elements from critical theory have been used to develop critical perspectives to explore the processes of medical travel. The main frameworks that have been used to study the use of travel to access care are critical medical anthropology, critical medical geography, critical ethics, post-colonial theory, and critical (im)mobilities.

Critical medical anthropology

Critical medical anthropology (CMA) recognises that both health and care are shaped by class, gender, age, and ethnicity. Health and access to care are highly political, in the sense that they are dependent on market and government policies, decisions on the distribution of resources, cultural representations of populations who are "deserving" and "undeserving" of care, and the histories of healthcare systems (Singer & Baer, 2018). Spatial and temporal arrangements of health and disease are analysed in relation to power differentials both inside and outside medical spheres (Armstrong, 1988; Frankenberg, 1992). These power differentials influence individuals' timely access to medical institutions, their navigation of the health system, their adherence to treatment regimes, and the possibility of maintaining a healthy lifestyle. CMA acknowledges that health and care inequalities are in constant transformation and tries to understand the role of individual actors in the negotiation of barriers to care (Singer & Baer, 2018).

CMA incorporates the anthropological, holistic approach and considers all aspects of human society when analysing particular treatments or healthcare models (Singer, 1995). This framework is based on the premise that medical knowledge and practice are neither homogeneous nor static and that "there exist institutional and situational openings for influence and activity at many points in health care systems" (Singer, 1995, p. 87). The recognition of historical backgrounds, contradictions in social relations, and imbalances of power in social categorisations (class, race, ethnicity, etc.) make CMA a good framework for understanding the factors that shape the treatment and movement experiences of patients at local and global levels.

Critical medical geography

The field of medical geography focuses on the spatial relationships between health and care. Different attempts of theoretical transformation within this field have led to a conceptual expansion where social interactionist or constructionist perspectives privileging the concern over meaning came to play a more important role (Gatrell & Elliott, 2009). An example is the concept of place, which has been defined as "an interactive relationship between daily experience of a (local) place and perceptions of one's place-in-the-world" (Kearns & Gesler, 1998). When applied to the examination of patients' access to medical services, the hospital where care is provided is subjected to a constant attribution of personal meaning. These ideas and perceptions of place influence the patient's treatment experience and are intrinsically linked to families' decisions to migrate (Kangas, 2002). Previous negative experiences, rumours, and intuition represent what medical geographers have called emotional geographies, where people, places, and emotions intersect to create personal attitudes towards specific locales (Davidson et al., 2005; Milligan, 2007).

Particular destinations, sometimes referred to as landscapes, are sought because they are believed to provide relief and healing (denoted as therapeutic landscapes) or avoided because they are associated with negative perceptions and feelings (landscapes of despair) (Gatrell & Elliott, 2009; Kearns & Collins, 2010). Therapeutic landscapes are those that "have achieved lasting reputations for providing physical, mental, and spiritual healing" (Kearns & Gesler, 1998, p. 8), including, for instance, spa towns, water springs, temples, gardens, etc. (Gesler, 1993, 1996;), and in the case of medical travel, medical facilities deemed worthy of providing high-quality care (Whittaker & Chee, 2015).

Critical perspectives have been incorporated in the field of medical geography to understand the uneven spatial development of health services and the impact of this unequal distribution on access to care, and, ultimately, the health of populations (Jenner, 2008). Individuals are able to negotiate these limitations demanding other forms of local care or bypassing local services and seeking care elsewhere (Ergler et al., 2011). However, some areas/populations receive fewer services or lower qualities of care than others (Warf, 2010), as global politics are reproduced in the delivery and access of medical services (Buzinde & Yarnal, 2012).

Critical ethics

Medical travel processes have also been analysed in the field of ethics, mainly through the concept of health as a universal human right and the exploration of equity in care (Smith, 2012). According to Pennings (2007), if access to healthcare is considered a universal human right, then access to services should be determined based on individual need and not on the capacity to pay for services. In practice, however, there is a constant interaction and tension between the representation of health as both a right and a commodity. These tensions are evident in the study of medical travel as health might be conceptualised as a commodity in some situations (i.e. when seeking cheaper services abroad), but not in others. The commodity/right tension is also present in the terminology used to describe processes of travel for medical services, where the term "medical tourism" has been widely used, yet it is frequently considered problematic as it equates to access to healthcare as optional and a luxury (Smith, 2012).

A critical ethics perspective highlights inequities in care, pointing to the ethical and moral dimensions of the distribution of services at a global scale (Whitehead, 1991). Pennings (2015) has presented an in-depth discussion of the concept of distributive justice, arguing that different theories of justice can be used to evaluate the current medical travel system across the world. For instance, individuals in destination countries can be considered in a state of exploitation as their work, bodies, and body parts are used to heal foreign patients (Cohen, 2015). Medical travel can be seen as an appropriation and domination of local medical services by the medical travel industry, so critical ethicists often raise the question of who has the moral obligation to address this domination. Should this be left to the destination areas or should medical travellers also play a role? (Pennings, 2015; Smith, 2012; Turner, 2007). Both Meghani (2011) and Snyder et al. (2013) have argued that medical travellers have a moral obligation to seek ways to reduce harm and ensure the care they seek abroad is not delivered at the expense of the care of local populations. Yet, global assertions of the moral responsibility and potential harm of specific flows of travelling patients across the globe are still missing (Pennings, 2015).

Postcolonial theory

A postcolonial perspective in medical geography views medical travel as a form of neocolonialism where structural relations of power maintain access to medical services for those in the core at the expense (and exploitation) of those in the peripheries (Buzinde & Yarnal, 2012). When using this lens, medical travel needs to consider the relationships between "sending" and "receiving" countries or regions and understand them in relation to a longstanding history of domination and resistance (Buzinde & Yarnal, 2012; Ormond, 2013). Medical travel can be seen as a new form of exploitation where countries who have dominated the geopolitical landscape take advantage of cheaper services, medical resources, and even body parts in "dominated" areas of the globe (Buzinde & Yarnal, 2012).

Critical (im)mobilities

The mobilities paradigm visualises social life as the production of constant flows of people, ideas, and objects (Urry, 2007). This paradigm presents a shift in the social sciences, where mobilities are studied in their own singularity and centrality and not as a result of studying other phenomena (D'Andrea et al., 2011). This shift entails reconceptualising processes that had been studied as static or sedentary, and developing terminology to account for a renewed focus on movement (Urry, 2002). It also means exploring a wide range of mobility forms and the factors that promote or hinder movement (Salazar et al., 2017).

The variability in the willingness and capacity to move became the focus of authors interested in integrating critical perspectives to the "mobilities paradigm" (Creswell, 2011; Hannam et al., 2006). A critical (im)mobilities framework has been developed to account for the role of asymmetries in power in the shaping of episodes of movement and stasis (Soderstrom et al., 2013). In other words, it seeks to identify the structures that allow some to move, while preventing others from doing so. This framework focuses on exploring how factors such as class, gender, and ethnicity contribute to the creation of particular types of movement or experiences of staying still. It also engages with inequalities operating at symbolic levels, such as emotions and the imagination, where we do not all have the same imagined possibilities, and the emotions we experience through travel might range from excitement and enchantment to frustration and fear.

This framework is relevant for medical travel research as medical travel is embedded in wider political and economic processes operating at a global scale, where not all healthcare systems have the same level of development and some patients have access to high-quality care for the sake of others. It can explore how these global processes are negotiated and reconfigured by individuals on a daily basis, as patients seeking medical services away from their place of origin must often bypass deficiencies in services and other barriers to care.

Implications for medical travel

The critical perspectives discussed above encourage us to view medical travel as complex processes shaped by political, economic, and cultural factors operating at global and local scales. These perspectives question key assumptions guiding the development of the medical travel industry and shed light on the impact of some of these developments on local populations and Low and Middle-Income Countries (LMICs). The main assumptions, critiques of these assumptions and future areas of research are discussed below.

Health as a commodity and the patient as a consumer

One of the guiding assumptions of medical travel is the development of this industry as a result of globalisation, where health is not seen as a public good but as a commodity that can be managed through international trade agreements (Cohen, 2010; Ormond, 2011, 2013). The medical traveller is often seen to epitomise the independent, discerning, and avid consumer who is empowered to review all available care options and make an informed and rational decision to travel for treatment (Runnels & Carrera, 2012). This assumption follows a neoliberal logic where patient choice emerges as a result of true emancipation from the market for medical travellers and their independent role as consumers (Ormond, 2011; Perfetto & Dholakia, 2010), becoming "patient-consumers" (Ormond, 2013). This concept of the medical traveller assumes that the main reason why patients travel for care is due to economic factors, where they seek to get the best value for money (Cohen, 2010). Furthermore, it assumes that all patients have a "choice"; they have the opportunity to make a decision to travel.

Assumptions on the freedom of movement for all afforded by globalisation have been critiqued, and empirical research has shown that not all who would like to travel elsewhere are able to do so (Ormond, 2011, 2013). These studies have questioned the idea of "choice", arguing that many patients do not have any option but to travel to save their lives (Cohen, 2010). Medical travel is not a homogenous industry, incorporated in the same way across the world. On the contrary, medical travel needs to be considered within local processes shaping healthcare delivery, such as the history of the privatisation of healthcare, where the representation of health and care has shifted from health as a universal right to health as a commodity (Ormond, 2013). Medical travel is incorporated and reworked into logics and structures at a policy level that has promoted the perception and implementation of health and care as commodities (Ormond, 2013).

Researchers have also queried the validity of the concept of the independent medical traveller who is emancipated from local and market constraints (Ormond, 2013; Perfetto & Dholakia, 2010; Smith, 2012). In their analysis of consumer agency and market emancipation in the case of medical travel, Perfetto and Dholakia (2010) found that, despite finding a potential escape from constraints in access to services, US "patient-consumers" continue to find themselves immersed in a medical travel market with its own social, political, and economic constraints, and a new set of rules and regulations they must learn and navigate. The market, then, reproduces inequalities in access to care.

Regulation

A central challenge for the medical travel industry is the regulation of healthcare facilities providing care to medical travel patients, medical travel facilitation agencies, and other intermediaries (Cohen, 2010; Connell, 2013; Hazarika, 2010; Kassim, 2009; Penney et al., 2011; Pocock & Phua, 2011; Smith et al., 2011). One way in which regulation has been approached is through the accreditation of medical facilities abroad (Turner, 2011). According to Connell (2010), this is the main way in which foreign medical establishments can convince potential medical travellers of the quality and reliability of the services they provide (see also Warf, 2010). Prestigious international accreditation agencies such as the Joint Commission International (JCI), Accreditation Canada, the Australian Council for Healthcare Standards, and the Society for International Healthcare Accreditation provide credibility to some medical facilities, but the proliferation of small-scale local accrediting organisations has cast doubt over accreditation processes as a whole (Connell, 2010, 2013; Crooks et al., 2013; Smith et al., 2011).

Even with fully accredited facilities, regulation of medical practice continues to be a challenge. Malpractice is tricky from a legal point of view as many patients will be unprotected and, in most cases, subjected to the laws of the place where they received treatment (Kassim, 2009). Countries like India and Thailand have limited malpractice laws (Smith et al., 2011), and many facilities in destination countries have little malpractice insurance costs (to maintain low prices) (Hopkins et al., 2010). Furthermore, some countries, such as Singapore and Malaysia, rely on having a confession to malpractice from local physicians before compensation can be awarded to the patient (Forgione & Smith, 2007), and other countries, such as Thailand, do not compensate for pain and suffering (Kassim, 2009). Many healthcare professionals in the place of origin feel uncomfortable treating patients with complications arising from procedures or therapies obtained abroad (Burkett, 2007; Hunter & Oultram, 2010; Martin, 2010; Parks, 2010; Storrow, 2005).

Benefits of medical travel "trickle down"

In theory, if health is seen as a good that can be traded, then it will generate profit. One dominant assumption here is the belief that medical travel (particularly in the case of foreign patients from affluent countries) will lead to local economic growth, as the revenue from this service trade will spill into other areas of the economy (i.e. hotels, transport) or the public sector (the education system, for instance) (Garcia-Altes, 2005; Lunt et al., 2014; Ormond, 2013; Ramirez de Arellano, 2007; Smith, 2012). In practice, however, research has shown that the relationship between the development of the medical travel industry in destination countries and "spillover" of the revenue into other areas of the economy and public services is not simple or linear (Chen & Flood, 2013). Adequate taxation systems are required to collect the income, but countries also require clear mechanisms for redistributing the funds to other areas, which are often missing (Helbe, 2011; Chen & Flood, 2013). Furthermore, facilities delivering care to medical travellers are often private and will have a certain degree of autonomy on how they decide to spend or invest the funds obtained from medical travel (Chen & Flood, 2013).

Medical travel as a limitless industry

The growth potential of this industry, originally portrayed as limitless, has been criticised, and existing figures on the numbers of patients seeking care away from home have been queried. In their exploration of the myths of medical travel, Lunt and colleagues (2014) have argued that most of the commonly used figures of medical travel activity, revenue and growth come from the medical travel industry itself, raising validity concerns. After analysing projections made over ten years ago on the growth of the medical travel industry, these authors found that the projected numbers of medical travellers have not been met (Lunt et al., 2014). They have also pointed to problems with the raw data and methods used to make the calculation of projections of the growth of the industry (Lunt et al., 2014).

Medical travel as a driver of medical innovation and raising standards of care

Another common assumption has been that some of the income (and potential income generated through taxation) would be used to improve existing healthcare facilities and the training of local healthcare staff, thus benefiting the local population seeking care in these facilities (Helbe, 2011; Ramirez de Arellano, 2007; Smith, 2012). This assumption is even more difficult to prove as the evidence has pointed to the opposite picture (Connell, 2006, 2013; Hopkins et al., 2010; Smith et al., 2011). Research from "hot-spots" of medical travel, such as India, Malaysia, and Thailand, has indicated that the local population is often faced with an increase in the cost of medical services, fewer care options (as these facilities become reserved for foreign private patients) and a decrease in access to healthcare professionals (Chen & Flood, 2013; Hazarika,

2010; Kassim, 2009). Several authors have highlighted the existence of two-tiered or multiple-tiered healthcare systems, where higher standards of care and better facilities are available for medical travellers and lower standards characterise the care delivered to the local population (Pocock & Phua, 2011; Smith, 2012).

Brain drain

Promoters of medical travel assumed that the development of the national healthcare system would help to reduce the brain drain of healthcare workers as these would be more willing to stay in the country due to more financial incentives and better opportunities for career development (Pocock & Phua, 2011). Internal brain drain has been documented in some of the "hot-spots" of medical travel (Wibulpolprasert & Pengpaibon, 2003). Increase in patient demand, financial incentives, and lower workloads in the private sector lead healthcare workers to migrate from medical facilities in rural areas to urban ones or from the public to the private sector (Pocock & Phua, 2011; Wibulpolprasert & Pachanee, 2008). In the case of Thailand, doctors experienced the greatest income gap between the private and public sectors, explaining why this is the professional group with the highest level of outflow in the country (Pannarunothai et al., 1998). Internal brain drain also poses questions in relation to the public funding used to train medical professionals who will then leave to work in the private sector (Pocock & Phua, 2011). Hopkins and colleagues (2010) have estimated, that, in the case of India, the annual value of public subsidies for the education of medical professionals is over $100 million.

In sum, the frequently advertised benefits of the medical travel industry need to be critically analysed and explored within the context of sending and destination countries, particularly in relation to the healthcare-seeking realities of local populations in destination countries. Medical travel flows also need to be understood in relation to the processes that have created and reinforced health inequalities, where medical travel might not be a choice, but a life-saving necessity.

Implications for research

An important part of the work on medical travel has emerged from clinical fields such as medicine and nursing, exploring the potential consequences of patients seeking care abroad, issues around the global regulation of care, malpractice, and dealing with complications when patients returned to their place of origin (Burkett, 2007; Hunter & Oultram, 2010; Martin, 2010; Parks, 2010; Pennings, 2004; Storrow, 2005). The main patient flows explored by this literature were those of the US or European patients seeking elective care in the Global South, and most of these journeys were explored from a macro-level point of view, without focusing on patients' experiences of care.

A later trend in medical travel research took an empirical turn as it became preoccupied with the generation of data on patient numbers, experiences of care, and descriptions of the ways in which care is delivered to foreign patients (Lunt et al., 2016). International travel was still the main focus, but there was an increase in the research focusing on intra-regional travel and cross-border care (Ormond, 2013, 2014; Inhorn, 2007). Several literature reviews were published, mainly exploring the information provided by medical travel facilitators (Cormany & Baloglu, 2011), the impact of medical travel (Johnston et al., 2010), and the state of existing knowledge on medical travel (Hopkins et al., 2010; Lunt & Carrera, 2010; Smith et al., 2011). Many ethnographies of medical travel, focusing on the experiences of patients seeking care away from home, were also developed (Ackerman, 2010; Aizura, 2010; Bergmann, 2011a; Edmonds, 2011; Green et al., 2016; Inhorn, 1996, 2003, 2007, 2008, 2015; Nolan et al., 2011; Sobo et al.,

2011; Song, 2010; Speier, 2011, 2016; Brage, 2018; Kangas, 2007, 2010; Vindrola-Padros, 2011, 2015; Whittaker, 2008).

A limited amount of research has engaged with the arrangements that need to be put in place by travelling patients and their families to seek care elsewhere. The few studies that have provided this level of detail have indicated that medical travel is a highly burdensome process, entailing great physical and emotional labour (Brage, 2018; Kangas, 2007, 2010; Vindrola-Padros, 2011, 2012, 2019). Additional work needs to be carried out to understand the financial implications of medical travel and how these expenses are normally covered. Other types of arrangements back home (i.e. employment, childcare, housework) as well as in the medical travel destination (i.e. accommodation, paperwork, other services), need to be explored.

Most of the research on medical travel focuses on international travel, thus neglecting other, more local, journeys for medical care. All types of travel entail material and symbolic processes that need to be taken into consideration in patients' quest for care. Internal and more localised forms of travel also have meaning and represent challenges for patients and families (Brage, 2018; Vindrola-Padros, 2011, 2019). The study of these, more localised forms of travel, could make important contributions to our examination of international medical travel as experiences of patients having to cross national borders could be compared with those who move within their regions (potentially crossing other types of borders).

There is also a lack of research on the experiences of those accompanying medical travellers. Some of the research on reproductive tourism engaged with the views of partners who travelled with the patient (Inhorn, 2015; Speier, 2016), but, on several occasions, partners were also receiving some form of intervention or diagnostic procedure. Ethnographies on travel for paediatric oncology treatment (Brage, 2018; Vindrola-Padros, 2011, 2012) and Kangas' work (2007, 2010) are probably the main texts to show the role played by accompanying family members. Future research would benefit from exploring the role of these companions, as they negotiate care for patients, expand their sense of loyalty and dedication beyond borders and experience movement with the patient to potentially unknown destinations.

Most of the research on medical travel has focused on successful journeys, that is, instances where patients were able to secure the medical services they required beyond their place of origin. A neglected area of research, then, is all of those cases where patients might have dreamed of seeking care in a different location and were not able to enact those journeys, or where they might have tried, but failed. These journeys are just as important as successful medical travel journeys and can shed light on barriers to care and the strategies attempted by patients and families to overcome them. In sum, the future development of the field of medical travel will depend on our capacity to explore experiences of travel from the point of view of travelling patients and their accompanying caregivers, document different types of travel (from international to intranational), and analyse the conceptualisation of medical travel in the imaginary, including those journeys that might be dreamed of and never enacted.

Conclusions

Medical travel has been studied under concepts such as medical tourism, cross-border care, return medical tourism, and, more recently, intra-regional and intra-national medical travel. Although extensive research has been carried out on medical travel, research that engages with theory, and more specifically, research that draws from critical perspectives is limited (Lunt et al., 2016). This chapter has provided an overview of the most common critical perspectives used to explore processes of medical travel and has aimed to demonstrate the contributions of these perspectives for identifying and critiquing the underlying assumptions guiding the development of this industry. The application of the main concepts emanating from these critical perspectives (the focus on the (re)production of inequalities in access to care, distributive justice, neocolonial models of care delivery across the globe, and the shaping of movement/stasis by power relations) to the empirical evidence on medical travel has also pointed to four gaps in knowledge and future areas of exploration: the logistics of travel and care, internal medical travel, the role and experiences of companions, and unsuccessful medical travel journeys. There is plenty of work ahead to generate a theoretically-rich and critical field of medical travel studies.

Bibliography

Ackerman, S. (2010). Plastic paradise: Transforming bodies and selves in Costa Rica's cosmetic surgery tourism industry. *Medical Anthropology, 29*(4), 403–423.

Agee, B., Funkhouser, E., Roseman, J., Fawal, H., Holmberg, S., & Vermund, S. (2006). Migration patterns following HIV diagnosis among adults residing in the nonurban Deep South. *AIDS Care, 18*(1) Supplement 1, S51–S58.

Aizura, A. (2010). Feminine transformations: Gender reassignment surgical tourism in Thailand. *Medical Anthropology, 29*(4), 424–443.

Alsharif, M. J., Labonte, R., & Lu, Z. (2010). Patients beyond borders: A study of medical tourists in four countries. *Global Social Policy, 10*, 315–335.

Armstrong, D. (1988). Space and time in British General practice. In M. Lock, and Deborah Gordon (Eds.), *Biomedicine examined* (pp. 207–225). Dordrecht: Kluwer Academic Publishers.

Bergmann, S. (2011a). Fertility tourism: Circumventive routes that enable access to reproductive technologies and substances. *Signs, 36*(2), 280–289.

Bergmann, S. (2011b). Reproductive agency and projects: Germans searching for egg donation in Spain and the Czech Republic. *Reproductive BioMedicine Online, 23*(5), 600–608.

Brage, E. (2018). "Si no fuera porque me vine...". Itinerarios terapéuticos y prácticas de cuidado en el marco de las migraciones desarrolladas desde el Noroeste y Noreste Argentino hacia la Ciudad Autónoma de Buenos Aires para la atención del cáncer infantil: Un abordaje antropológico. Tesis doctoral. Facultad de Filosofía y Letras, Universidad de Buenos Aires.

Burkett, L. (2007). Medical tourism: Concerns, benefits, and the American legal perspective. *Journal of Legal Medicine, 28*, 223–245.

Buzinde, C., & Yarnal, C. (2012). Therapeutic landscapes and postcolonial theory: A theoretical approach to medical tourism. *Social Science & Medicine, 74*, 783–787.

Chen, Y., & Brandon, C. F. (2013). Medical tourism's impact on health care equity and access in low-and middle-income countries: Making the case for regulation. *Journal of Law, Medicine and Ethics, 41*(1), 286–300.

Chen, Y. B., & Flood, C. (2013). Medical tourism's impact on health care equity and access in low-and middle-income countries: Making the case for regulation. *Journal of Law, Medicine, and Ethics, 41*(1), 286–300.

Cohen, E. (2010). Medical travel – A critical assessment. *Tourism Recreation Research, 35*(3), 225–237.

Cohen, G. I. (2015). *Patients with passports: Medical tourism, law and ethics.* Oxford: Oxford University Press.

Connell, J. (2006). Medical tourism: Sea, sun, sand and ... surgery. *Tourism Management, 27*(6), 1093–1100.

Connell, J. (2010). *Migration and the globalization of health care.* Cheltenham: Edward Elgar.

Connell, J. (2013). Contemporary medical tourism: Conceptualisation, culture and commodification. *Tourism Management, 34*, 1–13.

Cormany, D., & Baloglu, S. (2011). Medical travel facilitator websites: An exploratory study of web page contents and services offered to the prospective medical tourist. *Tourism Management, 32*, 709–716.

Cresswell, T. (2001). The production of mobilities. *New Formations, 43*, 11–25.

Crooks, V., Turner, L., Cohen, G., Bristeir, J., Snyder, J., Casey, V., & Whitmore, R. (2013). Ethical and legal implications for the risks of medical tourism for patients: A qualitative study of Canadian health and safety representatives' perspectives. *BMJ Open, 3*(2), 1–8.

Cresswell, T. (2011). Mobilities I: Catching up. *Progress in Human Geography, 35*(4), 550–558.

D'Andrea, A., Ciolfi, L., & Gray, B. (2011). Methodological challenges and innovations in mobilities research. *Mobilities, 6*(2), 149–160.

Davidson, J., Bondi L., & Smith, M. (2005). *Emotional geographies.* Aldershot: Ashgate.

Edmonds, A. (2011). Almost invisible scars: Medical tourism to Brazil. *Signs, 36*(2), 297–302.

Ergler, C., Sakdapolrak, P., Bohle, H., & Kearns, R. (2011). Entitlements to health care: Why is there a preference for private facilities among poorer residents of Chennai, India? *Social Science & Medicine, 72,* 327–337.

Frankenberg, R. (1992). "Your time or mine": Temporal contradictions of biomedical practice. In F. Ronald (Ed.), *Time, health and medicine* (pp. 1–30). London: SAGE.

Forgione, D. A., & Smith, P. C. (2007). Medical tourism and its impact on the US health care system. *Journal of Health Care Finance, 34,* 27–35.

Garcia-Altes, A. (2005). The development of health tourism services. *Annals of Tourism Research, 32*(1), 266–268.

Gatrell, A., & Elliott, S. (2009). *Geographies of health: An introduction.* Malden, MA: Wiley-Blackwell.

Gesler, W. (1993). Therapeutic landscapes: Theory and a case study of Epidauros, Greece. *Environment and Planning D: Society and Space, 11*(2), 171–189.

Gesler, W. M. (1996). Lourdes: Healing in a place of pilgrimage. *Health and Place, 2,* 95–105.

Green, S. (2013). Borders and the relocation of Europe. *Annual Review of Anthropology, 42,* 345–361.

Hannam, K., Sheller, M., & Urry, J. (2006). Editorial: Mobilites, immobilities and moorings. *Mobilities, 1*(1), 1–22.

Hazarika, I. (2010). Medical tourism: Its potential impact on the health workforce and health systems in India. *Health Policy and Planning, 25,* 248–251.

Helble, M. (2011). The movement of patients across borders: Challenges and opportunities for public health. *Bulletin of the World Health Organization, 89,* 68–72.

Hopkins, L., Labonte, R., Runnels, V., & Packer, C. (2010). Medical tourism today: What is the state of existing knowledge? *Journal of Public Health Policy, 31*(2), 185–198.

Horsfall, D., & Lunt, N. (2016). Medical tourism by numbers. In N. Lunt, D. Horsfall, & J. Hanefled (Eds.), *Handbook on medical tourism and patient mobility* (pp. 25–36). Cheltenham: Edward Elgar.

Hunter, D., & Oultram, S. (2010). The ethical and policy implications of rogue medical tourism. *Global Social Policy, 10,* 297–299.

Inhorn, M. (1996). *Infertility and patriarchy: The cultural politics of gender and family life in Egypt.* Philadelphia, PA: University of Pennsylvania Press.

Inhorn, M. (2003). *Local babies, Global science: Gender, religion and In-vitro fertilization in Egypt.* New York: Routledge.

Inhorn, M. (2007). Masculinity, reproduction and male infertility surgeries in Egypt and Lebanon. *Journal of Middle East Women's Studies, 3*(3), 1–20.

Inhorn, M. (2008). Islam, assisted reproductive technologies, and the Middle Eastern state. Babylon: Norwegian *Journal of the Middle East, 6,* 32–43.

Inhorn, M. (2011). Diasporic dreaming: Return reproductive tourism to the Middle East. *Reproductive BioMedicine Online, 23*(5), 582–591.

Inhorn, M. (2015). *Cosmopolitan conceptions: IVF sojourns in global Dubai.* Durham, NC: Duke University Press.

Jenner, E. (2008). Unsettled borders of care: Medical tourism as a new dimension in America's health care crisis. *Research in the Sociology of Health Care, 26,* 235–249.

Johnston, R., Crooks, V. A., Snyder, J., & Kingsbury, P. (2010). What is known about the effects of medical tourism in destination and departure countries? A scoping review. *International Journal for Equity in Health, 9*(24), 1–13.

Johnston, R., Crooks, V. A., & Snyder, J. (2012). "I didn't even know what I was looking for": A qualitative study of the decision-making processes of Canadian medical tourists. *Globalization and Health, 8*(3), 1–12.

Kangas, B. (2002). Therapeutic itineraries in a global world: Yemenis and their search for biomedical treatment abroad. *Medical Anthropology, 21*(1), 35–78.

Kangas, B. (2007). Hope from abroad in the international medical travel of Yemeni patients. *Anthropology and Medicine, 14*(3), 293–305.

Kangas, B. (2010). Traveling for medical care in a global world. *Medical Anthropology, 29*(4), 344–362.

Kangas, B. (2011). Complicating common ideas about medical tourism: Gender, class, and globality in Yemeni's international medical travel. *Signs, 36*(2), 327–332.

Kassim, P. (2009). Medicine beyond borders: The legal and ethical challenges. *Med Law, 28,* 439–450.

Kearns, R. (1993). Place and health: Toward a reformed medical geography. *The Professional Geographer, 45,* 139–147.

Kearns, R., & Collins, D. (2010). Health geography. In T. Brown, S. McLafferty, & G. Moon (Eds.), *A companion to health and medical geography* (pp. 15–32). Malden, MA: Wiley- Blackwell.

Kearns, R., & Gesler, W. (1998). Introduction. In R. Kearns & W. Gesler (Eds.), *Putting health into place: Landscape, identity, and wellbeing* (pp. 1–13). New York: Syracuse University Press.

Keckley, P. H., & Underwood, H. R. (2008). *Medical tourism: Update and implications.* Washington, D.C.: Deloitte Center for Health Solutions.

Knodel, J., & VanLandingham, M. (2003). Return migration in the context of parental assistance in the AIDS epidemic: The Thai experience. *Social Science and Medicine, 57,* 327–342.

Lunt, N. & Carrera, P. (2010). Medical tourism: Assessing the evidence on treatment abroad. *Maturitas, 66,* 27–32.

Lunt, N., Horsfall, D., & Hanefeld, J. (2016). Medical tourism: A snapshot of evidence on treatment abroad. *Maturitas, 88,* 37–44.

Lunt, N., & Mannion, R. (2014). Patient mobility in the global marketplace: A multidisciplinary perspective. *IJHPM, 2*(4), 155–157.

Martin, D. (2010). Ethical issues in medical travel for human biological materials. *Global Social Policy, 10,* 3.

Meghani, Z. (2011). A robust, particularist ethical assessment of medical tourism. *Developing World Bioethics, 11*(1), 16–29.

Milligan, C. (2007). Restoration or risk? Exploring the place of the common place. In A. Williams (Ed.), *Therapeutic landscapes.* Aldershot: Ashgate.

Nolan, J., & Schneider, M. (2011). Medical tourism in the backcountry: Alternative health and healing in the Arkansas Ozarks. *Signs, 36*(2), 319–326.

Ormond, M. (2011). Shifting subjects of health-care: Placing "medical tourism" in the context of Malaysian domestic health-care reform. *Asia Pacific Viewpoint, 52*(3), 247–259.

Ormond, M. (2013). *Neoliberal governance and international medical travel in Malaysia.* London: Routledge.

Ormond, M. (2015). En route: Transport and embodiment in international medical travel journeys between Indonesia and Malaysia. *Mobilities, 10*(2), 285–303.

Pannarunothai, S., et al. (1998). *Management of public and private hospitals: Financial and business opportunities for the autonomous hospitals.* Nonthaburi: Health Systems Research Institute.

Parks, J. (2010). Care ethics and the global practice of commercial surrogacy. *Bioethics, 24,* 323–332.

Penney, K., Snyder, J., Crooks, V., & Johnston, R. (2011). Risk communication and informed consent in the medical tourism industry: A thematic content analysis of Canadian broker websites. *BMC Medical Ethics, 12*(17), 1–9.

Pennings, G. (2004). Legal harmonization and reproductive tourism in Europe. *Human Reproduction, 19,* 2689–2694.

Pennings, G. (2007). *Ethics without boundaries: Medical tourism. Principles of health care ethics* (pp. 505–510). John Wiley & Sons.

Pennings, G. (2015). Ethics of medical tourism. In N. Lunt, D. Horsfall, & J. Hanefeld (Eds.), *Handbook on medical tourism and patient mobility* (pp. 341–349). Cheltenham: Edward Elgar Publishing.

Perfetto, R., & Dholakia, N. (2010). Exploring the cultural contradictions of medical tourism. *Consumption Market and Culture, 13*(4), 399–417.

Plotnikova, E. (2018). Governing mobility of health workers across borders: From local to global policy tools. In Vindrola-Padros, C., Pfister, A., & Johnson G. A. (Eds.), *Healthcare in motion: (Im)mobilities in health service delivery and access* (pp. 116–138). Oxford: Berghahn Books.

Pocock, N., & Phua, K. (2011). Medical tourism and policy implications for health systems: A conceptual framework from a comparative study of Thailand, Singapore and Malaysia. *Globalization and Health, 7,* 1–12.

Ramirez de Arellano, A. (2007). Patients without borders: The emergence of medical tourism. *International Journal of Health Services, 37*(1), 193–198.

Runnels, V., & Carrera, P. (2012). Why do patients engage in medical tourism? *Maturitas, 73,* 300–304.

Salazar, N. (2010). Towards an anthropology of cultural mobilities. *Crossings: Journal of Migration and Culture 1,* 53–68.

Salazar, N. B., & Smart, A. (2011). Anthropological takes on (im)mobility. In: N. Salazar & A. Smart (Eds.), *Identities: Global studies in culture and power* (pp. i–ix). London: Routledge.

Salazar, N., Elliot, A., & Norum, R. (2017). Studying mobilities: Theoretical notes and methodological queries. In A. Elliot, R. Norum, & N. Salazar (Eds.), *Methodologies of mobility: Ethnography and experiment* (pp. 1–24). Oxford: Berghahn Books.

Saniotis, A. (2007). Changing ethics in medical practice: A Thai perspective. *Indian Journal of Medical Ethics*, *4*(1), 24–25.

Singer, M. (1995). Beyond the ivory tower: Critical praxis in medical anthropology. *Medical Anthropology Quarterly*, *9*(1), 80–106.

Singer, M., & Baer, H. (2018). *Critical medical anthropology*. London: Routledge.

Smith, K. (2012). The problematization of medical tourism: A critique of neoliberalism. *Bioethics*, *12*(1), 1–8.

Smith, R., Martinez-Alvarez, M., & Chanda, R. (2011). Medical tourism: A review of the literature and analysis of a role for bi-lateral trade. *Health Policy*, *103*, 276–282.

Snyder, J., Crooks, V., Turner, L., & Johnston, R. (2013). Understanding the impacts of medical tourism on health human resources in Barbados: A prospective, qualitative study of stakeholder perceptions. *International Journal of Equity in Health*, *12*, 2–11.

Sobo, E., Herlihy, E., & Bicker, M. (2011). Selling medical travel to US patient-consumers: The cultural appeal of website marketing messages. *Anthropology and Medicine*, *18*(1), 119–136.

Soderstrom, O., Ruedin, D., Randeria, S., D'Amato, G., & Panese, F. (Eds.). (2013). *Critical mobilities*. London: Routledge.

Song, P. (2010). Biotech pilgrims and the transnational quest for stem cell cures. *Medical Anthropology*, *29*(4), 384–402.

Speier, A. (2011). Brokers, consumers and the Internet: How North American consumers navigate their infertility journeys. *Reproductive Biomedicine Online*, *23*(5), 592–599.

Speier, A. (2016). *Fertility holidays: IVF tourism and the reproduction of whiteness*. New York: New York University Press.

Storrow, R. (2005). Quests for conception: Fertility tourists, globalization and feminist legal theory. *Hastings Legal Journal*, *57*, 295–330.

Turner, L. (2007). First world care at third world prices: Globalization, bioethics and medical tourism. *Biosocieties*, *2*, 303–325.

Turner, L. (2011). Canadian medical tourism companies that have exited the marketplace: Content analysis of websites used to market transnational medical travel. *Globalization and Health,* *7*(40).

Urry, J. (2002). Mobility and proximity. *Sociology*, *36*(2), 255–274.

Urry, J. (2007). *Mobilities*. Cambridge: Polity Press.

Vindrola-Padros, C. (2011). *Life and death journeys: Medical travel, cancer and children in Argentina*. PhD. Department of Anthropology, University of South Florida.

Vindrola-Padros, C. (2019). *Critical ethnographic perspectives on medical travel*. London: Routledge.

Vindrola-Padros, C., & Brage, E. (2017). Child medical travel in Argentina: Narratives of family separation and moving away from home. In C. R. Ergler & R. A. Kearnes (Eds.), *Children's health and wellbeing in urban environments*. London: Routledge.

Vindrola-Padros, C., & Johnson, G. A. (2015). Children seeking health care: International perspectives on children's use of mobility to obtain health services. In A. White, C. Ni Laoire, & T. Skelton (Eds.), *Movement, mobilities and journeys* (pp. 289–306) [Geographies of children and young people series, Vol. 6.] Singapore: Springer.

Vindrola-Padros, C., & Whiteford, L. M. (2012). The search for medical technologies abroad: The case of medical travel and pediatric oncology treatment in Argentina. *Technology and Innovation*, *14*, 25–38.

Warf, B. (2010). Do you know the way to San Jose? Medical tourism in Costa Rica. *Journal of Latin American Geography*, *9*(1), 51–66.

Whittaker, A. (2008). Pleasure and pain: Medical travel in Asia. *Global Public Health*, *3*(3), 271–290.

Whittaker, A., Manderson, L., & Cartwright, E. (2010). Patients without borders: Understanding medical travel. *Medical Anthropology*, *29*, 336–343.

Wibulpolprasert, S., & Pengpaibon, P. (2003). Integrated strategies to tackle the inequitable distribution of doctors in Thailand: Four decades of experience. *Human Resources for Health*, *1*, 1–17.

Whitehead, M. (1991). The concepts and principles of equity and health. *Health Promotion International*, *6*(3), 217–228.

Whittaker, A., & Chee H. (2015). Perceptions of an "international hospital" in Thailand by medical travel patients: Cross-cultural tensions in a transnational space. *Social Science & Medicine*, *124*, 290–297.

Wibulpolprasert, S., & Pachanee, C. (2008). Addressing the internal brain drain of medical doctors in Thailand: The story and lesson learned. *Global Social Policy*, *8*, 12–15.

24

PLACE IN HEALTH, ILLNESS, AND HEALTHCARE

Robin A. Kearns and Gavin J. Andrews

Introduction

The experience of health and illness, as well as elements of the healthcare system, invariably *takes place* in both a bodily and locational sense. In considering this statement, we can read "take place" both in the conversational sense of "occurring", but also more literally as occupying or making a place – in a system or hierarchy as well as in specific sites. In this chapter our aim is to critically review ways in which "place" has been considered within studies of health and illness, granting particular attention to changing views of place within geography, the concept's disciplinary "home". In particular, we trace a movement from viewing place in largely locational terms to a contemporary openness to posthumanist and non-representational considerations. At the heart of our chapter is the idea that the "whereness" of place is a necessary, but not sufficient, aspect of the concept; that the connections to identity and felt place-in-the-world are indelibly etched into the experience of health and illness.

We aim to trace the evolution in thinking about place in health, illness, and healthcare in geography and more broadly in allied social sciences. First, we consider the shift from treating place as a literal location to the embrace of place as a meaningful and felt construct. The body is both a place in itself and the site from which all other places are known. Our second section therefore examines embodiment and the move towards posthumanist thinking about place. A third section considers "real world" examples of sites of healthcare such as clinics and waiting rooms, asking how these places are implicated for users in the experience of place-in the-world, or identity-formation. In a last substantive section we take a wider view, considering the structural influences upon health experience and the merits of assemblage theory in further developing place-thinking in health.

From literal to felt place

The field of medical geography is arguably the subdiscipline with the longest history of researching the potency of places in health and illness. However, until recently place has been implicitly reduced to location with key elements of a healthcare system (from bodies to hospitals) regarded as spatial nodes. Reduced to point-form, locations lend themselves to mapping and the characteristics of elements of interest such as diseased bodies and medical clinics have been analysed to establish their location relative to other sites of care. Other factors of concern to researchers have included residential coordinates of patients and their socio-demographic characteristics. This spatial-analytic perspective held sway as the status quo until the 1980s and remains a robust expression of quantitative health geography. It provides a powerful set of tools for addressing concerns such as medical workforce availability as well as patient accessibility and utilisation (Joseph & Phillips, 1984).

Scholarship in this spatial-analytic vein has tended to treat medical personnel and facilities as static. This "spatial fixing" invariably is extended to patients as well as personnel and infrastructure with data sets "freezing" residential locations in time and space. Reliance on census data is one explanation for why this immobilisation has occurred. Census information is collected in regular cycles every few years. Yet this data is widely used by researchers in the years between counts, often with the tacit assumption that people still reside where they were most recently enumerated. Work in this tradition has illuminated the role of place-as-location in influencing the utilisation of clinics and hospitals by patients, behaviour described as "revealed" accessibility. In other words, people reveal how accessible a place is to them by going there, rather than it only being *potentially* accessible because of, for instance, proximity to place of residence (Joseph & Phillips, 1984).

The question of accessibility of healthcare services was one of a range of concerns that led to a questioning of the primacy of place-as-location within medical geography (Kearns, 1993). Consideration of accessibility has commonly commenced by focussing on distance. However, a straight line between a clinic location and a patient's residence seldom reflects either the journey travelled or the obstacles encountered (Hays et al., 1990). Rather, accessibility to a place of care is multidimensional. According to Penchansky and Thomas (1981) accessibility can include the influences of service quality (*is a clinic regarded as good enough?*), its temporal availability (*do opening hours suit?*), affordability (*what is the cost?*), continuity (*is it reliably available?*), connectivity (*is the clinic connected to other and often higher-order services?*), and acceptability (*is the care offered acceptable?*). This last aspect of acceptability is the most subtle (Kearns & Neuwelt, 2009). Indigenous peoples may well, for instance, postpone or completely avoid contact with a clinic even when it is located within their own community if traditional beliefs are demeaned or overlooked such that the place and the services it offers become "culturally unsafe" (Neuwelt et al., 1992; Wepa, 2015).

A socio-ecological model of health inspired much early work connecting health with an enlarged view of place. This model expressed the connectedness of elements of place through being, symbolically, an eco/echo-system in which disruptions to everyday experience reverberated around the system. This way of seeing health helped geographers move away from under the shadow of medicine and the orthodoxy of spatial analysis (Kearns, 1993). A further influence towards change was the "humanistic turn" in geography, which, in the late 1970s and early 1980s, was both a reaction against place being reduced to location and a quest to embrace a broader spectrum of place-based human experience (Ley & Samuels, 1978). Acknowledging how human senses influence the experience of place was a key driver with, for instance, terms like "smellscape" entering the vocabulary (Porteous, 1985). This incorporation of embodied capacities like smell or hearing, and later emotion, into the interpretive lens constituted a significant departure from the disembodied rational actors implicitly seen by many of those seeing place from a spatial-analytic perspective.

Heideggerian thinking about dwelling influenced Eyles (1985), a humanistic geographer who introduced the idea of a recursive relationship between on-the-ground places and people's experience of identity of "place-in-the-world". By way of example, if someone occupies unhealthy housing not only are they at risk of physical illness, but the compromised living conditions may lead to a reluctance to have visitors and a general decline in morale; hence, someone's identity is linked to health. This deepened understanding of the dynamics of places that preoccupied geographers in the 1990s was informed by a range of philosophies such as phenomenology and led researchers to focus on the meanings of places through the application of methods such as observation, in-depth interviews and focus groups (Baxter & Fenton, 2016). A growing embrace of more broadly-defined *health* rather than medical concerns emerged and coincided with attentiveness to the "health for all" imperatives of the Alma Ata Declaration (Kearns & Moon, 2002). Two decades on, it is arguably some version of Deleuzian thinking that is most likely to be at the vanguard of new articulations of place and health. This is because of the inherently indeterminate place of feelings and experience associated with health and well-being (Kearns, 2016). We explore this edge of scholarship further in the next section in which we connect health, illness experience, and place through a focus on bodies and wellbeing.

Bodies and place

An acknowledgement of the embodied place of wellbeing experience is relatively new within the longer trajectory of geographical thought. Yet elsewhere in the social sciences and humanities, scholars have noted that the body is surely the beginning of any consideration of health and illness as well as occupying the central place in the journey to and through care. As Longhurst (1994) has noted, the body is the "geography closest in", an intimate place or landscape from which vitality can emerge and upon which trauma can be etched or augmentation undertaken.

Humanistic and social constructionist research focussed on embodiment has grown since the 1990s. Key questions have become not only how but "*where* does the body as a corporeal presence serve as a surface for the assignment of personal meaning and an organising principle for social interaction"? (Gubrium & Holstein, 1999, p. 520). Hence, the body is not only a place unto itself but is also granted meaning through the places in which it dwells. For instance, the nursing home is a common institutional basis for everyday life and the maintenance of wellbeing for many older people. Here, the body becomes a surface of signs, monitored for evidence of varied concerns for stakeholders – from the residents' own maintenance of identity to family members who retain custodial responsibility after placement of their loved one.

More recently a posthumanist research emphasis has decentred and de-privileged the "sovereign human subject" – the single human body and mind – in favour of a processual approach incorporating a broad sweep of human and nonhuman actors and forces in health contexts. This does not mean, however, that the body has been placed on the side-lines in research. Rather the body has been understood in new ways. In particular, there is an emphasis on what a body and bodies "can do". On one level this perspective has arisen in response to an emphasis on how and what the body feels. Hence, body openness and sensing are of central importance; how touch, hearing, sight, taste, and smell lead to powerful forms of knowledge. This knowledge is not consciously learned, but achieved processually through the body and its hundreds of receptors and interactions. On another level, this perspective has arisen through an emphasis on the practices and performances of bodies singularly and collectively, specifically, on human movements and qualities such as their lines of action, spacing, and velocity. These movements and qualities are powerful forms of productivity, agency, expression, and communication that often do not involve full contemplation or verbalisation. On a final level this shift in vantage point has arisen in response to an emphasis on the relations bodies undergo and the energetic results of these relations. Specifically, human bodies are recognised as changing in step with, and through their encounters with, other biological and material actors. Deleuzian articulations of "affect" have been key to this movement in understanding. As suggested by Philo et al. (2015, p. 41):

affect is identified as a sensation which "moves" between peoples and perhaps other life-forms, a flow of possibilities for feeling "something" differently which circulates in the "atmosphere" of a given place, preceding its localisation in an individual's emotional register

Affects then are transferences, and collective sharings, of less-than-fully conscious, yet placed, "feeling states" between bodies. Those affected not only enjoy a new inter-body solidarity but also experience moving from one state to another. Depending on the type of affect, this movement can be either energising and strengthening or sapping and weakening (Deleuze, 1988). To return to the example of a nursing home, on a "good day" meals taste nice, the staff are happy and smiling, music is playing in the background, the early summer sun is shining through the windows, and people are talking enthusiastically. This collective sharing of affects in the particularity of a healthcare setting results in a positive atmosphere. It is something difficult to pin down, yet it is both palpable and obvious.

In healthcare institutions, affects might arise as the energetic physical engagements and interpersonal engagements of professional healthcare work (Ducey, 2007). Alternatively, affects might arise more widely as part of the way hospitals are designed and marketed to provide a feeling of competency, to lure potential clients, or appeal to particular constituencies (Kearns & Barnett, 1999; Soloman, 2011). Research also shows affect to be important in the production of community and public places. Here they might arise in numerous contexts such as atmospheres of mental-health recovery, social engagement, belonging (Duff, 2016), as a source of animal–human relations (Gorman, 2019), or in movement activities such as walking/talking support groups for visually impaired people (Macpherson, 2008). Affects are generated by, within, and between bodies. Hence there is an inescapable need to recognise bodies as both the beginning and end of any consideration of the links between place, health, and wellbeing.

Health and the human significance of place

With the addition of equipment and professional visitors, homes can take on medical functions. So too, sites ranging from clinics to hospitals can serve more than only medical purposes, becoming socially significant to their constituent communities of interest. Drawing on Heidegger's understanding that human existence is only possible through "being" in the world, contemporary cultural geography understands being – and the countless practices and experiences this involves – to be necessarily related to place (in other words, to be necessarily "emplaced") (Crang, 2002). In an early demonstration of this perspective, community clinics in the Hokianga district of northern New Zealand were shown to act as *de facto* community centres, attracting not only patients (i.e. people with a self-acknowledged need to see a doctor or nurse) but also other residents just "dropping in" to talk. Across all clinics, this observational research showed waiting room conversations as revealing a strong emphasis on matters of community interest (Kearns, 1991). Clearly this evidence of conviviality suggests that people need to feel some of what Penchansky and Thomas (1981) call "acceptability" in a clinic reception area in order to engage in a relaxed manner. Although loyalty to medical professionals has long been documented (e.g. Platonova et al., 2016), the novelty of this study was the idea that place attachment (Manzo & Perkins, 2006) is relevant in the micro-geographies of healthcare places themselves. This is especially the case in areas such as rural districts where there can be a high level of at least *de facto* community ownership.

Primary care clinics, such as in the Hokianga study, are ultimately more than simply parts of a community's institutional fabric; rather, they are fundamentally relational places whose importance, like schools, is most acutely felt when under threat of closure (Witten et al., 2003). Building on this recognition, we can say that clinics are, potentially at least, more than the buildings they occupy and the services they provide. Rather, they are informally constituted by the social relations they produce (Kearns & Neuwelt, 2009). However, it is unlikely to be the medical consultation itself that does this work. Rather, the reception area is the more public face and place of the clinic. The waiting room is an under-examined location in the primary care system. In the language of Foucault, it is a place where the gaze is paramount; a benign panopticon in which patients are told to "take a seat" under the watchful eye of the receptionist, and where patients themselves are observed by other patients who may well inwardly wonder the reasons for each other's visits.

As significant healthcare places, clinics have undergone transformation in an increasingly digital age of medicine. Developments over recent decades, for instance, have seen a range of technologies labelled "telehealth" begin to dissolve some of the otherwise tenacious access barriers (e.g. distance, precipitous terrain) between patients and clinics, especially in rural areas (Hanlon & Kearns, 2016). These interventions can facilitate clinical, educational, administrative, and research-related services so that populations with limited access to healthcare professionals can benefit from expertise that would otherwise have to be encountered in person (Cutchin, 2002). What is moved in such transactions is information rather than people. Hence, in the language of the mobilities paradigm (Hannam et al., 2006), we witness a relaxing of the ties of both patients and professionals being "moored" to a clinic.

Attempts to understand the acceptability of places of healthcare reflect the way geographers and others have increasingly placed themselves more self-consciously in the field of inquiry through qualitative methodologies (Baxter & Fenton, 2016). Through considering the implications of their place within the relations of research, researchers have recognised that fieldwork invariably involves the co-production of knowledge; through place-sensitive research, understandings of health both literally and metaphorically takes place. This entanglement of researcher and participant in knowledge production is highlighted by Eggleton and colleagues (2017). In their study, the lead author employed a sketching method whereby by both he and patients in primary care waiting rooms drew images depicting their feelings about the space. Discussing these drawings of the reception area then allowed a better understanding of the power dynamics within this port of entry to primary healthcare. It became evident that this seemingly neutral waiting space was perceived by some as firmly controlled and confronting. Through the researcher placing himself within the field of inquiry, aspects of the acceptability of the waiting room became clear. For some, it led to feeling anxious and self-conscious, while others felt comfortable and at home. For another set of occupants of this space – receptionists – the waiting area is a workplace where multiple tasks are undertaken: greeting arrivals, responding to phone calls, booking appointments, and receiving payments. As a space of transition, waiting rooms lie between the public spaces of the outside world and the private interior site of clinical consultation. They are places on the way to somewhere else, in which embodied identities experience a pause in the passage from the everyday world to the clinical encounter (Neuwelt et al., 2015).

Under the influence of more recent posthumanist thinking the significance of place, and specifically healthcare places such as waiting rooms and clinics, can be thought about in new ways, bringing on board more-than-human actors and experiences. The *meaning of place*, for example, is not considered a product of individual cognitive processes but rather mind, discourse, and representation are understood to be locked together with physical materiality. Hence, *place identity* is no longer only about self or externally attributed conscious association; rather, it is also concerned with forms of less-than-fully conscious association attained through senses and physicality (that may or may not lead to conscious association). According to Deleuzian theory, any mental stability and continuity comes from a dynamic bodily relation and repetition between difference and sameness. Place identity is therefore in the first instance about levels of the body's "attunement" to things that surround and interact with it in a place (social constructions, if they occur, always being based on these ever-constructing basic states). By way of example, in her work with people with sight impairment, Bell (2019) demonstrates how walking and talking together leads to place-based exploration producing a sense of freedom that, in turn, develops a sense of wellbeing. In another application of this approach, Pitt (2014) explores therapeutic community gardening. Her participants became sufficiently involved in the flow of their activity that only later did they develop an opinion on what it, and the garden, actually meant to them.

Structuring and assembling places of health

Whether one is experiencing the body as a difficult, disabled place or a health-seeking vehicle in the quest for wellbeing, our conduct does not take place under conditions of our own choosing. Rather, the constraints of time and space may be beyond the control of individual actors (Dyck & Kearns, 2015). This recognition of the emplaced constraints to human action has a history in geography. Pred (1984), for example, worked with Giddens' critical engagement with time geography in tracing how the material contingencies of everyday life are fundamental to understanding place as an unfolding process. An associated attempt to achieve a firmer binding of structure and agency occurred through the work of Dear and Moos (see Dyck & Kearns, 2015). These writers were among the first geographers to both unravel the language of Giddens' structuration theory *and* apply it in an empirical study (in their case, of mental-health care and the so-called "boarding house ghetto"). The value of embracing the tension between structure and agency, whether invoked through the language and concepts of structuration theory, or through a more generalised recognition of the complex links between the individual and society operating at different scales, has informed work attempting to link culture, place and health (Gesler & Kearns, 2002).

A more fluid sense of place has recently been embraced by researchers with an interest in assemblage thinking (e.g. Brenner et al., 2011; Baker & McGuirk, 2017). Perhaps unhelpfully, assemblages are neither consistently defined nor identified. However, Anderson and McFarlane (2011) identify a number of typical processes that are built on this "posthumanist" perspective on place: gathering, coherence, and dispersion in the assembly and reassembly of socio-material practices. A fundamental position of posthumanism is its rejection of humanism's separation of the self and other. Instead, human, biological, and material entities are considered to be on the same level of existence (i.e. are of the same "ontological type"), and co-evolve in together. A further understanding is that social realities emerge through the generative capacities of assemblages composed of these entities. Overall, as a concept, assemblage has offered a way to interpret the social dimensions of places that can reveal their content, order, and how they are produced through the ways in which the world is arranged and bound. It is an approach that is not deterministic as is the case with many others that seek to establish single or multiple "causality" for a phenomenon (as is commonly the case in health research).

While descriptions vary, one helpful account of an assemblage is a "gathering of heterogeneous elements consistently drawn together as an identifiable terrain of action and debate" (Li, 2007, p. 266). Such placing and gatherings of elements have been observed in domains of scholarship ranging from social policy to economic production. Yet, as Baker and McGuirk (2017) describe, there are common threads to assemblage thinking that include emphases on a *multiplicity* of elements, *processes* rather than products, forms of contributing *labour* and the *uncertainties* of trajectories and outcomes. Assemblage thinking allows such focus on emergent conditions –

situations in which otherwise often disparate activities and entities become mutually entangled but nonetheless have potential agency beyond those interactions (Anderson et al., 2012; Muller, 2015). Assemblages are essentially geographical in that they are always in places, comprise places, and/or encompass more than one place. Moreover, they are almost always networked in a complex manner, connecting other places further afield at various scales. In short, they always occur and work out on the ground (DeLanda, 2016).

There have been instances of geographers examining the occurrence and movement of healthcare's materialities (e.g. equipment, buildings; Baker, 1979; Kearns et al., 2005). However, only recently has the idea of "assemblage" entered discussions of health and places of health significance. A recent study of postage stamps as a vehicle for health promotion is one example of employing assemblage thinking an interpretive lens (Kearns et al., 2019). This study viewed stamps as material artefacts connecting and portraying places that reflect ideologies relating to nationhood. In an annual New Zealand series in support of children's health camps, the depicted images (e.g. of children at play; endemic biodiversity) are health-related. An analysis of their changing themes over the years of their issue (1929–2016) revealed evolving understandings of health and the character of healthy places. This recognition allowed the authors to regard health stamps as a vehicle for health promotion and part of a mobilised assemblage. This assemblage comprised temporally and spatially-specific practices involving not only trained practitioners but also designers of postage stamps, their users, and collectors, as well as the stamps themselves as highly mobile nonhuman actors.

In sum, assemblage theory leads scholars to ask fundamental questions such as: *What is in-situ? What is arriving or leaving? What is passive or active? What is interacting with what and how?* (Andrews, 2018). Although assemblages often bridge communities and institutions, they can originate or be experienced in one or the other. The aforementioned questions are hence being asked in place-based research such as studies of assemblages in movement and fitness activities (Barratt, 2012; Middleton, 2010); baths and bathing (Foley, 2014); caring assemblages for disabilities (Stephens et al., 2015); enabling assemblages for mental healing and recovery (Duff, 2012); and urban assemblages of drug use (Duff, 2016). They are also asked in institutionally-based research, for example, in studies of the role of hospitals in global health assemblages (Sullivan, 2012), the role of schools in the production of surveillant anti-obesity assemblages (Richs, 2010), and the role of classroom assemblages in school-based therapeutic interventions (Atkinson & Scott, 2015). What is clearly evident from this literature, then, is the variety, and that different assemblages do quite different work with regards to the place health and illness.

Conclusion

In concluding, we note that 2020 was the 25th anniversary of the founding of the journal *Health & Place*, whose mandate is to publish work that coequally considers these two constructs and their interactions. Its lifespan has been an era in which geographers as well as other social scientists and applied humanities scholars have increasingly seen place as an "operational and living construct which 'matters' as opposed to being a passive 'container' in which things are simply recorded" (Kearns & Moon, 2002, p. 587). Place, we have argued in this chapter, is both a vital and generative context for health and illness and an ontological condition; identity and location are recursively connected. If the spatial-analytic focus on place-as-location reduced the human to two dimensions, then the humanistic impulse in geography introduced a third. Informed by phenomenology, humanistic approaches recentred the focus firmly on in-place experience and the human condition in all its sensory and emotional capacities. We also introduced a posthumanist health geography which, in its subtlety and nuance, brings in a fourth dimension: affect.

This approach to place and health is inspiring inquiries into a range of questions such as the nature of therapeutic places (Gastaldo et al., 2010), walkability (Macpherson, 2008), and well-being (Pitt, 2014). What remains to be seen is how this new field brings a fresh perspective to established fields of inquiry in health social sciences, such as urban health, rural health, environmental health, ageing and health, global health, formal and informal care, and indigenous health.

If there is a limitation to recent posthumanist work linking place and health, it is the lack of attention to "ill-health" and its contexts. As Philo (2017) notes, while much effort has been paid to what grows, adds to, pushes, amplifies, frees, enchants, attracts, and involves humans psychologically and physically, there is an equally extensive, opposite side of the coin to explore. What stunts, detracts from, silences, confines, disenchants, repels, and excludes humans psychologically and physically? As Philo adds, what nags, pokes, and prods away at people over time, gradually breaking their spirit and resilience. Health geography does have some record here (e.g. Andrews, 2019; Bissell, 2010), particularly if sub-disciplinary parameters on wellbeing are stretched to include Harrison's recent theoretical considerations of instances of vulnerability, fatigue, hesitancy, and deterioration (Harrison, 2008, 2009, 2015). Thus, despite the "new" health emphases in social science and the positive valences of endeavours like health promotion, geographers, and interdisciplinary colleagues must also confront the emplaced experience of disease, trauma, worry, symptoms, side effects, and even death.

Our chapter has suggested a trajectory in place-related health research that is moving towards what Dewsbury (2003) describes as "witnessing": a disposition of critical awareness of our complicity in the co-production of our world. This term seems useful for its sense of engagement in the time and place of our co-dwelling and encounter with others. To be a witness is to be involved, by virtue of being present and in-place, and not just observing places at a distance.

References

Anderson, B., Kearnes, M., & McFarlane, C. (2012). On assemblages and geography. *Dialogues in Human Geography*, *2*(2), 171–189.

Anderson, B., & McFarlane, C. (2011). Assemblage and geography. *Area*, *43*(2), 124–127.

Andrews, G. J. (2018). *Non-representational theory & health: The health in life in space-time revealing*. London: Routledge.

Andrews, G. J. (2019). Spinning, hurting, still, afraid: Living life spaces with Type I Chiari Malformation. *Social Science & Medicine*, *231*, 13–21.

Atkinson, S., & Scott, K. (2015). Stable and destabilised states of subjective wellbeing: Dance and movement as catalysts of transition. *Social & Cultural Geography*, *16*(1), 75–94.

Baker, S. R. (1979). The diffusion of high technology medical innovation: The computed tomography scanner example. *Social Science & Medicine – Part D Medical Geography*, *13*(3), 155–162.

Baker, T., & McGuirk, P. (2017). Assemblage thinking as methodology: Commitments and practices for critical policy research. *Territory, Politics, Governance*, *5*(4), 425–442.

Barratt, P. (2012). "My magic cam": A more-than-representational account of the climbing assemblage. *Area*, *44*(1), 46–53.

Baxter, J., & Fenton, N. (Eds.). (2016). *Practising qualitative methods in health geography*. London: Routledge.

Bell, S. L. (2019). Experiencing nature with sight impairment: Seeking freedom from ableism. *Environment and Planning E: Nature and Space*, *2*(2), 304–322.

Bissell D. (2010). Placing affective relations: Uncertain geographies of pain. In B. Anderson & P. Harrison (Eds.), *Taking place: Non-representational theories and geography* (pp. 79–98). Aldershot: Ashgate.

Brenner, N., Madden, D. J., & Wachsmuth, D. (2011). Assemblage urbanism and the challenges of critical urban theory. *City*, *15*(2), 225–240.

Crang, M. (2002). Qualitative methods: The new orthodoxy? *Progress in Human Geography*, *26*(5), 647–655.

Cutchin, M. P. (2002). Virtual medical geographies: Conceptualizing telemedicine and regionalization. *Progress in Human Geography*, 26, 19–39.

DeLanda, M. (2016). *Assemblage theory*. Edinburgh: Edinburgh University Press.

Deleuze G. (1988). *Spinoza: Practical philosophy*. San Francisco, CA: City Lights Books.

Dewsbury, J. D. (2003). Witnessing space: "Knowledge without contemplation". *Environment and Planning. Part A, 35*(11), 1907–1932.

Ducey, A. (2007). More than a job: Meaning, affect, and training health care workers. In P. Clough & J. Halley (Eds.), *The affective turn: Theorizing the social* (pp. 187–208). Durham, NC: Duke University Press.

Duff, C. (2012). Exploring the role of "enabling places" in promoting recovery from mental illness: A qualitative test of a relational model. *Health & Place, 18*(6), 1388–1395.

Duff, C. (2016). Assemblages, territories, contexts. *International Journal of Drug Policy, 33*(6), 15.

Dyck, I., & Kearns, R. (2015). Structuration theory: Agency, structure and everyday life. In S. C. Aitken & G. Valentine (Eds.), *Approaches to human geography: Philosophies, theories, people and practices* (2nd ed.) (pp. 79–90). London: SAGE.

Eggleton, K., Kearns, R., & Neuwelt, P. (2017). Being patient, being vulnerable: Exploring experience of general practice waiting rooms through elicited drawings. *Social and Cultural Geography, 18*(7), 971–933.

Eyles, J. (1985). *Senses of place*. Warrington: Silverbrook Press.

Foley, R. (2014). The Roman-Irish bath: Medical/health history as therapeutic assemblage. *Social Science & Medicine, 106*, 10–19.

Gastaldo, D., Andrews, G., & Khanlou, N. (2010). Therapeutic landscapes of the mind: Theorizing some intersections between health geography, health promotion and immigration studies. *Critical Public Health, 14*(2), 157–176.

Gesler, W. M., & Kearns, R. A. (2002). *Culture/place/health*. London: Routledge.

Gorman, R. (2019). Thinking critically about health and human-animal relations: Therapeutic affect within spaces of care farming. *Social Science & Medicine, 231*, 6–12.

Gubrium, J., & Holstein, J. (1999). The nursing home as a discursive anchor for the ageing body. *Ageing & Society, 19*, 519–538.

Hannam, K., Sheller, M., & Urry J. (2006). Mobilities, immobilities and moorings. *Mobilities, 1*(1), 1–22.

Hanlon, N., & Kearns, R. (2016). Health and rural places. In M. Shucksmith & D. Brown (Eds.), *Routledge international handbook of rural studies* (pp. 62–70). London: Routledge.

Harrison, P. (2008). Corporeal remains: Vulnerability, proximity, and living on after the end of the world. *Environment and Planning. Part A, 40*, 423–445.

Harrison, P. (2009). In the absence of practice. *Environment and Planning D: Society and Space, 27*, 987–1009.

Harrison, P. (2015). After affirmation, or, being a loser: On vitalism, sacrifice and cinders. *GeoHumanities, 1*, 285–306.

Hays, S., Kearns, R. A., & Moran, W. (1990). Spatial patterns of attendance at general practitioner services. *Social Science & Medicine, 31*, 773–781.

Joseph, A. E., & Phillips, D. R. (1984). *Accessibility and utilization: Geographical perspectives on health care delivery*. London: Harper & Rowe.

Kearns, R. A. (1991). The place of health in the health of place: The case of the Hokianga special medical area. *Social Science & Medicine, 33*, 519–530.

Kearns, R. A. (1993). Place and health: Towards a reformed medical geography. *The Professional Geographer, 45*, 139–147.

Kearns, R. (2016). Conclusion. In J. Baxter & N. Fenton (Eds.), *Practising qualitative methods in health geography* (pp. 257–262) London: Routledge.

Kearns, R. A., & Barnett, J. R. (1999). To boldly go? Place, metaphor and the marketing of Auckland's Starship Hospital. *Environment and Planning D: Society and Space, 17*, 201–226.

Kearns, R. A., & Moon, G. (2002). From medical to health geography: Theory, novelty and place in a decade of change. *Progress in Human Geography, 26*, 587–607.

Kearns R. A., & Neuwelt, P. M. (2009). Within and beyond clinics: Primary health care and community participation. In G. Andrews & V. Crooks (Eds.), *Primary health care: People, practice, place*. (pp. 203–220). Aldershot: Ashgate.

Kearns, R. A., Coleman, T., & Edmeades, J. (2019). New Zealand children's health stamps: Ideological artefacts linking health and place. *Social Science & Medicine, 229*, 38–46.

Ley, D., & Samuels, M. (1978). *Humanistic geography: Progress and prospect*. Chicago, IL: Maaroufa Press.

Li, T. M. (2007). Practices of assemblage and community forest management. *Economy and Society, 36*(2), 263–293.

Longhurst, R. (1994). The geography closest in – the body…the politics of pregnability. *Geographical Research, 32*, 214–223.

Macpherson, H. (2008). "I don't know why they call it the Lake District they might as well call it the rock district!" The workings of humour and laughter in research with members of visually impaired walking groups. *Environment and Planning D: Society and Space, 26*(6), 1080–1095.

Manzo, L. C., & Perkins, D. D. (2006). Finding common ground: The importance of place attachment to community participation and planning. *Journal of Planning Literature, 20*, 335–350.

Middleton, J. (2010). Sense and the city: Exploring the embodied geographies of urban walking. *Social and Cultural Geography, 11*, 575–596.

Müller, M. (2015). Assemblages and actor-networks: Rethinking socio-material power, politics and space. *Geography Compass, 9*(1), 27–41.

Neuwelt, P., Kearns, R. A., & Browne, A. (2015). The place of receptionists in access to primary care: Challenges in the space between community and consultation. *Social Science & Medicine, 133*, 287–295.

Neuwelt, P. M., Kearns, R. A., Hunter, D. J. W., & Batten, J. (1992). Ethnicity, morbidity and health service utilisation in two Labrador communities. *Social Science and Medicine, 34*, 151–160.

Penchansky, R., & J. Thomas. (1981). The concept of access: Definition and relationship to consumer satisfaction. *Medical Care, 19*, 127–140.

Philo, C. (2017). Less-than-human geographies. *Political Geography, 60*, 256–258.

Philo, C., Cadman, L., & Lea, J. (2015). New energy geographies: A case study of yoga, meditation and healthfulness. *Journal of Medical Humanties, 36*, 35–46.

Pitt, H. (2014). Therapeutic experiences of community gardens: Putting flow in its place. *Health & Place, 27*, 84–91.

Pred. (1984). Place as historically contingent process: Structuration and the time-geography of becoming places. *Annals of the Association of American Geographers, 74*(2), 279–297.

Platonova, E., Kennedy, K. N., & Shewchuck, R. M. (2016). Understanding patient satisfaction, trust, and loyalty to primary care physicians. *Medical Care Research and Review, 65*, 696–712.

Porteous, J. D. (1985). Smellscape. *Progress in Human Geography, 9*(3), 356–378.

Rich, E. (2010). Obesity assemblages and surveillance in schools. *International Journal of Qualitative Studies in Education, 23*(7), 803–821.

Stephens, L., Ruddick, S., & McKeever, P. (2015). Disability and Deleuze: An exploration of becoming and embodiment in children's everyday environments. *Body & Society, 21*(2), 194–220.

Sullivan, N. (2012). Enacting spaces of inequality: Placing global/state governance within a Tanzanian hospital. *Space and Culture, 15*(1), 57–67.

Wepa, D. (Ed.). (2015). *Cultural safety in Aotearoa New Zealand* (2nd ed.). Melbourne, VIC: Cambridge University Press.

Witten, K., Kearns, R., Lewis, N., Coster, H., & McCreaor, T. (2003). Educational restructuring from a community viewpoint: A case study from Invercargill, New Zealand. *Environment and Planning C: Government and Policy, 21*, 203–223.

25

COMMERCIALISATION

The role of unhealthy commodity industries

Peter J. Adams

While the efforts of public health researchers have led to assembling a strong evidence base for a range of effective policy interventions for reducing the harm from unhealthy commodities, governments around the world have repeatedly turned their backs on such interventions and, if they do decide to act, tend to opt for demonstrably less effective interventions such as consumption awareness campaigns and school education. The driver for this avoidance tracks back clearly to the efforts of unhealthy commodity industries to influence policymakers, which, in turn, prompts the question, how do these industries pursue their interests in the domains of policy and regulation? This question beckons us to look further upstream, further upstream than the focus of traditional public health; it calls us to look for the causes of the causes, to look beyond the social and economic determinants of health and to begin exploring some of the commercial determinants. Behind each of these unhealthy commodities stands the corporations that profit from their consumption and, since several of the most important consumptions are addictive by nature, their potential for profits are immense. Also, the corporations themselves are not easily circumscribed; they refer to an industrial complex of producers, retailers, hospitality enterprises and ancillary professionals, such as advertising agencies and legal and accounting firms.

A focus on commercial determinants is particularly important in understanding what drives levels of noncommunicable diseases (NCDs). For higher-income countries, particularly the 36 countries belonging to the Organization for Economic Cooperation and Development (OECD), around 85% of the burden of disease is attributable to NCDs, with three of top four risk factors being tobacco use, unhealthy diet, and harmful alcohol use (Lopez et al., 2006; Beaglehole et al., 2011). Public health researchers have long recognised the importance of these risky consumptions and considerable effort has gone into identifying upstream causes and to trial interventions likely to make a difference. Their research has consistently identified four effective ways of reducing harmful consumptions, namely, manipulations of pricing (e.g. tax increases), decreases in availability (e.g. prohibiting sales to minors), constraints on marketing (e.g. banning television advertising), and designing less harmful products (e.g. lowering alcohol content). As can be seen, each of these call on governments to take an active role in policy and legislation (World Health Organization, 2017).

Unfortunately, despite the high quality of research evidence, governments have displayed a reluctance to act. For example, from the 1950s when tobacco was first recognised as carcinogenic, industry stalling, and diversion tactics successfully delayed effective legislation in high-income countries by another 50 years. This achievement drew on a complex and organised series of tactics and strategies which have enlisted a wide range of actors who have helped in stalling policy interventions (Friedman, 2009; Saloojee & Dagli, 2000). It was only after the major legal battles in the United States led to the Master Settlement Agreement that full appreciation of the use of these strategies was revealed. Government efforts – at least in high-income countries – have steadily constrained their use thereby freeing them up to put in place effective legislation. However, for low- and middle-income countries, tobacco consumption has continued to rise, with little sign of governments engaging seriously in constraining industry tactics (Savell, Gilmore, & Fooks, 2014).

This chapter seeks to provide an overview of the commercial determinants of NCDs and to explore ways in which the influence of unhealthy commodity industries on health policymakers might be constrained.

Chains of influence

In the book *Moral Jeopardy: Risks of Accepting Money from the Alcohol, Tobacco and Gambling Industries* (Adams, 2016), I focus on the ways such industries invest profits in activities aimed at stalling, diverting, obscuring, and blocking health policy initiatives that threaten consumption of their products. The book points out that industry organisations have only a limited number of ways of directly influencing policymakers because any visible attempt to do so is likely to be perceived as exploitative and corrupt. Instead, they seek channels of influence by means of organised arrays of paid intermediaries such as lobbyists, researchers, community groups and industry front groups. The involvement of intermediaries can be conceptualised as operating along three chains of influence: the public good chain, the knowledge chain, and the political chain.

The public good chain

The public good chain of influence is the most visible of the three because it seeks to advance corporate interests by pushing key messages in the public mind and, by that route, influencing policymakers. The first key message is that unhealthy commodity industries are positively impacting on public good by contributing visibly to economic development, employment, and charitable causes. For example, corporate social responsibility programmes (CSR) have become, for industries in general, a well-established mechanism of advancing the positive image of corporations, as occurs when the coffee-maker Starbucks invests in local community projects (Garriga & Melé, 2004; Tesler & Malone, 2008). Tobacco and alcohol corporations have followed suit and typically invest, with considerable press coverage, in high public anxiety initiatives – such as HIV epidemics and environmental threats (Fooks & Gilmore, 2013; Yoon & Lam, 2013). Such initiatives have been criticised as primarily aimed at reinforcing industry legitimacy and at diverting attention away from their ethically questionable relationship regarding health concerns (Baumberg et al., 2014; Leung & Snell, 2017).

The second key message is that corporates profiting from unhealthy commodities are actually doing something significant in addressing the harm. This provides a further boost to their corporate image but, more importantly, it reassures governments that, for those few people who are experiencing harms, responsible providers are doing their level best to ameliorate the damage. These measures include industry funded awareness campaigns and behavioural interventions but, for alcohol and gambling at least, most effort has gone into host responsibility programmes. These programmes typically consist of a suite of measures – such as training staff, brochures, and warning labels – aimed at recognising and intervening with hazardous drinkers and problem gamblers. The main criticisms of these approaches are their poor evidence of effectiveness (Babor et al., 2018; Rintoul, Deblaquiere, & Thomas, 2017) and that they are intended more as window dressing rather than serious attempts to intervene with troubled consumers (Adams & Rossen, 2012; Jones, Wyatt, & Daube, 2016).

The third and arguably most important message along the public good chain claims that the downsides of consuming negatively originate from individuals and not from the systems and environments in which the consumption takes place. If only consumers could learn to consume more responsibly, then most harms could be avoided. This message is reinforced by industry and government initiatives targeting individual attitudes and behaviours such as public awareness, behaviour change, and brief intervention initiatives. It is further advanced through industry communications such as government submissions, advertising, and industry statements in the media. The emphasis is on mobilising individualised perspectives which serve to divert attention away from effective public health interventions (Hawkins & Holden, 2014; Livingstone & Woolley, 2007).

The knowledge chain

The processes by which we acquire and legitimate knowledge, including research, scholarship and other forms of enquiry, play an active role in shaping policy decisions.

The way evidence is generated and communicated requires a complex chain of connections that include those who set research agendas, those who fund projects, those who judge the quality of the work, and those who interpret and communicate this knowledge. At each point along this chain actors from unhealthy commodity industries have opportunities to influence and manipulate what goes on. Strategies include industry input into defining priorities, biased funding and review processes, selection of industry-naïve or industry-compliant panels and reviewers, and the disguising of industry links by transferring funds via intermediaries such as industry front groups or government agencies (Adams, 2011; Cassidy, 2014; Grüning, Gilmore, & McKee, 2006).

Behind these distorting processes, the primary reason for the ability corporates have in manipulating relevant knowledge stems from the willingness of researchers to accept money either directly or indirectly from industry sources (Chapman & Shatenstein, 2001; Livingstone & Adams, 2016). Researchers themselves might justify taking the money because they see the funding source as having little influence over what they are planning to achieve. However, this misses out on the broader picture. For example, interest in further funding from the same source can shape decisions on what research questions to concentrate on, what methods to use and the way results are disseminated. On a wider front, researchers can find themselves becoming complicit in industry agendas that aim to divert attention away from effective public health measures and perhaps in providing industry friendly advice to policymakers. Entry into these processes might start with naïve acceptance of industry funding for a small project, followed by more funding, then perhaps acceptance of a large programme grant followed later by enlistment into communicating pro-consumption viewpoints to key advisory bodies and to policymakers. The increasing neoliberalisation of universities also plays a role in pushing researchers in the direction of industry funding.

An interesting case example of these processes can be seen in the career of a prominent Canadian psychologist, Hans Selye. His seminal research on stress spawned many spin-offs in terms of strategies for people to adapt to the pressures of modern living and in the development of stress management programmes in clinical practice. Selye's tobacco industry involvements began in 1958 with him approaching the American Tobacco Company for funding. While they turned him down, he was soon receiving small amounts of tobacco money for court memorandums, court testimony, and papers on smoking and stress (Petticrew & Lee, 2011). By 1969, his relationship with tobacco companies had resulted in regular funding for his University of Montreal stress research and by 1972 the industry front group Council for Tobacco Research was providing "special project" funding of US$50,000 per year for three-year periods. Also, in 1972, Selye was a key player in the influential San Martin Conference funded by Philip Morris and subsequently his work on tobacco as a stress-relieving activity was used by tobacco companies in Britain, Australia, New Zealand, Ireland, and Brazil. While on the surface his research appeared unrelated to tobacco, in hindsight the links are more obvious in that by emphasising the role of stress, smoking is positioned as a stress relaxant thereby offering an alternative explanation to nicotine addiction and for relapse in smoking cessation. His funding was assured because of his willingness to allow tobacco corporations to use his work to divert attention away from the real drivers of tobacco addiction.

The political chain

The political chain of influence is a low visibility chain along which industry executives seek to build relationships of mutual obligation with policymakers. The key links along this chain include the coordinating strategies of global corporates, the local activities of producer and retail associations, and the brokering of relationships by lobbying and public relations firms. Attempts to expose what is going on is fraught with difficulty because many of the processes occur under the radar and in ways that are purposely difficult to detect. For example, some studies have attempted to monitor corporate donations to political parties and election campaigns, but obtaining accurate information has proved very challenging (Holden & Lee, 2009; Kypri et al., 2019). Recent studies in the United Kingdom have exposed some of the ways in which alcohol industry corporations penetrate government contexts (Gornall, 2014; Lyness & McCambridge, 2014) and have highlighted how activities typically involve long-term investment in relationship building, which include the targeting of opposition politicians (McCambridge, Hawkins, & Holden, 2013; McCambridge, Hawkins, & Holden, 2014). However, our knowledge of activities along the political chain remains meagre because enquiry into this politically sensitive but important area is under-developed (Babor, Robaina, & Jernigan, 2015; Drope & Chapman, 2001; Young & Markham, 2015).

Central in the building and consolidation of relationships are the use of various forms of interpersonal exchange such as sharing of gifts or granting favours. In everyday life we share in this way with a variety of purposes in mind. Gifts are commonly used to acknowledge achievements, to convey affection, and to symbolise the importance of a particular relationship. The sharing of even small gifts can turn into acts of high cultural salience. For example, an unexpected gift from an acquaintance can foster a sense of obligation to return the favour at a later point. To fail to do so would be more than impolite; it would signal rejection of an attempt to establish a meaningful relationship. This understanding of the importance of reciprocity is embedded deeply and, arguably, unconsciously within how we form and maintain most of our relationships. Politicians are likely to see themselves as unaffected by favours that occur within their relationships with industry actors or, at least, capable of keeping them at arm's length. But their confidence misses out on the powerful symbolic potential of gifting and favours. For example, ways of gaining influence are not limited to exchanges of money, such as those involved in advertising or paying political lobbyists (Bond, Daube, & Chikritzhs, 2009). Benefits can include appointments (e.g. of retired politicians to boards), cross-board memberships (e.g. company executives on government advisory committees), exchanges in kind (e.g. contributing to a hospital with an understanding of looser regulations), and currying public favour (e.g. funding local sporting or cultural events).

Tactic synergies and specialities

Now, with some of the broader processes described, let's take a closer look at common tactics and illustrate them with reference to specific consumptions. While each of these industries have developed and refined particular strategies, they all tend to employ combinations of the main tactics to varying degrees.

Tobacco: knowledge manipulation

In the 1950s, with evidence accumulating on the carcinogenic potential of smoking, tobacco corporations started seeing researchers not only as a threat to business but also as an opportunity for cultivating influence. Researchers could assist in generating and packaging industry friendly research to both governments and the public. For instance, between 1954 and 1999 the Council for Tobacco Research, based in the US, provided over US$225 million to around 1,000 researchers for contributions intended to counter or confuse negative health science (Gundle, Dingel, & Koenig, 2010). The recruitment of scientists by tobacco companies reached its peak in the late 1980s when the tobacco corporation *Philip Morris* launched its consultants programme in Europe, Asia, and Latin America – otherwise known as their "Project Whitecoat" (Drope & Chapman, 2001). They invested over US$16.5 million in recruiting scientists to restore smoker confidence in the face of mounting evidence of the effects of second-hand smoke (Muggli et al., 2001; Muggi, Forster, Hurt, & Repace, 2001). Their action-plan outlined how scientists should be:

> appropriately encouraged to prepare papers, participate in scientific societies with relevant areas of interest, and take active roles in scientific conferences. Where possible, without compromising a scientist's effectiveness, they should be encouraged to provide statements or testimony for use before government commissions and information to the media.
>
> *(Barnoya & Glantz, 2006, p. 72)*

Taking care to keep the operation secret and with assistance from the Washington DC based law firm Covington and Burling, they managed to recruit 81 prominent scientists into the project from around the world. They also made use of the tobacco front group, the Centre for Indoor Air Research, to keep these activities at arm's length.

Besides serving to obscure the evidence, researchers also help in diverting attention away from worrying findings. As described earlier with Hans Selye's stress research, tobacco corporations have funded research aimed to distract policymakers from alarming evidence. For example, between 1997 and 2002 the China branch of British American Tobacco funded the Beijing Liver Foundation (later called Beijing Health Promotion Society in 1999) as a way of diverting government attention from second-hand smoke. They pointed out in internal documents that health issues other than tobacco "should be of greater significance … including hepatitis which is very prevalent in China" and, accordingly they funded liver research in order that the Chinese government would "re-prioritise health issues" (Muggli et al., 2008, p. 1731). In a similar vein, Philip Morris funded Federal Focus to conduct educational seminars on science and policy with

US government officials and funded the Ventilation Task Force for work on ventilation systems in workplaces to reduce harm from second-hand smoking.

Alcohol: front groups

Front groups, variously referred to as "third party" or "social aspect and public relation" organisations, are industry funded groups that engage in activities that on the surface appear to be addressing harm but in reality seek to divert attention away from legislative change and towards individualistic understandings of what is going wrong (Miller, de Groot, Mckenzie, & Droste, 2011; Petticrew, Maani Hessari, Knai, & Weiderpass, 2018). While tobacco corporations first pioneered front groups, in the last 20 years alcohol corporations have embraced them and overtaken tobacco corporations in their widespread use. Examples include Alcohol in Moderation in Britain, the Working Group for Alcohol and Responsibility in Germany, Fundacion Alcohol y Sociedad in Spain, Enterprise & Prévention in France, Forum-psr in the Czech Republic, Mature Enjoyment of Alcohol in Society in Ireland, The Sense Group in Malta, the Foundation for Advancing Alcohol Responsibility in the United States, Fundacion de Investigaciónes Sociales A.C. in Mexico, Responsible Alcohol Drinks Companies Association in Kenya, the Thai Foundation for Responsible Drinking, the Hong Kong Forum for Responsible Drinking, the Korean Alcohol Research Foundation, the Taiwan Beverage Alcohol Forum, and Drinkwise in Australia. By-and-large, these industry funded organisations seek to mimic health agency responses to alcohol-related harm through a range of programmes where the focus is squarely on individual responsibility. Typical programmes include host responsibility, alcohol awareness, underage drinking, drink-driving, and brief intervention (Babor et al., 2018). This individual focus serves to divert attention away from more effective policy interventions such as restrictions on availability and advertising.

The highly visible charm offences of front groups give them a prominent place on the public good chain particularly in conveying the impression of corporations being good corporate citizens and doing something about the problems. Their activities also contribute to links on the other two chains. For example, some front groups, such as The Portman Group and the International Center for Alcohol Policies (replaced in 2015 by the International Alliance for Responsible Drinking) are more focused on relationship building with political actors and policymakers. Similarly, some have ramped up their activities along the knowledge chain by conducting or commissioning their own research. Front groups such as Drinkaware in the UK and the Korean Alcohol Research Foundation have steadily increased their involvement with researchers (McCambridge et al., 2014; McCambridge, Mialon, & Hawkins, 2018).

Gambling: community capture

In most high-income economies, in the short period of two-to-three decades, gambling has moved from a dispersed cottage industry to a high-volume consumer enterprise – an industrial revolution on a worldwide scale. As a cottage industry, it took the form of relatively low consumption occurring in specific social venues such as racetracks or bingo halls. Then, at the forefront of this industrialisation, 8 million gambling machines found their way to various locations throughout the world: in the US onto riverboats, reservations, and casinos; in Australia into bars and sports clubs; in Europe into bars and state casinos; and in Asian nations into the rising number of large casinos and the pachinko parlours of Japan. This epidemic of machines has expanded alongside steady improvements to their electronic and psychological technologies. The dominance of gambling machines has swept aside the positive aspects of small-scale gambling in favour of high-volume consumption with social engagement and cultural dimensions reduced to a minimum (Schüll, 2012). And yet, in many people's minds, gambling is still associated with the virtues of a cottage industry: moderate fun-oriented consumption, social involvement, and community fund-raising. But the realities of mass consumption are very different. Where machines are present, rates of problem gambling average around 2% of populations with a range of other serious consequences for home income, family relationships, employment, mental health, and crime (Australian Productivity Commission, 2010; Williams, Volberg, & Stevens, 2012).

Gambling industries have adopted many of the same tactics as tobacco and alcohol, but, because of gambling's history as a source of charitable funding, gambling has developed a particularly strong focus on the deployment of charities in gaining political influence (Thomas et al., 2016). For example, Berdahl and Azmier (1999) surveyed Canadian non-government organisations who had received grants from gambling and found 20% had received over half their annual revenues from gambling grants and, of these, half rated gambling grants as their top funding source. Many also stated they would not be able to survive without these grants. In in-depth interviews, board members declared how their commitment to the mission of their organisation mattered more than ethical concerns. They described accepting profits from gambling sources as a "compromise" or a "necessary evil".

The potential for community capture is amply illustrated with gambling in New Zealand. There the regulatory framework for gambling has been established with benefits to communities as a central purpose. Two of the five main forms of gambling, lotteries and gambling machines, were set up to return significant amounts of money to community groups. Unsurprisingly, it did not take long for many charities, sports clubs, churches, schools, arts groups, and other recipients to begin viewing this funding source as vital for their survival. Moreover, once hooked into a long-term dependence on these profits, many community groups were transformed into active players in the political gambling arena. Their outcries could be heard far-and-wide whenever the slightest dips in gambling consumption led to reductions in their funding. This converted many community organisations into vociferous advocates for gambling, and they were not shy in voicing their support in the media, at government consultation committees and within community forums. Added to this, these allegiances penetrated deep into universities, research organisations, hospitals, and community health services; places from which, in normal circumstances, voices of concern would normally be heard regarding community reliance on addictive consumptions. In this way the New Zealand community landscape was transformed into a hostile environment for public health solutions, particularly solutions that might lead to reductions in gambling consumptions and related profits (Adams & Rossen, 2012; Adams, 2007b).

Unhealthy food: diversion tactics

The high availability of unhealthy food products, including sugary beverages and fast food, generates the sorts of profits that motivate food corporates to invest in discouraging consumption-reducing regulations such as sugar taxes or product restrictions. Accordingly, some corporates have adopted many of the same tactics mentioned earlier, including manipulations of science (Kearns, Glantz, & Schmidt, 2015; Mialon, Swinburn, & Sacks, 2015) and the infiltration of agencies that advise governments on nutrition (Gornall, 2015; Nestle, 2007).

A strategy that has proved particularly effective has involved efforts to divert attention away from the way their products are supplied and towards individual behavioural options, particularly the promotion of physical exercise. This is achieved by bringing together nutrition scientists, government agencies, and health promotion experts in initiatives designed to divert attention away from eating in favour of physical activity. In 1978 Coca-Cola helped establish the International Life Sciences Institute (ILSI), which, supported later by companies such as Nestlé, McDonald's, and Pepsi, sought to guide governments on physical activity responses to obesity. For example, during the mid-2000s, as China began to recognise their increasing challenges with obesity, ISLI-China and its team of obesity experts, under the banner of "healthy active lifestyles", pushed a focus on physical activity that would eventually overshadow concerns about unhealthy food and beverages (Greenhalgh, 2019). In another example, Nason Maani Hessari and colleagues analysed 86 emails between Coca-Cola staff and the US Centers for Disease Control and Prevention and were able to identify attempts at building relationships, framing debates and advocating for industry friendly policies (Maani Hessari, Ruskin, Mckee, & Stuckler, 2019).

Of some concern is the active contribution of nutrition scientists to the success of such tactics (Freudenberg, 2014; Nestle, 2001). For example, in 2003, McDonald's set up its Global Advisory Council on Balanced, Active Lifestyles with 15 members that included nutrition experts from leading universities. By calling on nutrition scientists, they bring a level of credibility to the refocusing on physical activity and help disguise the shift away from worrying about products. What's more, such diversion is reflected in distortions in food science. For example, Lesser et al. (2007) reviewed 206 studies looking into whether the funding sources are associated with conclusions that favour food industry interests. When they combined the results, they concluded that food industry funded articles were over seven times more likely to provide favourable conclusions than those not funded by industry.

Other commodities: Mix and match

Other industries profiting from unhealthy commodities adopt various combinations of tactics depending on the type of influence they are seeking. These industries include fossil fuels (Miller Gaither & Gaither, 2016), guns (Freudenberg, 2014), cosmetic surgery (Pitts-Taylor, 2007), and lead and vinyl chloride industries (White & Bero, 2010). For example, the National Rifle Association (NRA), a gun front group based in the US, has adopted many of the same tactics as tobacco and alcohol front groups, including funding research, emphasising individual responsibility, and building relationships with political actors. Cagle and Martinez (2004) examined how NRA undermined the public health focus on firearm control of the US CDC by refocusing research funding on traumatic brain injuries. As with alcohol and tobacco, such tactics shift the centre of attention from wider determinants – such as access and promotion – to individual factors – such as poor skills or mental stability. In another industry with potential for harm, cosmetic surgery, Tahiri et al. (2012) examined 1,706 articles on cosmetic surgery and found that those not disclosing funding sources were also those with lower standards of evidence.

Pharmaceutical industries have also exploited tactics commonly used on all three chains of influence. For example, along the public good chain, companies have for many decades engaged doctors in various forms of gifting. These have included purchasing lunches with company representatives, funding publications, honoraria and travel support to attend conferences, sponsoring recreational activities, and contributions to medical student teaching. Ashley Wazana (2000) reviewed the literature on these practices and concluded that doctors generally endorsed their interactions with company representatives and continued to meet with them about four times per month. These meetings were, despite what doctors thought, also associated with changes in prescribing practices (Fickweiler, Fickweiler, & Urbach, 2017).

Pharmaceutical industry manipulation of the knowledge chain has attracted considerable attention over the last ten years (Gray, 2013; Katz, Caplan, & Merz, 2010). Tactics commonly used include the use of non-equivalent comparison or control groups, no or poor disclosure of industry funding, biased reporting of positive results, and inaccurate reporting of adverse events (Goldacre, 2012; Law, 2006). One example which illustrates several of these occurred with the drug company Roche when, in the 1990s, it developed Tamiflu and managed to convince governments around the world to spend billions stockpiling it. However, the science on the drug was called into question when a Japanese paediatrician, Keiji Hayashi, posted an online comment noting that evidence of the effectiveness of Tamiflu tracked back to one paper, "The Kaiser paper", which summarised the findings of ten trials, only two of which had been published. The Cochrane Collaboration – which conduct systematic reviews on health interventions – then took up the case and challenged Roche to provide them with access to their data. This led to three years of stalling and diverting, with the Cochrane editors becoming increasingly concerned about the lack of sufficient data and, for what they did have, the presence of worrying inconsistencies in terms of how adverse events were being reported and the use of healthy participants rather than typical flu patients. So, in 2009, the Cochrane Library published their review without using the Kaiser data. Roche responded by releasing some data, but this only highlighted more inconsistencies and prompted more requests for access to a complete set of data. Roche then adopted a variety of stalling tactics, including attacking the Cochrane reviewers (Loder, Tovey, & Godlee, 2014).

Weakening the links

The combined effect of industry tactics has served to impede and sometimes completely block effective public health responses to NCDs. To conclude this overview, the following looks at three counter-strategies aimed at combating the headway corporates are making in promoting unhealthy consumptions.

Self-assessment of risk

A key difficulty to forming ethical decisions regarding associations is the likelihood of being caught off-guard by sudden opportunities. Once a funding offer has been presented and the money is immediately available, it becomes very difficult to pull away; the momentum of one's own ambition drives acceptance forward. For example, a researcher in psychology who receives a letter from a casino offering $150,000 to support her research in an area she has been wanting to pursue for several years is likely to have difficulty seriously deliberating whether to take it. She may have some nagging ethical doubts, but the immediacy of the resource and her ambition to proceed is likely to nudge her into acceptance. It would be simply too churlish to stand in the way of what her and her research colleagues are seeking to achieve. For her, the prospect of forming a well-considered ethical position is far more likely should her deliberations have occurred well before being faced by an actual offer. Similar to the way planning for emergencies, such as hurricanes or earthquakes, is best undertaken in advance of the actual event, so it is more prudent to talk through the various issues associated with industry funding well before any money appears on the table. Moreover, once the organisation's position is clarified, it becomes easier to steer clear of sources that are not acceptable and thereby avoid situations where offers sneak up and catch one off-guard.

I have developed an approach, called a "PERIL analysis", which aims at assisting individuals and organisations to assess the risks of associations, particularly financial associations (Adams,

2007a; Adams, 2012; Adams, 2016). It guides people through a series of steps that facilitate their self-assessment of the level of overall risk involved in accepting funding from industry sources. The process is based around five PERIL indicators as signalled in the first letters of Purpose, Extent, Relative harm, Identifiers, and Link:

1. *Purpose* (the degree to which purposes between funder and recipient diverge):

    Discussion here seeks to clarify the primary purpose of recipients and compare it with the primary purpose of the funding source. If one of the primary purposes of the recipient is the advancement of public good – particularly for those attempting to advance social wellbeing, health, and welfare – then receiving funds from an unhealthy consumption industry will conflict with this purpose; pursuing good for society and profiting off harmful products are simply not consistent. For example, a child health organisation will have credibility difficulties in commenting on child poverty when they themselves are seen to be receiving significant funds from a local brewery.

2. *Extent* (the degree to which the recipient is reliant on this source):

    As the proportion of income increases, it becomes more difficult for groups to maintain independence from what is expected of them by the source. This can build up slowly, sometimes even without people being aware. For example, a cancer treatment fund might start out receiving only 2% of its funding from alcohol industry sources; two years later, the proportion may have crept up to 5%; two years after that, as the relationship matures, the proportion may have risen to 10%. The question then becomes, at what point would they perceive themselves as reliant on this funding? Is it at 5%? … 10%? … 30%? … There will be point at which the proportion of industry funding will be sufficient for people to perceive the money as essential for survival.

3. *Relevant harm* (degree of harm associated with this form of consumption):

    The level of harm generated by different forms of consumption will vary. For example, lower potency products – such as lottery tickets or low alcohol beer – are, on the whole, less likely to lead to problems than more potent products – such as gambling machines or spirits and liqueurs. To assess relevant harm, the group may need to access summaries of the research literature on the harmfulness of the product or particular variants of that product. An estimate of relative harm will need to take on board the wider impacts of a product. Furthermore, environments can make a difference; venues that encourage binge drinking are more likely to lead to harm than venues with an accent on socialising and moderate consumption.

4. *Identifiers* (the degree to which the recipient is visibly identified with the funder):

    For relationships on the public good chain, funders are unlikely to contribute anonymously because for them the whole point of the exercise is to form a visible association with good causes for the purpose of image-building. They are, therefore, more than likely to insist on having their logos displayed prominently on an opera programme, on the side of a hospital extension, and across a footballer's jersey. While this certainly suits industry interests, the linkage is likely to have negative implications for the recipient depending on how prominently it is displayed; the more visible the identifier, the greater the association.

5. *Link* (nature and directness of the link between recipient and donor):

    The more direct the link, the stronger the influence and the more visible the association. For example, accepting money directly from a tobacco company would involve significant exposure that could involve the company insisting on certain provisions and potentially refusing further funding should these provisions not be satisfied. However, the influence is, arguably, less when funding is received via an independent intermediary agency, such as a government funding body. As long as there are no major conflicts of interest for the intermediary agency, the separation reduces the likelihood that recipients will feel obligations to the source.

People in relevant roles in organisations or governance boards are encouraged to talk through the risks associated with each of these criteria then to aggregate these into a combined judgement of the level of risk. The process of talking through these issues and their final judgement provides them with a reference point for an informed decision on industry future offers of support.

Increasing visibility

A second approach to weakening the chains involves shining a light on activities that rely on secrecy to be effective. Initiatives on the public good chain are obscured by hiding and disguising involvements such as industry donations and gifting; the recruitment of researchers on the knowledge chain is also kept hidden, and, on the political chain, contacts involving industry actors, lobbyists, and politicians are definitely kept as secret as possible.

The antidote to silence and secrecy is disclosure. When what is hidden becomes known, the motive force for silence no longer applies. However, when disclosures do surface they tend to take the form of confessions provided a considerable time after the event. Such retrospective disclosures are not that useful because the damage caused by accepting industry money occurs in real-time; the power in the chains drives influence on what is currently happening in policy and legislation. To reduce the potency of non-disclosure, what is really needed are systems that accelerate our access to detailed information on industry links. Happily, such systems do already exist and they are beginning to be used to monitor industry tactics.

Database systems with internet access are ideally suited as platforms for facilitating disclosures on financial ties. For example, the Legacy Tobacco Documents Library now provides internet access to over 13 million internal documents – letters, memos, reports – which have been used as a base for research into industry tactics. A second example is the "Dollars for Docs" website developed by ProPublica in New York. This website exploits requirements under the Physicians Payment Sunshine Act that obliges manufacturers of drugs, devices, and biological products to annually report to the US Centers for Medicare and Medicaid Services all payments of over US$10. By 2014 the Dollars for Docs website contained US$4 billion of disclosed payments based on information from 17 pharmaceutical companies making up an estimated half of the market share. Its information enables users to look up how much money or other forms of benefits their own doctors have been receiving from pharmaceutical companies.

Despite these important examples, much of these corporate financial transactions with intermediaries, such as public relations companies, lobbyists, advertisers, researchers, and politicians, tend by-and-large to remain undisclosed or, at best, only partially disclosed, which, in the end, has the same effect because the missing bits with partial disclosures are usually the bits that matter. Indeed, very little information is available on the scope of these financial exchanges at local, national, or international levels. Occasionally, the information does surface. For example, in 2011, operators of gambling machines in New South Wales clubs claimed to have put aside A$40 million (US$31.1 million) for a campaign opposed to Australian government gambling reforms – a campaign rewarded at the end of the year by the government stepping away from proposed reform measures (Johnson & Livingstone, 2020). But such disclosures are rare. The money transacted remains, on the whole, undisclosed, which, accordingly, means there is little available data to fuel internet-based observatories.

Positional stances

Another promising intervention focuses on the adoption of ethical codes of conduct to act as beacons or benchmarks for how people in an organisation or association should behave. For example, Jang Singh (2011) surveyed 101 Canadian corporations about their use of codes of ethics and how effective they found them. His results indicated a strong relationship between use of a code and its perceived effectiveness, particularly when corporates backed it up with training, episodic updates and ongoing internal and external communication. Now, it certainly does not follow that when an authority sets an ethical standard, those subject to the standard will automatically abide by that position. The research literature on professional codes of conduct highlights how, for many practitioners, personal morality can override statements of professional morality (Somers, 2001). Nonetheless, a strong statement of adherence to ethical principles sets the scene for a range of measures that are likely to impact on behaviour. Most importantly, it provides the key ingredient in a process that enables decisions on whether and to what degree a body allows its constituents to enter into certain types of relationship. For instance, if a bank adopts a principle that insists on all their branches pursuing ethical relationships, then it follows that guidance would be provided to managers on not accepting money from cartels trading in illicit drugs.

The open and visible statement of ethical positions by a particular body – whether that be a government, a corporate, a community group or a university – achieves several important ends. First, it declares an expectation: "We as a collective entity stand by this value ..." The position is out there, solid and real, and this, in turn, puts the onus on the reader of the message to consider how they are positioned relative to that statement. Second, the statement provides a benchmark for how individuals are expected to behave with each other within a particular work context. It sets the tone for all interactions, both internal and external. Third, it provides a reference point for assessing how individuals or organisations measure up to the stated ideal. This, of course, is double-edged because once a body declares a position, it, and the people associated with it, will be vulnerable to judgements of how truly they hold to the stated intentions. Finally, the statement of an ethical principle from those high up in leadership positions opens up the legitimacy of speaking out about ethical dilemmas. It breaks the silence in such a way that it becomes easier and more permissible for people to speak about ethical issues and perhaps to challenge unethical behaviour.

The World Health Organisation has produced two important documents that identify standards for public health responses to NCDs, namely their Framework Convention on Tobacco Control (WHO, 2003) and their Global Strategy to Reduce Harmful Use of Alcohol (WHO, 2010). These have provided guidance to governments in devising their response to tobacco and alcohol-related harm. However, such charters or conventions have proved challenging with other consumptions. I was involved with a group of researchers concerned about the extent to which gambling corporations fund the bulk of gambling research (Adams, 2011; Livingstone et al., 2018). In one article we called on gambling researchers to support a set of ethical principles aimed at reducing industry influence (Livingstone & Adams, 2016). These principles included: not accepting money from industry sources, research priorities being set independently of the beneficiaries of gambling, not attending conferences and other events influenced by industry, and full disclosure of conflicts of interest. However, without the support of international bodies and government agencies, researchers have chosen to ignore our call and these practices have continued unabated.

Conclusion

The organised study of processes of influence with NCDs is at an early stage of development. Initial effort has gone into highlighting that these tactics are taking place and that they are successfully blocking effective health reforms (McCambridge, Kypri, Sheldon, Madden, & Babor, 2020). But those of us involved recognise this as a new field of enquiry that is leading us away from theories and methods that are normally applied in health. First, what is needed is a more sophisticated understanding of key concepts such as "industry", "influence", and "gifting". Second, new theoretical frameworks are required that draw on understandings from political science, economics, and sociology. Third, new applications of research methods need refining that draws on disparate fields such as investigative journalism and ethnography. And, finally, we need to find ways of incorporating understandings from legal, global, and governance studies. This is a new and exciting field which I am sure will look a lot different in another ten years.

References

Adams, P. J. (2007a). *Gambling, freedom and democracy* (Volume 53 in Routledge Studies in Social and Political Thought). New York: Routledge.

Adams, P. J. (2007b). Assessing whether to receive funding support from tobacco, alcohol, gambling and other dangerous consumption industries. *Addiction, 102*(7), 1027–1033.

Adams, P. J. (2011). Ways in which gambling researchers receive funding from gambling industry sources. *International Gambling Studies, 11*(2), 145–152.

Adams, P. J. (2012). Should addiction researchers accept funding derived from the profits of addictive consumptions? In A. Campbell (Ed.), *Genetic Research on Addiction: Ethics, the Law and Public Health* (pp. 122–138). Cambridge: Cambridge University Press.

Adams, P. J. (2016). *Moral Jeopardy: The risks of accepting money from tobacco, alcohol and gambling industries*. Cambridge: Cambridge University Press.

Adams, P. J., & Rossen, F. (2012). A tale of missed opportunities: Pursuit of a public health approach to gambling in New Zealand. *Addiction, 107*(6), 1051–1056.

Australian Productivity Commission. (2010). *Gambling: APC report no. 50*. Canberra, ACT: Productivity Commission. Retrieved from http://www.pc.gov.au/projects/inquiry/gambling-2009/report

Babor, T. F., Robaina, K., Brown, K., Noel, J., Cremonte, M., Pantani, D., … Pinsky, I. (2018). Is the alcohol industry doing well by "doing good"? Findings from a content analysis of the alcohol industry's actions to reduce harmful drinking. *BMJ Open, 8*(10), e024325.

Babor, T. F., Robaina, K., & Jernigan, D. (2015). The influence of industry actions on the availability of alcoholic beverages in the African region. *Addiction, 110*(4), 561–571.

Barnoya, J., & Glantz, S. A. (2006). The tobacco industry's worldwide ETS consultants project: European and Asian components. *European Journal of Public Health, 16*(1), 69–77.

Baumberg, B., Cuzzocrea, V., Morini, S., Ortoleva, P., Disley, E., Tzvetkova, M., … Beccaria, F. (2014). *Corporate social responsibility* (Deliverable 2, Work Package 11). Addiction and Lifestyles in Contemporary Europe: Reframing Addictions Project (ALICE RAP): Deliverable 2, Work Package 11.

Beaglehole, R., Bonita, R., Horton, R., Adams, C., Alleyne, G., Asaria, P., … Watt, J. (2011). Priority actions for the noncommunicable disease crisis. *The Lancet, 377*(9775), 1438–1447.

Berdahl, L. Y., & Azmier, J. (1999). *Summary report: The impact of gaming upon Canadian non-profits: A 1999 survey of gaming grant recipients*. Calgary, AB: Canada West Foundation. Retrieved from http://cwf.ca/pdf-docs/publications/July1999-Summary-Report-The-Impact-of-Gaming-Upon-Canadian-Non-Profits.pdf

Bond, L., Daube, M., & Chikritzhs, T. (2009). Access to confidential alcohol industry documents: From "Big Tobacco" to "Big Booze". *Australian Medical Journal, 1*(3), 1–26.

Cagle, M. C., & Martinez, J. M. (2004). Have gun, will travel: The dispute between the CDC and the NRA on firearm violence as a public health problem. *Politics & Policy, 32*(2), 278–310.

Cassidy, R. (2014). Fair game? Producing and publishing gambling research. *International Gambling Studies, 14*(3), 345–353.

Chapman, S., & Shatenstein, S. (2001). The ethics of the cash register: Taking tobacco research dollars. *Tobacco Control, 10*(1), 1–2.

Drope, J., & Chapman, S. (2001). Tobacco industry efforts at discrediting scientific knowledge of environmental tobacco smoke: A review of internal industry documents. *Journal of Epidemiological Community Health, 55*, 588–594.

Fickweiler, F., Fickweiler, W., & Urbach, E. (2017). Interactions between physicians and the pharmaceutical industry generally and sales representatives specifically and their association with physicians' attitudes and prescribing habits: A systematic review. *BMJ Open*, 7(9), e016408.

Fooks, G. J., & Gilmore, A. B. (2013). Corporate philanthropy, political influence, and health policy. *PLoS ONE*, 8(11), e80864.

Freudenberg, N. (2014). *Lethal but legal: Corporations, consumption, and protecting public health*. New York: Oxford University Press.

Friedman, L. C. (2009). Tobacco industry use of corporate social responsibility tactics as a sword and a shield on second-hand smoke issues. *Journal of Law and Medical Ethics*, 37(4), 819–827.

Garriga, E., & Melé, D. (2004). Corporate social responsibility theories: Mapping the territory. *Journal of Business Ethics*, 53(1), 51–71.

Goldacre, B. (2012). *Bad pharma: How drug companies mislead doctors and harm patients*. London: Fourth Estate.

Gornall, J. (2014). Under the influence: 3. Role of parliamentary groups. *British Medical Journal*, 348(f7571).

Gornall, J. (2015). Sugar: Spinning a web of influence *British Medical Journal*, 350, h231.

Gray, G. C. (2013). The ethics of pharmaceutical research funding: A social organisation approach. *Journal of Law, Medicine & Ethics*, 41(3), 629–634.

Greenhalgh, S. (2019). Making China safe for Coke: How Coca-Cola shaped obesity science and policy in China. *BMJ*, 364, k5050.

Grüning, T., Gilmore, A. B., & McKee, M. (2006). Tobacco industry influence on science and scientists in Germany. *American Journal of Public Health*, 96(1), 20–32.

Gundle, K. R., Dingel, M. J., & Koenig, B. A. (2010). "To prove this is the industry's best hope": Big tobacco's support of research on the genetics of nicotine addiction. *Addiction*, 105, 974–983.

Hawkins, B., & Holden, C. (2014). "Water dripping on stone"? Industry lobbying and UK alcohol policy. *Policy & Politics*, 42(1), 55–70.

Holden, C., & Lee, K. (2009). Corporate power and social policy: The political economy of the transnational tobacco companies. *Global Social Policy & Society*, 9, 328–325.

Johnson, M., & Livingstone, C. (2020). Measuring influence: An analysis of Australian gambling industry political donations and policy decisions. *Addiction Research & Theory, Early View*. doi: 10.1080/16066359.2020.1766449

Jones, S. C., Wyatt, A., & Daube, M. (2016). Smokescreens and beer goggles: How alcohol industry CSM protects the industry. *Social Marketing Quarterly*, 22(4), 264–279.

Katz, D., Caplan, A. L., & Merz, J. F. (2010). All gifts large and small: Toward an understanding of the ethics of pharmaceutical industry gift-giving. *American Journal of Bioethics*, 10(10), 11–17.

Kearns, C. E., Glantz, S. A., & Schmidt, L. A. (2015). Sugar industry influence on the scientific agenda of the National Institute of Dental Research's 1971 National Caries Program: A historical analysis of internal documents. *PLoS Medicine*, 12(3), e1001798.

Kypri, K., McCambridge, J., Robertson, N., Martino, F., Daube, M., Adams, P., & Miller, P. (2019). "If someone donates $1000, they support you. If they donate $100 000, they have bought you". Mixed methods study of tobacco, alcohol and gambling industry donations to Australian political parties. *Drug and Alcohol Review*, 38(3), 266–233.

Law, J. (2006). *Big pharma: How the world's biggest drug companies control illness*. New York: Carroll & Graf.

Lesser, L. I., Ebbeling, C. B., Goozner, M., Wypij, D., & Ludwig, D. S. (2007). Relationship between funding source and conclusion among nutrition-related scientific articles. *PLoS Medicine*, 4(1), e5.

Leung, T. C. H., & Snell, R. S. (2017). Attraction or distraction? Corporate social responsibility in Macao's gambling industry. *Journal of Business Ethics*, 145(3), 637–658.

Livingstone, C., Adams, P., Cassidy, R., Markham, F., Reith, G., Rintoul, A., … Young, M. (2018). On gambling research, social science and the consequences of commercial gambling. *International Gambling Studies*, 18(1), 56–68.

Livingstone, C., & Adams, P. J. (2016). Clear principles are needed for integrity in gambling research. *Addiction*, 111(1), 5–10.

Livingstone, C., & Woolley, R. (2007). Risky business: A few provocations on the regulation of electronic gaming machines. *International Gambling Studies*, 7(3), 361–376.

Loder, E., Tovey, D., & Godlee, F. (2014). The Tamiflu trials. *British Medical Journal*, 348, g2630.

Lopez, A. D., Mathers, C., Ezzati, M., Jamison, D., & Murray, C. (Eds.). (2006). *Global burden of disease and risk factors*. Washington, DC: World Bank.

Lyness, S., & McCambridge, J. (2014). The alcohol industry, charities and policy influence in the UK. *European Journal of Public Health*, 24(4), 557–561.

Maani Hessari, N., Ruskin, G., Mckee, M., & Stuckler, D. (2019). Public meets private: Conversations between Coca-Cola and the CDC. *Milbank Quarterly, 97*(1), 74–90.

McCambridge, J., Hawkins, B., & Holden, C. (2013). Industry use of evidence to influence alcohol policy: A case study of submissions to the 2008 Scottish Government Consultation. *PLoS Medicine, 10*(4), e1001431.

McCambridge, J., Hawkins, B., & Holden, C. (2014). The challenge corporate lobbying poses to reducing society's alcohol problems: Insights from UK evidence on minimum unit pricing. *Addiction, 109*(2), 199–205.

McCambridge, J., Mialon, M., & Hawkins, B. (2018). Alcohol industry involvement in policymaking: A systematic review. *Addiction, 113*, 1571–1584.

McCambridge, J., Kypri, K., Sheldon, T. A., Madden, M., & Babor, T. F. (2020). Advancing public health policy making through research on the political strategies of alcohol industry actors. *Journal of Public Health, 42*(2), 262–269.

Mialon, M., Swinburn, B., & Sacks, G. (2015). A proposed approach to systematically identify and monitor the corporate political activity of the food industry with respect to public health using publicly available information. *Obesity Reviews, 16*(7), 519–530.

Miller, P. G., de Groot, F., Mckenzie, S., & Droste, N. (2011). Alcohol industry use of social aspect public relations organisations against preventative health measures. *Addiction, 106*(9), 1560–1567.

Miller Gaither, B., & Gaither, T. K. (2016). Marketplace advocacy by the U.S. fossil fuel industries: Issues of representation and environmental discourse. *Mass Communication and Society, 19*(5), 585–603.

Muggli, M. E., Forster, J. L., Hurt, R. D., & Repace, J. L. (2001). The smoke you don't see: Uncovering tobacco industry scientific strategies aimed against environmental tobacco smoke policies. *American Journal of Public Health, 91*(9), 1419–1423.

Muggli, M. E., Lee, K., Gan, Q., Ebbert, J. O., & Hurt, R. D. (2008). "Efforts to reprioritise the agenda" in China: British American Tobacco's efforts to influence public policy on second-hand smoke in China. *PLoS Medicine, 5*(12), e251.

Nestle, M. (2001). Food company sponsorship of nutrition research and professional activities: A conflict of interest? *Public Health Nutrition, 4*(05), 1015–1022.

Nestle, M. (2007). *Food politics: How the food industry influences nutrition, and health.* Berkeley, CA: University of California Press.

Petticrew, M., Maani Hessari, N., Knai, C., & Weiderpass, E. (2018). The strategies of alcohol industry SAPROs: Inaccurate information, misleading language and the use of confounders to downplay and misrepresent the risk of cancer. *Drug and Alcohol Review, 37*(3), 313–315.

Petticrew, M. P., & Lee, K. (2011). The "father of stress" meets "Big Tobacco": Hans Selye and the tobacco industry. *American Journal of Public Health, 101*(3), 411–418.

Pitts-Taylor, V. (2007). *Surgery junkies: Wellness and pathology in cosmetic culture.* New Brunswick, NJ: Rutgers University Press.

Rintoul, A., Deblaquiere, J., & Thomas, A. (2017). Responsible gambling codes of conduct: Lack of harm minimisation intervention in the context of venue self-regulation. *Addiction Research & Theory, 25*(6), 451–461.

Saloojee, Y., & Dagli, E. (2000). Tobacco industry tactics for resisting public policy on health. *Bulletin of the World Health Organization, 78*(7), 902–910.

Savell, E., Gilmore, A. B., & Fooks, G. (2014). How does the tobacco industry attempt to influence marketing regulations? A systematic review. *PLoS ONE, 9*(2), e87389.

Schüll, N. D. (2012). *Addiction by design: Machine gambling in Las Vegas.* Princeton, NJ: Princeton University Press.

Singh, J. B. (2011). Determinants of the effectiveness of corporate codes of ethics: An empirical study. *Journal of Business Ethics, 101*(3), 385–395.

Somers, M. J. (2001). Ethical codes of conduct and organizational context: A study of the relationship between codes of conduct, employee behavior and organizational values. *Journal of Business Ethics, 30*(2), 185–195.

Tahiri, Y., Kanevsky, J., Vorstenbosch, J., Mok, E., & Gilardino, M. (2012). Disclosure of funding source and conflict of interest: Exposure of biases affecting evidence and clinical utility of plastic surgery publications. *European Journal of Plastic Surgery, 35*(6), 457–462.

Tesler, L. E., & Malone, R. E. (2008). Corporate philanthropy, lobbying, and public health policy. *American Journal of Public Health, 98*(12), 2123–2133.

Thomas, S. L., David, J., Randle, M., Daube, M., & Senior, K. (2016). Gambling advocacy: Lessons from tobacco, alcohol and junk food. *Australian and New Zealand Journal of Public Health, 40*(3), 211–217.

Wazana, A. (2000). Physicians and the pharmaceutical industry: Is a gift ever just a gift? *JAMA, 283*(3), 373–380.

White, J., & Bero, L. (2010). Corporate manipulation of research: Strategies are similar across five industries. *Stanford Law & Policy Review, 21*, 105–133.

WHO. (2003). *Framework convention on tobacco control*. Geneva: World Health Organisation. Retrieved from http://www.who.int/tobacco/framework/WHO_FCTC_english.pdf

WHO. (2010). *Global strategy to reduce harmful use of alcohol*. Geneva: World Health Organization. Retrieved from http://www.who.int/substance_abuse/alcstratenglishfinal.pdf?ua=1

Williams, R. J., Volberg, R. A., & Stevens, R. M. G. (2012). *The population prevalence of problem gambling: Methodological influences, standardized rates, jurisdictional differences, and worldwide trends*. Toronto, ON: Report prepared for the Ontario Problem Gambling Research Centre and the Ontario Ministry of Health and Long Term Care. Retrieved from http://hdl.handle.net/10133/3068

World Health Organization. (2017). *Tackling NCDs: "Best buys" and other recommended interventions for the prevention and control of noncommunicable diseases*. Geneva: World Health Organization, No. WHO/NMH/NVI17.9.

Yoon, S., & Lam, T. H. (2013). The illusion of righteousness: Corporate social responsibility practices of the alcohol industry. *BMC Public Health, 13*, 630.

Young, M., & Markham, F. (2015). Beyond disclosure: Gambling research, political economy, and incremental reform. *International Gambling Studies, 15*(1), 6–9.

26

TOWARDS A CRITICAL SOCIAL SCIENCE OF CLIMATE CHANGE AND HEALTH

Sara MacBride-Stewart

Introduction

Climate change has been described as one of the most defining problems of our generation, with implications for the health of existing and future generations (White, 2017). For health academics and practitioners, climate change refers to the impacts caused by raised greenhouse gases in the atmosphere. The health consequences of climate change include increased mortality rates, direct and indirect exposure to extreme climate-related events, or a lack of preparedness of health and other public or social services (WHO, 2018). Chronic or enduring health problems associated with climate change, are found at higher rates (Franchini & Mannucci, 2015).

At first glance, identifying the effects of environmental change on human health, seems relatively straightforward. Yet climate change has the potential to disrupt many of the social processes, public services, and economic activities, on which a healthy society depends (Baker, 2015). So severe are these human-caused impacts, that scientists have proposed that the earth has entered a new geological epoch – the anthropocene. This is the period in which human activity exceeds the natural drivers of environmental change. It is also the first geological epoch in which the primary geological force has the potential to be conscious of its geological role (Pálsson et al., 2013, p. 8). While the most recent Intergovernmental Panel on Climate Change (IPCC) report (2018) identified that an increase in human-led global warming of 1.5°C will exponentially increase risks to health, livelihoods, food security, water supply, human security, and economic growth, and the impact on disease and illness as global warming reaches 2°C is potentially catastrophic. At this point, the capacity of technological, scientific, and societal resources to manage anthropogenic disturbance are likely to have been exceeded, resulting in unpredictable or unsuccessful solutions (Richardson, Steffen, & Liverman, 2011).

With growing awareness of how climate change shapes and transforms human health, the social sciences, and humanities have helped improve understandings about the societal conditions impacting the environment, including the drivers of and barriers to human health. Public health and health psychology, drawing on (Dewey) functionalist and behaviourist schools of thought, describe the mental processes and behaviour that shape health outcomes related to climate change. They emphasise the need for adaptation to the environment, despite the impacts of climate change being identified as diverse, far-reaching, cumulative, and abrupt (Okereke & Charlesworth, 2014).

Slowing down the accumulated impact of human activities means understanding what is creating the conditions for climate change, and considering the objectives and means by which society achieves health (Rapport, 2007). A key question emerges: how we can achieve positive health outcomes in a way that neither negatively impacts on society nor exacerbates environmental degradation? For while social and economic development contributes to positive health outcomes, it can negatively impact on the environment. To engage critically with these ideas, there is a need to integrate societal and environmental perspectives, and provide some analysis of what this integration can achieve in the pursuit of health (Baker, 2015).

Critical health studies was conceived to confront the increasingly normative goals of contemporary health problems. It is inspired by thinking about how conventional distinctions between biomedical and social perspectives, processes, and health outcomes have the potential to be broken down when diseases and illness are considered beyond their form and content, to include practices, cultures, and institutions (Lyons & Chamberlain, 2017). This recognises a complementarity between social and other physical processes (i.e. environmental ones), and seeks to understand how knowledge about each is shaped by structures of power (Foucault et al., 2006). Critical health studies, therefore, is helpful for assessing how climate change is constructed, and for problematising human health that is being achieved at the expense of planetary health (Baker, 2015).

In this chapter, critical health studies is employed as a lens to explore this "turn" to environment and health. It does this by outlining major developments in the field of health studies that contribute to understandings about health in the context of climate change: ecohealth, one health, and planetary health. The chapter explains their critical potential for understanding the complex interdependencies between the concepts of the environment and society (Rapport, 2007). It seeks to communicate a sense of dynamism and reciprocity when addressing environmental change in the anthropocene. It sets the context first, by explaining how the concepts of health, inequality, and sustainable development are mobilised in the climate change debate. Finally, the chapter highlights how the concept of resilience exemplifies some of the fundamental contradictions in discussions about climate-related health. The chapter concludes with a consideration of how climate change is transforming our understanding of human health through our relationship to the natural world.

Core ideas

Conceptualising health

Recent decades have witnessed a steady and progressive improvement in health. This is due to better provision and access to a range of social, structural, and economic resources at the global, regional, and national level (UNFCCC, 2017; WHO, 2018). While some health conditions could reasonably be expected to benefit from climate change (e.g. reduction of cold-related deaths in some regions), its overall global impact is reflected in an increase in mortality. The European Commission, for example, calculated 150,000 deaths caused by climate change annually (Forzieri et al., 2018). Heat-related deaths and malnutrition caused by failing crops and poor soil fertility have increased, as have rates of infectious diseases (Franchini & Mannucci, 2015; Liang & Gong, 2017; McMichael, 2013) and chronic ill health (e.g. asthma, respiratory disease), while reported wellbeing has lowered (Whitmee et al., 2015). The most vulnerable groups in society are particularly susceptible, to the toxicities and infectious diseases caused by environmental change (Benevolenza & DeRigne, 2019).

The changing rates of disease and ill health has provided an insight into the effects of climate change on groups and populations (IPCC, 2018; McMichael, 2013). Social determinants of health have recorded both the direct climatic influences on the environment or society (i.e. increased disease risk or traumatic stress), and those that are more indirect, like water shortages, or poor weather that cause disruptions to food production and supply chains, or other dislocations, and human conflicts (McMichael, 2013). The response from health psychology can be largely distinguished between a focus on individual behaviour, cognitions, and lifestyles – and their role in mitigating the health impacts of climate change (Clayton et al., 2015; Reser, Morrissey, & Ellul, 2011) – and the social and structural dimensions of health (Gifford, 2011; Haines, Kovats, Campbell-Lendrum, & Corvalán, 2006). Research on the latter is also interested in the processes that lend themselves to societal-level adaptations to climate change (Kjellstrom & Weaver, 2009). More recent work from psychosocial studies considers how human cognitions and affects mediate the relationship between everyday life, social conditions, and environmental changes (Adams, 2016; Frosh, 2003; MacBride-Stewart, 2019). These latter perspectives provide the backdrop for the critical studies of health; while these have received relatively less attention in climate change research than those involving individuals they are largely the focus of the second part of this chapter.

Critical theorists commenting on these developments in health psychology have argued that climate change is an opportunity to rethink the concept of health, and its understanding of our relationship with the natural world (Huber et al., 2011). The concept of health reified by the WHO (1986) is defined as the state of complete physical, social, and mental wellbeing. This definition has become nearly ubiquitous in describing and explaining health in public policy and discourse. Yet, it does not fully describe the human need for ecosystems or the planet also to be healthy, to achieve a sense of wellbeing (Charron, 2012; Huber et al., 2011; MacBride-Stewart, 2019). This view misses a sense of consciousness about nature, or how the construct of health itself is sustained and reproduced, maintaining the status quo where nature is considered separately from humans. This is also the case for the fields of environmental psychology (Wells, Evans, & Cheek, 2016) and eco-psychology (Hanna et al., 2019), which even though distinctively framed operate without the substantive involvement of environmental constructs (e.g. conservation or the environmental impacts of lifestyles) that can potentially alter understandings about how psychological behaviours and characteristics mediate relationships between the environment and the social world.

Critical approaches to health studies, then, reflect a deepening of our understanding of the scope of influences on the social world (MacBride-Stewart, 2019). This includes identifying those social structures that are directly pertinent to the natural environment, that shape, for example, how people are affected by or have access to environmental resources (Dakubo, 2013). When viewed dynamically, health is a complex of interdependent influences, shaped by policy, infrastructures, cultures, capacities, needs, and habits. The environment too – whether considered to be social or natural, or both – matters. For climate change, this myriad of factors can contribute to or mitigate its effects, whether social support, financial resource, leadership, technology, or physical infrastructure (e.g. housing or parks) (MacNaughton, 2003). It is in this broad understanding of the multiple processes and contexts that shape health that the environment–health relationship comes alive. This plurality adds a degree of complexity to each dimension. The social world, for example, can be represented across many levels of society or groups (community, city, state, or nation along with individuals, groups, institutions, or governments, Charron, 2012, p. 1). Similarly, scalar descriptions of the natural world, from species to ecosystem and landscape, add to the endless possibilities for relationships that they promote. Conventional understandings of health can be reconsidered in light of these webs of relationships between the social and natural world, which deepen the discourses, domains, and theoretical base through which new ways of thinking about climate change and health emerge.

Neither critical health scholars nor climate scientists take human health for granted. Conceiving of climate change as a consequence of accumulated, large-scale human activity has implications for how natural and health scientists engage with the complexity of the social world (Stott et al., 2010). Globalisation, urbanisation, deforestation, and agricultural intensification processes produce climate change, and while the timescales for these processes are diffuse, for natural scientists the human health effects may be less directly obvious than those generated by extreme events (Charron, 2012). Both recognise the need to untangle environmental paradoxes – as human societies and health outcomes improve, ecosystem health (for climate scientists), and health inequalities (for health scholars) worsen (Raudsepp-Hearne et al., 2010). It is possible, for example, to see how this paradox played out in the emergence and spread of COVID-19, where consumption and travel patterns created the conditions for the rapid distribution of a severely infectious disease, which in turn is a consequence of human activity (land-use change and deforestation). Furthermore, this disease has had the greatest impact on the most vulnerable in society, not just for those people living in places with the weakest health systems, and people with pre-existing and poverty-related health conditions, but for those with the most polluted and degraded environments (Ferreira, Sá, Martins, & Serpa, 2020). Making a serious contribution to the health agenda means drawing on perspectives that frame climate change as an environmental and social problem, related to human progress and societal development. While integrative approaches are not new to critical health psychology, sustainable development, and the intimate interdependencies it considers between economics, society, and the environment, are. This chapter turns briefly to consider the insights provided by a sustainable development approach and its contribution to the discussion about health (McLaren & Hawe, 2005).

Sustainable development

Sustainable development as promoted by the UN Brundtland Report (World Commission on Environment and Development [WCED], 1987) saw climate change as a uniquely global project, where it was the responsibility of different groups (including governments) to establish appropriate mechanisms towards international global action, with the goal of ensuring that social wellbeing did not reduce, and might even improve (Baker, 2014). Its stated approach was to integrate environmental, social, and economic dimensions of policy and practice in order to achieve sustainable futures, including for health, and also to address unjust causes of unsustainable development, including those that produce health inequalities (Baker, 2015). Also recognised as a model of change, the concept of sustainable development has sought to influence understandings of what development means, the equality principles that drive it (i.e. environmental justice), and the societal, economic, and environmental mechanisms and transformations necessary for change to occur.

For health, sustainable development is also about achieving health benefits that take account of ecological limits, and the need to place limits on economic growth (for a review, see Moldan, Janoušková, & Hák, 2012). For example, when considering the use of environmental resources for fuel, or housing, or for meeting any number of human needs, the expectation is that efforts are made to greatly reduce any effects on people or the environment, either by finding ways to support social and ecological forms of resilience or by efforts to mitigate actions and reduce the impact of increased human activity in the environment. It also recognises that the resources that the earth has to support human health are limited. Due to existing inequalities in the distribution of resources, some groups are more likely to benefit than others. It is therefore founded on the recognition that greater social and environmental equality improves the health of those who are most vulnerable, and reduces the overall health impacts of climate change (Cushing, Morello-Frosch, Wander, & Pastor, 2015). Thus sustainable development can be used for driving thinking around new health inequalities emerging in the context of climate change.

Yet, long-standing knowledge about climate risks has largely come from epidemiological studies that promote a linear one-way process for explaining disease progression. This approach identifies, for example, El Nino weather systems that affect food yields and water supplies with negative outcomes for physical health, or that link the loss of forest ecology to transmissible diseases (Chowdhury & Haque, 2013; Gislason, 2013; McMichael, 2013). As health is more complex than this, a focus on a multiple causality has led to an emphasis on how to improve the conditions across a range of social and environmental forces that drive it, relying sometimes on a level of abstraction to understand the health and societal effects that result from it. Yet, for critical health theorists, the emphasis it places on social analysis and complexity, rather than description and linearity, has been welcomed (Kaijser & Kronsell, 2014).

Variability, too, in how sustainable development has been conceived means it has not been widely endorsed in critical health studies. Baker (2015) refers to sustainable development as a continuum where the rationale for mitigating the effects of climate change varies between the necessity to preserve human wellbeing (anthropocentric) and to protect nature (for) itself (eco-centric). The focus on nature as the provider of human wellbeing, the time spent in nature for physical and mental health (Maller, Townsend, Brown, & St Leger, 2002), or a lack of access to nature (categorised as a "nature deficit disorder"; Louv, 2009) are examples of an anthropocentric view of nature. An alternative ("deep ecology") view of sustainable development suggests that nature should not be interfered with and that an anthropocentric, extractive approach to nature should be avoided. This view is commensurate with indigenous perspectives of nature (Bradshaw et al., 2020), but also with biological conservationists who argue for the protection of 50% of nature ("*nature needs half*"). For "deep ecologists", social equity can fundamentally conflict with efforts to reduce the degradation of ecological environments, and even placing some level of concern for disadvantaged groups ahead of conservation efforts "ultimately sees nature as just a 'resource' for humans" (Kopnina, Washington, Gray, & Taylor, 2018, p. 142). In other examples, we are reminded how the mechanisms for promoting environmental and social equity are no longer universal, and the benefits may be diffuse: substituting small-scale farming for intensive farming may require biotechnologies or informal markets to improve biodiversity, yields, or profits (Mincyte, 2011), or replacing local bus transport with carbon-efficient systems can lead to job loss and precarity (Pulido-Martinez, 2008). While seeking to balance multiple demands on the environment, in practice sustainable development has generated considerable debate over its ability to deal with competing socioeconomic benefits and environmental costs.

Much of the debate about sustainable development relates to managing trade-offs, but as shown, its terms are not ethically neutral (Hayward, 2012). In making the case for sustainable development, the different perspectives and assumptions about health can lead to different tools for action and questions over who has responsibility for bearing the burden of mitigating climate change (Braveman, 2010). One approach to managing this complexity is asking what principles should be applied across peoples and environments, so that a range of conceptual approaches that focus on the ecological health of nonhuman elements such as trees or soil can be considered (Gislason, 2013). It may involve identifying the related principles, values, and norms that sustainable development and critical health psychology approaches share. One of these is the concern about health inequality, to which this chapter turns.

Health inequality

Research on health inequalities has changed very little over the past decades. However, the sustainable development literature adds a new dimension by considering the need to generate (sustainable) growth to reduce poverty and health inequality. This can also increase environmental impacts through raised consumption, so there is a need to better understand the role of cooperation and inequality in efforts to mitigate climate change (Kitting, 2014). For example, ensuring that homes are properly heated or cooled can lead to an increase in energy consumption and air pollution, while creating the optimal household thermal conditions for pathogens (Vardoulakis & Heaviside, 2012).

Climate change poses a major burden to vulnerable populations (UNFCCC, 2017). The UN Climate Change and Health committee reports that climate change is expected to exacerbate health problems like infectious diseases and malnutrition, and that these impacts are worsened by existing inequalities. These inequalities may be spatial and economic – for example, communities that have a poor basic infrastructure for water supply, sanitation, and transport are those most badly hit by climate change, and least likely to recover quickly after extreme events (see Benevolenza & DeRigne, 2019; Charron, 2012). Poverty and economic deprivation put these communities at the greatest risk of having to rely on already degraded ecosystems, which can combine with a lack of alternatives, leading to over-reliance and further degradation. Alternately, the rich and those who live in the developed world have a greater capacity to protect themselves against climate-related health impacts. This can include having better protection against diseases produced by climate conditions (e.g. respiratory diseases) or resources to protect against the health effects of displacement, and food and water insecurity caused by floods and drought (Patz, Campbell-Lendrum, Holloway, & Foley, 2005).

Climate change raises issues of gender and racialised inequality. Women, for example, are more likely to be affected because of their social and economic roles. In circumstances of drought, women may have to walk further to collect water (Baker, 2015), be less-able swimmers, and be more likely to be working on land when flooding occurs (Vincent, Cull, & Archer, 2010). In areas of economic development where parks or nature spaces have become scarce resources, women may have their leisure time reduced relative to men, reducing the positive benefit they may receive to their health (MacBride-Stewart, Gong, & Antell, 2016; Vincent et al., 2010). Furthermore, the experiences of women vary depending on their economic and geographic location. It must be noted too that efforts to address climate injustice risk reinforcing and normalising gender inequalities if gender roles are not properly considered (MacGregor, 2009). For example, economic incentives can perpetuate women's roles as household growers or caretakers of household finances, if not directed towards local food systems or public decision-making (see further work on structural vulnerability; Moran, Hollenbeck, & Phoenix, 2013).

Addressing inequality on a global scale requires cooperation. Yet, the major economies of the Global North have significantly higher levels of consumption and a greater proportion of emissions per person compared to the global south. This asymmetry of economics and political power between richer and poorer nations produces disparities in exposures to climate change (Cushing et al., 2015; in relation to COVID-19, see Foster & Suwandi, 2020). Sustainable development has been used as a conceptually pragmatic approach for addressing cooperation, for example, through efforts to redress the "ecological debt" (owed by the Global North) by targeting resources at regions or areas that are the most vulnerable to climate change. Due to the complex interactions between inequality and the scale at which climate change occurs, efforts to address health inequality need to be cognisant of how it can act differently in different contexts. For example, improvements at the household level that include fuel, water, sanitation, and food have the greatest effect on the most vulnerable communities. Once basic household-level needs are addressed, improvements at the community (e.g. air quality) and the global level, become more important for tackling environmental health problems (UNDESA, 2013). In addition, models of public health development that work closely with local communities are also regarded as more successful than those that intervene without community involvement (Nading, 2014).

This chapter has so far explained how human health is negatively affected by both extreme climate change events and ongoing human-led processes of ecological change. Conceptualising health connects back to sustainable development: economic, social, and environmental determinants of health can be integrated in the effort to reduce climate-related health inequalities. In this context, health is also understood as part of an environmental paradox where, as humans increasingly use nature for health, so their potential contribution to climate change also increases. For critical health theorists, the need to drive better health outcomes based on these interdependencies requires a closer understanding of how inequalities contribute to the degradation of the environment and create disparities in environmental health, with disproportionate impacts on the most vulnerable in society. Despite a long history of health research on the socioeconomic contributions to health inequalities and efforts to address social injustice, the need for a cooperative or integrative approach, is identified is a way forward (Campbell & Jovchelovitch, 2000).

Towards ecological health approaches

Frumkin (2016) identified three main developments towards the emergence of a modern field of environmental health research. The first was research into chemical hazards (as described in the seminal work of Rachel Carson's (1962) *Silent Spring*) and the second was the subfield of environmental psychology that, drawing from cognitive approaches, considered human perceptions of the natural environment. The latter led to concepts such as "biophilia" (Wilson, 2017) and "topophila" (Tuan, 1990), which have been used respectively to describe the innate and socially-constituted emotional ties that people have with the environment. The third development was the continued integration of ecological approaches with human health. This development built on advances in the natural sciences, while seeking to better understand the relationships between humans and ecological systems. This section sets out three ways in which ecological approaches have been integrated into perspectives on human health (ecohealth, one health, and planetary health). The explanation of each of these approaches takes up the themes discussed in the previous section and offers an explanation for each about how the relationship between the environment and health has been conceived.

Notably, a properly ecological conceptualisation of health requires something of a paradigm shift, in that ecology is an approach that avoids reducing the relationship between human health and the environment to a series of linear, mechanistic, cause–effect relationships (MacNaughton, 2003). In that way it is more aligned to a critical health psychology approach, which is informed by conceptualisations of health that acknowledge the interplay of societal, psychological, and biological processes (Murray, 2014). While critical health approaches are broad enough in scope to resist definition they share an interest in how the experiences and meanings of health are connected to these larger domains of human relationships, action and power (Parkes & Horwitz, 2016). At the core of both a critical health and an ecological approach is the desire to attend to the plurality of meanings and structures that inform our understanding of the role of health in a changing world.

Ecohealth/ecosystem health

An ecohealth or ecosystems health approach is an interdisciplinary approach that links health thinking in the social and health sciences to that of the natural sciences (McLaren & Hawe, 2005). At the heart of its conceptualisation is the natural ecosystem. Using concepts and metaphors from natural systems thinking, it helps describe interdependencies between ecosystem and human health (Dakubo, 2013). With health represented in this way, this approach is an alternative to the linearity inherent in medical or biological models of disease and illness (Roger et al., 2016). However, its tendency to prioritise thinking about the component parts of the system, over the relationships and evolving processes that constitute the system as a whole, can lead to reductionism, and is one of the main barriers against its acceptance within critical psychology.

Notably, systems thinking has a long history in medicine where biological systems describe the disease as a breakdown in "networks of interacting components – such as the coordination of internal systems (nervous, endocrine, respiratory, etc.) with gene and gene product expression and behavioural and environmental factors" (Federoff & Gostin, 2009, p. 994). Systems thinking has been useful for the health sciences where health has been described as "a fundamental property of life at all levels of organization, from cells to the biosphere ... [where] at each level, health can be compromised ... and complex systems can break down" (Rapport & Singh, 2006, p. 79). Rather than rejecting systems approaches, the diverse processes that they describe may promote an understanding of health as a set of reciprocal yet functional processes (Chowdhury & Haque, 2013; Rapport & Singh, 2006).

Ecosystems approaches have emerged to make it easier to identify those aspects needed to repair a breakdown in the system. Where the breakdown refers to disease, it approaches the patient as a collection of visceral organs or as a nervous system. This has been critiqued by critical health scholars because of the way the ecosystems approach advances specific domains of scientific knowledge (e.g. neurology or gynaecology) over that of patient experiences and beliefs (pain, distress), normative ideologies, or the relationships of power that shape the relationship between the two (Lyons & Chamberlain, 2017). Ecosystem health approaches may address the gap in considering the environmental drivers of health, by providing a context for understanding how the relationships in the physical, natural, nonhuman world contribute to human health across different domains of knowledge (Charron, 2012; Sheiham, 2009). However, it remains the case that critical attention needs to be given to how health is being shaped by these relationships, in an ongoing way.

Notably, in the field of health – where two ideas about the environment dominate: the environment where people live, work, and recreate; and the environment as nature or the "wild" – a key concern has been the social environment (Fox & Alldred, 2016). Bronfenbrenner's (1979) ecological systems theory is a conceptual model that draws attention to a range of environmental influences on individual health. Pictured as five layers of nested circles, it provides a visual representation of the various levels of social influence that extend from the individual to those further away from the centre, from microsystem of family/peers, to the macrosystem (or attitudes, culture, ideologies), and the exosystem (neighbours / public sphere). Similarly, it also provides an understanding of how possible interventions, when introduced at one level (e.g. changing city streets), may influence and shape health at another level (e.g. encouraging individuals to participate in active travel). The "turn to nature" that has been occurring in the social sciences has the potential to offer a more critical approach to ecosystem health, focusing on the dynamic flows of information and power relations that support the "system", noting that as the ecosystem is made of diverse worldviews, ideologies, and discourses, there is a need to be attuned to the presence of potential conflicts between different elements (Grove, 2015).

A qualitatively new idea of an ecosystem is emerging here to explain thinking about connections between the health of humans and the state of the environment (Rapport & Singh, 2006). For McShane (2004), this development can be understood across a spectrum. At one end is the functionalist approach using traditional ecological systems thinking that represent health as a complex entity, with "a structure and functioning parts just [like] organisms, but on a larger scale" (McShane, 2004, p. 87). The other end is based on an ecocentrist view that the nonhuman world is much more of a space of socio-ecological interconnection.

Building on this, an ecosystem health approach has three main conceptual elements:

i)   it borrows from natural systems thinking to represent and explain the relationships between social, ecological, and economic aspects that shape health, taking seriously the view that human health is consequential on ecological and not just social or economic aspects (Dakubo, 2013);

ii) it views nature and health as a set of reciprocal relationships among living and non-living things, with no distinction made between human and nonhuman elements (Nguyen-Viet et al., 2015); and

iii) it can also be represented as an ecological whole, in which the health of the entire system (also known as a "biome") itself is more important than its constituent elements (McShane, 2004).

Biopower is highly relevant to understanding how ecohealth has the potential to align itself with a critical health approach. Biopower has been used to describe regulatory forces that shape the social and medical systems that human health is ultimately part of, and which influence our understanding of risk and uncertainty under conditions that establish what is possible for individual lives (and human populations) to achieve (Foucault et al., 2006). However, while traditional ecosystem approaches are shaped by the idea that systems can be self-organising and adaptive in response to external forces, for critical health scholars this biological aspect of the model (and its orientation towards ideas about equilibrium and stasis) is less important (Grove, 2015). Rather, a critical understanding of an ecosystems approach mobilises a discussion about various socio-political processes – for example, resilience and productivity – that contribute to the normative shaping of the relations between human health and ecological processes (Rapport, 2007).

Where an explicit goal of an ecohealth approach has been to rethink health through a consideration of their sustainability and value for human health (Baker, 2015; Bunch, 2016), contemporary research from critical health studies approaches health as a socio-ecological issue that regards ecosystems as loosely and contingently defined. Not only does such an approach take seriously the broadening of the concept of the environment to include its natural, physical, cultural, and social aspects (McLaren & Hawe, 2005). It also involves a rethinking of the concept of the social to consider its effects on the wellbeing of "ecological communities", of which humans are now just a part (Gislason, 2013). A socio-ecological perspective on health changes our sense of what health is. Health is the effect of our dependence on intersubjective and ecological wellbeing, informed by relationships that are politically and socially constructed, yet dependant on familiar images or metaphors of the natural world to explain complex processes (McLaren & Hawe, 2005).

Socio-ecological approaches are starting to be utilised by critical health scholars. For example, they may be used to explore the relations and processes that shape of understandings of water quality and health, which may involve the motility of bacteria and parasites, the socio-cultural shaping of the biodiversity of a watershed, and the physical and infrastructural resilience to storms and other natural events. Simultaneously – because ecohealth takes into account the involvement of multiple social dimensions, including the role of public health, cultural practices around water, the contribution to sustainable livelihoods, and the multiple mechanisms of water governance – ecohealth then is taking seriously the idea that human health is the result of dynamic interactions between multiple elements, between ecosystems and social and economic activities. The overall ecosystem health model is one that draws on the discursive goal of working towards equilibrium in, or adaptation to, the environment to produce human health. This largely anthropocentric approach to health is distinguishable from other ecological health models that conceive of health as something that also encompasses nonhumans (animals or ecosystems) (one health), and planetary systems (planetary health).

One health

Constructing health through approaches that integrate the human social world with the ecological or the biological provides rich frameworks for thinking about the relationships between humans, and between human and nonhumans. The contemporary one health approach:

> recognises that the health of humans, animals, and ecosystems is intimately connected and involves a coordinated, collaborative, interdisciplinary, and cross-sectoral approach to addressing a wide range of risks at the animal–human–ecosystem interface.
>
> *(Zinsstag, 2012, p. 371)*

The roots of this approach comes from the integration of veterinary and public health sciences, which is distinct from the engineering science base of the ecosystems health model. It has been strengthened in recent times through contributions from broad disciplinary areas, including environmental health, microbiology, and health economics (Lerner & Berg, 2017). While ecosystem health does address animal health, it is mostly in the context of diseases transmitted from animals to humans, and the impacts of ecosystem change on human health. one health on the other hand expands focuses mainly on "issues squarely at the nexus of human and animal health", including the impacts of ecosystem changes on animal health (Zinsstag, 2012, p. 372).

One health has traditionally dominated in the management of disease threats to humans from animals. It is interested in how human and animal health are linked through climate change, where zoonotic diseases (SARS, MERS, Ebola, H1N1, and now COVID-19), for example, are indicators of climate change. Rather than just tracking their effects, its potency is the development of animal-based (often bio-technological) solutions that benefit both humans and animals (and here it is more aligned to the planetary health approach discussed next). In COVID-19, for example, the genomic mapping of influenza viruses in animal populations was one of the first scientific discoveries of the origins of the disease, which has been critical in the development of a vaccine and for identifying the processes on its ongoing development (or mutation) (Amanat & Krammer, 2020; Enjuanes et al., 2008). More recently, it has extended to developing nature-based solutions for human health. It is a field with broadening interests, for example, from antimicrobial resistance (e.g. bees) to food issues (e.g. nutritional quality and water supplies) and light/noise pollution (e.g. birds and insects), where animal responses are used either as indicators for, or solutions to, both animal and human health.

Despite their differences, calls have been made for the better integration of ecohealth and one health approaches (Morand, Guégan, & Laurans, 2020). This is based on the understanding that nonhumans profoundly shape human societies through disease and other ecological processes, and that a consideration of the nonhuman perspective means engaging with the social, political, and economic dimensions of both natural and social environments. Ecohealth in particular has benefited from the contributions from one health, having taken up the view that human health is an important outcome of effective ecosystem management, particularly where local issues may have an impact at a wider scale (e.g. infertility in fish stocks caused by microplastics also reflects a larger issue of waste disposal and human consumption). More than this, giving substance to this integrative logic would facilitate, in particular, how to consider the potential for not only human agency (in the management and control of illness) but for opening up questions that allow for forms of "ecological agency". Here, plants, animals, and organisms are conceived as active participants in the shaping of the environment and the social world.

However, despite the one health concept generating new research topics that are very different to those in the veterinary sciences and human infectiology, it is clear that some of the integrative potentialities described here remain at the margins of this approach (Zinsstag et al., 2020). One health is arguably less interdisciplinary than ecohealth and has been represented as more of an "umbrella" concept, sometimes presented as deriving from a "holistic" linking of some specialised approaches (Morand et al., 2020). Rather than seeing health as being the product of socio-ecological aggregations, systems, and processes, one health segregates and often distinguishes between the social and environmental determinants of human and nonhuman disease. The value of improving integrated and cooperative understanding in this field may still be driven by more practical concerns – leading to biomonitoring and biosecurity – than conceptual approaches, which are more often linked to ecohealth.

Planetary health

Building on the work of sustainable development and a recognition of the anthropogenic crisis caused by climate change, the planetary health approach focuses on achieving an attainable and sustainable standard of human health and places particular value on nature for health. The proponents of planetary health state that: "*put simply, planetary health is the health of human civilisation and the state of the natural systems on which it depends*" (Horton & Lo, 2015). Due to its focus on human wellbeing but also on the use of natural resources for health (Whitmee et al., 2015) some authors make the claim that planetary health is distinct from one health and ecohealth. However, this critique does not consider the full spectrum of sustainable development approaches introduced earlier (Baker, 2015). In light of an ecocentrist (or deep ecological) viewpoint and arguments in support of maintaining the integrity of ecological systems, a planetary health approach might otherwise be more closely aligned to ecohealth.

planetary health was recently conceived jointly by the Rockefeller (USA) and Lancet (UK) foundations (Horton et al., 2014). Its aim is to meet the aspirations of a global and transdisciplinary public health approach, taking into account present systems of governance and institutions of knowledge. The concept has been largely promoted by academics in international public health and epidemiology, but also by global health bodies, such as the International Red Cross and UN. This prefiguration is why the dominant rationale for health remains a predominantly human one (see Baker, 2015). While the goal is to achieve interdisciplinarity, much of the struggles around this approach emerge from efforts to define and distinguish the concept of health being planetary (to include social as well as ecological layers like landscapes, "biomes", "critical zones"). The alternative is to integrate with socio-ecological thinking to support a concrete willingness to combine the medical, animal health, and ecological dimensions in order to analyse and understand the problems of climate change (Morand et al., 2020).

Where one health, ecohealth and planetary health are aligned is in their understanding of the potential for developments in biotechnology, science, and information systems (also known as "technological modernisation") to address environment-related health problems (Pellow & Brehm, 2013). Notably, the first two approaches identify a role for multiple nature-based, socio-ecological technologies that improve environmental quality and human health, respectively. Planetary Health provides the impetus for grounding these developments in a critical understanding of the science-driven and centralised discourses associated with top-down climate monitoring and mitigation techniques implemented at global scales. It is an approach that seeks to respond to the market-driven approach used to produce these technologies and encourage health. It does this by aligning with globalised as well as civic society practices of healthcare delivery, by focusing on the expansion and the saturation of the concept of health itself, to include the governance of individuals, populations, as well as natural environments. This approach has been devised in light of concerns about economic growth, scare resources, and ecological destruction (Baker, 2015). Thus planetary health represents a shift from national to global health issues (understood in its broadest sense), with particular attention given to the generation of new medical technologies, new health markets, and new actors (see also Barry, 2007). The emphasis is on innovative research and methodological steering towards nature-based, human–animal solutions and "planetary" conscious practices.

For critical health scholars, planetary health represents the acceleration of medical innovation (e.g. new plant-based drugs or other technologies), and the need to address ethical issues (e.g. about the exploitation of resources, including those belonging to indigenous communities). It seeks to question the normative expression of planetary health's proposals about what health research *should* do, whom it should include and how health is being constituted. It recognises the drivers for this include the loss of efficiency of existing medical resources and the general slowing down of health gains in the context of climate change, particularly because of the consequences of health consumption and the re-emergence of a focus on biological processes in the model has not been critically addressed.

Despite disagreement over the merits of planetary health as conceptually able to address the main challenges it has identified as maintaining and enhancing human health (i.e. imagination, research, and information and governance), planetary health offers the opportunity for a "global and national" strategy of reform of policies and practices (Whitmee et al., 2015, p. 1973). Its strengths lie in its potential to encompass one health and ecohealth, while appealing to health professionals who are already working on a broad agenda for climate change. Similarly, it proposes a range of solutions which in the context of food provision, for example, range from the reduction of food spoilage, to biofortification of foods and the promotion of healthy, low environment impact diets, along with interventions at the city or health system level (e.g. sustainable cities). Some of its most innovative thinking is at the intersection of socio-ecological approaches, where research into impacts of land-use changes (for mining or transport) has identified increases in malaria, and similarly forest conservation has been shown to reduce malarial disease. This focus on extending medicine towards tackling environmental health challenges, has allowed for planetary health to become the approach of choice for health funders in the UK and USA in recent times.

The critical potential of ecological health approaches

The concept of ecological health has proven very helpful for understanding how society is addressing the challenges of climate change. First, health researchers have proposed different approaches (described above) using different conceptualisations of the relationships between society and the environment for the maintenance and protection of health. Second, sustainable development is implicit in each approach. In this final section, the critical potential of ecological approaches is considered in their effectiveness of having implemented a discursive and material shift in addressing the vulnerability of human health in the context of climate change.

Resilience, and the limits of lifestyle thinking and behavioural change

The most problematic aspect of environmental and public health responses to climate change is that health problems are still often attributed to peoples' "reckless behaviours and inappropriate land-use practices" (Dakubo, 2013, p. 28). Viewed through a critical lens, lifestyle and behaviour have been incorporated also into the logic of an environment that has been constructed as a resource or commodity for health. Lifestyles have become lived cultures that people use to express their capacity to manage or adapt to the pressures of the environment (Blackman, 2005). In turn, the ecological contexts and human efforts, are arranged through the discourse of adaptation, and the opportunities it offers people for managing health in the context of a damaged environment (EASAC, 2019).

Ecological approaches have introduced new social and environmental relational complexities in the efforts to address climate change impacts, which also lends itself to resilience thinking (Methmann & Oels, 2014). In a social context, the concept of resilience might consider how the economic "livelihoods of communities may be able to buffer the changes in economic conditions within a particular system or landscape" or the resilience of cultural traditions within the context of their capacity to be transferred through one generation to the next (Rapport, 2007, p. 81). Within a health context, resilience may refer to the capacity of a population to "cope with" endemic disease or the risk of it. This may involve managing the disease but also the social and economic processes that may be affected by, for example, loss of work through illness from a malarial or dengue disease, or a necessary change in household practices to prevent the storage of water-breeding sites.

The latest IPCC report states from the outset that there while there are a range of strategies for adaptation that can reduce the risks of climate change that there are some limits to adaptations and humans' resilience once planetary temperatures reach 1.5°C (IPCC, 2018, p. 10). Due to the tendency to construct resilience in ecological terms where it is understood as a return to stasis after a disruption, Urry (2009) has argued that the assumption that systems naturally seek out equilibrium needs to be rethought in the context of existing practices of economic growth, where feedback loops produce ever more drain on existing and limited resources.

Resilience therefore can be used at both individual and societal levels to describe either psychological qualities or structural solutions, as well as their limits. The ecological approaches explored here have initiated a discursive shift towards integration and critical thinking, where responses to climate change are presented as a more contextualised story of the health of a community and of animals, plants, ecosystems, and the planet. As such, dealing with climate change requires a thorough appraisal of how these processes are structured by dominant expectations about how different people (should) act in relation to the environment. The ecological approaches here could be used to explore the many links between vulnerable communities, nonhumans, development, and environmental quality. Accordingly, complementing these efforts with sustainable development narratives has encouraged a conversation about how communities with more capacities to withstand shocks, or longer-term climatic changes, have better health outcomes than those where these capabilities have been undermined (Hobden, 2014). Efforts then at improving the health of diverse communities are increasingly challenged by the need to understand how resilience and capacity discourses are also dependant on political decisions, policies, and practices negotiated in the context of sustainable development.

Conclusion

Climate change will contribute to major health consequences which we must address. This chapter has so far explained how it may be necessary to reject a traditional focus on human health that does not give proper attention to the argument that there are natural limits to human activities and environmental resources. The role of health in climate change represents a paradox in which human health is improving as environmental processes are degrading, which in turn is leading to health gains being stalled or reversing. For critical health studies, existing critiques concerning claims about the unlimited possibilities for human health (Rose, 2001) may also need to consider how to address these environmental limits identified by climate change. Accepting the existence of environmental limits means either accepting that there are difficult trade-offs between competing social and environmental priorities that have to be accommodated, or that there needs to be a redistribution of priorities, to achieve human health (Baker, 2015).

A conceptual approach to how thinking about human health and the natural environment can be redistributed is provided jointly by ecological health models. This chapter has outlined three key ecological health approaches that offer a meaningful picture of how health is understood and conceptualised in the context of climate change. Comparing these approaches can be misleading, given their varied conceptual and methodological descriptions. Yet, it has also been possible to also explain how sustainable development discourses are at the core of how climate change effects are being considered, and the challenges facing the critical health research community in their efforts to finding effective and equitable solutions. Furthermore, since health challenges can both be immediate (i.e. in response to climate shocks), or long term, taking account of the diffuse health effects of climate change can be difficult.

One important contribution from ecological health has been its role in encouraging solutions requiring critical health scholars to work with other disciplines and fields of knowledge. The complex intersection between climate change and sustainable development also provides the space for a strong critique of existing patterns of health inequalities focused largely on socioeconomic determinants. This is because the effects of climate change are mediated through social, cultural, and economic structures and processes that are unevenly distributed for some communities. The opportunity for social analysis (rather than description) has been welcomed (Kaijser & Kronsell, 2014). In particular, critical theorists argue that climate change is an opportunity to rethink both the concept of the health of, and our relationship with, the natural world.

References

Adams, M. (2016). *Ecological crisis, sustainability and the psychosocial subject.* London: Palgrave Macmillan.

Amanat, F., & Krammer, F. (2020). SARS-CoV-2 vaccines: Status report. *Immunity, 52*(4), 583–589.

Baker, S. (2014). Governance. In C. Death (Ed.), *Critical environmental politics* (pp. 100–110). London: Routledge.

Baker, S. (2015). *Sustainable development.* London: Routledge.

Barry, J. (2007). *Environment and social theory.* London: Routledge.

Benevolenza, M.A., & DeRigne, L. (2019). The impact of climate change and natural disasters on vulnerable populations: A systematic review of literature. *Journal of Human Behavior in the Social Environment, 29*(2), 266–281.

Blackman, S. (2005). Youth subcultural theory: A critical engagement with the concept, its origins and politics, from the Chicago school to postmodernism. *Journal of Youth Studies, 8*(1), 1–20.

Bradshaw, R. E., Bellgard, S. E., Black, A., Burns, B. R., Gerth, M. L., McDougal, R. L., … Winkworth, R. C. (2020). Phytophthora agathidicida: Research progress, cultural perspectives and knowledge gaps in the control and management of kauri dieback in New Zealand. *Plant Pathology, 69*(1), 3–16.

Braveman, P. (2010). Social conditions, health equity, and human rights. *Health and Human Rights, 12*(2), 31–48.

Bronfenbrenner, U. (1979). *The ecology of human development: Experiments in nature and design.* Cambridge, MA: Harvard University Press.

Bunch, M. J. (2016). Ecosystem approaches to health and wellbeing: Navigating complexity, promoting health in social–ecological systems. *Systems Research and Behavioral Science*, *33*(5), 614–632.

Campbell, C., & Jovchelovitch, S. (2000). Health, community and development: Towards a social psychology of participation. *Journal of Community & Applied Social Psychology*, *10*(4), 255–270.

Carson, R. (1962). *Silent spring*. Boston, MA: Houghton Mifflin Harcourt.

Charron, D. F. (2012). EcoHealth: Origins and approach. In D. F. Charron (Ed.), *Ecohealth research in practice: Innovative applications of an ecosystem approach to health* (pp. 1–32). Ottawa, ON: Springer.

Chowdhury, P. D., & Haque, C. E. (2013). Why is an integrated social-ecological systems (ISES) lens needed to explain causes and determinants of disease? A case study of dengue in Dhaka, Bangladesh. In M. K. Gislason (Ed.), *Ecological health: Society, ecology and health* (pp. 217–239). Bingley: Emerald.

Clayton, S., Devine-Wright, P., Stern, P. C., Whitmarsh, L., Carrico, A., Steg, L., … Bonnes, M. (2015). Psychological research and global climate change. *Nature Climate Change*, *5*(7), 640–646.

Cushing, L., Morello-Frosch, R., Wander, M., & Pastor, M. (2015). The haves, the have-nots, and the health of everyone: The relationship between social inequality and environmental quality. *Annual Review of Public Health*, *36*, 193–209.

Dakubo, C. (2013). Towards a critical approach to Ecohealth research, theory and practice. In M. K. Gislason (Ed). *Ecological health: Society, ecology and health* (pp. 23–43). Bingley: Emerald.

Death, C. (2014). Critical, environmental, political: An introduction. In C. Death (Ed.), *Critical environmental politics* (pp. 1–12). London: Routledge.

EASAC. (2019). *The imperative of climate action to protect human health in Europe: Opportunities for adaptation to reduce the impacts, and for mitigation to capitalise on the benefits of decarbonization*. Jagerberg: German National Academy of Sciences Leopoldina.

Enjuanes, L., DeDiego, M. L., Álvarez, E., Deming, D., Sheahan, T., & Baric, R. (2008). Vaccines to prevent severe acute respiratory syndrome coronavirus-induced disease. *Virus Research*, *133*(1), 45–62.

Federoff, H. J., & Gostin, L. O. (2009). Evolving from reductionism to holism: Is there a future for systems medicine? *Jama*, *302*(9), 994–996.

Ferreira, C. M., Sá, M. J., Martins, J. G., & Serpa, S. (2020). The COVID-19 contagion–pandemic dyad: A view from social sciences. *Societies*, *10*(4), 1–19.

Forzieri, G., Bianchi, A., e Silva, F. B., Herrera, M. A. M., Leblois, A., Lavalle, C., … Feyen, L. (2018). Escalating impacts of climate extremes on critical infrastructures in Europe. *Global Environmental Change*, *48*, 97–107.

Foster, B. J., & Suwandi, I. (2020). COVID-19 and catastrophe capitalism. *Monthly Review*. Retrieved from https://monthlyreview.org/2020/06/01/covid-19-and-catastrophe-capitalism/

Foucault, M., Lagrange, J. E., Burchell, G. T., Ewald, F. E., Fontana, A. E., & Davidson, A. I. (2006). *Michel Foucault: Psychiatric power: Lectures at the Collège de France, 1973–1974*. London: Palgrave Macmillan.

Fox, N. J., & Alldred, P. (2016). *Sociology and the new materialism: Theory, research, action*. London: SAGE Publications.

Franchini, M., & Mannucci, P. M. (2015). Impact on human health of climate changes. *European Journal of Internal Medicine*, *26*(1), 1–5.

Francois, R., Caron, A., Morand, S., Pedrono, M., Michel De Garine-Wichatitsky, Chevalier, V., Tran, A., Gaidet, N., Figuié, M., Marie-Noël, D.V. And Binot, A. (2016). One health and EcoHealth: The same wine in different bottles?. *Infection Ecology & Epidemiology*, *6*(1), 30978.

Frosh, S. (2003). Psychosocial studies and psychology: Is a critical approach emerging? *Human Relations*, *56*(12), 1545–1567.

Frumkin, H. (2016). Introduction to environmental health. In H. Frumkin (Ed.), *Environmental health: From global to local* (pp. 12–27). San Francisco, CA: John Wiley & Sons.

Gifford, R. (2011). The dragons of inaction: Psychological barriers that limit climate change mitigation and adaptation. *American Psychologist*, *66*(4), 290–302.

Gislason, M. K. (2013). Expanding the social: Moving towards the ecological in social studies of health. In M. K. Gislason (Ed.), *Ecological health: Society, ecology and health* (pp. 3–22). Bingley: Emerald.

Grove, K. (2015). Biopolitics. In C. Death (Ed.), *Critical environmental politics* (pp. 22–30). London: Routledge.

Haines, A., Kovats, R. S., Campbell-Lendrum, D., & Corvalán, C. (2006). Climate change and human health: Impacts, vulnerability and public health. *Public Health*, *120*(7), 585–596.

Hanna, P., Wijesinghe, S., Paliatsos, I., Walker, C., Adams, M., & Kimbu, A. (2019). Active engagement with nature: Outdoor adventure tourism, sustainability and wellbeing. *Journal of Sustainable Tourism*, *27*(9), 1355–1373.

Hayward, T. (2012). Climate change and ethics. *Nature Climate Change, 2*(12), 843–848.

Hobden, S. (2014). Postmodernism. In C. Death (Ed.), *Critical environmental politics* (pp. 175–184). London: Routledge.

Horton, R., Beaglehole, R., Bonita, R., Raeburn, J., McKee, M., & Wall, S. (2014). From public to planetary health: A manifesto. *The Lancet, 383*(9920), 847.

Horton, R., & Lo, S. (2015). Planetary health: A new science for exceptional action. *The Lancet, 386*(10007), 1921–1922.

Huber, M., Knottnerus, J. A., Green, L., van der Horst, H., Jadad, A. R., Kromhout, D., … Schnabel, P. (2011). How should we define health?. *BMJ, 343*, d4163.

Intergovernmental Panel on Climate Change (IPCC). (2018). *Special report: Global warming of 1.5°C*. Retrieved from https://www.ipcc.ch/sr15/ (accessed 12 May 2019).

Kaijser, A., & Kronsell, A. (2014). Climate change through the lens of intersectionality. *Environmental Politics, 23*(3), 417–433.

Kitting, G. (2014). Limits. In C. Death (Ed.), *Critical environmental politics* (pp. 145–155). London: Routledge.

Kjellstrom, T., & Weaver, H. J. (2009). Climate change and health: Impacts, vulnerability, adaptation and mitigation. *New South Wales Public Health Bulletin, 20*(2), 5–9.

Kopnina, H., Washington, H., Gray, J., & Taylor, B. (2018). The "future of conservation" debate: Defending ecocentrism and the nature needs Half movement. *Biological Conservation, 217*, 140–148.

Liang, L., & Gong, P. (2017). Climate change and human infectious diseases: A synthesis of research findings from global and spatio-temporal perspectives. *Environment International, 103*, 99–108.

Lerner, H., & Berg, C. (2017). A comparison of three holistic approaches to health: One health, EcoHealth, and planetary health. *Frontiers in Veterinary Science, 4*, 163.

Louv, R. (2009). Do our kids have nature-deficit disorder. *Educational Leadership, 67*(4), 24–30.

Lyons A. C., & Chamberlain, L. (2017). Critical health psychology. In B. Gough (Ed.), *The Palgrave handbook of critical social psychology* (pp. 533–555). London: Palgrave Macmillan UK.

MacBride-Stewart, S. (2019). Atmospheres, landscapes and nature: Off-road runners' experiences of wellbeing. *Health, 23*(2), 139–157.

MacBride-Stewart, S., Gong, Y., & Antell, J. (2016). Exploring the interconnections between gender, health and nature. *Public Health, 141*, 279–286.

MacGregor, S. (2009). A stranger silence still: The need for feminist social research on climate change. *The Sociological Review, 57*(2_suppl), 124–140.

MacNaughton, P. (2003). Embodying the environment in everyday life practices. *Sociological Review, 51*(1), 63–84.

Maller, C., Townsend, M., Brown, P., & St Leger, L. (2002). *Healthy parks, healthy people: The health benefits of contact with nature in a park context: A review of current literature*. Melbourne, VIC: Parks Victoria, and Deakin University Faculty of Health & Behavioural Sciences.

McLaren, L., & Hawe, P. (2005). Ecological perspectives in health research. *Journal of Epidemiology & Community Health, 59*(1), 6–14.

McMichael, A. J. (2013). Globalization, climate change, and human health. *New England Journal of Medicine, 368*(14), 1335–1343.

McShane, K. (2004). Ecosystem health. *Environmental Ethics, 26*(3), 227–245.

Methmann, C., & Oels, A. (2014). Postmodernism. In C. Death (Ed.), *Critical environmental politics* (277–286). London: Routledge.

Mincyte, D. (2011). Subsistence and sustainability in post-industrial Europe: The politics of small-scale farming in Europeanising Lithuania. *Sociologia Ruralis, 51*(2), 101–118.

Moldan, B., Janoušková, S., & Hák, T. (2012). How to understand and measure environmental sustainability: Indicators and targets. *Ecological Indicators, 17*, 4–13.

Moran, R., Hollenbeck, J., & Phoenix, C. (2013). Structural vulnerability and narrative: Sensitising concepts for understanding the health impacts of climate change. In M. K. Gislason (Ed.), *Ecological health: Society, ecology and health* (pp. 109–126). Bingley: Emerald.

Morand, S., Guégan, J.-F., Laurans, Y. (2020). From one health to Ecohealth, mapping the incomplete integration of human, animal and environmental health. *Iddri, Issue Brief, 04/20*.

Murray, M. (2014). Introducing critical health psychology. In M. Murray (Ed.), *Critical health psychology* (pp. 1–16). Basingstoke: Palgrave Macmillan.

Nading, A. M. (2014). *Mosquito trails: Ecology, health, and the politics of entanglement*. Oakland, CA: University of California Press.

Nguyen-Viet, H., Doria, S., Tung, D. X., Mallee, H., Wilcox, B. A., & Grace, D. (2015). Ecohealth research in Southeast Asia: Past, present and the way forward. *Infectious Diseases of Poverty, 4*(1), 5.

Okereke, C., & Charlesworth, M. (2014). Environmental and ecological justice. In C. Death (Ed.), *Advances in international environmental politics* (pp. 328–355). London: Palgrave Macmillan.

Pálsson, G., Szerszynski, B., Sörlin, S., Marks, J., Avril, B., Crumley, C., ... Buendía, M. P. (2013). Reconceptualizing the "anthropos" in the Anthropocene: Integrating the social sciences and humanities in global environmental change research. *Environmental Science & Policy, 28*, 3–13.

Parkes, M. W., & Horwitz, P. (2016). Ecology and ecosystems as foundational for health. In H. Frumkin (Ed.), *Environmental health: From global to local* (pp. 27–58). San Fransico, CA: John Wiley & Sons.

Patz, J. A., Campbell-Lendrum, D., Holloway, T., & Foley, J. A. (2005). Impact of regional climate change on human health. *Nature, 438*(7066), 310.

Pellow, D. N., & Brehm, N. H. (2013). An environmental sociology for the twenty-first century. *Annual Review of Sociology, 39*, 229–250.

Pulido-Martinez, H. C. (2008). *On psychology, work and the production of the subject: The case of the urban passenger transport system in Bogota, Columbia.* Cardiff: Cardiff University.

Rapport, D. J. (2007). Sustainability science: An ecohealth perspective. *Sustainability Science, 2*(1), 77–84.

Rapport, D. J., & Singh, A. (2006). An ecohealth-based framework for state of environment reporting. *Ecological Indicators, 6*(2), 409–428.

Raudsepp-Hearne, C., Peterson, G. D., Tengö, M., Bennett, E. M., Holland, T., Benessaiah, K., ... Pfeifer, L. (2010). Untangling the environmentalist's paradox: Why is human wellbeing increasing as ecosystem services degrade? *BioScience, 60*(8), 576–589.

Reser, J. P., Morrissey, S. A., & Ellul, M. (2011). The threat of climate change: Psychological response, adaptation, and impacts. In I. Weissbecker (Ed.), *Climate change and human wellbeing* (pp. 19–42). New York: Springer-Verlag.

Richardson, K., Steffen, W., & Liverman, D. (2011). *Climate change: Global risks and decisions.* Cambridge: Cambridge University Press.

Rose, N. (2001). The politics of life itself. *Theory, Culture & Society, 18*(6), 1–30.

Sheiham, A. (2009). Closing the gap in a generation: Health equity through action on the social determinants of health. A report of the WHO Commission on Social Determinants of Health (CSDH) 2008. *Community Dent Health, 26*(1), 2–3.

Stott, P. A., Gillett, N. P., Hegerl, G. C., Karoly, D. J., Stone, D. A., Zhang, X., & Zwiers, F. (2010). Detection and attribution of climate change: A regional perspective. *Wiley Interdisciplinary Reviews: Climate Change, 1*(2), 192–211.

Tuan, Y. F. (1990). *Topophilia: A study of environmental perceptions, attitudes, and values.* New York: Columbia University Press.

United Nations. (2012). *Futures we want: Outcome document.* Retrieved from https://sustainabledevelopment.un.org/futurewewant.html (accessed 12 May 2019).

United Nations Department of Economic and Social Affairs (UNDESA). (2013). *World economic and social survey 2013: Sustainable development challenges.* New York: UN.

United Nations Framework Convention on Climate Change (UNFCCC). (2017). *Climate change impacts human health.* Retrieved from https://unfccc.int/news/climate-change-impacts-human-health (accessed 13 August 2019).

Urry, J. (2009). Sociology and climate change. *The Sociological Review, 57*(2_suppl), 84–100.

Vardoulakis, S., & Heaviside, C. (2012). *Health effects of climate change in the UK 2012.* London: Health Protection Agency.

Vincent, K., Cull, T., & Archer, E. R. (2010). Gendered vulnerability to climate change in Limpopo province, South Africa. In I. Dankelman (Ed.), *Gender and climate change: An introduction* (pp. 160–167). London: Routledge.

Wells, N. M., Evans, G. W., & Cheek, K. A. (2016). Environmental psychology. In H. Frumkin (Ed.), *Environmental health: From global to local* (pp. 203–290). San Fransico, CA: John Wiley & Sons.

White, J. (2017). Climate change and the generational timescape. *The Sociological Review, 65*(4), 763–778.

Whitmee, S., Haines, A., Beyrer, C., Boltz, F., Capon, A. G., de Souza Dias, B. F., ... Horton, R. (2015). Safeguarding human health in the anthropocene epoch: Report of The Rockefeller Foundation–Lancet Commission on planetary health. *The Lancet, 386*(10007), 1973–2028.

WHO. (1986). *Ottawa charter for health promotion.* Geneva: World Health Organization.

WHO. (2018). *COP24 special report health & climate change*. Geneva: World Health Organization.

Wilson, E. O. (2017). *Biophilia*. Cambridge, MA: Harvard University Press.

World Commission on Environment and Development (WCED). (1987). *Our common future*. Oxford: Oxford University Press.

Zinsstag, J. (2012). Convergence of ecohealth and one health. *EcoHealth*, *9*, 371–373.

Zinsstag, J., Schelling, E., Crump, L., Whittaker, M., Tanner, M., & Stephen, C. (Eds.). (2020). *One health: The theory and practice of integrated health approaches* (2nd ed.). Wallingford: CABI International.

27

GLOBALISATION AND HEALTH

Angelina Taylor and Johanna Hanefeld

Introduction to globalisation

This chapter introduces *globalisation* as an important concept for understanding health. As the world becomes more interconnected and interdependent, globalisation is increasingly relevant to all aspects of health. More than ever, people are travelling and moving across the globe; pathogens can spread within a matter of days or weeks to almost all continents; multinational companies are based in almost every country worldwide, and the internet and mass media connect the world's population to just a small set of channels and platforms. Lifestyles, exposures, and identities cut across country borders. The most recent prominent shifts for globalisation and health relate to our social identities, with the way in which we see ourselves and relate to each other becoming an increasingly shared and uniform experience worldwide. Politics and the internet are playing decisive roles in this change, with 45% of the world's population using social media at the beginning of 2019 (Statista, 2020) and a wave of divided politics sweeping across the globe.

Globalisation is a complex cross-cutting issue, and the other chapters in this handbook, such as those on migration and commercialisation, can be described as examples of globalisation topics. This chapter is written from the perspective that globalisation is fundamental in its own right to our understanding of planetary health today.

This chapter includes several sections to illustrate the breadth of the topic. This includes the section "Introduction to globalisation", which covers a discussion of its definition and history. The section "Globalisation as a health topic" describes why globalisation is an important but to date little researched public health topic and why a *planetary health* perspective of globalisation is particularly useful. The section "Global coordination, health policies and governance" describes the value of increasingly global coordination beyond individual countries, along with the changing nature of the actors and governance architectures. "Climate change, the environment and communicable diseases" highlights the substantial impact that climate change and environmental are having and are predicted to have on health. The section "Trade, commercialisation and noncommunicable diseases" describes the role that economic globalisation is playing in changing diets and lifestyles, including tobacco use, and the shift worldwide to a predominance of noncommunicable diseases. Finally, the section "Global communication, changing politics and their roles in health" draws attention to changes in social identities worldwide, potentially the most recently area of globalisation to emerge.

What is globalisation?

Globalisation can be understood as the intensification of the global exchange of technological, cultural, economic, institutional, social, and environmental activities. These include increased global trade and flows of capital, concomitant global exchange of information and cultures, as well as large-scale environmental changes such as climate change. These processes are transforming societies, relationships, lifestyles, and identities worldwide.

Definitions and views on globalisation are often divergent. Some definitions focus on the sociological and anthropological aspects, describing it as the formation of a *global village*, the idea that people are creating a sense of a shared global experience and an "intensification of worldwide interconnectedness" (McGrew, 2017, pp. 15–30). This is often seen as the result of *cultural diffusion*, the spread of cultural ideas from one culture to another, as well as the weakening of ties between a particular culture and place, termed *de-territorialisation*. Other definitions emphasise the economic aspect and the emergence of a global marketplace, focusing on it as "a process of greater integration within the world economy … that leads increasingly to economic decisions being influenced by global conditions" (Jenkins, 2004).

These changes are taking place at different levels, which can be described as *spatial, temporal,* and *cognitive* (Hanefeld & Lee, 2015, pp. 1–13).

Spatial change describes the movement of humans, products, and services. People are travelling the world more frequently than in the past for a variety of reasons, either temporarily, for work or leisure, for example; or longer term. We are therefore much more interconnected than previously. According to the International Organization for Migration, 272 million people (3.5% of the world's population) today are international migrants (2019, pp. 19–56).

Temporal change describes our changing experience and perception of time. Many processes are automated and technology is much more powerful and faster, which can be perceived as time speeding up and saving time. Writing an email in comparison to sending a letter in the post is one example of this.

Cognitive change is about how we are thinking of ourselves and the world differently and creating new norms. Social and mass media, advertising, and various political and social movements and groups are globally spreading and shifting identities, beliefs, values, and knowledge, creating a rapid amalgamation and spreading of cultures (Lee, 2005, pp. 3–12). The *Black Lives Matter* movement is one example, which started in 2013 in protest against violence and police brutality against Black people in the United States of America, and which led to prominent protests in at least 60 countries during 2020.

Depending on the definition of globalisation, the present process of globalisation can be traced back to the 18th century, with colonial governments funding public health measures in colonised countries to prevent the spread of communicable diseases to their own countries (Labonté, Mohindra, & Schrecker, 2011). In many cases, the focus on the perceived health threat from Low-and Middle-Income Countries (LMICs) to High-Income Countries (HICs) continues today. Globalisation has been critiqued as a continuation of the colonisation of LMICs (Mikander, 2016), with the persistence of economic and cultural forms of dominance by some HICs over others, termed *neocolonialism* (Bhandal, 2018; Owens, Baylis, & Smith, 2017, pp. 1–14).

Definitions of globalisation are political in nature, with often contested and conflicting views on its meaning and how to address or advance it. The extent of integration and globalisation and to whom it is happening and why continues to be discussed; the impacts, benefits and costs to health are particularly debated (Lee, 2004). For some critics, for example, the costs of globalisation are too high, while for others the focus is placed on its benefits. It is a topic with few easy answers, a broad scope, and which holds relevance to everyone, making it particularly ripe for political discussion and divergent views.

It has also been posited that the effects of globalisation on health (and health systems) cannot be described as either universally good or bad, but rather as context-specific (Martin, 2005). As argued by Lee (2004), it is therefore important for those working in health – from the doctor who may be considering working in another country, to the policymaker looking to develop health policies fit for the future – to be informed and to critically engage on this topic in order to ensure the genuine promotion of good health.

Globalisation as a health topic

Globalisation is central to individual and population health, shaping it at every level: from the environments that we live in, the types of healthcare we receive, our diseases, even to our biological make up, and the interaction between these different factors. It is causing complex and dynamic changes to every aspect of planetary and human health, bringing with it both risks and negative impacts, as well as benefits and opportunities.

To date, globalisation has been little explored and framed in relation to health. This is likely due to its conceptual complexity, its political nature, and the challenge of researching a phenomenon with interconnected causal pathways. Pulling all of the research relevant to globalisation and health together would also a challenge, since it is often not labelled such, and the determinants relevant to globalisation and possible health effects would be difficult to comprehensively identify.

Recognising globalisation as a health topic and its impacts is essential for having a real-world understanding of health and of global health governance and national health systems. Addressing and adapting to the changes that come with globalisation requires an understanding of systems, complexity, and the *social* and *commercial determinants of health* to understand the multiple influences of health (Huynen, Martens, & Hilderink, 2005; McMichael, 2013). The social determinants of health describe the conditions in which people are born and live that affect health states and outcomes, such as the school an individual is able to attend, the home they live in, and their economic position and so forth; while the commercial determinants of health refer to the extent to which health is shaped by commercial actors, such as for example the alcohol and the food industry. Globalisation is a topic that highlights other areas not traditionally associated with health and medicine, such as trade, economics, and sustainability. It challenges those working in health to move beyond a clinical view and to critically question what really shapes good population health and to question the extent to which our currently prevailing economic and political approaches support this.

Understanding globalisation and health is, however, not just a conceptual and knowledge exercise; it can also guide decision-making and efforts to ensure multi-sectoral coordination. For example, it could help a ministry of health weigh up the potential health impacts and opportunities of a new trade agreement with another country and contribute to this decision. Globalisation is not an unstoppable or unamenable process, and the health community can play a role in ameliorating it and managing its planetary health impacts, including ensuring that the benefits are sustainable and are shared equitably.

At its core, globalisation can be described as a *planetary health* topic. This term describes "the health of human civilisation and the state of the natural systems on which it depends" (The Lancet Planetary Health, 2019). It broadly describes the health and sustainability of the whole planet and appreciates the interconnectedness of all systems, with nothing taking place in isolation. It is a fairly new term, popularised in 2015 by the Rockefeller Foundation-Lancet Commission on planetary health (The Lancet, 2015), but has conceptual foundations in the

Gaia theory. This theory was developed by the chemist James Lovelock in the 1970s, where *Gaia* is defined as "the global ecosystem, understood to function in the manner of a vast self-regulating organism, in the context of which all living things collectively define and maintain the conditions conducive for life on earth" (Radford, 2019).

Global health is generally a useful term for understanding collective human processes and action to improve and impact on human health worldwide, and which emphasises the role of transnational organisations and other international bodies in these shared efforts. However, globalisation impacts the health of the whole planet, including humans, animals, and the environment. Thinking of globalisation in these terms requires a systems perspective in order to recognise the need to care for the planet as a whole and helps to illustrate the causal pathways involved. Planetary health is arguably the broadest definition and conceptual understanding of health efforts to date, helpful for appreciating the complexity, interconnectedness, and brevity of the scope of globalisation and health. Globalisation will therefore be framed in relation to planetary health throughout this chapter. All other related terms are intentionally used in line with their definitions, such as *health system* (which includes all aspects of the provision of health services and care within a country), *population health* (the health of a population) and *global health* (global efforts to improve health).

Over the past 25 years, researchers have increasingly focused on different pathways through which globalisation affects health. Some of these are better explored than others. For example, the reach and global penetration of tobacco corporations and its direct effects on the rise of noncommunicable diseases, on health promotion efforts and on health regulation and their governance is fairly well analysed and understood. This serves as an example of how the economic processes of globalisation (such as enabling transnational commercial actors, greater trade), changes in social norms, and global actors (in this case the tobacco corporations on the one side and health regulators on the other) interplay to produce health outcomes for individuals and at a population level. However, for many aspects of "globalised life" and how these affect health, pathways are yet to be analysed and fully understood.

The next sections provide examples of some causal pathways, focusing in particular on the emerging shift in social identities as a result of mass communication and changes to social and political contexts. These are illustrative to help understand how social processes relating to globalisation increase interconnectedness and the extent to which these influence our health.

Global coordination, health policies, and governance

Health issues increasingly require structures, goals and efforts that reach beyond individual states. The COVID-19 pandemic is an example of this. It is a borderless issue, which led to substantial global cooperation and information and evidence sharing between states in order to prevent and contain the virus. Without this level of shared effort and cooperation, the health outcomes relating to the virus would be unrecognisably different.

Globalisation can enable improved coordination through rapid information exchange on emerging communicable diseases and the surveillance of health states and risk factors through central databases and electronic methods of communication. The European Centre for Disease Prevention and Control (ECDC), a European Union agency, is one organisation set up to allow for information sharing amongst members in order to have more effective responses. The speed of information sharing and scientific discovery could be seen as an example of *temporal change*.

Global health issues are also addressed through governance in the global public health domain, which has been defined along three political spaces: "Global health governance" describes institutions and processes of governance that explicitly have a health mandate, such as the WHO. "Global governance for health" describes the institutions and processes of global governance that do not necessarily have explicit health mandates, but have a direct and indirect health impact, such as the World Trade Organization. "Governance for global health" refers to the institutions and mechanisms at the national and regional level that contribute to global health governance and/or to governance for global health (Kickbusch & Szabo, 2014). It is useful to categorise using these terms in order to understand the purpose, roles and contributions of specific institutions and processes in the overall governance of global health domain, as well as to understand the interplay between these actors and their interests.

Over the past 30 years, the complexity of governance in global health has increased, with many new actors entering the field. Traditionally, the WHO as a normative organisation in global health has played a core role in setting standards and coordinating global action on health. However, the global health architecture has changed substantially in recent years, with the WHO becoming a less prominent actor as a number of new actors entered the field of global health. These include non-governmental organisations (NGOs), civil society organisations (CSOs) and the private sector (Kruk, 2012), as well as private foundations, such as the Bill and Melinda Gates Foundation and public–private partnerships such as the Global Vaccine Initiative (GAVI). These partnerships describe a formal agreement between public and private actors. They play an increasingly large role in funding and determining the prioritisation of global health issues, as well as contributing towards the coordination and delivery of healthcare, the development of new drugs and vaccines, and the financing of interventions. GAVI is, for example, a highly influential actor in the governance space, and is praised by some for using this position to drive innovations and supporting significant health benefits globally, such as preventing an estimated 12.23 fewer under-5 deaths per 1,000 live births (Jaupart, Dipple, & Dercon, 2019). However, others have questioned the legitimacy of these actors and GAVI is criticised for its dominance in global agenda-setting and driving an increasing focus on technical solutions in global health (Storeng, 2014).

The Millennium Development Goals and the subsequent Sustainable Development Goals (SDGs) were set up in recognition that globalisation contributes to a range of global issues that need to be globally managed and agreed on (Kruk, 2012). The SDGs commit member states to "take urgent action to combat climate change and its impacts" (SD13), "ensure healthy lives and wellbeing for all at all ages" (SDG3), and "strengthen the means of implementation and revitalize the global partnership for sustainable development" (SDG17), amongst others. The agreements to these goals were significant and signalled a shift in the global governance approach to globalisation and remain relevant for shaping the activities of the global health community.

Climate change, the environment, and communicable diseases

Globalisation, and in particular the economic expansion that is captured by the term, is associated with causing unprecedented and irreversible changes to the environment. The scale and intensification of economic activity, such as international trade and consumption of products from global brands, are putting substantial pressures on the environment. This is resulting in environmental degradation and erosion, loss of biodiversity, resource depletion, and climate change. Many of the processes in these global production chains and so forth form part of the *spatial change* happening as part of globalisation and is central to the concerns of planetary health.

Climate change poses a significant threat to human health, both directly and indirectly, and is linked to a number of communicable diseases. Infectious diseases require three components: A *pathogen*, a *host*, and a particular environment for *transmission* (the ability to spread from one infected individual to another). These three components require specific climate conditions to survive and transmit. Changes to climate have been linked to an extended geographical reach and changes to the seasonality of some infectious diseases (Wu, Lu, Zhou, Chen, & Xu, 2016). Malaria is one example of this. The *Anopheles* mosquito, a pathogen host, tends to be more active in warmer temperatures, and climate change is therefore predicted to increase the length and geographical range of its transmission. The WHO has predicted that climate change is expected to cause an additional 60,000 deaths per year between 2030 and 2050 due to malaria (World Health Organization, 2020a). Similarly, the *Aedes* mosquito, which transmits dengue, Zika, and yellow fever, is very sensitive to climate (The Lancet Infectious Diseases, 2017) and climate change could well extend its range and impact. However, predicting the impact of climate change is challenging, the interactions between climate change and communicable diseases are poorly understood, and the evidence does not present an entirely clear picture. More research taking a systems perspective and consideration of additional factors that modulate disease risk, such as socioeconomic status and land use, is required (Franklinos, Jones, Redding, & Abubakar, 2019).

Communicable diseases will also be affected by indirect and multi-factorial effects of climate change, such as through rising sea levels and erosion of soils. Water-borne diseases and pathogen hosts, including insects, snails, and other cold-blooded animals, are strongly affected by climate, and flooding can increase the spread of water-borne diseases. Migration of people through droughts, famines, and natural disasters will have further far-reaching effects on the health of societies.

Improved health surveillance, better infrastructures, and coordinated global efforts can all support populations dealing with the health impact of these changes. However, not all populations are and will be geographically, socioeconomically, and demographically affected equally by climate change. Due to the impacts of climate change, 1 billion refugees are expected by 2100 (Geisler & Currens, 2017), which has a range of implications for health, likely including access issues to healthcare and psychological distress. Other disproportionately affected populations include those living in coastal areas, polar and mountainous regions, and megacities. Children and elderly people as well as those with pre-existing health conditions are more vulnerable to climate change. Populations in areas with weaker infrastructures and reduced ability to respond to the effects of climate change are also likely to be disproportionately affected, as well as people who are socioeconomically disadvantaged and with poorer access to resources to mitigate the effects (World Health Organization, 2020a).

Antimicrobial resistance

Antimicrobial resistance (AMR) is a cross-cutting example of globalisation and the impact of environmental changes on communicable diseases. AMR is the loss of the effectiveness of anti-microbials, a group of medicines including antibiotics, to bacteria, viruses, fungi or parasites. It is sometimes termed *drug-resistance infections*. While resistance is a natural evolutionary process, it is being sped up at an alarming rate by over- and misuse of antimicrobials in the agricultural, environmental, veterinary and health sectors. It is now a question of when all of the current antibiotics will become entirely ineffective, not whether. Drug-resistant infections are estimated to cause at least 700,000 annual deaths globally (O'Neill, 2014). Resistance is a significant global challenge, threatening modern medicine entirely. Alongside *excess* use of antimicrobials, AMR is an issue of *access* to medicines for millions of people around the world.

Globalisation plays a role in AMR through different environmental pathways, such as intensi-fied economic pressures, and the need to increase crop yield for export leads some farmers to use antimicrobials as fertilisers and growth promoters. With climate change likely leading to an increase in communicable diseases, this may result in increased treatment with antimicrobials. The spread of meat-rich "Western diets" worldwide means that more antimicrobials are used to rear and treat animals. An increase in the movement of people and traded products across borders is more likely to spread resistant pathogens. The global pharmaceutical sector has strict rules on the trade of antimicrobials, which results in both established global trading of medicines as well as informal markets in some low-resource settings. These are often associated with the sale of counterfeit or poor-quality medicines, which contribute to AMR.

In order to tackle this borderless issue, the global governance of AMR has developed in recent years through strengthened cooperation between the animal health sector represented by the World Organisation for Animal Health (OIE), agriculture through representation from the Food and Agriculture Organisation (FAO), human health through representation from WHO, and environment through representation from the UN Environment Programme (UNEP). This partnership reflects a planetary health approach to addressing AMR.

Trade, commercialisation, and noncommunicable diseases

Economic globalisation, through intensification of trade, increased Foreign Direct Investment (FDI), and greater integration of global markets are structural factors that are increasingly recognised for their role in influencing the environments people live in, the habits they are able to adopt and the structural factors that guide people's nutritional status and health outcomes.

Overall economic globalisation and trade liberalisation have led to an increase in global production and Gross Domestic Product (GDP). However, the benefits of this economic growth have been unequal and inequality has increased significantly over the past 30 years, including inequalities in health. Industrial wages and household income inequality were found to increase with globalisation, particularly among countries that are part of the Organisation for Economic Co-operation and Development (OECD), which tend to be HICs (Dreher & Gaston, 2008).

There have also been effects on nutrition. The intensification of economic activity across borders has played an important role in making calorie-dense, highly processed foods with a high proportion of saturated fats and simple carbohydrates cheaply available in most reaches of the world, and this availability has been linked to global changes in dietary patterns and obesity and overweight. For example, there was a 12.5% rise in processed food consumption in urban areas in India after tariffs were reduced following economic globalisation reforms in the 1990s; the soft-drink sales per capita grew in Vietnam 4.6 litres per annum faster following their economic globalisation reforms than compared to the Philippines, which did not reform at the time (Barlow, McKee, Basu, & Stuckler, 2017; Cuevas García-Dorado, Cornselsen, Smith, & Walls, 2019). Alongside changes to diets, changes to more sedentary work and lifestyles are additional factors increasing people's risk for noncommunicable diseases, including coronary heart disease, diabetes mellitus and hypertension (World Health Organization, 2003).

Obesity, overweight, and noncommunicable diseases often co-exist with micronutrient deficiencies and undernutrition, called the *double* or *triple burden of nutrition* (The Lancet, 2019). Many LMICs have been undergoing a significant shift in the burden of disease in the last two decades, from predominantly communicable diseases to a higher burden of noncommunicable diseases, accounting for 80% of deaths from noncommunicable diseases in LMICs, called the *epidemiological transition*. These could all be described as *spatial*, *temporal* and *cognitive changes*. They impact not only the health of populations but the whole planet – from over-use of packaging to unsustainable farming and distribution approaches.

Global tobacco control

Global tobacco control is an example of the contribution of economic globalisation to population health. Tobacco has been aggressively marketed for a number of years, with the tobacco industry shifting its focus from HICs to LMICs in more recent years (Collin, 2002). Children, young people, and women have been particularly targeted. For many years, tobacco companies denied the harmful risks associated with consumption, and prevented the WHO from delivering tobacco control efforts (Zeltner, 2002). Free trade and tobacco-related FDI have been strongly linked to increased tobacco consumption (Bettcher, 2001).

The Framework Convention on Tobacco Control introduced in 2003 brought together state and non-state actors in agreeing the first international public health law. It aims to protect present and future generations from the consequences of tobacco consumption and exposure by stating the dangers of tobacco and limiting its use through taxation, advertisements, and other means. While it is seminal in its global reach, it has been criticised by some people in the global health community, amongst others, for not taking trade considerations into account in its wording. This has allowed challenges from the tobacco industry on the introduction of plain packaging for cigarettes, for example, since the industry claims that this intervention is not consistent with the rules of the World Trade Organisation (WTO), the intergovernmental body responsible for international trade. These challenges led to some countries being wary of implementing measures to reduce tobacco consumption and exposure.

Global communication, changing politics, and their roles in health

Global communication describes the forms of communication across borders. The increase in global communication is contributing towards a significant shift in societal and individual identities. The internet, social media, and music are examples of media that are contributing to what has been described as "hybrid" global identities, the combination of more than one cultural identity, particularly among younger generations (Bhavsar & Bhugra, 2008). The shift in global identities has also seen a rise in a divided politics, many of which have been characterised by anti-globalisation or national *protectionism* (the restriction of imports from other countries). The election of Donald Trump to the US Presidency in 2016, the exit of the United Kingdom from the European Union, and populist anti-immigration support in Europe can all be seen as examples of this. These could be described as examples of *cognitive and temporal changes* and are contributing to a change in how we see ourselves and relate to each other. These are emerging areas to consider when thinking about the connection between globalisation and health.

Social media, mental health, and wellbeing

Social media platforms, such as Instagram and Facebook, allow users to create their own online identities. Social media has the ability to deliver images to millions of people within seconds across the globe, often reinforcing a narrow version of beauty and norms. Coupled with idolisation of global celebrities, the small range of popular media channels, and newspapers that are owned by a limited number of companies, globalisation may be contributing to a greater homogenisation of online and offline identities.

Greater social media use amongst 14-year olds is related to online harassment, poor self-esteem, and poor body image, such as body weight dissatisfaction, and these are all related to higher depressive scores. The link between higher social media use and increased depressive scores is stronger amongst girls than boys (Kelly, Zilanawala, Booker, & Sacker, 2018). Teenage years are a particularly vulnerable time in the development of depression and some other mental health problems, and with social media being an increasingly important form of communication for this age group worldwide, this presents a global mental health challenge.

Some researchers have suggested that the simultaneous influences and pressures to conform to both global and local (more traditional) identities can be a source of stress, confusion, and uncertainty. For example, a group of young professionals in India were conflicted around their engagement with the global world in their work and traditional expectations in the home (Bhavsar & Bhugra, 2008). These changing identities can also create widening differences between the generations and between different communities within countries, such as those in urban and rural areas.

Loneliness, social isolation, and globalisation

Globalisation has been linked to changes in family and community structures, as a result of changes to working patterns, locations, migration, use of technology, and social media, and shifts in identities. Some of these changes have led to more people living alone and feeling isolated (the amount of contact with others) and lonely (the amount and quality of contact with others), another example of a cross-cutting issue in globalisation. In HICs, around one-third of people are thought to be affected by loneliness (Cacioppo & Cacioppo, 2018). Loneliness can have adverse impacts on mental health, including depression, anxiety, schizophrenia, suicide, and dementia and Alzheimer's disease. People experiencing poor health are most likely to report being lonely. Good, strong social relationships and networks are important for health and wellbeing and to prevent loneliness.

Loneliness and social cohesion have not been addressed at the global level, but instead tend to be small community-based efforts. Social prescribing is one example of a healthcare-based treatment, which is the referral of patients to non-health treatments, such as gardening or other social and community-based activity. Outside of health, community organising, the coordinating of cooperative efforts amongst a community and which are often led by trained community organisers, can help to empower and strengthen community and social ties.

The internet, knowledge, and sense of empowerment

While the internet may contribute to a narrower bandwidth of popular views and identities, the online world simultaneously allows a much greater number of voices to be expressed and connected with those on other sides of the world with similar views and experiences than previously. This may help people have a greater sense of agency and empowerment. It can also provide a sense of connection, shared identity and belief, a sense of belonging and solidarity, potentially promoting a sense of wellbeing.

Increased knowledge via global communication can be beneficial for health. Social media and online forums can also be a very positive source of social support and information (Thornicroft et al., 2016). This can be true for the general public, as well as for people with mental health conditions or marginalised groups. For people with mental health conditions, such as depression or bipolar disorder, online communities can be an important means of connection with friends or peers with similar conditions and for feeling less alone. Family members can also access their own support, information, and self-help programmes (The Lancet, 2018). The internet can also help to organise action to change health services and the social determinants of health, such as protecting and restoring the environment. These are potentially an important part of a shift to an increased democratisation of health, moving the power to citizens and away from traditional authorities on medicine and health.

The anti-vaccination movement and misinformation

Vaccinations are an essential public health measure: They prevent 2–3 million deaths per year and an additional 1.5 million deaths could be avoided with improved global coverage of vaccinations. Over 1 billion children were vaccinated in the last decade worldwide and fortunately the uptake of new and underused vaccines is increasing (World Health Organization, 2020b). However, vaccine coverage targets are still not being reached globally, with an estimated 19.7 million children under the age of one year not receiving basic vaccines. *Vaccine hesitancy*, the reluctance or refusal to vaccinate, presents an additional challenge to this. The effectiveness of the vaccination programme relies on collective and cooperative efforts to achieve herd immunity.

Vaccine hesitancy can fluctuate a great deal, varies worldwide (de Figueiredo, Simas, Karafillakis, Paterson, & Larson, 2020) and is also dependent on the type of vaccine. The reasons for hesitancy also vary. For example, low confidence in the measles vaccine is in many cases due to the disproven belief that the vaccine causes autism, contributing to a 30% increase in measles cases in recent years. Broadly, however, the anti-vaccination movement can be seen as an example of the rejection of evidence-based medicine, a core principle of modern medicine. This can be understood within the wider context of a wave of protectionism, individualism (promotion of one's independence and freedoms), a rise in populism (a political moment that rejects the idea of an "elite"), and reduced international cooperation, which have been described as anti-globalisation (Kennedy, 2019; Macgregor-Bowles & Bowles, 2017). Some of the supporters of these movements have experienced social and economic inequalities that can be attributed to globalisation (Globalization Knowledge Network, 2007). This in turn can influence the rejection of "expert" knowledge and the dominance of some forms of knowledge, such as evidence-based medicine, over others.

While vaccine hesitancy is not new, the scale and range of people now being reached and engaged by this anti-vaccination movement has grown in recent years. Vaccine hesitancy is one of the WHO's top ten threats to global health (World Health Organization, 2019) and is an issue in HICs and LMICs alike. Social media and news channels have played a central role in the spread of misinformation on vaccines in recent years (Burki, 2019). Social media platforms have struggled to regulate users' exposure to anti-vaccination groups, but some have increased efforts in recent years (Burki, 2019). This is particularly relevant in the efforts to vaccinate against COVID-19 worldwide.

Conclusions

This chapter sought to illustrate how globalisation is important for anyone seeking to understand health, why certain health events – such as pandemics – occur, and why specific health policies or regulations succeed or fail.

The first section introduces the concept of globalisation and describes the three types of changes that are conceptualised as spatial, temporal, and cognitive changes, which are having profound effects on the health of people and the planet. The colonial origins of globalisation are highlighted, and we describe the political nature of the topic, which has led to divergent views on its definition and the extent of its value to health. The section concludes by emphasising that the advantages and disadvantages of globalisation and its role should be weighed up with context in mind.

The chapter highlights why we need to examine globalisation and health together – stating that globalisation helps to identify the political nature of health, including the reasons why we see certain outcomes and effects in population health, health systems, and other activities that influence our health globally. Planetary health is a valuable framing for understanding the impact of globalisation on health, as it emphasises the interconnectedness of concepts in health as well as human and animal health along with the environment.

Global information exchange, cooperation, and governance are becoming increasingly important, as has been underlined again by the COVID-19 pandemic. The governance of global health is changing, and this section describes the increasing prominence of public–private partnerships, the proliferation of new actors, and the attempts of the SDGs to bring actors together around a set of global agreements.

Finally, the chapter sets out the complex cognitive impact of processes of globalisation on the health of people. While social media and the internet may promote a feeling of being more connected to each other than ever, this may also contribute towards a new shift of separation, less integration, less trust, and protectionism in other areas. These present new challenges for globalisation and for health.

Globalisation plays a significant role for planetary health. In order to promote health, it is important to understand the contexts in which globalisation is occurring. A nuanced conceptual understanding of globalisation and critical engagement with the topic is essential for everyone working in health – from frontline healthcare professional to policymaker – to support decision-making that promotes planetary health for all.

References

Barlow, P., McKee, M., Basu, S., & Stuckler, D. (2017). The health impact of trade and investment agreements: A quantitative systematic review and network co-citation analysis. *Globalization and Health, 13*(1), 13–13. doi:10.1186/s12992-017-0240-x

Bettcher, D. (2001). *Confronting the tobacco epidemic in an era of trade liberalization.* Retrieved from Geneva: https://www.who.int/tobacco/publications/industry/trade/confronting_tob_epidemic/en/

Bhandal, T. (2018). Ethical globalization? Decolonizing theoretical perspectives for internationalization in Canadian medical education. *Canadian Medical Education Journal, 9*(2), e33–e45.

Bhavsar, V., & Bhugra, D. (2008). Globalization: Mental health and social economic factors. *Global Social Policy, 8*(3), 378–396. doi:10.1177/1468018108095634

Burki, T. (2019). Vaccine misinformation and social media. *The Lancet Digital Health, 1*(6), e258–e259. doi:10.1016/S2589-7500(19)30136-0

Cacioppo, J. T., & Cacioppo, S. (2018). The growing problem of loneliness. *The Lancet, 391*(10119), 426. doi:10.1016/S0140-6736(18)30142-9

Collin, J. (2002). Think global, smoke local: Transnational tobacco companies and cognitive globalization. In Lee, K. (Ed.), *Health impacts of globalization: Towards global governance* (pp. 61–85). London: Palgrave Macmillan.

Cuevas García-Dorado, S., Cornselsen, L., Smith, R., & Walls, H. (2019). Economic globalization, nutrition and health: A review of quantitative evidence. *Globalization and Health, 15*(1), 15–15. doi:10.1186/s12992-019-0456-z

de Figueiredo, A., Simas, C., Karafillakis, E., Paterson, P., & Larson, H. J. (2020). Mapping global trends in vaccine confidence and investigating barriers to vaccine uptake: A large-scale retrospective temporal modelling study. *The Lancet.* doi:10.1016/S0140-6736(20)31558-0

Dreher, A., & Gaston, N. (2008). Has globalization increased inequality?★. *Review of International Economics, 16*(3), 516–536. doi:10.1111/j.1467-9396.2008.00743.x

Franklinos, L. H. V., Jones, K. E., Redding, D. W., & Abubakar, I. (2019). The effect of global change on mosquito-borne disease. *The Lancet Infectious Diseases, 19*(9), e302–e312. doi:10.1016/S1473-3099(19)30161-6

Geisler, C., & Currens, B. (2017). Impediments to inland resettlement under conditions of accelerated sea level rise. *Land Use Policy, 66*, 322–330. doi:10.1016/j.landusepol.2017.03.029

Globalization Knowledge Network. (2007). *Towards health-equitable globalisation: Rights, regulation and redistribution final report to the commission on social determinants of health.* Retrieved from Ottowa: https://www.who.int/social_determinants/resources/gkn_report_06_2007.pdf

Hanefeld, J., & Lee, K. (2015). Introduction to globalization and health. In J. Hanefeld (Ed.), *Globalization and health* (pp. 1–13). London: Open University Press.

Huynen, M. M. T. E., Martens, P., & Hilderink, H. B. M. (2005). The health impacts of globalisation: A conceptual framework. *Globalization and Health, 1*(1), 14. doi:10.1186/1744-8603-1-14

International Organization for Migration. (2019). *Chapter 2 - Migration and migrants: A global overview.* Retrieved from Geneva: https://publications.iom.int/books/world-migration-report-2020-chapter-2

Jaupart, P., Dipple, L., & Dercon, S. (2019). Has Gavi lived up to its promise? Quasi-experimental evidence on country immunisation rates and child mortality. *BMJ Global Health, 4*(6), e001789–e001789. doi:10.1136/bmjgh-2019-001789

Jenkins, R. (2004). Globalization, production, employment and poverty: Debates and evidence. *Journal of International Development, 16*(1), 1–12. doi:10.1002/jid.1059

Kelly, Y., Zilanawala, A., Booker, C., & Sacker, A. (2018). Social media use and adolescent mental health: Findings from the UK millennium cohort study. *EClinicalMedicine, 6*, 59–68. doi:10.1016/j.eclinm.2018.12.005

Kennedy, J. (2019). Populist politics and vaccine hesitancy in Western Europe: An analysis of national-level data. *European journal of public health, 29*(3), 512–516. doi:10.1093/eurpub/ckz004

Kickbusch, I., & Szabo, M. M. C. (2014). A new governance space for health. *Global Health Action, 7*, 23507–23507. doi:10.3402/gha.v7.23507

Kruk, M. E. (2012). Globalisation and global health governance: Implications for public health. *Global Public Health, 7*(sup1), S54–S62. doi:10.1080/17441692.2012.689313

Labonté, R., Mohindra, K., & Schrecker, T. (2011). The growing impact of globalization for health and public health practice. *Annual Review of Public Health, 32*(1), 263–283. doi:10.1146/annurev-publhealth-031210-101225

Lee, K. (2004). Globalisation: What is it and how does it affect health? *Medical Journal of Australia, 180*(4), 156–158. doi:10.5694/j.1326-5377.2004.tb05855.x

Lee, K. (2005). Introduction to global health. In K. Lee & J. Collin (Eds.), *Global change and health* (pp. 3–12). Maidenhead: Open University Press.

Macgregor-Bowles, I., & Bowles, D. C. (2017). Trump, Brexit, right-wing anti-globalisation, and an uncertain future for public health. *AIMS Public Health, 4*(2), 139–148. doi:10.3934/publichealth.2017.2.139

Martin, G. (2005). Globalization and health. *Globalization and Health, 1*(1), 1. doi:10.1186/1744-8603-1-1

McGrew, A. (2017). Globalization and global politics. In J. Baylis, S. Smith, & P. Owens (Eds.), *The globalisation of world politics: An introduction to international relations* (pp. 15–30). Oxford: Oxford University Press.

McMichael, A. J. (2013). Globalization, climate change, and human health. *New England Journal of Medicine, 368*(14), 1335–1343. doi:10.1056/NEJMra1109341

Mikander, P. (2016). Globalization as continuing colonialism: Critical global citizenship education in an unequal world. *Journal of Social Science Education, 15*(2). doi:10.4119/UNIBI/jsse-v15-i2-1475

'Neill. (2014). *Review on antimicrobial resistance: Tackling a crisis for the health and wealth of nations.* Chaired by Jim O'Neill. Retrieved from London: https://amr-review.org/sites/default/files/AMR%20Review%20Paper%20-%20Tackling%20a%20crisis%20for%20the%20health%20and%20wealth%20of%20nations_1.pdf

Owens, P., Baylis, J., & Smith, S. (2017). Introduction: From international politics to world politics. In J. Baylis, S. Smith, & P. Owens (Eds.), *The globalization of world politics: An introduction to international relations* (pp. 1–14). Oxford: Oxford University Press.

Radford, T. (2019). James Lovelock at 100: The Gaia saga continues. *Nature, 570*, 441–442.

Statista. (2020). *Number of social network users worldwide.* Retrieved from https://www.statista.com/statistics/278414/number-of-worldwide-social-network-users/

Storeng, K. T. (2014). The GAVI alliance and the "Gates approach" to health system strengthening. *Global Public Health, 9*(8), 865–879. doi:10.1080/17441692.2014.940362

The Lancet (Producer). (2015). Safeguarding human health in the anthropocene epoch: Report of The Rockefeller Foundation–Lancet Commission on planetary health. *Commissions from the Lancet Journals.*

The Lancet (Producer). (2018). The Lancet Commission on global mental health and sustainable development. *Commissions from the Lancet Journals.* Retrieved from https://www.thelancet.com/commissions/global-mental-health

The Lancet (Producer). (2019). The double burden of malnutrition. *Series from the Lancet Journals.* Retrieved from https://www.thelancet.com/series/double-burden-malnutrition

The Lancet Infectious Diseases. (2017). Climate change: The role of the infectious disease community. *The Lancet Infectious Diseases, 17*(12), 1219. doi:10.1016/S1473-3099(17)30645-X

The Lancet Planetary Health. (2019). The bigger picture of planetary health. *The Lancet Planetary Health*, *3*(1), e1. doi:10.1016/S2542-5196(19)30001-4

Thornicroft, G., Mehta, N., Clement, S., Evans-Lacko, S., Doherty, M., Rose, D., … Henderson, C. (2016). Evidence for effective interventions to reduce mental-health-related stigma and discrimination. *The Lancet*, *387*(10023), 1123–1132. doi:10.1016/S0140-6736(15)00298-6

World Health Organization. (2003). *Globalization, diets and noncommunicable diseases*. Retrieved from Geneva: https://apps.who.int/iris/bitstream/handle/10665/42609/9241590416.pdf?sequence=1&isAllowed=y

World Health Organization. (2019). *Ten threats to global health in 2019*. Retrieved from https://www.who.int/news-room/feature-stories/ten-threats-to-global-health-in-2019

World Health Organization. (2020a). *Climate change and health*. Retrieved from https://www.who.int/en/news-room/fact-sheets/detail/climate-change-and-health

World Health Organization. (2020b). *Immunization coverage*. Retrieved from https://www.who.int/news-room/fact-sheets/detail/immunization-coverage

Wu, X., Lu, Y., Zhou, S., Chen, L., & Xu, B. (2016). Impact of climate change on human infectious diseases: Empirical evidence and human adaptation. *Environment International*, *86*, 14–23. doi:10.1016/j.envint.2015.09.007

Zeltner, T. (2002). *Tobacco industry strategies to undermine tobacco control activities at the World Health Organization*. Report of the Committee of Experts on Tobacco Industry Documents. Retrieved from Geneva: https://www.who.int/tobacco/publications/industry/who_inquiry/en/

INDEX